HIV and the Pathogenesis of AIDS

SECOND EDITION

JAY A. LEVY

Department of Medicine and Cancer Research Institute
University of California, School of Medicine
San Francisco, California

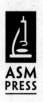

Washington, D.C.

ASM
PRESS

HIV and the Pathogenesis of AIDS

SECOND EDITION

Cover: Detail from "The Cell #2," painting by George Habergritz (dedicated to Maya)

Copyright © 1998 American Society for Microbiology
1325 Massachusetts Ave., NW
Washington, DC 20005-4171

Library of Congress Cataloging-in-Publication Data
Levy, Jay A.
    HIV and the pathogenesis of AIDS / by Jay A. Levy.—2nd ed.
      p.   cm.
    Includes bibliographical references and index.
    ISBN 1-55581-122-1
    1. HIV (Viruses) 2. HIV infections—Pathogenesis. I. Title.
    [DNLM: 1. Acquired Immunodeficiency Syndrome—etiology.
    2. Acquired Immunodeficiency Syndrome—physiopathology. 3. HIV—
    pathogenicity. WC 503.3 L668h 1998]
    QR201.A37L48 1998
    616.97′92—dc21
    DNLM/DLC
    for Library of Congress   97-42731
                                                CIP

To Sharon, for her continual support and encouragement

Contents

Preface

Friends, colleagues, and other readers of the first edition encouraged me to update this book. This task involved rereading many articles and evaluating over 2,000 new papers related to the human immunodeficiency virus (HIV) and the acquired immune deficiency syndrome (AIDS). During this work, it became increasingly evident that over the past three and a half years, research in both basic and clinical science has provided important changes in our understanding of HIV and its ability to cause disease. One noteworthy observation was the large number of articles on antiviral therapies and vaccine development. This volume of literature necessitated assigning each topic a separate chapter. Among the advances made in the pursuit of understanding HIV pathogenesis, I would cite the following:

1. Throughout the world, many more HIV-1 clades (or viral genotypes) in the M (or main) category, going up to J, were recognized, and those from the outlying (O) clade can now be found in several parts of the world, including the United States. Not as much progress has been made in identifying new HIV-2 clades (Chapter 7).

2. It is now a proven observation that needle exchange programs can reduce the risk of HIV infection in users of illicit intravenous drugs. Such programs thus decrease the number of deaths from AIDS and the costs for treatment in this population (Chapter 2).

3. Zidovudine (AZT) therapy for pregnant mothers can greatly reduce the transmission of HIV to newborn children (Chapter 2). While first cited in the 1994 edition of this book, the evidence for this effect is now well established, and the incidence of HIV transmission to newborns in the United States has dramatically decreased.

4. The basic research that defined the crystal structure of reverse transcriptase (RT) and protease has led to the development of several new antiviral drugs that have shown promise in clinical trials. In particular, the administration of protease inhibitors along with effective anti-RT therapies has reduced plasma viremia to undetectable levels and brought clinical benefits to many individuals now receiving these drugs (Chapter 14). Whether such effective attacks upon the virus will maintain control of the infection and substantially prolong life remains an unanswered question. The enhanced ability to detect viral RNA in blood has helped greatly in the management of therapy for infected people (Chapter 2).

5. More emphasized than previously is the fact that HIV can remain in certain reservoirs, such as the brain and testes, that may not be affected by antiretroviral therapy (Chapter 14). Thus, these sites for viral replication need to be approached if continual control of HIV infection is to be achieved.

6. Coreceptors that HIV uses to enter macrophages and T-cell lines have been identified (Chapter 3). These newly recognized virus entry sites are chemokine receptors and are important in the early steps of virus:cell interaction. Individuals lacking expression of these coreceptors appear to show some resistane to HIV infection. this discovery was made during studies on natural immune factors produced by $CD8^+$ cells that block HIV infection (Chapter 11).

7. Natural immune anti-HIV factors have received increased attention, primarily because of the finding that chemokines, released by lymphocytes as well as by other cells, can block HIV infection in vitro. The focus on natural immune factors has brought new emphasis on $CD8^+$ cell noncytotoxic antiviral responses which appear to be mediated by a $CD8^+$ cell antiviral factor (CAF) (Chapter 11). The data indicate that CAF is not a chemokine; this important mechanism for controlling HIV infection remains to be elucidated.

8. Apoptosis continues to be emphasized as a potential process for $CD4^+$ cell loss during HIV infection (Chapter 6). Most important, the controversy over whether HIV directly causes $CD4^+$ cell loss or induces it indirectly through a variety of phenomena has not been completely resolved. However, most studies suggest that primarily uninfected cells die by apoptosis. This finding may bring greater attention to finding therapies to prevent apoptosis.

9. In the field of cancer research, the discovery of the human herpesvirus 8 associated with Kaposi's sarcoma and body cavity-associated B-cell lymphomas has quickened the pace of research on these two malignancies (Chapter 12). Attention is being given to defining whether this new herpesvirus is oncogenic and how it could cause transformation of endothelial cells and B cells.

10. The use of DNA as an approach for HIV vaccines has received increased attention (Chapter 15).

11. Primate models for testing antiviral therapies and vaccines have been further developed, particularly those employing SIV/HIV (SHIV) virus chimeras (Chapter 15).

12. Further evidence on the inability to productively infect resting cells has been reported (Chapter 5). In particular, new data have indicated that HIV can enter resting lymphocytes but does not undergo complete reverse transcription, and the infection in a truly quiescent cell is abortive, With monocytes, HIV does not appear to enter unless the cells are in a differentiated state.

While this list indicates that several new insights in a variety of fields have been provided over the last three and a half years, certain areas of study have not progressed at the same pace. I would include in the latter category the process of viral latency in cells (Chapter 5), the potential proteolytic activity involving gp120 that appeared a few years ago to be important for virus entry (Chapter 3), and the cellular host range of HIV (Chapter 4). Most of the latter studies seemed to have been completed by 1993. In addition, a better definition of HIV pathogenesis in the brain and in the bowel, and in endocrine organs such as the testes, has not been achieved and merits further study. A focus on the role of antigen-presenting cells (APC) (particularly dendritic cells) in HIV pathogenesis must be encouraged. APC are very important in eliciting appropriate immune responses and may be the common denominator for the immune deficiencies observed in HIV infection (Chapter 13). Only recently has attention been given to the detrimental effects of HIV on the thymus and the thymic epithelium. The need for immune reconstitution, particularly of thymus-derived cells, for complete recovery from an HIV infection also warrants further focus. A section of the book is now devoted to this topic (Chapter 14). Likewise, while the concept of autoimmunity as playing a potential role in HIV pathogenesis (Chapter 10) has been considered for several years, new evidence implicating this process in HIV pathogenesis has not been provided.

Work in vaccines, while generating many publications and new approaches, has led to conflicting comments on the feastibility of various directions. In most cases, the controversies involve the value of trials with subunit vaccines. Some investigators believe that the results in animals, particularly chimpanzees, warrant clinical trials in humans. Others, concerned with the costs involved in what would appear to be fruitless experiments, argue against using subunit vaccines without further evidence of promising results in animals or in the limited studies using humans. In this regard, the recent encouraging results with prime/boost approaches and DNA vaccines may affect the direction in this field (Chapter 15).

The next few years should witness an increased intensity in research on vaccines, particularly because of the greater attention given recently by the U.S. government to vaccine development. Some of this impetus may come from the current belief that anti-HIV treatment (i.e., with combination therapy) has been working and we should now focus more on prevention. It is, however, still too early to know how long the present antiviral drugs will control HIV. In any event, the challenge of an HIV vaccine remains the same as the challenge of cancer: the affected cell (see Conclusions). One must be able to eliminate the incoming infected cell and the resident infected cells if approaches to prevent established infection are to be successful.

Since 1993, the pandemic of HIV infection has continued to soar, with several new countries (e.g., India, China, Korea) realizing the speed with which this infection can spread. In the United States, 68,473 new cases of AIDS were reported in 1996, 47% higher than reported in 1993. The total number of cases since AIDS was recognized in 1981 has now reached close to 600,000 (1). Since 1992, non-Hispanic blacks, Hispanics, and women have accounted for increasing proportions of AIDS cases (1). In 1996, represented 20% of all adult cases reported (1). Currently, nearly half of the reported AIDS cases in the United States are from transmission by homosexual and bisexual men, followed by intravenous drug use (26%) and heterosexual contact (12%). This last source of transmission rose to the highest proportion during 1996 (19%) (1).

By June 1996, the established prevalence of AIDS was 223,000 in U.S. residents older than 13 years. This number reflects increases of 10% and 65% since mid-1995 and January 1993, respectively (1). Until 1996, AIDS in the United States was the leading cause of death of young people, both male and female, between 25 and 44 years of age (Figure A). Recently, death from AIDS has decreased because of the success of antiviral therapies. In the first edition of this book, 1 in 250 Americans was estimated to be infected by HIV, including 1 in 100 males and 1 in 800 females. That number has not changed, indicating that either the prediction in 1993 was too high or the rate of new infections has stabilized. However, the total number of cases worldwide has reached over 20 million (2164), with the largest number of cases of HIV infection now in Asia and sub-Saharan Africa (Table A, Figure B). Noteworthy is the rapid spread of HIV-1 and HIV-2 in India, where 10 years ago the virus infection was rarely encountered. Fears of similar epidemics in countries like China and Indonesia are surfacing. As reported in the first edition, it is estimated that a new infection takes place in the world every 13 seconds and a death from HIV infection occurs every 9 minutes. By the year 2000, over 100 million individuals could be infected by HIV-1 or HIV-2 (1660). Education is the immediate approach needed, and a vaccine is a vital necessity.

In this second edition, I have attempted to control the growing bibliography of this book by selecting first those references in which the earliest observation on a given topic was made. Then, where appropriate, I have included a reference that supports this evidence and, finally, a recent reference updating the finding. Part of the effort to reduce citations is to provide readers with a preferential set of references as well as some historical citations and reviews on the subject. Thus, several references from the first edition have been dropped but can be found in that volume. However, many more recent ones have been added, particularly with the new topics addressed. Papers published on HIV and AIDS have increased at a fast rate.

Table A   Prevalence of HIV infection (1996)[a]

India	2–3 million
South Africa	1.8 million
Uganda	1.5 million
Nigeria	1.2 million
Zimbabwe	1.2 million
Kenya	1.1 million
USA	900,000
Thailand	800,000

[a] Source: UNAIDS Program.

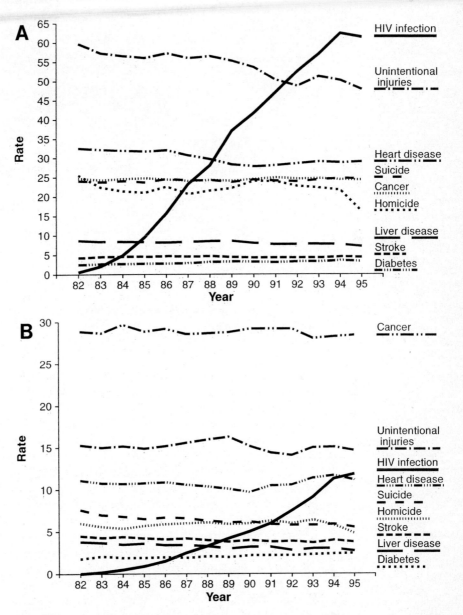

Figure A   Leading causes of death among men (A) and women (B) 25 to 44 years of age in the United States, by year, from 1982 to 1995 (based on underlying cause of death reported on death certificates, using final data for 1982–1994 and preliminary data for 1995). A steady rise in deaths secondary to HIV infection is apparent (386a). (Figures courtesy of R. Selik.)

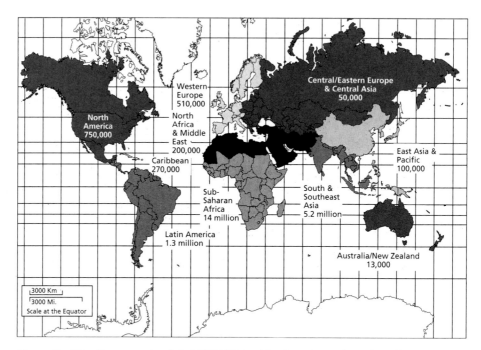

Figure B   New figures on the global HIV/AIDS epidemic. Estimated number of persons living with HIV infection or AIDS, by region, at the end of 1996. (Source: UNAIDS–Joint United Nations Program on HIV/AIDS, December 1996.)

Since the initial report on AIDS in 1981 (383), a total of 140,072 articles have been written on this subject through September 1997. The number of papers published on HIV and AIDS peaked at 19,721 in 1996 (1907a). For this book (updated through October, 1997), about 3,100 have been cited.

To add a personal touch to the challenge of AIDS research, I have asked several of the early pioneers in this field—those who were very active from 1981 through 1984—to provide photographs of themselves for inclusion in this book. These individuals form the nucleus of others who were involved with HIV and AIDS at the time. Many of these researchers and clinicians are the mentors of present leaders in AIDS research.

Readers are recommended to read the Preface to the First Edition and refer to the criteria for AIDS as defined by the Centers for Disease Control (Appendices I and IV) (376). In this edition, the term HIV is again used to reflect properties shared by HIV-1 and HIV-2, unless otherwise stated. I hope this revised text will continue to be of help to investigators, health care providers, and students who are joining in the efforts to find a solution to this devastating disease.

The research conducted by the author and his coworkers was supported by grants from the National Institutes of Health, the California State Universitywide Task Force on AIDS, and the American Foundation for AIDS Research. In addition to my gratitude to those who provided helpful suggestions and advice on the initial text in *Microbiological Reviews* and the first edition of this book, I want to thank for their assistance on the present edition the following individuals: Donald Abrams,

Edward Barker, Susan Barnett, Karen Beckerman, David Blackbourn, Michael Busch, Irwin Chen, Cecilia Cheng-Mayer, David Cooper, Lawrence Corey, Steven Deeks, Anthony Fauci, Robert Garry, Francisco Gonzalez-Scarano, Barton Haynes, Brian Herndier, James Hoxie, Barbara Klencke, Carla Kuiken, Christopher Locher, Paul Luciw, Allen Mayer, Alan Landay, H. Clifford Lane, Alexander Levine, Nancy Padian, Lynn Pulliam, W. Edward Robinson, Gene Shearer, Haynes Sheppard, Gregory Spear, Leonidas Stamatatos, Mario Stevenson, Frederick Siegal, Bruce Torbett, Dean Winslow, and Susan Zolla-Pazner. I acknowledge as well the careful editing of the chapters by Mary McKenney. I thank Ann Murai for her assistance with the manuscript and especially Christine Beglinger for her close attention, helpful advice, and overall handling of this second edition.

Preface to the First Edition

This book reviews the history, background, and current studies of the human immunodeficiency virus (HIV) and the pathogenic pathways leading to the development of the variety of diseases now known as AIDS. The text was originally written as a review for *Microbiological Reviews* and has been updated with further references and new topics, including a chapter on AIDS-associated malignancies. The book aims to define the important events surrounding this relatively recent public health and medical challenge, which introduces new concepts in viral pathogenesis and demands new approaches for control and prevention of an infectious disease. The onset of AIDS appears to reflect events that have occurred over many years, including economic distress, the breakdown of borders with migrations of populations from low endemic areas to uninfected regions, and the ease of travel worldwide. Whether the causative agent, HIV, is a virus recently transmitted to humans or one that has been present in human populations for thousands of years is not yet known. Certainly its emergence is an indication of how, in the future, the world may be plagued by other infectious agents resulting from a variety of natural, political, and economic factors (1436s).

My personal involvement with AIDS began in August of 1981 when Paul Volberding, who had just left my laboratory as a postdoctoral fellow, called me to see a young homosexual man with Kaposi's sarcoma at San Francisco General Hospital. The question was whether this unusual tumor in a young individual might offer us the opportunity to find a viral cause of a human cancer. Later that year, immune deficiency was found to be the underlying disorder in such patients and others with certain malignancies (e.g. B-cell lymphomas) and opportunistic infections (e.g., *Pneumocystis carinii* pneumonia, toxoplasmosis).

The search for the etiologic agent of AIDS forms the fist chapter of this book.

In retrospect, immune deficiency-causing viruses, similar to HIV, had already been described in a variety of animal systems. However, the possibility of a lentivirus occurring in humans, even after the discovery of the AIDS virus, took time to be recognized. This facet of the research merely reflects how certain ideas and preconceptions can delay discoveries that in hindsight appear so obvious.

Over the past 10 years since the discover of HIV, much progress has been made in understanding the virus, but many previously established concepts have now been changed and replaced by others. These early concepts include the initial conclusions that the virus only infects $CD4^+$ lymphocytes; that it only uses the CD4 molecule as its receptor; that it only undergoes productive infections; that it either can or cannot be neutralized by antibodies (i.e., enhancement was not considered a reality); that in the face of an immune-compromising agent, a cellular immune response would not be present and control HIV replication (e.g., $CD8^+$ antiviral cells); that the clinical course would be short (not, as is currently known, 10 years for 50% of patients to develop AIDS); and that all HIV strains would be similar in their biologic, serologic, and molecular features. On this latter point, beside the recognition of two types, HIV-1 and HIV-2, the diverse and constantly changing properties of each HIV strain are now recognized and present challenges to antiviral therapy and vaccines.

All these features of HIV pathogenesis need to be considered, including the viral effects on specific tissues, such as the brain, the bowel, the lungs, and perhaps the endocrine system. Moreover, the same HIV strain is now known to evolve within the host, and eventually these mutations make it more "virulent" and perhaps "home out" into specific tissues, causing disease.

The underlying conclusion from this past decade of research is that AIDS presents a unique challenge to researchers, physicians, health care workers, and public health officials throughout the world. The present rate of HIV spread, as noted in Conclusions, reflects a disease that is moving faster in the world than any other known agent in this half century, and the difficulty of controlling HIV reflects its manner of transmission: no sexually transmitted disease has ever been controlled. Moreover, its ability to integrate its genetic information within the infected cell and spread by cell-to-cell transfer as well as cell replication presents difficulties for its elimination and certainly for finding a cure for the infected host. The challenge of HIV resembles that of cancer in that both diseases involve an affected cell that must be destroyed. Thus, a vaccine against cancer or AIDS could have relevance for both disease processes.

Identification of the different facets of HIV pathogenesis comes through studies by investigators throughout the world. The early recognition that AIDS transmission patterns linked the causative agent to the blood and genital fluid is a tribute to the fine epidemiological studies conducted in the initial periods of this infection. Furthermore, the extensive molecular studies have brought new insights into novel intracellular events as well as new concepts in retrovirology: HIV is probably the most investigated infectious agent in history. During 1993, in the United States about 100,000 new cases of AIDS were reported, compared to 47,000 in 1992 and 45,000 in 1991. The total number of cases of AIDS has now reached 360,000. The increase in new cases recently reflects in part a change in the AIDS definition (see below). About one-half of the reported AIDS cases (55%) were associated with

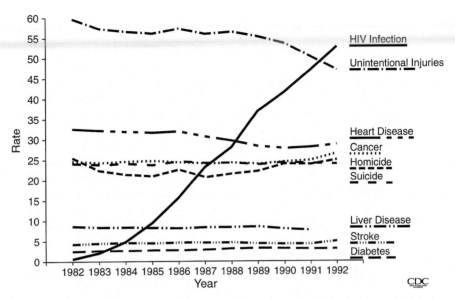

Figure A   Leading causes of death among persons 25 to 44 years of age in the United States from 1982 to 1992. A steady rise in deaths secondary to HIV infection is apparent (1826). Figure courtesy of R. Selik.

HIV transmission in homosexual or bisexual men, and the statistics indicate an increasing prevalence among both male and female intravenous drug users (28%) (229). As of December 1993 in the United States, 1 in 250 individuals was estimated to be infected by HIV. Based on gender distribution of AIDS cases, this number suggests that 1 in 100 males and 1 in 800 females were HIV-infected (229a). AIDS is rapidly becoming the leading cause of death among persons 25 to 44 years of age in the United States (Fig. A) (1826). Concern has been raised about its spread to even younger people, including adolescents (1501a). This year along, 40,000 to 80,000 new cases of HIV infection are expected in this country (1095). IN the world today, 13 million people are infected, most of them in sub-Saharan Africa. It is estimated that a new infection takes place every 13 s and that a person dies from HIV every 9 min. By the year 2000, 30 to 100 million people worldwide will have been infected by HIV-1 or HIV-2; 10 million will be children (1095). The number of reports written on the subject peaked at 16,860 in 1993, with a total through April 1994 of 97,098 citations since the initial reports in 1981 (125a).

Clearly the number of citations on this virus since its discovery in 1983 attests to the fact that much research has been dedicated to understanding the nature of the agent and its pathogenic processes. Of the over 90,000 references published up to May 1994, this book has selected about 2,100 that either solely or with other publications support the various statements cited. Nevertheless, as noted above, established concepts are often quickly replaced by new ones as further work on HIV is completed. Just as the infectious virus has proved to be a moving target, threatening populations throughout the world, it continues also to defy approaches in the laboratory to uncover ways in which it can be suppressed in the host. Moreover, the study of the transmission and epidemiology of HIV requires a further understanding of various behavioral and cultural differences in the world that can influence successful approaches to preventing and halting its spread.

In this book, readers are recommended to refer to the criteria for HIV infection and the 1993 revised classification system established by the Centers for Disease Control (Appendix I) (222). This expanded surveillance case definition for AIDS, used universally, should make some of the studies referring to clinical state more consistent in the future. Most noteworthy is the recent addition of invasive cervical carcinoma (Chapter 10), pulmonary tuberculosis, and recurrent pneumonia as conditions defined as AIDS. Moreover, the inclusion of CD4$^+$ cell counts of less than 200/µl and less than 14% is an important new definition of AIDS (see Appendixes I to IV, Categories A, B, and C). In general, in the book the term HIV is used to indicate properties shared by both HIV-1 and HIV-2. Where specific points related to HIV-1 or HIV-2, that distinction has been made in the text.

It is hoped that this book, reviewing HIV and its pathogenesis, will provide the foundation for future work that will find the solution to this devastating problem.

The research conducted by the author and coworkers was supported by grants from the National Institutes of Health, the California State Universitywide Task Force on AIDS, and the American Foundation for AIDS Research. I would like to thank the following for their helpful suggestions and advice on the initial text published in *Microbiological Reviews:* A. Allison, E. Barker, J. Bradac, C. Cheng-Mayer, D. Cooper, E. Engleman, L. Evans, T. Folds, R. Gaynor, H. Golding, N. Haigwood, A. Hoffman, J. Hoxie, S.-L. Hu, S. Kliks, S. Kohl, A. Landay, J. Laurence, S. Levy, J. Lifson, D. Littman, C. Mackewicz, S. McDougall, D. Nixon, J. Nelson, M. Peterlin, L. Pulliam, E. Robinson, E. Sawai, H. Sheppard, L. Stamatatos, K. Steimer, G. Van Nest, C. Walker, C. Weiss, A. Werner, R. Yarchoan, and M. Zeiger, I thank the following for their critical review of chapters in this book: E. Barker, S. Barnett, B. Herndier, S.-L. Hu, S. Kliks, A. Landay, S. Levy, A. Lifson, J. Palefsky, L. Pulliam, R. Pomerantz, E. Sawai, L Stamatatos, P. Volberding, and C. Weiss. I gratefully acknowledge the assistance of Ann Murai in the preparation of this book. I thank Leslie Compere for her valuable and excellent help with the graphics. I give tribute to Christine Beglinger for her tremendous efforts in the overall organization and presentation of the text and references, and for her encouragement and support. Finally, I thank Patrick Fitzgerald for asking me to write this book. I hope it will serve as a valuable reference for investigators and students in the field.

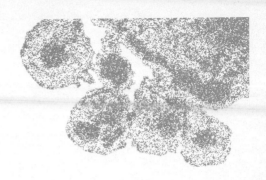

Discovery and Origin of HIV

LENTIVIRUSES CONSTITUTE A SEPARATE GENUS OF THE *Retroviridae* family, which includes many different viruses infecting a diverse group of animal species (Table 1.1) (490, 980, 1496). The human immunodeficiency virus (HIV), the subject of this book, is a lentivirus that was recognized relatively recently because of its association with the acquired immune deficiency syndrome (AIDS). This clinical syndrome, characterized by a marked reduction in the number of $CD4^+$ cells and the development of infections and cancers (Table 1.2) (1676), results from the persistent replication and spread of HIV (see Preface). In this monograph, historical aspects of the lentivirus group and the discovery of HIV will be covered. Features of HIV pathogenesis, including aspects of the virus itself, the cells it infects, the consequences of this infection, and the host immune response to HIV, will be discussed. Finally, potential approaches to therapy and a vaccine for the prevention of HIV infection and AIDS will be considered.

Ironically, one of the first viruses identified in nature was a lentivirus, the equine infectious anemia virus, discovered in 1904 (2747). It induces episodic autoimmune hemolytic anemia in horses, with devastating effects on the equine population in many parts of the world, particularly Japan. This agent, although initially

Table 1.1 Lentiviruses

Virus	Host infected	Primary cell type infected	Clinical disorder
Equine infectious anemia virus	Horse	Macrophages	Cyclical infection in the first year; autoimmune hemolytic anemia; sometimes encephalopathy
Visna/maedi virus	Sheep	Macrophages	Encephalopathy/pneumonitis
Caprine arthritis-encephalitis virus	Goat	Macrophages	Immune deficiency; arthritis; encephalopathy
Bovine immune deficiency virus	Cow	Macrophages	Lymphadenopathy; lymphocytosis; central nervous system disease (?)
Feline immunodeficiency virus	Cat	T lymphocytes	Immune deficiency
Simian immunodeficiency virus	Primate	T lymphocytes	Immune deficiency and encephalopathy
Human immunodeficiency virus	Human	T lymphocytes	Immune deficiency and encephalopathy

demonstrating some characteristics of a retrovirus (1503), was only later identified as an RNA virus containing reverse transcriptase (RT) and as a member of the *Lentivirus* genus (405). Similarly, lentiviruses of sheep (visna/maedi virus) and goats (caprine arthritis-encephalitis virus) have been known for many years to be associated with a long illness and clinical symptoms not generally characteristic of retrovirus infection (409, 537, 980, 1496). Instead of malignancies, they can cause pathologic entities such as autoimmunity, pneumonitis, and brain and joint disorders (Table 1.1).

If, in hindsight, AIDS researchers had looked for an agent that would cause first an immune disorder in humans and later neurologic syndromes, certainly a lentivirus would have emerged as a prime candidate. Instead, the search for the cause of AIDS in the early 1980s focused on a variety of viruses, including not only retroviruses but also parvoviruses and herpesviruses, which are known to cause immune deficiency (1947, 2293). Even after HIV was discovered, its classification as a lentivirus took almost a year (Table 1.3) (442, 907, 1512, 2175).

Table 1.2 Average CD4$^+$ cell count at diagnosis of an AIDS-defining condition[a]

Opportunistic infection	CD4$^+$ cell count/μl
Non-Hodgkin's lymphoma	240
Primary cerebral lymphoma	<50
Kaposi's sarcoma	220
Pneumocystis carinii pneumonia	120
Toxoplasmic encephalitis	98
Cryptococcal meningitis	73
Mycobacterium avium complex infection	<50
Cytomegalovirus retinitis	<50

[a] Reprinted from reference 1676 with permission.

Table 1.3 Characteristics common to lentiviruses

Clinical
1. Association with a disease with a long incubation period
2. Association with immune suppression
3. Involvement of the hematopoietic system
4. Involvement of the central nervous system
5. Association with arthritis and autoimmunity

Biological
1. Host species specific
2. Exogenous and nononcogenic
3. Cytopathic effect in certain infected cells, e.g., syncytia (multinucleated cells)
4. Infection of macrophages, usually noncytopathic
5. Accumulation of unintegrated circular and linear forms of viral cDNA in infected cells
6. Latent or persistent infection in some infected cells
7. Morphology of virus particle by electron microscopy: cone-shaped nucleoid

Molecular
1. Large genome ($\geq$9 kb)
2. Truncated *gag* gene; several processed Gag proteins
3. Highly glycosylated envelope gene
4. Polymorphism, particularly in the envelope region
5. Novel central open reading frame in the viral genome that separates the *pol* and *env* regions

It is worth noting that the subsequent dedicated efforts to understand the AIDS virus have led to remarkable progress in our appreciation of its pathogenic counterparts in other animal species. HIV research has provided important contributions to veterinary medicine, including the discovery of the primate (simian immunodeficiency virus [SIV]) and cat (feline immunodeficiency virus [FIV]) lentiviruses (570, 2060). The study of HIV has also encouraged further work on the bovine lentivirus (908). Thus, the lentivirus field is one of limited examples in which work on a human virus has led to a better understanding of viruses in other animal species.

I. Discovery of the AIDS Virus

The first indication that AIDS could be caused by a retrovirus came in 1983, when Barré-Sinoussi, Chermann, Montagnier, and associates at the Pasteur Institute (146) recovered a virus containing RT from the lymph node of a man with persistent lymphadenopathy syndrome (LAS). At the time, some physicians suspected that this syndrome was associated with AIDS (6), but there was no conclusive evidence. Since enlarged lymph nodes are observed during several viral infections, many clinicians believed initially that LAS resulted from infection with a known human virus such as Epstein-Barr virus or cytomegalovirus. In addition, the characteristics described for the retrovirus recovered by the Pasteur Institute group (146) included some that were reported for the human T-cell leukemia virus (HTLV) (for a review, see reference 2610). Thus, many investigators believed initially that the lymph node isolate was a member of this recognized human retrovirus group. In support of this conclusion was the concomitant publication of a paper by Gallo and coworkers (835) on the isolation of HTLV from individuals with AIDS in the same issue of *Science* that reported the recovery of the LAS agent (146).

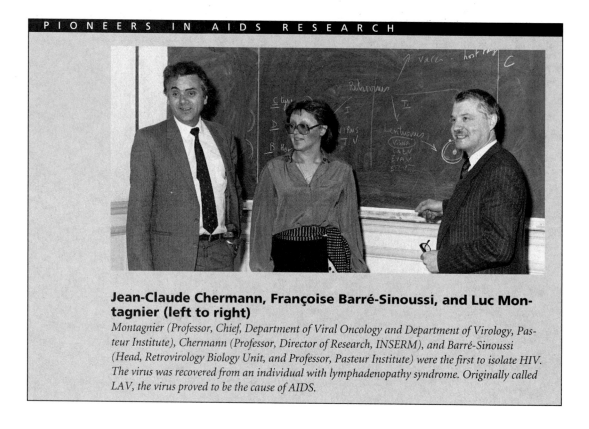

Jean-Claude Chermann, Françoise Barré-Sinoussi, and Luc Montagnier (left to right)

Montagnier (Professor, Chief, Department of Viral Oncology and Department of Virology, Pasteur Institute), Chermann (Professor, Director of Research, INSERM), and Barré-Sinoussi (Head, Retrovirology Biology Unit, and Professor, Pasteur Institute) were the first to isolate HIV. The virus was recovered from an individual with lymphadenopathy syndrome. Originally called LAV, the virus proved to be the cause of AIDS.

HTLV as the etiologic agent of AIDS, however, seemed unlikely because of its close cell association and its low-level replication in cells (1799, 2108, 2610). Since AIDS had been reported in hemophiliacs (382), how could this type of virus be transmitted by cell-free plasma products such as Factor VIII? HTLV is rarely found as a free virion in the blood. Moreover, HTLV does not kill lymphocytes; in fact, it often immortalizes them into continuous growth (1799). Thus, the characteristic loss of CD4$^+$ lymphocytes in AIDS patients (918, 1782, 2562) could not be explained by an HTLV infection (Table 1.4).

Further studies in 1983 by Montagnier and coworkers (1812) clarified these questions in relation to the LAS agent. Their results indicated that this human retrovirus, although similar to HTLV in infecting CD4$^+$ lymphocytes, had quite distinct properties. Their virus, later called LAV (lymphadenopathy-associated virus), grew to substantial titer in CD4$^+$ cells and killed them, instead of establishing the cells in culture as does HTLV. These observations on LAV provided important evidence supporting the potential etiologic role of a retrovirus in AIDS.

Several other laboratories were also searching for the agent responsible for this immune deficiency syndrome, and in early 1984, Gallo and associates reported the characterization of another human retrovirus distinct from HTLV that they called HTLV-III (834, 2122, 2359, 2425). It was isolated from the peripheral blood mononuclear cells (PBMC) of adult and pediatric AIDS patients. These workers noted the lymphotropic and cytopathic properties of the virus and reported that

Table 1.4 Comparison of HIV and HTLV

Characteristic	HIV	HTLV
Retrovirus genus	Lentivirus	HTLV/BLV
Genome size (kb)	9.8	9.0
Core morphology	Cone	Cuboid
Accessory genes	6	2
Infects CD4$^+$ lymphocytes	$+ +^a$	$+ +$
Infects CD8$^+$ lymphocytes	$-$	$+$
Wide tissue tropism	$+ +$	$+$
Causes syncytium formation	$+ +$	$+$
Cytotoxic	$+ +$	$-$
Transforms cells	$-$	$+ +^b$
Replicates to high titers	$+ +$	$-$
Mostly cell associated	$-$	$+ +$
Can exist in a latent state	$+$	$+$
Associated with immune deficiency	$+ +$	$+$
Associated with neurologic disorders	$+ +$	$+ +^c$

[a] Plus signs ($+$) indicate relative presence of each characteristic.

[b] T-cell leukemia.

[c] Tropical spastic paraparesis.

HTLV-III cross-reacted with some proteins of HTLV-I and HTLV-II, particularly the core p24 protein (834). Thus, they believed that it merited inclusion in the HTLV group, even though the newly isolated virus was cytolytic and did not induce an established cell line from infected lymphocytes.

Levy and coworkers (1510) also reported at that time the identification of retroviruses that they named the AIDS-associated retroviruses (ARV). These viruses were recovered from AIDS patients from different known risk groups, as well as from other symptomatic and some healthy people. Finding ARV in asymptomatic individuals indicated for the first time a carrier state for the AIDS virus. ARV showed some cross-reactivity with the French LAV strain when examined by immunofluorescence techniques (1510). Moreover, it grew substantially in PBMC, killed CD4$^+$ lymphocytes, and did not immortalize them. Thus, the three newly identified retroviruses had similar characteristics. Most importantly, infection by these viruses, as described in 1984, was not limited to AIDS patients. The viruses were also recovered from individuals with other clinical conditions, including lymphadenopathy. This latter observation supported the conclusion that LAS was part of the disease syndrome.

Within a short time, the three prototype viruses (LAV, HTLV-III, and ARV) were recognized as members of the same group of retroviruses, and their properties identified them as members of the *Lentivirinae* family (Table 1.3). Their proteins were all distinct from those of HTLV; their genomes showed only remote similarities to the genome of HTLV, no more than that of chicken retroviruses (2175). Thus, the initial cross-reactivity of HTLV-III with HTLV proved incorrect. The AIDS viruses had many properties distinguishing them from HTLV (Table 1.4). For all these reasons, in 1986 the International Committee on Taxonomy of Viruses recommended giving the AIDS virus a separate name, human immunodeficiency virus, or HIV (489).

In several studies, the HTLV-III strain was confirmed to be the same virus as the LAV strain (397, 433, 966). The Pasteur Institute group had sent LAV to the National Institutes of Health (NIH), where it appears to have contaminated a culture in the NIH laboratory (397, 995). This occurrence explains the unique molecular similarities between HTLV-III and LAV, in contrast to the sequence diversities observed with ARV-2 (now called HIV-1$_{SF2}$) and other strains (169, 305, 1512, 1871, 2193, 2351, 2804). Ironically, the French agent also was a contaminant in culture. At first considered an isolate from one patient (BRU), it was found to originate from a different individual (LAI). The LAI strain overgrew the BRU virus in a presumed mixed culture (397, 2805). Thus, HIV-1$_{LAI}$ is now the preferred name of the LAV and HTLV-III strains.

HIV isolates were subsequently recovered from the blood of many patients with AIDS, AIDS-related complex, and neurologic syndromes, as well as from the PBMC of several clinically healthy individuals (1521, 2337). Thus, the widespread transmission of this agent was appreciated, and its close association with AIDS and related illnesses strongly supported its role in these diseases. Soon after the discovery of HIV-1, a separate subtype, HIV-2, was identified in West Africa (462). Both HIV subtypes can lead to AIDS, although the pathogenic course of HIV-2 appears to be longer (see Chapter 7).

It is now known that some HIV-1-infected individuals can remain asymptomatic for up to 19 years and still have virus recoverable from their PBMC (308, 1491, 1539, 2311). Also noteworthy in these "long-term survivors," or "long-term nonprogressors" as some have called them (354, 2040), is the relative stability of the CD4$^+$ cell numbers, which are not necessarily decreased, as seen characteristically with HIV-induced disease (Chapter 13). The factors after HIV infection that influence this resistance to progression to AIDS are a major topic of this book.

About 3 years ago, the possibility of a new agent causing immune suppression in HIV-negative individuals (736, 2524) was suggested but not substantiated. In the few subjects reported with this syndrome of idiopathic CD4$^+$ T lymphocytopenia,

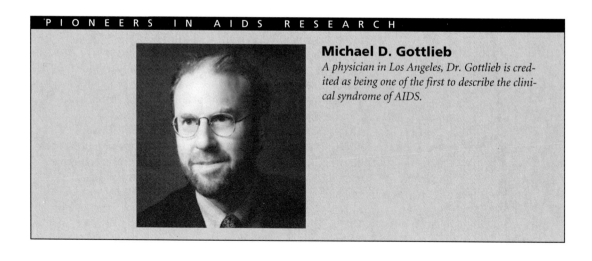

PIONEERS IN AIDS RESEARCH

Michael D. Gottlieb

A physician in Los Angeles, Dr. Gottlieb is credited as being one of the first to describe the clinical syndrome of AIDS.

the lymphopenia and CD4$^+$ cell reduction could be explained by measurement error or other known diseases (2588, 2680). In some instances, accelerated T-cell apoptosis has been observed but not explained (1445). Finally, while the role of HIV in AIDS has been challenged (670), the questions raised about a viral etiology have now been answered substantially, as detailed in the first edition of this book. The evidence has been substantiated even further by the additional data accumulated since May 1994.

II.	**The HIV Virion**

A.	**Structure**

Viewed by electron microscopy, HIV-1 and HIV-2 have the characteristics of a lentivirus, with a cone-shaped core composed of the viral p24 (or p25) Gag capsid protein (Figure 1.1). It was originally recommended that this capsid protein be referred to as p25 (1472), but common usage has led to the preferred terminology of p24. Inside this capsid, or nucleoid, are two identical RNA strands, with which the viral RNA-dependent DNA polymerase Pol, also called RT (p66 and p51), and the nucleocapsid proteins (p9 and p6) are closely associated. The inner portion of the viral membrane is surrounded by a myristoylated p17 core protein (MA), which provides the matrix for the viral structure and is vital for the integrity of the virion (861, 862) (Figures 1.1 and 1.2). MA appears to be required as well for incorporation of the Env proteins into mature virions (2948). Closely associated with the core are the Vif and Nef proteins (337, 1567, 2855). Estimates of 7 to 20 molecules of Vif per virion have recently been made (337). Also found within the virion and most probably outside the core is the viral accessory gene product Vpr (or Vpx for HIV-2) (1593, 2946). Recent data suggest that Tat may also be located inside virions (856a). The presence of all these viral proteins within the virion particles suggests that they play a role in early events of HIV infection. Certain cytoskeletal proteins (e.g., actin, ezrin, moesin, and coflin), perhaps cleaved by the HIV-1 protease, have also been detected within virions (1999); their role in infection, if any, is unknown.

The surface of the virus is characteristically made up of 72 knobs containing trimers or tetramers (679, 861, 2010, 2097, 2843) of the envelope glycoproteins. Electron microscopic pictures (861) and recent crystallization of the ectodomain of gp41 (393, 2849) suggest that the envelope protein is organized as a trimer. The envelope structures are derived from a 160-kDa precursor, gp160, which is cleaved inside the cell (most probably by cellular enzymes in the Golgi apparatus) into a gp120 external surface envelope protein and a gp41 transmembrane protein (1712). These proteins are transported to the cell surface, where part of the central and amino-terminal portion of gp41 is also expressed on the outside of the virion. The central region of the transmembrane protein binds to the external viral gp120 in a noncovalent manner, primarily at two hydrophobic regions in the amino and carboxyl termini of gp120 (1050). Some analyses suggest that a knob-and-socket-like structure is involved (2422) and that several envelope regions, including V1/V2 and the

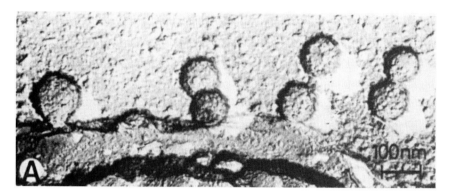

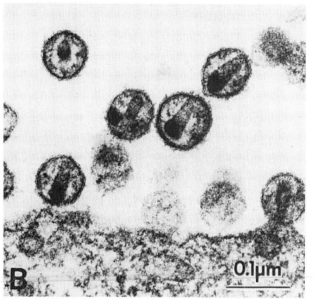

Figure 1.1 (A) Scanning electron micrograph of budding particles, most probably HIV, on the surface of a T lymphocyte. This process can incorporate cell surface proteins onto the surface of the virus and has been considered responsible in part for false-positive reactions in enzyme-linked immunosorbent assays (ELISA) (2372). Antibodies to normal T-cell proteins (e.g., HLA and CD4) could show a positive reaction. Photomicrograph courtesy of H. Gelderblom. (B) Transmission electron micrograph of HIV replicating in a T cell. Photomicrograph courtesy of R. Munn.

C2 and V3 domains of gp120, help stabilize the association (2614, 2885). In general, the virion has about 100 times more p24 Gag protein than it does envelope gp120 (1451, 1833) and 10 times more p24 than the polymerase molecule (1451).

The virion gp120, located on the virus surface, contains the binding site(s) for the cellular receptor(s) and the major neutralizing domains. Nevertheless, the external portion of gp41 and part of p17 have also been reported to be sensitive to neutralizing antibodies (400, 564, 1910, 2358) (see Chapter 10). The antibodies to p17 could indicate some protrusion of this core protein to the outside of the virion or on the surface of cells (2458). The specificity of these antibodies to p17 has been

Figure 1.2 An HIV virion with the structural and other virion proteins identified. The locations of Nef and Vif have not been well established. The abbreviated viral protein designations are those recommended (1472).

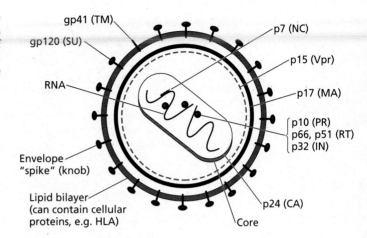

gp41 (TM)
gp120 (SU)
RNA
Envelope "spike" (knob)
Lipid bilayer (can contain cellular proteins, e.g. HLA)
p7 (NC)
p15 (Vpr)
p17 (MA)
p10 (PR)
p66, p51 (RT)
p32 (IN)
p24 (CA)
Core

challenged by some (2236). The antibodies could represent cross-reaction with anti-gp41 antibodies (318) (see Chapter 10).

B. Genomic Organization

The genomic size of HIV is about 9.8 kb, with open reading frames coding for several viral proteins (Table 1.5; Figures 1.3 and 1.4) (see also Chapter 5). The primary transcript of HIV is a full-length viral mRNA, which is translated into the Gag and Pol proteins (Figure 1.4). By proteolytic cleavage, the Gag precursor p55 gives rise to the smaller proteins, p24, p17, p9, and p6, cited above. The Pol precursor protein is cleaved into products consisting of the viral enzymes RT, protease, and integrase. Protease processes the Gag and Pol polyproteins; integrase is involved in virus integration. The Gag and Gag-Pol products are synthesized in a ratio of about 20:1 (1993). Splicing events producing many subgenomic messenger RNAs (mRNAs) are important for the synthesis of other viral proteins. The relative amounts of the unspliced to singly and multiply spliced mRNAs appear to be determined by the *rev* gene, which is itself a product of a multiply spliced mRNA (739, 2531) (see Chapter 5).

The envelope gp120 and gp41 proteins are made from a precursor gp160, noted above, which is a singly spliced message from the full-length viral mRNA. Gene products of other spliced mRNAs make up a variety of viral regulatory and accessory proteins that can affect HIV replication in various cell types (Figure 1.4). One regulatory protein is Tat, a transactivating protein that, along with certain cellular proteins, interacts with an RNA loop structure formed in the 3′ portion of the viral long terminal repeat called the Tat-responsive element. Tat is a major protein involved in upregulating HIV replication (for a review, see reference 2003).

Another viral regulatory protein, Rev (regulator of viral protein expression), interacts with a *cis*-acting RNA loop structure called the Rev-responsive element, located in the viral envelope mRNA (739, 2531). This interaction involves cellular proteins and multimers of the Rev protein and permits unspliced mRNA to enter the cytoplasm from the nucleus and give rise to full-length viral proteins needed for progeny production. Thus, Rev appears to affect the function of spliceosomes. Tat

Table 1.5 HIV proteins and their functions[a]

Protein	Size (kDa)	Function
Gag	p24 (p25)	Capsid (CA) structural protein
	p17	Matrix (MA) protein—myristoylated
	p6	Role in budding
	p7	Nucleocapsid (NC) protein; helps in reverse transcription
Polymerase (Pol)	p66, p51	Reverse transcriptase (RT); RNase H—inside core
Protease (PR)	p10	Posttranslational processing of viral proteins
Integrase (IN)	p32	Viral cDNA integration
Envelope	gp120	Envelope surface (SU) protein
	gp41 (gp36)	Envelope transmembrane (TM) protein
Tat[b]	p14	Transactivation
Rev[b]	p19	Regulation of viral mRNA expression
Nef	p27	Pleiotropic, can increase or decrease virus replication
Vif	p23	Increases virus infectivity and cell-to-cell transmission; helps in proviral DNA synthesis and/or in virion assembly (?) (2333, 2793)
Vpr	p15	Helps in virus replication; transactivation (?)
Vpu[b,c]	p16	Helps in virus release; disrupts gp160-CD4 complexes (2884)
Vpx[d]	p15	Helps in infectivity
Tev[b]	p26	Tat/Rev activities

[a] See Figure 1.3 for location of the viral genes on the HIV genome.

[b] Not found associated with the virion. Tat may be present in the virion (856a).

[c] Only present with HIV-1. Expression appears regulated by Vpr.

[d] Only coded by HIV-2. May be a duplication of Vpr.

and Rev are RNA binding proteins that interact with cellular factors for optimal activity.

Another protein, Nef (negative factor), appears to have a variety of potential functions, including cell activation and perhaps down-regulation of viral expression by some alleles. It was for this latter reason that this viral protein received its name (see Chapter 5). Its activity, however, is pleiotropic and also seems to require interactions with cellular proteins involved in signal transduction and cell activation (2368). How this effect influences HIV replication is under study. In addition, the accessory HIV gene products, Vif (2793), Vpr, and Vpu/Vpx, affect events such as assembly and budding, as well as infectivity during the production of infectious viruses (Table 1.5) (2003, 2081). Some studies suggest that the accessory genes, *vpr*, *vpu*, and *nef*, may be more important for replication of HIV-1 in macrophages than in CD4$^+$ lymphocytes (129).

As described in reviews on the molecular features of these viral gene products (2003, 2081), the regulation of virus expression involves the interplay of many viral proteins, leading to either high or low production of HIV or even the establishment of a latent state. For example, production of Rev in the later phases of the viral replicative cycle can down-regulate its own expression as well as that of Tat and Nef

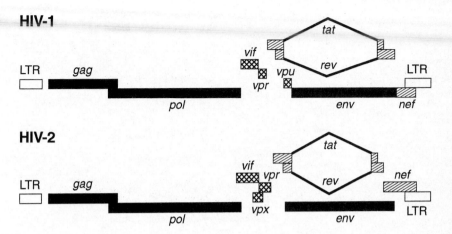

Figure 1.3 Genomic maps of HIV-1 and HIV-2. Note the unique presence of Vpu in HIV-1 and Vpx in HIV-2. Reprinted from reference 1494 with permission.

(see Chapter 5). Virus replication would then be limited. Finally, as with other retroviruses (1505), HIV strains have demonstrated selective incorporation of specific lipid domains from the host cell membrane during viral budding, as reflected in the molar ratio of cholesterol to phospholipid (50).

It is noteworthy that HIV codes for three major enzymes that function at different times during the replicative cycle. As expected, they have been prime targets for approaches to antiviral therapy (see Chapter 14). The RNA-dependent DNA polymerase (with its RNase H function) (i.e., RT) acts in the early steps of virus replication to form a double-stranded DNA copy (cDNA) of the virus RNA. The integrase functions inside the cell nucleus to integrate the viral cDNA into the host chromosomal DNA. The protease acts during the maturation of the viral particle, either at the cell surface or in the budding virion, by processing the Gag and Gag-Pol polyproteins (2081).

III.   Origin of HIV

One hypothesis on the origin of HIV links all human and simian viral sequences to a common ancestor existing 600 to 1,200 years ago (691). Others have proposed that the virus, as we currently know it, entered the human population as early as 30 to 100 years ago (1471, 1891, 1892), or perhaps several thousand years ago (for reviews, see references 1471 and 2464). The first documented evidence of HIV infection in humans can be traced to an African serum sample collected in 1959 (1899). However, other samples taken from many parts of Africa up to the mid-1970s have not shown evidence of HIV infection (for a review, see reference 1888). Thus, how and when this virus emerged and evolved into various sequence subtypes (or clades), including the outliers (clade O), remains a mystery. Several possibilities have been presented, such as frequent transfers from animal reservoirs to humans, but that suggestion seems unlikely with the recent recognition of at least 11 HIV-1

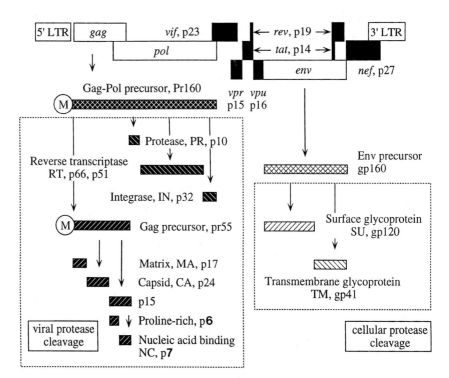

Figure 1.4   Processing of viral proteins. Some HIV-1 proteins, which are translated from 10 distinct viral transcripts, are further processed by viral and cellular proteases. From nine translated proteins, which include Tev (not diagrammed), 16 viral proteins are made. They form the virion structure, direct viral enzymatic activities, and serve regulatory and accessory functions. The Gag-Pol precursor of 160 kDa is processed by the viral (aspartyl) protease into seven proteins, which include four Gag proteins (MA, p17; CA, p24; proline-rich, p6; NC, p9), protease (P, p10), reverse transcriptase/RNase (RT, p66, p51), and integrase (IN, p32). The Env precursor (gp160) is processed by a cellular protease into the surface glycoprotein (SU, gp120) and the transmembrane glycoprotein (TM, gp41). Viral regulatory and accessory proteins—which include Tat (p14), Tev (p26), Rev (p19), Nef (p27), Vif (p23), Vpr (p15), and Vpu (p16)—are not processed. M, myristoylated. Figure courtesy of M. Peterlin.

clades (see Chapter 7). HIV could have evolved into a distinct clade through independent derivation after entry into a country, but this hypothesis suggests that changes in the virus can occur within selected populations after a limited amount of trafficking (or distribution) (1888). Why, then, is there only one major clade in North America, where the virus has existed for more than 10 years? Perhaps certain parts of Africa have been evolving the virus over time but the clades were recognized only as the disease became apparent. This possibility seems remote, since all of these independent events would have had to occur around the same time in this century. Conceivably, a viral sequence might also result from a lack of divergence from a common preexisting virus (1888).

Several investigators favor the conclusion that HIV came from primates. A connection between SIV and HIV-2 provides the most compelling evidence, although it is not conclusive. A laboratory worker was found to be infected by SIV (1284), and the future course of this infection, which is now clinically silent, could influence the thinking on this possibility. Other evidence in support of an origin of HIV-2 from SIV is the detection of an SIV-like HIV-2 strain in an individual in Liberia (838). Moreover, SIV strains in monkeys originating in West Africa are genetically more related to HIV-2 (1674). Nevertheless, the genomic heterogeneity among SIV and HIV-2 strains, which continues to be appreciated as more viruses are isolated and sequenced, brings into question the conclusion that HIV came directly from the nonhuman primate lentiviruses (774, 1872, 2723).

Along with the lentiviruses from other animal species (Table 1.1), the simian and human viruses could have evolved independently from a progenitor lentivirus that entered the animal kingdom many thousands of years ago. A primate counterpart to HIV-1 has not been identified, except perhaps for isolates from chimpanzees (SIV_{CPZ}) (1133, 2061). The relation of the SIV_{CPZ} to the transmission of HIV-1, however, is not clear, and the two viral types differ substantially (see Chapter 7) (1133). A recent isolate from a wild chimpanzee from Zaire has been sequenced, and it comes from a highly divergent group of viruses that are equidistant from other chimpanzee isolates and the clade O HIV-1 viruses (2760) (see Chapter 7). The rarity of lentiviruses in chimpanzees and the divergence of strains do not support a common transfer of HIV-1 between humans and chimpanzees.

It would seem most likely that HIV has been present in small habitats in parts of Africa (mostly central Africa) for centuries and, once having emerged through recent social and economic changes, was allowed to spread and evolve among several human populations. Whether the genetic makeup of these other human populations influenced the evolution of the clades is not clear. The distribution of HIV, however, appears to have occurred recently and rather rapidly, considering the very quick recognition of several clades already circulating in the world. The emergence of HIV has alerted public health officials and governments worldwide to the constant threat of new infectious agents that can be spread rapidly through the present-day means of international communication. Research on this agent and approaches for its control should provide insights into any future challenges to the well-being of human and animal populations.

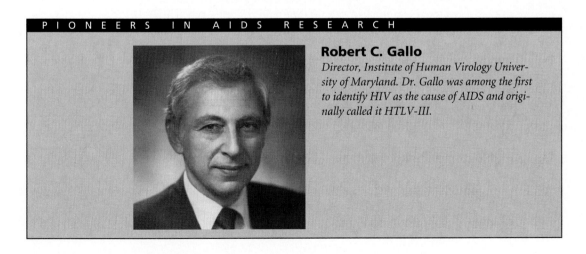

PIONEERS IN AIDS RESEARCH

Robert C. Gallo

Director, Institute of Human Virology University of Maryland. Dr. Gallo was among the first to identify HIV as the cause of AIDS and originally called it HTLV-III.

Chapter 1   SALIENT FEATURES

1. Human immunodeficiency virus (HIV), first identified in 1983, is the causative agent of AIDS. It is a member of the lentivirus genus of retroviruses.

2. The basic pathology in AIDS is a loss of $CD4^+$ lymphocytes and a variety of disorders in immune function.

3. AIDS is defined by a reduction in the number of $CD4^+$ cells (less than 200 cells/μl) and the onset of opportunistic infections (particularly *Pneumocystis carinii* pneumonia) and malignancies (e.g., Kaposi's sarcoma, B-cell lymphomas). Neurologic and gastrointestinal disorders are also commonly found in AIDS patients.

4. Development of disease results from a lack of control of HIV replication by the host immune system.

5. Two types of HIV exist in the world: HIV-1 and HIV-2. They can be distinguished particularly by their envelope glycoproteins.

6. Individual HIV-1 and HIV-2 isolates can be characterized by a variety of biologic, immunologic, and molecular features (see Chapter 7).

7. HIV can be recovered from the blood of asymptomatic people as well as those with symptoms of AIDS.

8. The HIV genome codes for two structural proteins (Gag and Env), three enzymes (polymerase, integrase, and protease), and six accessory genes that help to regulate virus replication (*tat, vif, vpu, vpr* [*vpx*], *nef,* and *rev*).

9. The replicative cycle of HIV involves reverse transcription of the viral RNA into a DNA copy and subsequent integration of the viral genome into the cell chromosome. Thus, the virus-infected cell is an important reservoir for HIV infection in the host.

10. The origins of HIV-1 and HIV-2 are unknown. Some investigators believe that HIV (particularly HIV-2) was transferred from primates to humans in the near-distant past. Others suggest that the viruses were derived from a progenitor virus that entered mammalian species thousands of years ago. The earliest documented case of HIV infection appears to be in 1959, and the epidemic phase became apparent in 1981.

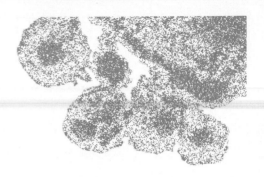

Features of HIV Transmission

THE TRANSMISSION FREQUENCY OF A VIRUS IS INFLUENCED BY THE amount of infectious virus in a body fluid and the extent of contact an individual has with that body fluid. Established infection depends on three points of a classic epidemiologic triangle (Figure 2.1): characteristics of the infectious agent (e.g., virulence and infectiousness), host-related factors (e.g., susceptibility, contagiousness, and immune response), and environmental factors (e.g., social, cultural, and political) (2300). The same features can influence disease development. Epidemiologic studies conducted during 1981 and 1982 first indicated that the major routes of transmission of AIDS were intimate sexual contact and contaminated blood (1182). The syndrome was initially described in homosexual and bisexual men and intravenous drug users (918, 1695, 1782, 2500), but its transmission through heterosexual activity was soon recognized as well (1020). High-risk sexual behavior early in the epidemic caused the rapid increase in HIV transmission (1713). Moreover, it became evident that transfusion recipients and hemophiliacs could contract the illness from blood or blood products (382) and that mothers could transfer the causative agent to newborn infants (61, 1979). These three principal means of transmission—blood, sexual contact, and mother-child—have

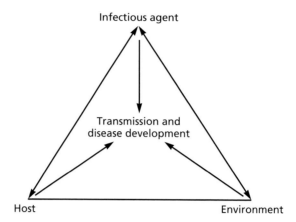

Figure 2.1 Epidemiology of infectious diseases. A variety of host and environmental factors, as well as characteristics of the infectious agent, determine the transmission of the agent and induction of disease (2300).

not changed (297, 2164) and can be explained to a great extent by the relative concentrations of HIV in various body fluids (Table 2.1).

The high virus load observed during acute HIV infection or the symptomatic period (Section I) might be expected to present the greatest risk of HIV transmission. Relative levels of virus in genital fluid at these times must be considered but are still somewhat inconsistent (Section II). The information could have important applications in campaigns to reduce the spread of HIV. Moreover, long-term or serial monogamous relationships, rather than concurrent multiple sexual contacts, could be emphasized (1132), since the risk of infection is lower. In this chapter, I review the evidence on the virus load in various body fluids and consider the findings in relation to virus transmission.

I.   HIV in Blood

Because of the great concern for the reported transmission of AIDS by blood, major efforts were made early in the study of HIV to quantify virus in this body fluid. The results indicated that both free infectious virus and infected cells were present in blood, and HIV-infected cells appeared to be more numerous than infectious virus. In blood, as well as other body fluids, noninfectious viruses and cells containing defective viral genomes detected by polymerase chain reaction (PCR) can be present in the largest quantities but do not represent sources of transmission.

A.   Infectious Virus

In the early studies of viremia, methods for detecting infectious virus had to be established and optimized. The initial data suggested that free infectious HIV was present in the blood of about 30 to 50% of infected individuals (729, 1776). However, improved virus detection procedures showed that most blood samples contain cir-

Table 2.1 Isolation of infectious HIV from body fluids[a]

Fluid	Virus isolation	Estimated quantity of HIV
Cell-free fluid		
Plasma	33/33	1–5,000[b]
Tears	2/5	<1
Ear secretions	1/8	5–10
Saliva	3/55	<1
Sweat	0/2	—[c]
Feces	0/2	—
Urine	1/5	<1
Vaginal-cervical	5/16	<1
Semen	5/15	10–50
Milk	1/5	<1
Cerebrospinal fluid	21/40	10–10,000
Infected cells		
PBMC	89/92	0.001–1%[b]
Saliva	4/11	<0.01%
Bronchial fluid	3/24	ND
Vaginal-cervical fluid	7/16	ND
Semen	11/28	0.01–5%

[a] For cell-free fluid, units are infectious particles per milliliter; for infected cells, percentage of total cells capable of releasing virus. Results from studies in the author's laboratory are presented. Abbreviation: ND, not determined.

[b] High levels associated with acute infection and advanced disease.

[c] —, None detected.

culating infectious virus whether the HIV-infected individual is asymptomatic or has AIDS (512, 1081, 2023, 2294, 2315). The quantity can reach 100 to 1,000 infectious particles (IP) per ml of blood. Importantly, the level is very low in healthy subjects and often undetectable in long-term survivors (354, 1520, 2040). To quantify optimally the level of free infectious virus in blood, the plasma needs to be tested within 3 h of venipuncture. Otherwise, neutralizing antibodies, complement (2612), and other undefined factors in the plasma (for a review, see reference 2541) reduce the infectivity of HIV (2023). An important procedure for detection of infectious virus in plasma is to allow at least a 24-h incubation with the target cells (1843, 2220a).

Infectious HIV is readily found during acute (primary) infection (461, 557, 823, 1512, 2023), but within weeks the level of free virus detected in the blood is markedly reduced (512, 715, 920, 1081, 2023, 2092, 2294). The reason for this decrease in viremia is most probably an active antiviral cellular immune response (see Chapter 11). Then, as disease develops with its characteristic loss of CD4$^+$ cells, the concentration of infectious HIV in blood rises substantially (Table 2.2), reflecting the increased virus load in peripheral blood mononuclear cells (PBMC) and lymphoid tissues (see Chapter 4) (512, 690, 1081, 1972, 2023, 2294). Thus, the risk of transmission of infectious HIV would seem to be highest in the early stage of infection and during the symptomatic periods. However, the risk at those times may exist only for blood; insufficient data are available concerning the levels of infectious virus in genital fluids at these times of high viremia (Section II).

Table 2.2 Titer of infectious HIV-1 recovered from plasma in relation to CD4$^+$ cell count[a]

CD4$^+$ cells/mm^3	No. of individuals	Range of HIV titer (TCID/ml)	Mean of HIV titer (TCID/ml)[b]
≥500	13	1–500	114
300–499	8	1–500	205
200–299	4	25–500	381
<200	8	25–5,000	1,466

[a] Abbreviation: TCID, tissue culture infectious dose.

[b] The trend of finding increased virus titer with lower CD4$^+$ cells counts was statistically significant (Kruskal-Wallis test; data from reference 2023).

B.   Viral Antigen and RNA

Other procedures that greatly increase the sensitivity for detection of HIV in blood and other body fluids have been developed. They include the measurement of viral p24 antigen (921), directly and after acid dissociation (244), and of HIV RNA by PCR (1100) and quantitative competitive (QC) PCR techniques (1754, 2092). QC PCR involves an internal control RNA template that serves as a measure of viral RNA quantity through a competitive mechanism. From 50 to 11 million virions per ml of blood have been detected by this method, and the amount correlates with disease stage and CD4$^+$ T-cell counts (2092) (Table 2.3). In these studies, a decrease in virus levels in plasma of more than 200-fold after seroconversion has been demonstrated (2092).

The most recent sensitive methods for detecting HIV RNA include reverse transcription-PCR and a procedure based on the attachment of branched oligodeoxyribonucleotides (bDNA) to viral RNA for subsequent signal amplification (625, 2738, 2751) (Figure 2.2). The sensitivity of these new procedures is similar to or higher than that of QC PCR. With these techniques, detection of viral RNA to levels of ~500 copies/ml or lower can be achieved (2174). These recently developed molecular approaches have proven to be the most sensitive for measuring the relation of viremia to the clinical condition and the response to therapy (353, 2448). They have provided an important advancement in handling the clinical approach to HIV infection (see Chapter 14). Importantly, whereas CD4$^+$ cell numbers can vary over a 24-h period (see Chapter 9, Section I.A), viral RNA levels appear to be relatively constant and show no diurnal pattern (610a). These procedures, however, do not distinguish between infectious and noninfectious virions. Moreover, the results can vary 20 to 30% in accuracy and may not detect certain HIV-1 isolates (e.g., clade A) (30). Improvements to these assays should resolve these problems.

With these techniques available, two groups of investigators, using antiretroviral drugs to suppress virus replication in vivo, calculated the potential kinetics of virus replication and time for removal of HIV from the peripheral blood (see also Chapter 14). These studies with symptomatic patients suggested that the half-life of HIV in plasma (measured by RNA) is about 6.5 h (1082, 2073, 2834). The data estimated that up to 10 billion virus particles could be present in the circulating blood in symptomatic patients (2073). This number was similar to that reported in previ-

Table 2.3 Plasma viremia and clinical stage[a]

Clinical stage	Viremia (virions/ml)
Acute (primary) infection	5×10^6
Asymptomatic	8×10^4
Early symptomatic	35×10^4
AIDS	2.5×10^6

[a] Summary of QC PCR data from reference 2092. Representative values are shown. Culturable infectious virus ranged from 100- to 100,000-fold less.

ous studies (2092). While the vast majority of these particles are noninfectious (see below), this level of circulating virions produced continuously was not expected.

In additional studies of infected individuals in different clinical states, various levels of virus were found. Large numbers correlated with progression of disease. In long-term survivors (those infected for $\geq$10 years, with normal $CD4^+$ cell counts and no symptoms) and several asymptomatic individuals (>500 $CD4^+$ cells/µl), free infectious virus and viral RNA were very scarce or undetectable in the blood (354, 843, 1520, 2040). Thus, the absence of viral RNA in plasma has been considered a good prognostic sign (see Chapter 13). This finding has sparked interest in beginning antiretroviral therapy in infected individuals at early stages in infection. The objective is to reduce the viral load to undetectable levels (now less than 200 copies of viral RNA/ml of blood) for long periods (see Chapter 14).

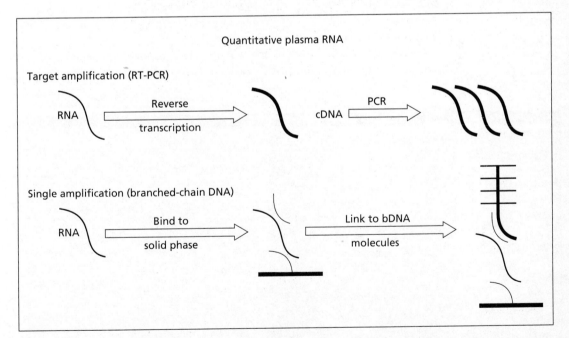

Figure 2.2 Schematic representation of the reverse transcription-PCR and branched-chain DNA techniques for amplification and quantitation of viral RNA in blood and body fluids. Adapted from reference 996a with permission.

The relation of data on viremia measured by these molecular procedures to the number of infectious particles, the potential source of HIV transmission, is important. It is estimated that up to 100,000 (average 60,000) more noninfectious virions than free infectious viruses are present in the plasma of seropositive individuals (1451, 2092). These noninfectious viruses would be the majority of virions detected by the quantitative antigen and RNA analyses cited above. Thus, in considering transmission, appreciation of the amount of infectious virus in the blood is obviously necessary. For prognosis, the extent of viral RNA production, as it reflects the overall clinical state, can be a valuable marker (see Chapter 13).

C.   Virus-Infected Cells

Despite this attention to free virus particles in the blood, their relationship to virus-infected cells remains an important question. In many cases, levels of free virus, even following antiviral therapy, have not consistently shown a correlation to virus numbers in PBMC (1461) or in the lymph node (496, 2284b) (see Chapter 14). The total number of HIV-infected cells has been estimated to be several hundred billion (696), a much greater number than that of the free virions found in blood (see Chapter 13). Moreover, studies have indicated that one infected cell can produce 200 to 1,000 particles per day (638, 1492, 1519, 2284b). Thus, the total number of infected cells responsible for the high viral RNA level in the blood could represent only a small fraction (10 to 20 million) of cells known to be infected (696, 1492, 1499). This observation emphasizes a concern about concluding that a block in de novo (fresh) virus infection by using antiretroviral drugs will give long-term benefit. Many virus-infected cells can remain in the body and be a continual source of new virions (1492, 1499) (see Chapters 13 and 14).

Several studies have indicated that virus-infected cells are more common in blood than is infectious virus. As with free virus, the number of infected cells is in-

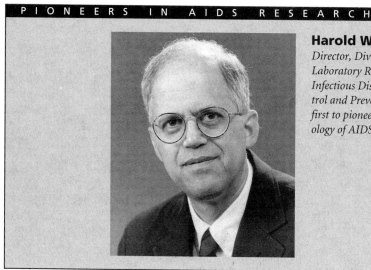

P I O N E E R S I N A I D S R E S E A R C H

Harold W. Jaffe

Director, Division of AIDS, STD and TB Laboratory Research, National Center for Infectious Diseases, Centers for Disease Control and Prevention. Dr. Jaffe was among the first to pioneer efforts at tracing the epidemiology of AIDS.

creased with symptomatic disease and reduced $CD4^+$ cell counts. Initially, the number of virus-infected cells detected by in situ hybridization techniques ranged from 1:10,000 to 1:100,000 PBMC (1015). Subsequent studies by PCR procedures increased this number to an average of 1 in 1,000 to 1 in 10,000 PBMC in healthy individuals and 1 in 10 PBMC in AIDS patients (1117, 2404, 2407). In studies by in situ PCR hybridization and flow cytometry, 1 in 10 PBMC were found infected in symptomatic patients (122, 2048). Most of the infected cells (50 to 90%) contained HIV in a latent (unexpressed, or "silent") state (2048).

The majority of cells showing HIV infection by these molecular techniques are $CD4^+$ lymphocytes (117, 122, 2048). Not many circulating macrophages are found to be infected (see Chapter 4). The nature of the virus in the unproductively infected cells is not well defined; it could be defective or in a latent state. Recent PCR analyses have provided some insight into this question (379) (see Chapters 4, 9, and 14). When the virus is latent, the factor that activates virus production in infected cells is important in HIV pathogenesis (see Chapter 5). Recently, by using a microculture assay, optimal procedures for measuring the number of infected cells were reported (2434). In studies in my laboratory, close to 50% of the virus-infected cells in lymphoid tissue from some infected individuals appeared to contain infectious virus (226).

For concerns about transmission and spread of virus in the host, the virus-infected cells become more important than the infectious virus load in the blood (Table 2.4). The total amount of free infectious virus in asymptomatic individuals can be 100 IP/ml of blood (1081, 2023), whereas the average number of virus-infected cells in these individuals is about 1 in 1,000 PBMC (117, 285, 1015, 1117, 2149, 2404, 2407) (see Chapter 4). Once again, total viral RNA (containing noninfectious virions) will be up to 100,000-fold higher but is not a factor in transmitting HIV. With at least 5×10^6 leukocytes/ml of blood, there can be about 5,000 infected cells/ml of blood in a healthy individual. From this total amount, one can estimate that at least 50% of these cells can release infectious virus (226). Thus, the number of infected cells in blood is at least 25-fold larger than the amount of free infectious virus. In addition, each cell could produce many infectious particles daily (638, 1519). During symptomatic infection, especially AIDS, the number of infectious viruses and infected cells is usually much larger (e.g., 1,000 IP/ml; up to 1:10 $CD4^+$ cells/ml) (117, 120, 866, 1117, 1502, 2404) (Table 2.2). Thus, the chance of trans-

Table 2.4   HIV pathogenesis: importance of the virus-infected cell with respect to free virus

1. Present at higher levels in the body (>200 billion cells) than free virus (1–10 billion particles)
2. Reservoir for persistent virus production (1,000 particles/day)
3. Transfers HIV to new cells more effectively than infection by free virus
4. Can induce apoptosis by cell-to-cell contact
5. Releases viral products that are toxic to the host (e.g., gp120, gp41, and Tat)
6. Releases toxic cellular products (e.g., tumor necrosis factor α and interleukin-6)
7. Present at higher levels (5–50 times) than free virus in genital fluids and blood
8. Remains viable in genital fluids and blood longer than free virus

mitting infection, particularly by cells containing HIV, could be even greater (1492, 1502). Furthermore, even if a latently infected cell were transferred, it could serve as a source of HIV transmission after its activation in the new host (1667).

HIV in Genital Fluids

General Observations

In the case of sexual transmission, the amount of virus in genital fluids is important. Generally, seminal and vaginal fluids have shown the presence of free infectious virus and/or virus-infected cells in 10 to 30% of specimens (68, 256, 1086, 1206, 1501, 1502, 2758, 2768, 2783, 2902, 2957; for a review, see reference 1868) (Figure 2.3). However, the levels of free infectious virus detected in these body fluids (estimated at 1 to 50 IP/ml) have not been reported from a large number of individuals, and the quantity of virus found can differ considerably (Table 2.1). Recently, measurements of viral RNA levels have shown a greater frequency of free virus in these fluids, but the risk of transmission will depend on the number of infectious virions

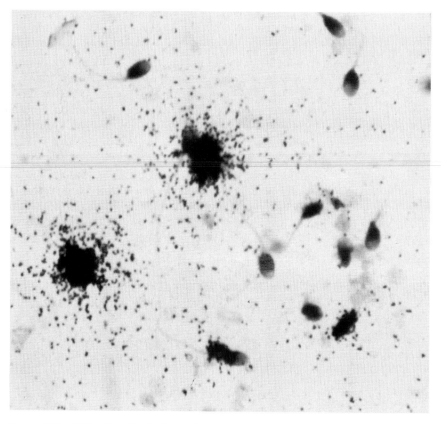

Figure 2.3 HIV-infected cells detected in seminal fluid by in situ hybridization. Magnification, ×40. Reprinted from reference 1501 with permission.

(for a review, see reference 1868). Moreover, the potential influence of anti-HIV antibodies in genital fluids (1932) on the risk of transmission merits further study. The biologic and epidemiologic factors that can influence virus shedding in the genital tract are listed in Table 2.5 (1868).

B.

HIV in Seminal Fluid

As noted above with virus in plasma, the largest amount of infectious virus in genital fluids might be expected in the acute phase of infection and during the symptomatic periods (Section I). In this regard, transmission has been found to be increased when the male partners with disease engage in heterosexual or homosexual activity (1995, 2356). In some reports, recovery of infectious virus from semen was highest from men with low $CD4^+$ cell counts (68, 2769). However, only a small number of subjects were studied, and virus was recovered primarily from infected cells.

Most studies suggest that the presence of infectious virus in seminal fluid does not correlate with clinical state (994, 1375). Both syncytium-inducing (SI) and non-syncytium-inducing (NSI) strains can be isolated from semen (2768). As reviewed in Chapter 7, the SI viruses are usually considered to be more "virulent." The quantity of HIV in semen also does not necessarily reflect the level of plasma viremia. In addition, the virus found in semen does not always show the same biologic phenotype as that in the blood (NSI versus SI) (2769). Similarly, no correlation of plasma

Table 2.5 Factors affecting HIV-1 shedding in the genital tract[a]

Status	Factors in:	
	Females	**Males**
Confirmed correlates[b]	Pregnancy Oral contraceptives Cervical ectopy Cervicitis	HIV disease stage $CD4^+$ lymphocyte count $CD8^+$ lymphocyte count Antiretroviral therapy Leukocytospermia Gonorrhea Urethritis
Potential correlates	HIV disease stage $CD4^+$ lymphocyte count Plasma viremia Viral phenotype or subtype Antiretroviral therapy Injectable contraceptives Nutritional deficiency states Specific cervical or vaginal STD Lactobacillus and H_2O_2 production Mucosal HIV antibodies Douching or drying agents	Plasma viremia Viral phenotype or subtype Vasectomy Circumcision status Nutritional deficiency states Nongonoccocal urethritis Mucosal HIV antibodies

[a] Adapted from reference 1868 with permission.

[b] The confirmed correlates listed are those which have been significantly associated ($P < 0.05$) with HIV-1 detection in genital tract fluids in one or more studies. STD, sexual transmitted disease.

viremia to viral levels (measured by reverse transcription-PCR) in semen or saliva was found when all three body fluids were examined (1570). Thus, direct infection (1756) or local inflammation in these various body compartments appears to be the important factor in determining the level of virus produced. Finally, in limited studies, virus has been detected in semen by cell culture or PCR techniques despite antiviral therapy (994, 1376, 2769). These findings probably reflect the inability of some drugs to penetrate the blood-testes barrier (see Chapter 14) (134).

The prevalence of virus-infected cells appears to be an important variable in genital fluids (1502, 2782, 2905) (Table 2.1). In seminal fluid, the number can range from 0.01 to 5% (1501) (Figure 2.3). Semen usually has over 1 million leukocytes/ejaculate (67, 1981, 2904), but levels and subsets of cells can vary widely from day to day in the same individual (2089a). Nevertheless, the HIV-infected cells ($>10^4$ in some cases) seem to be a greater source of transmission than free infectious virus. T cells appear to be most commonly infected, followed by macrophages (2162a). Moreover, if there is a sexually transmitted disease, many more inflammatory cells, and thus virus-infected cells, would be present in both seminal and vaginal fluids (Section V). In one study, HIV DNA was found in urethral cells during gonococcal urethritis, and the number of infected cells detected was decreased by treatment (1865).

The cellular source of HIV in seminal fluid is not well defined. By culture and in situ PCR hybridization procedures, HIV has been detected in large quantities in the testes of infected individuals. It has been found in urethral cells (1865), spermatogonia, spermatocytes, and occasionally in spermatids, but not in Sertoli cells (1955). Testicular atrophy can take place, limiting the detection of virus (1955). Low testosterone levels have also been noted in some HIV-infected men. These findings probably reflect the pathogenic effects of the virus in this tissue in some AIDS patients. The presence of HIV in spermatogonia could explain the puzzling finding of HIV DNA in the midportion of some spermatozoa, as noted by in situ PCR hybridization (116). Since only the head enters the egg during fertilization, a relevance of this finding to possible germ line transmission of HIV is unlikely. Nevertheless, a glycolipid resembling galactosyl ceramide on the middle portion of the sperm tail (294) could serve as an attachment site for HIV, as it does on some brain and bowel cells (see Chapter 3).

HIV has also been isolated from semen from vasectomized men (69), and after vasectomy, many lymphocytes can be found in the ejaculate (1981). Infectious virus has been recovered from preejaculatory fluid from infected men (1155, 2151). Thus, the virus and virus-infected cells must come from the urethra, prostate, and other secretory glands, as well as the testes (554, 1457). HIV has not been detected in the epithelia of the prostate, epididymus, seminal vesicles, or penis of men with AIDS by in situ PCR hybridization procedures (1955).

C. HIV in Vaginal Fluid

Vaginal fluid has been found to contain free infectious virus only rarely (1056, 2902); generally, infected cells are detected (1056, 2782, 2783, 2902), but the quantity has not been reported. Even by PCR analysis, HIV was found in cervicovaginal secretions of only 28% of infected women (1932). As with seminal fluid,

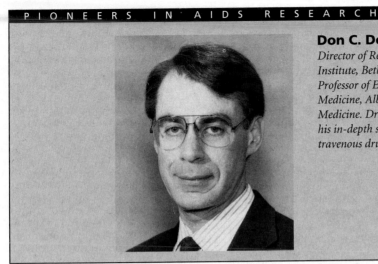

Don C. Des Jarlais

Director of Research, Chemical Dependency Institute, Beth Israel Medical Center, and Professor of Epidemiology and Social Medicine, Albert Einstein College of Medicine. Dr. Des Jarlais is well known for his in-depth studies of HIV infection in intravenous drug users.

plasma viremia does not correlate with virus shedding (1932, 2191). Moreover, the prevalence of free virus in cervicovaginal secretions does not reflect the clinical state, zidovudine (AZT) therapy, or risk group (1056, 2191). The prevalence of the virus, however, has been found to be significantly higher in pregnant women than in nonpregnant women (1056). It is also higher in women with cervical ectopy, abnormal vaginal discharge, or severe vitamin A deficiency (1206) and in those taking oral contraceptive pills (467; for a review, see reference 2300) (Table 2.4). A recent report showed a higher prevalence of virus in nonpregnant women compared to pregnant women, most probably reflecting present-day antiviral therapy for pregnant women (1932). Again, however, the number of subjects with infectious virus studied has been too small to draw definitive conclusions on these parameters.

In regard to viral subtypes, one report of recently infected Kenyan women revealed viruses in cervical secretions that differed genotypically from those found in the peripheral blood (2128). This recognition of tissue-specific variants supports the conclusion noted with seminal fluid that a different distribution (or evolution) of viruses can be found in the blood and genital tissues.

The source of HIV in vaginal fluid is not known but is most probably the secretory glands in the vagina or cervix, leukocytes in the uterine cavity, and, in some cases, menstrual blood. HIV has been detected in the cervix (2118), where, by in situ PCR hybridization procedures, it is found primarily in monocytes and macrophages (1956) and in the glandular epithelium in the zone of transformation between columnar and squamous cells (1956). The cervix is a more frequent source of virus than the vagina (467; for a review, see reference 2300).

In all these studies on genital fluids, detection of infectious virus was probably limited, since culturing of HIV can be technically difficult. These body fluids can be cytotoxic in culture, and survival of the virus can depend on the pH and potential antiviral factors present (1970). Moreover, a delay in assaying genital or other body fluids probably decreases the detection of virus, as noted with plasma samples (2023).

III.   ## HIV in Saliva and Other Body Fluids

Although blood and genital fluids can contain high levels of infectious virus or infected cells, other body fluids are not likely sources of HIV transmission (Table 2.1). Saliva, for example, yields infectious virus only on rare occasions (generally <10% of samples) and only in limited amounts (<1.0 IP/ml) (518, 916, 952, 1077, 1509). Both free virus and infected cells have been detected in saliva but only at a low level (916, 1509). By PCR techniques, virus-infected cells were rarely found, even in the presence of periodontal disease (2940), although in one report saliva-associated infected epithelial cells were detected in over 80% of seropositive subjects studied (2166). In another study, low levels of free HIV-1 genomes were detected by PCR in most saliva samples obtained from individuals with either high or low CD4$^+$ cell counts (1570). Nevertheless, as a source of transmission, it is the infectious virus titer that is important.

Because of the low level of infectious virus in this fluid, the risk of HIV infection following a human bite is extremely low. No infection was reported in over 600 incidents of bites treated in U.S. hospitals (2656), although one case of transmission by biting has been published (2773).

The low rate of recovery of infectious HIV from saliva could reflect not only a relatively low virus content but also direct antiviral properties of saliva fluid, such as the secretory leukocyte protease inhibitor (1743), or nonspecific inhibitory substances in the fluid (64, 78, 183, 518, 1651, 1898, 2607). The latter could be fibronectins, glycoproteins, and mucins (e.g., MG1), which come primarily from gingival and not parotid salivary glands (64, 183, 518, 2607). Like dextran sulfate (5, 107), MG1 blocks HIV infection at the cell surface (64) and could prevent cell-to-cell transfer of virus. Alternatively, saliva could aggregate HIV (1651) but not necessarily reduce infectivity unless these aggregates were removed. The presence of these inhibitory substances provides additional reasons to consider saliva an unlikely cause of transmission. Nevertheless, since infectious HIV has been recovered from the throats of infected children (1255), the question of antiviral activity in the saliva of children needs further study.

Urine, sweat, milk, bronchoalveolar lavage fluids, amniotic fluid, synovial fluid, feces, and tears have also been shown to contain none or only low levels of infectious HIV (608, 804, 1193, 1417, 1502, 1512, 1532, 1875, 2339, 2519, 2673, 2899, 2915, 2941, 2994) (Table 2.1), although viral RNA may be detected in some specimens (e.g., in feces) (2750). Thus, these fluids do not appear to be important sources of virus transmission. This conclusion is supported by the lack of HIV transmission in households or schools with infected children where there is exposure to body fluids (195, 799, 2266). Nevertheless, transfer of HIV to newborns by milk has been reported (675, 2748, 2749, 2987). In this regard, HIV-1 core antigen has been detected in 24% of milk specimens obtained from women within days after delivery but not in subsequent samples (2307). Moreover, by PCR procedures, virus-infected cells were detected in 58% of milk samples from over 100 infected African women. Whether these findings reflect viruses that can be transmitted by milk is the important question. Low CD4$^+$ cell counts and vitamin A deficiency were associated with the highest risk of having the virus-infected cells in milk (1911).

Transmission by milk carries the greatest risk when the mother is infected after birth (e.g., by blood transfusion). In this case, the infectious virus content in milk at the time could be high because of a lack of a substantial maternal antiviral immune response. Milk has also been reported to have antiviral substances that could be protective (1918); it is perhaps similar to that found in saliva (64, 78). Some researchers suggest that the antiviral effects come from α-lactalbumin and β-lactoglobulin A/B in milk (2620).

In contrast to the other body fluids described, cerebrospinal fluid contains large amounts of virus (e.g., 1,000 IP/ml), particularly in individuals with neurologic findings (1084, 1098, 1511, 2217, 2537; for a review, see reference 424) (see Chapter 9). Cerebrospinal fluid, however, would not be a natural source of transmission.

IV.   HIV Transmission by Blood and Blood Products

A.   Intravenous Drug Users

Among the first group of individuals showing evidence of HIV infection were intravenous drug users in the United States and Europe. The virus apparently entered this population in the mid-1970s and spread rapidly through 1983 (620, 621, 1863). The seroprevalence in this group is now estimated to be about 50 to 60% (622). The finding of AIDS in intravenous drug users further confirmed the presence of HIV in blood and the high risk of infection through shared needles and syringes (for a review, see reference 622). The provision of sterile injection equipment (through needle and syringe exchanges and pharmacy sales) and stable attendance at methadone clinics have been major means of decreasing HIV infection among intravenous drug users. Such programs have led to definite decreases in the risk of HIV infection in people who inject illicit drugs (622, 1142a, 1863).

B.   Transfusion Recipients and Hemophiliacs

Before the screening of blood and blood products (e.g., Factors VIII and IX), HIV could be transmitted to transfusion recipients and hemophiliacs. Screening of blood for anti-HIV antibodies has now reduced the chance of HIV transmission by transfusion in the United States to about 1 in 450,000 to 660,000 units (1395, 2412). Based on the known 12 million donations collected nationwide each year, it is estimated that about 18 to 27 units contain infectious virus (1395). New methods of screening should reduce this risk of HIV transmission even further.

For transfusion recipients, the potential risk of transmission depends on the virus load, defined as the number of free infectious virus or HIV-infected cells in the blood (324). As noted above (Section I), the amount of virus in the blood is greatest during acute infection and as an infected individual (as donor) advances to disease (Tables 2.2 and 2.3). In one study, the chance of infection was reported to rise substantially if the donor developed AIDS within 2 or 3 years (2075). Other studies have shown that individuals receiving blood from donors who subsequently develop AIDS within 29 months have a greater risk of progressing to disease than those who receive infected blood from donors who become symptomatic after 29 months (2823). Thus, these findings could reflect (i) the amount of virus present; (ii) the biologic properties of HIV in the donated blood (e.g., if it replicates rapidly and is cytopathic); (iii) the need for virus-infected cells to be activated to release virus; and (iv) the potential existence of a strong antiviral immune response (see Chapters 10 and 11).

In hemophiliacs without a history of blood transfusion, HIV transmission could be caused only by free virus and has been associated with the receipt of many vials of unheated clotting factors. The chance of an infectious HIV particle being present in the lyophilized product was thereby increased (724, 726, 897, 1332). Retroviruses can survive lyophilization (1508, 1517). Nevertheless, evidence of virus particles in old clotting factor preparations has been substantiated only by PCR analysis (2449, 2977), in which viral RNA was detected. Attempts to isolate infectious HIV from these sources have thus far been unsuccessful (1505a).

When present in a Factor VIII or Factor IX preparation, the quantity of infectious HIV particles must have been relatively low (estimated at <10 IP/vial). The products prepared during the time of HIV transmission came from concentrates of 2,000 or more plasma collections (1502), obtained during 1980 to 1983, before HIV was recognized and when virus prevalence was low (726, 1332). This assumption is supported by evidence showing that HIV infection in hemophiliacs is associated with receipt of multiple clotting-factor preparations (1332). Nevertheless, the amount of free virus needed to infect a human is not known; 4 IP administered intravenously to a chimpanzee caused infection (91). Moreover, studies of stored blood samples suggest that up to 50% of hemophiliacs were already infected by 1982 to 1983 (897). Serologic data in one report indicated that infection of hemophiliacs began in 1978, peaked in 1982, and declined by 1984. Very few infections occurred after 1987, but by that time, over one half of the hemophiliacs under study had become infected (1377b). Currently, heating Factor VIII and Factor IX to high temperatures (>60°C) either before (in the fluid phase) or after lyophilization (1517, 1518, 1720) has virtually prevented further infection of hemophiliacs.

C.   Needlestick Injuries

The estimated risk for HIV infection after percutaneous exposure to virus-infected blood is 1 in 300 to 400 (870, 2685). The potential for infection is increased if it is a deep injury, if there is visible blood on the device causing injury, if the device has been in contact with the infected person's blood vessel, and if the infected person died from AIDS within 2 months after the exposure (511). The risk from mucosal membrane and skin exposure to infected blood is approximately 1 in 1,000 or less (870) and is again influenced by the amount of blood and viral load. Precautions introduced into the hospital setting (e.g., sheathing devices for needles and prevention courses) should help reduce this risk.

V.   Sexual Transmission of HIV

A.   General Observations

AIDS was identified early as a disease most probably transmitted by a sexual route. A high prevalence among homosexual men was initially reported. Subsequent studies indicated spread by heterosexual activity, which now is responsible for the majority of infections worldwide (552, 1660, 1940, 2164; for a review, see reference 1703). As discussed above, the transmission of HIV by genital fluids is most likely to occur through virus-infected cells, since they can be present in larger numbers than free infectious virus in these body fluids. Moreover, cell culture studies suggest that the infected cells transfer HIV to epithelial cells most effectively when present in seminal fluid; cell:cell contact is most probably increased via factors (e.g., prostaglandins) in semen (2055) (Figure 2.4).

Several variables can be involved in the differences observed in virus transmission among sexual partners (for reviews, see references 1703 and 2300) (Figure 2.5). For example, as noted above (Section II), different levels of infected cells in the genital fluids can be an important factor. Thus, it is not unexpected to find a higher risk of transmission in individuals who have sexually transmitted diseases (99, 340, 1073, 1142, 1404, 2107), during which large numbers of inflammatory cells containing virus-infected cells are present in genital fluids. For example, nonulcerative sexually transmitted diseases (chlamydia, gonorrhea, trichomoniasis) are associated with an increased risk for HIV-1 transmission in women (1404). Moreover, treatment of sexually transmitted diseases reduces the number of infected cells in the seminal fluid (1865) (Section II). In reference to the potential impact of sexually transmitted disease, electron microscopic observations have suggested that herpesvirus lesions might increase HIV transmission by facilitating HIV infection of keratinocytes (1055). Moreover, HIV infection of macrophages in the lesions appears to make these cells susceptible to herpesvirus. The possibility that phenotypic mixing brought about these changes in cellular host range has been considered (see Chapter 3, Section IX, and Chapter 13) (1055) but seems unlikely in vivo.

A study of homosexual men showed a greater potential for transmission close to or after the onset of disease (1995), when virus levels in the blood are high (Section I). Contact with symptomatic male partners positive for p24 antigenemia or low $CD4^+$ cell counts also led to an increased risk of infection by heterosexual activity (1703, 2356). The relationship of these peripheral blood parameters to virus in genital fluids may be important. However, as noted above (Section II), a correlation between the level of virus in blood and genital fluids has not been consistently found. Therapy directed at the cellular source could be helpful. HIV-infected men treated with the antiviral drug AZT had a reduced incidence of heterosexual transmission compared to untreated men (1884), perhaps reflecting an effect of this drug on virus load in the genital fluid. AZT therapy, however, has not reduced virus levels considerably in vaginal fluid (Section II.C).

Some individuals do not become infected by HIV despite many unprotected exposures to the genital fluids of infected sexual partners (340, 2011, 2107). Other factors (e.g., immune response and virus subtypes) besides viral load may be involved in this lack of HIV transmission (see Chapters 11 and 13).

B.   ## Infection of the Receptive Partner

1. RISK OF TRANSMISSION

As is well known, during heterosexual or homosexual activity the receptive partner is more at risk for infection than the active partner. In some studies of heterosexual

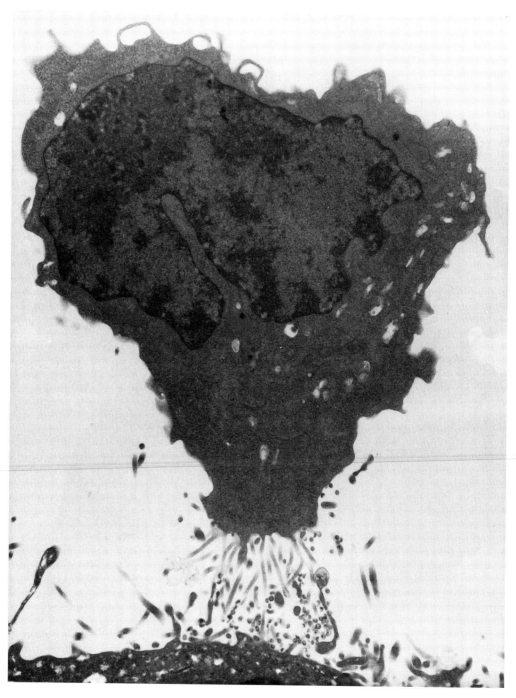

Figure 2.4   Transmission electron micrograph of an HIV-infected monocyte (U937 cell) 3 h after addition to the I-407 intestinal epithelial cell line (at bottom). Virus particles can be observed between the monocyte and the epithelial cell surface. Magnification, ×14,000. Reprinted from reference 264 with permission. Photomicrograph courtesy of D. Phillips.

Figure 2.5 Interconnected factors that influence the sexual spread of HIV. Adapted from reference 1703 with permission.

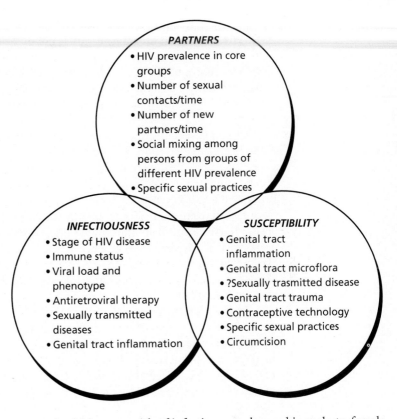

PARTNERS
- HIV prevalence in core groups
- Number of sexual contacts/time
- Number of new partners/time
- Social mixing among persons from groups of different HIV prevalence
- Specific sexual practices

INFECTIOUSNESS
- Stage of HIV disease
- Immune status
- Viral load and phenotype
- Antiretroviral therapy
- Sexually transmitted diseases
- Genital tract inflammation

SUSCEPTIBILITY
- Genital tract inflammation
- Genital tract microflora
- ?Sexually trasmitted disease
- Genital tract trauma
- Contraceptive technology
- Specific sexual practices
- Circumcision

activity, a two- to fivefold greater risk of infection was observed in male-to-female transmission (601, 2011) than in female-to-male transmission (2011). In heterosexual activity, female-to-male transmission appears to be increased during menses or when other bleeding is involved (2011). Not surprisingly, for a susceptible partner, transmission correlates directly with the number of exposures (2012), but transmission probably depends more on the number of different partners than the frequency of sexual contacts (658). As with mother-child transmission (Section VI.B), viral RNA levels in the plasma have correlated with transmission (755a), perhaps reflecting viral load in genital fluid (see below). The estimate of infection from one heterosexual contact with an infected male has been 500 to 1,000 (600, 2010a). With homosexual activity, infection in a high-prevalence community was estimated to be 1 in 10 partners (935; for a review, see reference 2300). The apparent efficiency rates of contact transmission differ among the cohorts studied because of the different variables involved (e.g., viral load in genital fluid and the presence of inflammatory diseases). Thus, estimates of transmission rates during heterosexual contact have ranged from 1 in 30 per contact to >1 in 1,000 per contact (600). Male-to-female transfer during heterosexual activity is more efficient than female-to-male transfer (1703).

Mathematical modeling has suggested that transmission from a person with primary infection can be 100- to 1,000-fold higher than that from a long-term asymptomatic person (1181). The evidence suggests that infectiousness is on the order of 1:10 to 1:20 per contact in the primary infection and 1:1,000 to 1:10,000 in the long asymptomatic phase; it then increases to 1:100 to 1:1,000 during the pre-AIDS phase (1181). If the transmission is not modeled according to a constant infectivity level, infection from a single contact with a randomly selected partner has been estimated to be about 0.17 (658). As noted above, these and other numbers estimating the risk of transmission, while useful for epidemiologic modeling (Table 2.6) (548), reflect only some of the variables that might be involved in contact with the virus.

These observations suggest a relation of the clinical state to viral load in genital fluid, but that correlation, as noted above, has not been conclusive (Section II); other factors may be involved. Importantly, while the risk of infection per contact can be estimated (Table 2.6), it is difficult to establish any accurate or even semi-accurate number because of the lack of information on variables that could influence HIV transmission. These variables include time of infection, extent of viral load, presence of sexually transmitted diseases, presence of erosions (cervical ectopy), menses, circumcision, number of leukocytes in genital fluids, and age of the partner during sexual intercourse (Figure 2.5). Each parameter could be different, depending on the time of contact and on whether the same or a different partner was involved (658).

For the receptive partner in sexual contact, early epidemiologic data suggested that HIV needed a point of entry in the anal canal or vagina. Abrasions at these sites presumably would increase transmission. This assumption helped to explain the high rate of heterosexual spread of HIV in Africa, where genital ulcers from venereal diseases (e.g., *Haemophilus ducreyi*) are associated with increased HIV seroprevalence (340, 1073, 2107). Some studies suggest that genital ulcers not only are a

Table 2.6 Estimates of risk of HIV transmission and global importance[a]

Type of exposure	Likelihood of infection after a single exposure (%)	Global total (%)
Sexual intercourse	0.01–1.0	70–80
Receptive vaginal	~0.01	60–70
Receptive anal	~1.0	5–10
Injecting drug use	0.5–1.0	5–10
Maternal transmission		
Pregnancy/delivery[b]	12–50	5–10
Breastmilk	12[c]	Not quantified
Medical interventions		
Blood transfusion	>90	3–5
Blood products	Not quantified	Not quantified
Organ transplantation	Not quantified	Not quantified
Artificial insemination	Not quantified	Not quantified
Health care worker (needlestick, etc.)	0.1–1.0	<0.01

[a] Reprinted from reference 548 with permission.

[b] Rate of infection diminished greatly by AZT therapy during pregnancy and neonatal period.

[c] Risk for continuous breastfeeding, not a single exposure.

possible point of entry for the virus but also could contain HIV and thus be the source of virus transmission (1055, 1373) (see above). Possibly, inflammation of the penis could explain the increased incidence of transmission associated with uncircumcised men (1141) (see below). Herpes simplex and syphilis infections in the United States have also been correlated with an increased risk of HIV transmission among heterosexuals (1105). Nevertheless, studies of biopsy tissues have shown that the bowel mucosa and perhaps the cervical and uterine epithelium can be infected directly by HIV (1047, 1112a, 1516, 1696, 1916, 2118) without the need for ulcerations.

2. INFECTION VIA THE BOWEL

The finding of HIV in the bowel mucosa (see Chapters 7 and 9) provides another reason, besides abrasions, for the high risk of transmission associated with receptive anal-genital contact. This risk would appear to be the same for both male and female partners. Direct contact of the bowel mucosa with HIV-infected cells in semen could be responsible (264, 2055, 2090) (Figures 2.3 and 2.4). Infection could occur after interaction of the virus with cellular receptors (2926) or attachment of virus-antibody complexes to Fc receptors on the mucosal cells (1144) (see Chapter 3). Another possible means of HIV entry could be via intestinal M cells present in the bowel epithelium (57). HIV infection of the mucosa also supports the epidemiologic data showing that douching of the anal canal before sexual contact increases the risk of infection (2894). Cleansing permits easier contact of infected cells with the mucosal epithelial cells. Thus, infection of the bowel mucosa could have been the portal of virus entry for many HIV-infected individuals. The number of sexual contacts with sufficient virus in the genital fluid could be the most important factor in determining sexual transmission.

3. INFECTION VIA THE FEMALE GENITAL TRACT

Because the columnar and squamous cell epithelium of the vagina can be a barrier to virus infection, ulcerations caused by sexually transmitted diseases might be a prerequisite for infection at this site. Nevertheless, transmission of HIV has been reported in a chimpanzee inoculated in the vaginal canal with high doses of the virus in culture fluid (806). The factors involved in this infection, however, could be different from those in the natural state (i.e., via semen). In some cases, infection of cells in the cervix might take place (467, 1112a, 1956, 2118, 2638). In this regard, recent studies have shown that epithelial and stromal cells from the uterus, fallopian tube, and cervix can be infected in vitro with HIV-1, but not cells derived from the vagina (1112a). Observations on HIV-1 infection of vaginal cells remain controversial; studies in animal models suggest that this tissue can be infected (806). In situ studies of vaginal cells in HIV-infected women are warranted. Cervical ectopy (erosion) is associated significantly with HIV transmission to women (1864). Moreover, cell culture procedures have shown transmission of HIV from infected lymphocytes and macrophages to cervix-derived epithelial cells (2638) (Figure 2.6).

Some studies have suggested that Langerhans cells in the vagina or cervix might serve as targets for HIV (2539). In particular, certain virus strains associated with heterosexual transmission (e.g., clade E) (1386) have been reported to be more infectious

Figure 2.6 HIV-infected HUT 78 cell (top) cocultivated for 1 h with an ME180 cervix-derived epithelial cell (bottom). Virus can be seen at the cell-cell interface (2638). It is noteworthy, as observed in the legend to Figure 2.4, that virus is produced by the T-cell line only at the point of contact with the epithelial cells. A role of cytokines in this localized induction of virus production should be considered. Magnification, ×10,000.

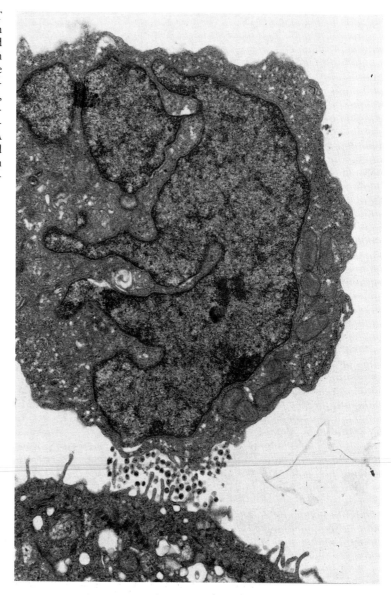

for these cells. However, these observations have been challenged by recent findings (641a, 2120a) (see Chapter 7). The CD4$^+$ dendritic cells are found within the superficial epithelial layers of the vagina and the foreskin but are rare in the upper third of the oral epithelium and in the urethra and rectum (1145, 1326). In one study, the foreskin and the cervicovaginal epithelium contained CD4$^+$ Langerhans cells that could be susceptible to HIV infection. The urethral epithelium had Fc receptors that could mediate infection by HIV-antibody complexes. The oral cavity, however, lacked CD4$^+$ Langerhans cells and Fc receptors, thereby making transmission by this route more difficult (1145). In this regard, rhesus macaques inoculated intravaginally with a chimeric simian/human immunodeficiency virus (SHIV) showed the presence of the virus within 2 days in the vagina, uterus, and pelvic and mesentery lymph nodes. By 4 days, virus-infected cells were present in spleen and thymus, and by day 15, loss of $CD4^+$ cells was evident in the peripheral blood. A similar spread of virus replication and $CD4^+$ cell loss was noted in an animal inoculated orally with the virus (1203a). All of these findings need confirmation before they can be cited as reasons to explain differences in susceptibilities to HIV infection at various sites in the body (see Chapter 9). Finally, a factor that can stimulate HIV replication has been found in cervicovaginal lavage samples. This factor could affect sexual or vertical transmission of HIV-1 (2541a).

Recently, increased heterosexual transmission in women has been linked to contraceptive therapy. Apparently, the female hormones (particularly progestin) make the vaginal lining cells thinner and more susceptible to erosion, as shown in studies of the SIV system (1686). The possibility that this observation explains why these women are more susceptible to virus infection is under study.

HIV transmission to women via the vaginal canal seems most likely if virus-infected cells in the semen gain entry into the uterus through the cervical os and infect resident lymphocytes, macrophages, and perhaps uterine epithelial cells susceptible to HIV. This risk for HIV infection is particularly high during or shortly after menses, before the re-formation of the mucosal plug (1502). Some studies have indicated that women whose sexual partners are uncircumcised have a threefold-increased risk of HIV infection (2300, 2731). This finding could reflect the increased infection rate in uncircumcised males (340, 1374) (see below) and/or HIV transmission from infected cells associated with the foreskin (1787). In the case of HIV transmission associated with artificial insemination (2599), virus-infected cells, along with spermatozoa, gained entry to the uterus when injected through the cervical os. Alternatively, infection of the cervix could have occurred from the presence of erosion (or ectopy) or during inflammatory conditions in the vagina (650). In one limited study, uninfected women, when inseminated with semen processed to remove free virus and infected cells, gave birth to infants who were all HIV seronegative (2450).

C.   Infection of the Insertive Partner

The insertive partner in sexual contact carries a relatively low risk for infection, although it is not minimal (2894). As noted above, lack of circumcision in males has correlated in some studies with increased risk of infection (up to twofold) (340, 1374). Transmission could take place through infection of macrophages or lymphocytes in the foreskin or along the urethral canal. Virus could be transferred to the penis from infected cells (mostly macrophages or Langerhans cells) in the cervix (1956) or in the intestinal mucosa (1916). In heterosexual contact, the infected woman could be most contagious during menses (2011). In macaques, the macrophages associated with the foreskin or urethral canal are found to be infected with SIV (1787). In this case, sexually transmitted diseases involving the foreskin could increase the chance of infection of inflammatory cells associated with the foreskin. Moreover, the mucosal lining cells of the foreskin could be susceptible to HIV infection. Obviously, in all participants of sexual contact, an increased number of virus-infected cells in the genital fluids (e.g., resulting from sexually transmitted disease) would increase both transfer and receipt of the infectious virus.

D.   Oral-Genital Contact

Oral-genital contact could also lead to HIV infection of either partner, albeit at a low frequency (1542, 2348, 2382, 2894). In a recent study, adult macaques exposed nontraumatically to high doses of SIV through the oral route developed AIDS (109). In other studies, however, chimpanzees receiving virus by the oral route were not infected (806).

E.   Summary: Preventive Measures

All these observations on HIV transmission emphasize the importance of barrier techniques during sexual activity. The most common method is the use of condoms, which have been demonstrated by both in vitro and epidemiologic studies to be effective in preventing the passage of virus (503, 1923). In this regard, the recommendation of using spermicidal products (e.g., nonoxynol-9) against HIV is being reconsidered. Some studies have demonstrated that vaginal and cervical irritations associated with the use of certain doses of these compounds might increase virus transmission (1934). In one report, nonoxynol-9 was not effective in preventing heterosexual transmission (1372). Female condoms (903), vaginal microbicides, and compounds that inhibit HIV adsorption and cell : cell contact (e.g., polycations) need further evaluation. Moreover, the use of a diaphragm in women might be helpful if, indeed, transmission occurs mostly by virus entry through the cervical os. This approach would be particularly useful in countries in which women need to protect themselves without the consent of their partners. Approaches for preventing sexual transmission have met with some success, including the 100% condom policy in Thailand and the management of sexually transmitted diseases in Tanzania and Uganda (for a review, see reference 2300). Moreover, if one can avoid sexual encounters during primary infection and have monogamous rather than multiple sequential contacts, transmission can be reduced. Finally, environmental factors, such as mood-altering drugs and alcohol, can affect mental capacity and increase the risk of infection.

VI.   Mother-Child Transmission of HIV

A.   Prevalence of Transmission

The transmission of HIV from mother to child is believed to occur in 11 to 60% of children born to HIV-positive mothers (19, 228, 1146, 1919, 2006, 2288, 2380; for reviews, see references 2056 and 2375). This prevalence is based primarily on PCR and virus culture studies; diagnosis by serologic testing is difficult because maternal antibodies are present in infants at birth (for reviews, see references 2006 and 2265). The reason for the wide variation in virus transmission rates is not known, and the answer could provide approaches for prevention. Nevertheless, some estimates on the risk of infection by mother-child transmission have been reported (Table 2.6).

Determining infection in the newborn can be difficult. Serologic evaluation at birth is not possible unless IgA antibodies are measured (1418, 1680, 2165, 2835). IgA does not pass the placenta and thus does not confer seropositivity to neonates, as other maternal antibodies do. Generally, maternal antibodies decline to background levels by 6 to 18 months (2042); IgG antibody synthesis in an infected infant has been estimated to occur 3 months after birth (2042). Anti-HIV IgA production should be specific for HIV infection in the newborn and could be explained in part by the swallowing of maternal blood or secretions by the infant in utero or during birth.

Another proposed serologic procedure for detecting an infected newborn is the induction of anti-HIV antibody production in the newborn's PBMC cultures by using a B-cell mitogen (2016). Both this evaluation method and the measurement of IgA antibody production require further study. The two most helpful methods for detecting infection in newborns are PCR analysis for viral RNA and virus isolation procedures (597, 1377, 1919, 2380). However, PCR can lack specificity, and virus culture can be time-consuming and difficult to conduct routinely.

Most recent studies suggest that the diagnosis of HIV infection in a child is best made by analyzing two blood samples in a single assay or in a combination of virus culture and PCR. By this protocol, two negative DNA-PCR results on two consecutive blood samples at 6 months of age would establish a lack of infection (2050). The latter conclusion may be misleading, as noted above, if no circulating infected lymphocytes or macrophages can be detected but virus is still present in lymphoid organs such as the liver or spleen. Recently, RNA-PCR has been reported to be a more reliable assay for the detection of perinatal infection than is DNA-PCR (2593).

B.   ## Factors Influencing Mother-Child Transmission

The factors influencing transfer of virus from the mother to the newborn are not conclusive, but several possibilities have been suggested (Table 2.7). Transmission has been reported to correlate with low levels or an absence of antibodies to the viral envelope, especially the third variable region (V3 loop) of gp120 (898, 2289) and, as recently noted, to the carboxyl region of gp41 (2735), in the mother. Several reports have correlated transmission with a low $CD4^+$ cell count, high virus load (particularly measured by PCR), and p24 antigenemia in the mother at the time of delivery (598, 600, 632, 898, 2289, 2380) and with illicit drug use (1419, 2259).

Neutralizing antibodies in maternal serum and, in some studies, inflammation of placenta membranes have been correlated with protection from transmission (1322, 2376, 2560) (see below). A long duration of membrane rupture before delivery can increase mother-child transmission (1379). These observations suggest that the level of free infectious virus in the maternal blood could predict the infectious status of the newborn. In developing countries, maternal vitamin A deficiency has been associated

Table 2.7 Possible factors associated with mother-child transmission[a]

1. Absence of anti-gp120 (V3 loop) antibodies in the maternal serum
2. Low $CD4^+$ cell count in the mother
3. High virus load (p24 antigenemia) in the mother at time of delivery
4. Lack of neutralizing antibodies in the maternal serum
5. Enhancing antibodies in the maternal serum
6. High-replicating (syncytium-inducing) virus in the maternal blood

[a] The importance of each of these parameters is under further evaluation (see Section VI.B).

with increased risk of infection of the newborn (1206, 2446), perhaps resulting from reduced epithelial cell function in the gastrointestinal tract (1932). Encouraging results have been reported in blocking mother-child transmission with AZT treatment (386, 759). However, in some cases, AZT-treated women with high HIV-1 levels have transmitted AZT-sensitive virus to newborns (632). Nevertheless, the universal use of AZT (or other antiviral drugs) in HIV-seropositive pregnant women has the potential to reduce or even eliminate HIV transmission by the maternal route.

| C. | ## Time of Transmission |

The source of virus and the time of infection of the newborn are controversial. Transmission appears to occur either in utero or during or after delivery (1615, 2288). Support for intrauterine transmission comes from the detection of HIV in placentas and fetuses by in situ hybridization, PCR, and immunohistochemical studies (534, 584, 1528, 1662, 2532). In some studies, the presence of HIV-1 proviral DNA in the placenta has correlated with the detection of virus in the cord blood of newborns, but HIV-positive cord blood can also be found in the absence of infection in the placenta (583, 584). Besides its isolation from cord blood, infectious HIV has been found in amniotic fluid and in placental and fetal tissues (396, 1214, 1701, 1875, 2288, 2556). Neonatal monocytes and macrophages may have an increased susceptibility to HIV-1 infection (2548). Furthermore, placental cells, either expressing or lacking CD4 protein, have been infected in vitro by virus or virus-infected cells. In one report examining the possible role of the Fc receptor on placental cells, infection was achieved with an antibody-virus complex but only low-level replication took place (58, 655, 1701, 2695, 2952). Thus, the relevance of these findings to the in vivo state is not clear.

Recovery of HIV from cord blood or within 48 h of delivery certainly infers infection before delivery and has been estimated to occur in up to one-half of the infections of newborns (597, 1615). Nevertheless, the exact time and source of the infection are not known. It could occur late in pregnancy, when maternal cells are most frequently found in the blood of the newborn and can carry HIV (583). It is estimated that 1 cell out of 500 fetal cells can be of maternal origin (583). Despite the reports of HIV detection in placentas and fetuses, the frequency of HIV infection of fetal tissues in utero has not been well documented. Some investigators have found no virus in early-term fetal tissues (58). In certain reports, but not others, cesarean delivery has been associated with decreased HIV transmission (1380, 1920, 2697; for a review, see reference 2288). Perhaps interferon or female hormones produced by trophoblast cells help to prevent infection (263). In summary, transfer of virus or virus-infected cells to the developing fetus via the placenta requires further evaluation.

Observations suggesting a high rate of perinatal (intrapartum) or postdelivery infection have received increased attention (1223). HIV is often not isolated from cord blood but is recovered from virus-infected infants at 2 to 4 weeks of age (319, 597, 613a, 689, 1377, 1377a). In a study of 100 fetal thymuses from HIV-1-positive pregnancies, only 2 were infected (298). Moreover, the virus has been detected in gastric aspirates (1932). All these findings suggest that perhaps up to half the infant infections occur during birth through contact with the genital secretions or blood of the mother. Such a route of infection could explain the increased risk of transmission when the fetal membrane ruptures more than 4 h before delivery (1419). HIV transmission at the time of delivery could also explain how only one monozygotic twin would be infected (1753) and why the first-born of twins is at higher risk of infection (896). The infected newborn twin could have been exposed to a higher concentration of virus.

After delivery, in certain cases, HIV infection could result from infected milk (1074, 1231, 2019, 2749, 2987), particularly from mothers who acquired HIV postnatally (for a review, see reference 675). This route of transmission has been associated with the presence of virus-infected cells and the absence of anti-HIV IgM and IgA antibodies in breast milk (2748) and is considered uncommon (1074, 2749).

The factors that protect the newborn from infections could be studied in relation to SIV infection. This primate virus appears to be transmitted primarily when the animals are sexually active and not during pregnancy or at birth (1707). Information on transmission of the other human pathogenic retrovirus, HTLV, might also have relevance to HIV. HTLV is not passed readily in utero (2362). This virus is transferred primarily from breast milk and genital fluids, most probably via infected cells (1072). Moreover, in one study on HTLV transmission, approximately 22% of the placentas but only 7% of the infants were found to be infected. This observation suggests a defense mechanism at the maternal-fetal interface (805), which may also be operating in HIV infection. Perhaps this event is reflected in the inflammation of the placenta membrane that correlates with protection from HIV transmission (2560).

D. Characteristics of the Transmitted Virus

An important parameter in transmission could be the type of virus transferred from the mother (see also Chapter 4). Some studies suggest that maternal and newborn viruses can be distinguished by molecular and serologic properties (1319a, 1322, 1409, 1410, 2378, 2910). The transferred virus, for example, could be a more virulent fast-replicating strain found at low frequency in the mother but readily transferred to the newborn. Maternal viruses with high replication kinetics and cytopathic properties associated with the SI phenotype have been considered risk factors in transmission (see below and Chapter 7) (1322, 2377–2379). However, in one report, a predominance of macrophage-tropic NSI viruses that replicated in the child's target cell was noted in transmitters (1983). In another study, all HIV-1 isolates from four infants were of the NSI phenotype (2547). Nevertheless, apparently, both SI and NSI viruses can be transmitted (1322, 2377–2379). In these cases, perhaps replicative ability and not SI capacity is the major determinant (1322). These latter findings counter some suggestions that a noncytopathic, macrophage-tropic strain is primarily transmitted because it can infect placental macrophages (250). This route would be involved only in infections in utero.

As cited above, some findings (1319a, 2910) suggest the selection in the newborn of a minor virus variant from the mother with specific virologic properties (detected by sequence or serologic differences) (1322). This observation, however, was not made in another study (2378). Moreover, in examining V1 and V2 envelope heterogeneity, multiple maternal HIV-1 genotypes were found to be transmitted to the infants (1410). The frequency of this latter finding, based on the present literature, would appear to be low.

In our laboratory, a virus resistant to maternal antibodies or sensitive to enhancing antibodies in the mother's serum has been detected in newborns (1322). The presence of enhancing antibodies could explain the reports of increased transmission of HIV from mother to child in the presence of high levels of maternal antibodies to the V3 region of gp120 and the immunodominant domain of gp41 (1406, 1672). Thus, not only the level of viremia but also specific features of various HIV strains and antiviral antibodies present in the mother could determine whether transmission occurs. Furthermore, as noted above, the time at which HIV-1 is transferred might determine the particular virus strain transmitted to the newborn.

E.   Clearance of Infection by the Newborn

A noteworthy finding has been the apparent clearance of HIV infection by infants who are infected during the perinatal period. In these cases, children who had at least two positive PCR assays for HIV in blood specimens, or by culture of PBMC, seroreverted and have remained free of antibodies and detectable virus in their blood (307, 2277). The reason for this phenomenon is not known. Recurrent hepatosplenomegaly in two children may indicate the presence of virus in the liver and spleen. The rarity of the virus clearance event has put into question whether indeed the seronegative children contained virus in their blood at birth and what mechanism would have removed the HIV from a presumably immunologically immature host (274, 1708). Nevertheless, it seems feasible that in some children, a transmitted virus does not establish infection, either because of the inherent resistance to the infection by infant leukocytes or because of an early anti-HIV response (see Chapters 10 and 11). Moreover, maternal lymphocytes that carry the virus may not remain in the newborn circulation long enough to transfer the virus or to be activated to release virus into the child.

The extent of virus clearance and its importance are not known. In some instances, we have noted CD8$^+$ cell antiviral responses in uninfected children of seropositive mothers (1491, 1511a). These observations suggest that there was exposure to virus or to viral proteins some time in the fetal or perinatal periods but that infection was not established. Similar findings have been made with cord blood lymphocytes from some uninfected infants; the cells proliferated after exposure to viral envelope peptides (482). Whether these observations reflect protection from HIV by cell-mediated immune responses remains to be determined (see Chapter 11).

F.   Conclusions: Preventive Measures

In summary, maternal transmission seems to occur in association with parameters observed during a poor clinical state: high virus load, fast-replicating HIV strains, and low CD4$^+$ cell numbers. If the factors influencing maternal transmission of HIV can be ascertained, approaches to avoid virus transfer could be better targeted. Besides antiviral therapy, methods could include monitoring the mother during labor, cleansing the vaginal canal, and rapidly removing genital secretions and maternal blood from the newborn. In one report, cleansing of the birth canal before delivery did not significantly affect the risk of HIV transmission (208). Nevertheless, some of these procedures might at least reduce the transfer of HIV in the perinatal period. Importantly, administration of antiretroviral therapy shows the most promise in decreasing virus transmission substantially.

| *Chapter 2* | **SALIENT FEATURES** |

1. The risk of HIV transmission is increased with high levels of virus in the body fluids and the number of contacts an individual has with a body fluid.

2. Blood has the highest level of infectious virus that could serve as a source of transmission. The number of infectious viruses in body fluid is usually 1 in 60,000 to 1 in 100,000 of the virus particles detected. The amount of infectious virus in blood is smaller than the number of virus-infected cells that could transfer virus to an individual.

3. Generally, HIV-infected cells in genital fluids are the major source of transmission by the sexual route. Sexually transmitted diseases enhance the risk of virus transmission to either partner by increasing the presence of virus-infected cells.

4. The receptive partner in sexual transmission is most at risk. The infection can involve bowel mucosal cells or lymphocytes and macrophages present in the rectum. In women, cells in the cervix or within the endometrium can be infected. The insertive partner may be infected by cells along the urethral canal or associated with the prepuce.

5. Saliva, which contains HIV-inhibitory substances and only small amounts of infectious virus, is not a major source of transmission. Tears, urine, sweat, and other body fluids are not sources of virus infection.

6. The risk of HIV infection via blood depends on the level of infectious virus in this body fluid. Heating has eliminated the risk of infection from blood products. The estimated risk for HIV infection from needlestick injuries is 1 in 300 to 400, with deep injury carrying the greatest chance of infection. Risk from mucosal membrane and skin exposures is approximately 1 in 1,000 or less and is influenced by the amount of blood and viral load.

7. Condoms, male and female, should serve as efficient barrier techniques for sexual transmission of virus. Compounds that irritate the vaginal canal should be avoided.

8. Transmission of virus from mother to child appears to involve direct infection of the fetus or, during birth, exposure of the newborn to maternal blood and secretions. A variety of factors can influence this transmission, in particular, the level of infectious virus in the mother at the time of delivery.

9. Maternal milk can serve as a source of virus transmission to the newborn, but this fluid also contains substances that can block virus infection.

10. Antiretroviral therapy and other preventive measures can greatly reduce the risk of mother-child transmission.

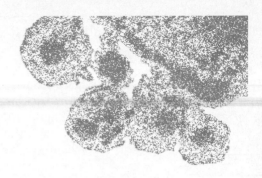

Steps Involved in HIV:Cell Interaction and Virus Entry

3

T RANSMISSION OF HIV REQUIRES THE SUCCESSFUL INTERACTION OF the virus with receptors on a cell surface. Subsequent processes facilitate the final penetration of the viral nucleocapsid through the cell membrane into the cell. The sites on the virus and on the cells that are involved in this interaction, and the events required for viral entry, are reviewed in this chapter.

I.   CD4 Receptor

A.   Virus Attachment Site

One of the first breakthroughs in studies of HIV was the discovery that its major cellular receptor was the CD4 molecule. The reason for preferential growth of HIV in CD4$^+$ lymphocytes was explained by its attachment to the CD4 protein on the cell surface (563, 1310, 1311). Subsequent studies have indicated that the D1 region of the CD4 molecule (particularly involving the Phe-43 amino acid in the complementarity-determining region 2 [CDR2] domain) (Figure 3.1) is involved in virus binding (87, 265, 464, 1183, 1800; for reviews, see references 357 and 2621).

When the crystal structure of CD4 was determined (2314, 2819), the binding site for the viral surface envelope protein gp120 was located on a protuberant ridge along one face of the D1 domain (Figure 3.1). Initially, the viral attachment site appeared to be separate from the major histocompatibility complex (MHC) binding site of CD4 (768, 1407), but the location has been delineated further by using viral mutants and high-resolution CD4 atomic structure (1804). These studies indicate that the class II MHC binding site appears to include the same CD4 region. Thus, this overlap might affect the use of inhibitors of the CD4:gp120 interaction.

On HIV, a major CD4 binding region (amino acids 413 to 447) is in the fourth conserved portion (C4) near the carboxyl-terminal end of the viral gp120 (1434, 1960; for reviews, see references 357 and 2621). The conformation of gp120 is important for CD4 binding (1719) (see also Chapter 8), and other noncontiguous regions of gp120 are now known to interact with sites on the CDR2 domain of the CD4 molecule (Figure 3.1). The CD4 binding domain on gp120 appears to be a complex folded structure with sites from several regions coming in contact with the CD4 molecule (for a review, see reference 1838). Among these could be two hydrophobic domains in the conserved C2 and C4 regions of gp120 as well as hydrophilic domains in the C3 and C4 regions (1366, 1982, 2126; for reviews, see references 1838 and 2583) (Color Plate 1, following p. 188) (see Chapter 10, Section II, for a

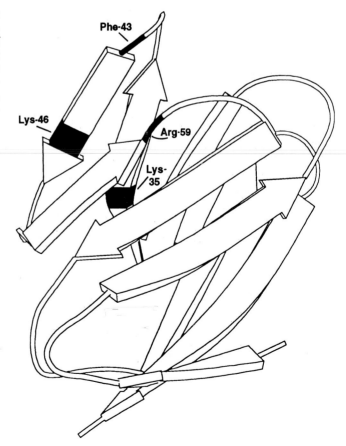

Figure 3.1   The gp120 binding sites on the CD4 molecule as determined by mutational analysis, displayed on this model of domain 1 (D1). The consensus is that Phe-43 and Arg-59 are likely contact sites for gp120, but there are different conclusions regarding Lys-35 and Lys-46. Reprinted from reference 1838 with permission.

definition of viral envelope structure). In support of the involvement of an envelope conformational structure, several studies indicate that small changes in various regions of the HIV envelope can affect virus binding to the CD4 molecule and tropism (526, 527, 1982, 2497) (see also Chapter 8). In this regard, two highly conserved aspartic acid residues in the C4 and C5 domains of gp120 (in a predicted groove of this protein) contribute substantially to the binding (1982) (Color Plate 1).

The CD4 molecule could also play a role in viral infection aside from its binding to the HIV envelope (339, 1031, 2717). For example, conformational changes in CD4 as a result of virus attachment could help in HIV entry (2815) (for reviews, see references 357, 1838, and 2621) (see below). The participation of CD4 in virus:cell fusion, perhaps by means of flexibility in the D2-D3 hinge region (2314, 2819), has been suggested (2132). Furthermore, certain domains of CD4 could be selectively involved in cell:cell fusion (1547, 2132, 2717) (see Chapter 6).

Another potential factor in the CD4:gp120 interaction is the glycosylation pattern of gp120 (1700, 1846), which can also affect envelope conformation. Although glycosylation was initially reported to have no influence on the gp120/160:CD4 interaction (745), other studies have indicated that nonglycosylated envelope gp120 does not bind well to CD4 (2583).

B.   ## Studies with Soluble CD4

Biologic studies with soluble forms of CD4 (sCD4), produced in mammalian cells by molecular techniques, have revealed some potentially important findings on the gp120:CD4 interaction, with differences noted among HIV isolates (see Chapter 7). The experiments suggest that the particular HIV envelope and its conformational changes are important factors that determine the result of this interaction. After being mixed with sCD4, many HIV-1 strains are inactivated to various extents (2845). Some, particularly macrophage-tropic isolates, are relatively resistant (see below). Certain HIV-2 strains, especially the SIV_{agm} isolates, show an increase in infectivity, notably when low sCD4 concentrations are used (46, 458, 2860). In some studies, this interaction with sCD4 permits HIV-2 infection of $CD4^-$ human cells and nonhuman primate cells (see Chapter 4) (458). Moreover, sCD4 at low concentrations enhances infection of $CD4^+$ cells by some primary HIV-1 isolates (2613).

Although the reason for these diverse observations is not clear, a possible explanation for these different reactions to sCD4 is that sCD4 has differing affinities for the various gp120s. With the inactivation of HIV, the sCD4 molecule apparently attaches to the viral envelope region and blocks receptor binding. Some experiments suggest that it causes removal of gp120 from the virus. Thus, gp120 displacement (or shedding) and/or gp120:CD4 binding causes a loss of infectivity (1027, 1833, 1834, 1992) (Section II).

In contrast, with certain HIV-2 strains, SIV_{agm}, and some HIV-1 isolates, sCD4 might bind at low affinities and gp120 is not displaced on the virion. In this case, conformational changes could have occurred in the viral envelope, thereby permitting virus:cell interactions. The latter possibility has been suggested by studies with monoclonal antibodies (Section II) (1731, 2364). A lower affinity of sCD4 for binding to these viruses has been documented (2366), but other evidence supports the concept that a strong association of SIV_{agm} envelope gp120 with the transmembrane protein gp36 plays the major role in this lack of sCD4 inactivation (47, 2366). A similar conclusion has been drawn with sCD4-resistant HIV strains (see below).

Most studies do suggest that the conformation of the viral envelope is altered by its association with sCD4 and that the fusion domain on gp41 (Section III) probably becomes exposed and can now interact with the cell. Infection subsequently takes place and might even be enhanced. Such an event could occur during natural infection after HIV binds to the cell surface CD4 (2364, 2571). A conformational change in the envelope takes place, permitting virus fusion and entry. During this process, a subsequent cleavage of the envelope V3 loop may increase the rate of infection (Section II.B).

In perhaps related observations, some freshly isolated HIV-1 strains, usually macrophage tropic, have shown reduced susceptibility to sCD4 inactivation (93, 556, 904). The reason for this resistance is not well defined. It is reflected in some isolates by the need for up to 1,000-fold-higher concentrations of sCD4 for inactivation. As noted above, the findings could reflect less efficient binding of virus to sCD4 and/or lack of gp120 shedding or displacement following the interaction with sCD4 (1832, 1992). Similar suggestions have been made to explain the relative effectiveness of antibody neutralization and enhancement (see Chapter 10). One proposed explanation for the resistance of primary virus isolates to sCD4 inactivation is their selection in the host to resist neutralizing antibodies to the CD4 binding site (1838). Another suggestion is that a large amount of gp120 on the virion surface prevents sCD4 binding (1832, 1967). This possibility has not been supported by studies showing that neither envelope glycoprotein spike density nor stability determines sCD4 resistance (1243).

In regard to the role of sCD4 binding in neutralizing HIV, studies with soluble monomeric gp120 do not link resistance of sCD4 inactivation of primary virus isolates to a low affinity of attachment (93, 283, 1838). Postbinding events, including a strong gp120:gp41 interaction within the virion, appear to be involved (1992, 2728). Nevertheless, most importantly, when whole virus is used in these experiments, a low-affinity binding of sCD4 is observed (1832, 1992, 2570) and could be responsible for the resistance to inactivation. These results emphasize the problems involved in using soluble proteins instead of the whole virus when studying HIV:cell interactions.

This resistance of certain HIV-1 strains to inactivation by sCD4 has been mapped in some studies to the V3 region of the virus envelope (1148, 1963). In other studies with different HIV-1 strains, sites outside the V3 loop but in the nearby regions (e.g., C2) appear to be responsible (2570) (see Chapter 8). Since none of these portions of gp120 binds to CD4, the envelope conformation influencing this process seems to be involved (see Chapter 8). Some mutations in gp120, including those within the V3 region that impair cell:cell fusion by some strains, do not affect sCD4 inactivation and HIV gp120 shedding (179, 2665). Therefore, the shedding of gp120 induced by sCD4 cannot be a common indication of conformational changes in the HIV-1 envelope proteins needed for virus infection or syncytium formation. Moreover, gp120 displacement cannot be a general explanation for sCD4 inactivation (2665). Nevertheless, spontaneous shedding of gp120 and the sensitivity to sCD4 inactivation appear to correlate with a high efficiency of infection when T-cell lines are used (1832, 2570, 2886).

It seems reasonable that one explanation for the different effects of sCD4 on primary isolates might be a greater avidity of the macrophage-tropic virus strains for the cell surface CD4 receptors than for sCD4 (1172, 2570). Conceivably, culturing strains in vitro leads to the emergence of viruses with increased affinity for sCD4 or decreased affinity for CD4 (1369). However, most importantly, as mentioned earlier, studies of gp120:CD4 interactions should measure the affinity for the cellular CD4 protein, not sCD4, and for the entire envelope of the virus, not just soluble gp120 (1114, 1838). The conformation of the monomeric gp120 can be quite different from that of the gp120/gp41 oligomer on the virus or infected cell surface. In this regard, binding of several gp120 oligomers (and not monomers) to CD4 molecules takes place simultaneously (678), and this event could be important in the initial phases of the infection process. Nevertheless, in evaluating virus:cell interactions, the relative resistance of certain HIV-1 isolates to sCD4 is a property that can reflect a characteristic envelope conformation (see Chapter 8).

II.   Postbinding Steps in Virus Entry

A.   Envelope Displacement

The HIV envelope gp120 can be involved in steps other than binding during virus infection of a cell. Some reports have suggested, as noted above, that after attachment to the CD4 molecule, the gp120 is displaced, leading to the uncovering of domains on the envelope gp41 that are needed for virus:cell fusion (Figure 3.2) (1833, 1834, 1992, 2364). This displacement appears to result from a dissociation of a "knob-and-socket"-like structure involving the carboxyl-terminal region of gp120 and the central portion of gp41 (2422). It may involve gp120 cleavage (see below).

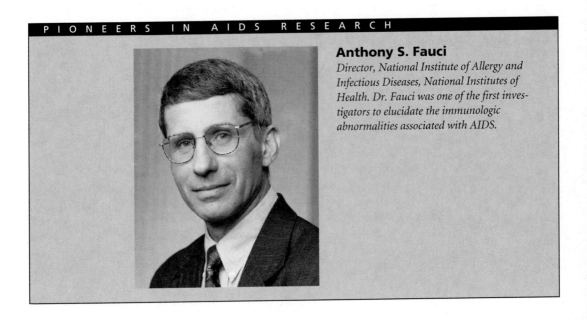

PIONEERS   IN   AIDS   RESEARCH

Anthony S. Fauci

Director, National Institute of Allergy and Infectious Diseases, National Institutes of Health. Dr. Fauci was one of the first investigators to elucidate the immunologic abnormalities associated with AIDS.

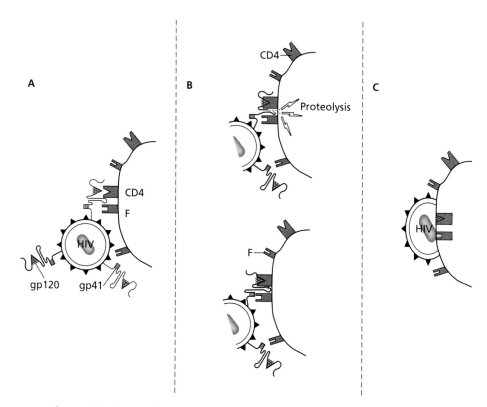

Figure 3.2 Proposed processes involved in HIV infection of cells. (A) HIV approaches a cell. A region on the viral surface envelope protein, gp120, interacts with a domain on a cell surface receptor (e.g., CD4). (B) Top: The interaction causes a conformational change in the gp120 (and perhaps CD4), potentially resulting in a proteolytic cleavage of the gp120, most likely in the V3 loop. Bottom: This process results in an interaction of the external portion of gp41 (fusion domain) with a proposed fusion receptor (F) on the cell surface. (C) HIV fuses with the cell. Alternatively, the interaction of gp120 with CD4 could lead to removal of gp120, with subsequent exposure of gp41 to the cell surface (Section II.A).

Multimeric CD4 binding may be important for this release (678), which can be demonstrated with sCD4 (Section I) and is related to specific CD4 binding to gp120 (178, 1027, 1833). Support for this phenomenon comes from the demonstration that certain V3 monoclonal antibodies can neutralize HIV-1 only in the presence of sCD4; the V3 epitope is exposed by this gp120:CD4 interaction (1731, 2364).

Whether a complete dissociation of gp120 from gp41 takes place during HIV infection is not clear. Shedding does not appear to occur (637) or to be necessary as long as the fusion domain on gp41 is exposed (2364). In this connection, the sCD4-induced shedding of gp120 from viruses observed in vitro has not correlated well with virus entry or with the syncytial properties of the viral envelope (179, 2665). It is now known that cell tropisms are determined only in part by the relative extent of gp120 displacement resulting from the virus interactions with cellular CD4. The extent of interactions of the viral envelope with coreceptors can be important (Section II.C).

B.   ## Envelope Cleavage

Another possible event in virus infection, evaluated some years ago, is cleavage of the HIV envelope gp120 prior to HIV entry into cells. Certain studies of gp120 revealed sites within the V3 loop that could be sensitive to selected cellular proteolytic enzymes (1033, 1286, 1339, 1878). These protease-sensitive sites included sequences (e.g., GPGR) that resembled trypsin inhibitors. Other aspartic-protease cleavage sites have also been identified in the HIV-1, HIV-2, and SIV envelope regions (466). Moreover, HIV-1 gp120 has been found to bind to a TL2-trypsin-like protease (1287). These observations suggested that these enzymes, when present on the cell, cleave the gp120 after binding to CD4. This event could facilitate a conformational change in the envelope so that a viral region (e.g., on gp41) can subsequently fuse with the cell membrane (2364) (Figure 3.3). Thus, some CD4$^+$ cells that cannot be infected by certain HIV strains might lack the necessary cellular proteases to cleave that particular virus envelope region when it is exposed.

The importance of envelope cleavage in infection gained some support from evidence demonstrating that gp120 can be digested by proteases and that this activity can be blocked by neutralizing antibodies (466). Other studies showed that exposure of purified HIV to sCD4 leads to cleavage of gp120 by proteolytic activity (Figure 3.3) (2859). This phenomenon can be blocked by monoclonal antibodies to the GPGR-containing regions of the V3 loop (2859). The cleavage therefore appears to involve the crown of the V3 loop. The explanation given for this observation is that an initial conformational change in gp120 (and perhaps CD4) takes place after attachment of gp120 to CD4 and that this event exposes the V3 loop to the enzymatic activity. The source of the protease is not known but is most probably a cellular protein that copurifies with the virus.

The importance of the proteolytic process to virus entry remains to be clarified. The fact that macrophage-tropic strains are relatively resistant to the cleavage of gp120 (962, 2566, 2859) raises the question of the universality of this process for virus infection. Some researchers are considering whether the lack of gp120 cleavage is a characteristic needed by a virus to infect monocyte/macrophages (962). In this regard, when a non-macrophage-tropic virus (e.g., HIV-1$_{SF2}$) is inoculated onto T-cell lines, the residual virus in the culture fluid shows cleavage in the enve-

Figure 3.3   Purified HIV-1$_{SF2}$ was mixed with soluble CD4 and incubated for 1 to 8 h at 37°C. Subsequently, the viral envelope protein gp120 was extracted and examined by immunoblot procedures. Lanes 1 and 8, virus preparation without sCD4 incubated for 8 h; lane 2, virus preparation mixed with 1 μg of sCD4 at time zero; lanes 3 to 7, virus and sCD4 mixed for 0.5, 1, 2, 4, and 8 h, respectively. After incubation with sCD4, the cleavage of the envelope gp120 into 50- and 70-kDa proteins is evident, and this process continues over time. The site of cleavage appears to be in the V3 loop (2859).

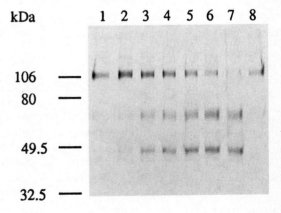

lope. In contrast, the same virus inoculated onto macrophages does not undergo proteolytic cleavage. Macrophage-tropic viruses handled in the same way do not undergo cleavage after inoculation on either cell type. Moreover, HIV-1$_{SF2}$ incubated with culture fluid from T-cell lines is not cleaved (2569a). Thus, it appears that virus:cell interaction is needed for this process to take place, that macrophages do not demonstrate this proteolytic activity, and that macrophage-tropic strains are not very sensitive to cleavage of gp120.

Whether envelope cleavage is needed for virus entry has also been studied by introducing mutations into the proteolytic cleavage site on the V3 loop (2423). In these studies, although cleavage appeared to be important for infectivity of T-cell lines, resistance to this process did not prevent infection by all mutants. Moreover, some mutant viruses with cleavable V3 loops were not infectious, although other modifications in the viral envelope structure might have been present. Other studies have indicated that viruses that have lost the trypsin-sensitive cleavage site can retain infectivity (2015), but whether other regions in the loop that could be cleaved were involved in the infection is not known. It seems likely that proteolytic sites for several cellular enzymes will be found in the envelope of various HIV strains. Thus, cleavage at certain sites may be required for entry of specific viral strains, but this possibility has not been demonstrated. Moreover, the envelope sequence linked to proteolysis can be separated from the sequences that determine T-cell line and macrophage tropisms (see Chapter 8) (2570). Nevertheless, since cleavage-resistant macrophage-tropic HIV-1 strains readily infect CD4$^+$ lymphocytes, the importance of this process in infection is not clear (Section VIII). Very little new information on the role of this process in virus infection has been reported recently.

C. Secondary Receptors for HIV Infection

1. GENERAL OBSERVATIONS

Several studies examining the role of the CD4-virus interaction involved in HIV infection indicated that the CD4 receptor alone is neither sufficient nor the sole means for viral entry (Table 3.1) (Section VI). Some human cells expressing high levels of the CD4 protein, including undifferentiated CD4$^+$ monocytes (see Chapter 5, Section IV), were not susceptible to HIV infection (434, 720, 1288). Some animal cells, derived through molecular or somatic hybrid techniques to express human CD4 on the cell surface, could not be infected (457, 1640, 2660). Studies with somatic cell hybrids, using human:human and human:CD4$^+$ rodent cells, suggested that another cell surface factor on certain human cells, besides CD4, is needed for HIV en-

Table 3.1   Evidence suggesting another cellular receptor for HIV

1. CD4$^+$ lymphocyte cell lines can be resistant to infection by HIV (1288).
2. Animal cells expressing human CD4 are not infectable by HIV (1640).
3. CD4$^-$ cells can be infected by HIV (427, 2648).
4. Some viruses incubated with soluble CD4 or antibodies to CD4 are not blocked from infecting certain CD4$^+$ and CD4$^-$ cell lines (2219).
5. A glycolipid, galactosyl ceramide, has been detected as an alternative virus receptor on CD4$^-$ brain- and bowel-derived human cells (1010, 2926).

try (292, 660, 1018, 2660). Furthermore, studies with cells expressing various constructs of CD4 showed that the D1 region does not appear to be the only portion of CD4 involved in the entry process (2132). In addition, antibodies to CD4 have not blocked infection of some CD4$^+$ cells by certain HIV-1 strains (2219). Finally, brain- and bowel-derived cells have an alternative receptor for HIV (Section VI).

On the basis of the above observations, several investigators began searching for secondary cellular attachment sites for HIV on human cells. Cell surface proteins reacting with regions of gp41 or gp36 (of HIV-2) were described (682, 1052, 2167, 2875). In addition, V3 loop binding proteins were identified on MOLT-4 cells (1879). One of these proteins could be the presumed fusion receptor molecule (see below) (Figure 3.2). The potential role of CD26, an aminopeptidase, as a secondary receptor for HIV was considered (336). Entry of HIV-1 or HIV-2 into T lymphoblastoid and monocytic cell lines, as measured by the intracellular concentration of p24, was inhibited by antibodies to the CD26 molecule. Moreover, murine cells expressing human CD4 were permissive for virus infection only after expression of human CD26 (336). However, antibodies to CD26 did not block cell-to-cell fusion and infection (2569), and CD26$^-$ T lymphocytes appear to be most susceptible to HIV infection (232). Thus, CD26 does not appear to be a coreceptor for HIV infection.

2. CHEMOKINE RECEPTORS AS CORECEPTORS

In searching for a coreceptor for HIV infection, Berger and coworkers found a human cDNA clone that expressed a protein, formerly called fusin (or LESTR), that mediated fusion in the mouse-human CD4$^+$-cell model. When introduced into HIV-resistant mouse cells expressing human CD4, the fusion-inducing molecule made the cells susceptible to HIV infection (743). This molecule, now called CXCR-4, has been shown to act as a coreceptor for HIV strains that are T-cell-line tropic and usually have an SI phenotype (194, 652; for an overview, see references 177a and

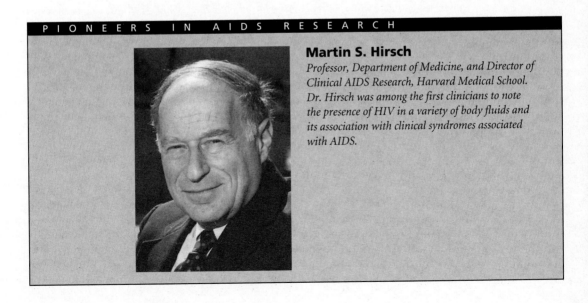

P I O N E E R S   I N   A I D S   R E S E A R C H

Martin S. Hirsch
Professor, Department of Medicine, and Director of Clinical AIDS Research, Harvard Medical School. Dr. Hirsch was among the first clinicians to note the presence of HIV in a variety of body fluids and its association with clinical syndromes associated with AIDS.

1495). The receptor permits a close interaction between the virus and the cell surface (194, 743, 1495) (Color Plate 2, following p. 188). The association of CXCR-4 with a CD4-gp120 complex in human cells has been demonstrated by immuno-precipitation studies (1429). These data provided further evidence of the physical attachment of these three molecules on the cell surface.

The amino-terminal domain of CXCR-4 is involved in virus binding, and intracellular signaling does not play an important role in HIV entry (2130). However, the particular region of CXCR-4 needed for viral infection appears to be determined by the virus strain involved. Mutations introduced into the amino-terminal extracellular domain of CXCR-4 affected infection by some, but not all, HIV-1 strains (2094). In general, multiple CXCR-4 domains appear to interact with HIV but especially the second extracellular loop structure (1595).

The natural ligand for CXCR-4 is the chemoattractant stromal-cell-derived factor 1 (SDF-1) (233, 1974), and this cytokine can block HIV infection of T-cell lines (1974). SDF-1 is a member of a family of low-molecular-weight cytokines called chemokines that mediate inflammation by recruiting immune cells to the site of injury (1985, 2603) (Table 3.2). The specific region of the viral envelope interacting with the CXCR-4 chemokine coreceptor has not yet been fully elucidated but appears to involve the V3 loop (2545a) (see Chapter 8).

CXCR-4 was identified as the receptor that assists HIV infection of the CD4$^+$ murine cells shortly before other investigators began examining chemokine receptors as possible coreceptors for HIV infection. The latter research was initially sparked by the observation that the β-chemokines RANTES, macrophage inflammatory protein 1α (MIP-1α) and MIP-1β, in combination, efficiently blocked HIV-1 infection of CD4$^+$ lymphocytes (487). The possibility was further supported once CXCR-4 was recognized as a chemokine receptor.

Working with molecular clones of the β-chemokine receptors, particularly CCR-5 but also CCR-3 and CCR-2b, several investigators showed that these molecules help macrophage-tropic NSI strains of HIV enter cells (45, 444, 618, 652, 661). These receptors are not used by the T-cell-line-tropic SI strains (for review, see reference 177a) (Table 3.3). The block of HIV infection by β-chemokines occurs at an early binding step in the infection process, presumably by competitive interaction at the coreceptor site. These cytokines do not inhibit virus production in chronically infected cells (1986). The early inhibitory events can include internalization of the chemokine receptor (55a, 76a). In this regard, several years ago, exposure of monocytes to HIV or the viral envelope glycoprotein was found to downregulate certain chemotactic ligand receptors and reduce the recruitment of peripheral blood monocytes to areas of inflammation (2800). These early studies, therefore, already suggested how chemokines could affect HIV infection if the chemokine receptor was involved.

The region of CCR-5 that participates in the interaction with the HIV-1 envelope (involving in part the V3 loop [2545a]) is the amino-terminal domain or the first extracellular region (488, 2303, 2710, 2920). The site on the receptor for HIV attachment has been found to be different from that involving the β-chemokines (98). Since chemokine receptors are G-protein-coupled molecules, this distinction in binding site and recent studies with mutant viruses indicate that signal transduction is not required for CCR-5 to act as an HIV coreceptor (913). Thus the role of

Table 3.2 List of some of the chemokines associated with hematopoietic system[a]

Receptors[b]: for C-X-C the receptor subcolumns are C-X-CR (1, 2, 3, 4) and Duffy Ag; for C-C the receptor subcolumns are CCR (1, 2a, 2b, 3, 4, 5) and Duffy Ag.
Chemoattracted cells subcolumns: N, Eo, Ba, Ma, T, B, NK, M, Dc, Ec, F.
Source[c] subcolumns: N, Eo, Ba, Ma, T, B, NK, M, Dc, Ec, F, Pl.

Chemokines	1	2	2a	2b	3	4	5	Duffy Ag	N	Eo	Ba	Ma	T	B	NK	M	Dc	Ec	F	N	Eo	Ba	Ma	T	B	NK	M	Dc	Ec	F	Pl
C-X-C (α)																															
IL-8	•	•							•	•	•	•	•		•			•	•								•		•	•	
Groα		•						•	•		•	•	•		•			•	•		•			•			•		•	•	
Groβ		•							•		•																•		•	•	
Groγ		•							•		•																•		•	•	
ENA-78		•							•																		•		•	•	
GCP-2		•							•																		•		•		
NAP-2		•							•		•					•			•												
PF-4									•			•																			•
MIG					•								•		•	•		•	•					•			•		•	•	
IP-10					•								•	•	•	•		•						•			•		•		
SDF-1α/1β						•			•				•						—[d]												
C-C (β)																															
MIP-1α	•			•		•	•		•	•	•	•	•	•	•	•	•			•		•	•	•		•	•	•		•	
MIP-1β	•					•	•		•	•	•	•	•	•	•	•	•		•	•				•		•	•	•		•	
RANTES	•		•		•	•	•	•	•	•	•	•	•	•	•	•	•	•		•				•		•	•	•	•	•	•
MCP-1			•	•				•		•	•	•	•		•	•	•	•		•							•		•	•	•
MCP-2			•	•						•	•	•	•		•	•		•	•	•							•				
MCP-3	•		•	•	•					•	•	•	•		•	•	•			•							•			•	
MCP-4			•		•					•	•	•	•			•				•							•				
I-309											•				•			•												•	
Eotaxin					•					•	•	•	•		•	•				•			•	•		•	•		•	•	
C(γ)																															
Lymphotactin																				•						•					

[a] Receptors for these chemokines, the cells affected by the chemokine (chemoattractant cells), and the source of the chemokine are also provided. Abbreviations: N, neutrophil; Eo, eosinophil; Ba, basophil; Ma, mast cell; T, T lymphocyte; B, B lymphocyte; NK, natural killer cell; M, monocyte; Dc, dendritic cell; Ec, endothelial cell; F, fibroblast; Pl, platelets. Information provided by G. Greco.

[b] HIV receptors are in boldface type.

[c] Only cells of the hematopoietic lineage are indicated.

[d] Bone marrow stromal cells.

Table 3.3 Coreceptors for HIV-1 infection of CD4$^+$ lymphocytes

Receptor	Phenotype	Tropism
CCR-5	NSI	Macrophage
CXCR-4^a	SI	T-cell line
CCR-3^b	NSI	Macrophage
CCR-2b	SI	Dual-tropic
Bonzo/ STRL33^b	NSI	Macrophage
BOB/GPR15^b	NSI	Macrophage

^{a} Major receptor for some HIV-2 strains.
^{b} Some isolates.

CCR-5 in chemotactic responses can be separated from its function as an HIV coreceptor (76a). This virus:cell interaction therefore resembles that involving CXCR-4 (see above). Nevertheless, infection of CD4$^+$ cells by NSI strains can enhance cell proliferation (938a), suggesting an ability of these viruses to activate the β-chemokine receptor pathway. Several domains in gp120 (2710) and CCR-5 (98) could participate in HIV entry. Also, differences among viral strains in their interaction with CCR-5 have been noted (2303), as was observed with CXCR-4 (see above). In this regard, several unrelated viruses can use CCR-5 for entry (e.g., HIV-1, HIV-2, and SIV). Furthermore, the sensitivity of NSI viruses to β-chemokines can vary up to 100-fold (1633a, 1826). Thus, in general, the interaction of HIV with its coreceptors must be complex, as is observed with the CD4 receptor (Section I). Finally, in one study of SIV/HIV chimeras, the coreceptor also appeared to participate in some way with a postbinding step needed for virus entry (389). Perhaps the Gag protein is involved (Section IV).

Several studies of viruses from different clades have further confirmed the role of CCR-5 as a coreceptor for the macrophage-tropic NSI strains (425, 1187, 1630, 2973) and CXCR-4 as a coreceptor for the T-cell-line-tropic SI strains (2973) (Table 3.3). Moreover, dual-tropic HIV isolates that are both macrophage tropic and T-cell-line tropic (NSI and SI) can use either receptor (652, 2509a). Some evidence suggests that the viral envelopes of these isolates interact with the first and second extracellular loops of CRCR-4 as well as the amino-terminal domain of CCR-5 (1595). All these findings indicate the promiscuity of HIV for cell surface receptors and the fact that multiple regions on the viral envelope can be involved in virus infection (see Chapter 8).

The observation on CCR-5 usage by macrophage-tropic viruses is curious since some studies indicate that β-chemokines do not block infection of macrophages by macrophage-tropic viruses (661, 2395) despite the presence of CCR-5 on the cell surface (1847). In fact, in certain studies, these cytokines appeared to enhance replication in macrophages (2395). However, primary macrophages from individuals who do not express CCR-5 on the cell surface (see below) are resistant to infection by both macrophage-tropic and T-cell-line-tropic viruses (508, 2181) but not dual-tropic viruses (2181). Importantly, the most recent studies indicate that HIV infection of primary macrophages and microglia (brain-derived macrophages) can be blocked by β-chemokines (136a, 1039, 2766). Furthermore, SIV$_{mac}$ isolates that replicate in T-cell lines can infect human macrophages expressing or lacking the CCR-5 receptor (417). Finally, studies with envelope mutant viruses indicate that the use of a particular chemokine receptor does not always correlate with cell tropism. For example, viruses that can use CCR-5 are not always macrophage tropic (641), and whereas macrophages express CXCR-4, they are not highly infectable by SI viruses (1738).

These observations indicate that virus entry into macrophages can involve CCR-5 but probably also another, unidentified receptor (425, 641, 1847) (see below). In this regard, a 75-kDa receptor has been considered a potential site for HIV-1 entry (1059) (Section VI.C). In addition, intracellular factors can influence the extent of virus replication (Chapter 5, Section II.B).

For both SI and NSI viral phenotypes, the coreceptor seems necessary to ensure binding by viruses to cells that have a small quantity of CD4 expressed (i.e., for NSI strains) or by viruses that bind weakly to CD4 (i.e., T-cell-line tropic viruses) (1369) (Color Plate 2, following p. 188). Since additional chemokine receptors (CCR-2b, CCR-3, Bonzo/STRL33, BOB/GPR15) can also serve as coreceptors (444, 618, 618a, 652, 784a, 1537a), still other sites for HIV interaction with the cell surface may soon be identified. For example, SI-type viruses have been found that use a variety of chemokine receptors such as CCR-3 and CCR-2b in addition to CXCR-4 (221a). In this regard, antibodies to CXCR-4 have not blocked infection of T-cell lines by some HIV-1 and HIV-2 strains (1738), suggesting strain differences in the use of this receptor or infection by a different coreceptor. Moreover, CXCR-4 itself can act as a primary receptor (without the need for CD4) for infection of CD4$^-$ cells by certain strains of HIV-2 (702). When this receptor was transferred to CD4$^-$ mink lung and feline kidney cells, infection by HIV-2 took place. The findings raise the possibility that the enhancement of infection of HIV-2 strains, when mixed with sCD4 (Section I.B), reflects a more efficient expression of the ligand on gp120 that interacts with CXCR-4.

A genetic variant involving a 12-bp deletion in CCR-5 (and thus no expression of the protein) has been linked to resistance to HIV infection (607, 1568, 2346). About 1 in 100 Caucasian people appear to be homozygous for this allele, but it is rarely detected in other racial groups (e.g., the black population from Western and Central Africa and the Japanese population) (2346) (Table 3.4). In this regard, peripheral blood mononuclear cells (PBMC) obtained from two high-risk uninfected individuals, homozygous for the mutant chemokine receptor allele, were found to be resistant to infection with macrophage-tropic viruses (508, 1568, 2181). In some studies, a delay in progression to disease in individuals who are heterozygous for the allele has also been suggested (607, 1568, 2346) but needs to be confirmed (2) (see Chapter 13, Section V).

Table 3.4   Genotype frequencies of CCR-5[a]

Ethnic group	No. of subjects	Genotype frequency (%)		
		+/+	+/Δ32	Δ32/Δ32
Caucasian	235	75	23	2
African American	238	97	3	<1
Hispanic	205	95	5	0

[a] Data from S. Y. Chang, Roche Molecular Systems.

These findings are very provocative but raise other questions about resistance to HIV infection. It seems remarkable that the individuals homozygous for the deletion allele have not come into contact with a T-cell-line-tropic virus, since these viruses are transmitted by the sexual route (for a review, see reference 919) (see Chapter 2). Perhaps these individuals were initially infected by an NSI macrophage-tropic strain that could not become well established in the host but elicited cellular immune responses against HIV. Subsequently, this immune response would have been able to ward off infections by other virus strains (e.g., SI phenotype) that might have the capacity to grow in the CD4$^+$ cells of these individuals (see Chapters 10 and 11). This possibility can be examined by studying anti-HIV cellular immune responses in these people. Recently, individuals homozygous for the CCR-5 deletion were found to be infected by HIV-1 (218, 1962, 2669). In these cases, SI viruses were recovered. However, since SI viruses are often associated with primary infection (see Chapter 4), factors other than coreceptor expression must be involved in this host resistance to HIV infection (see Chapters 10 and 11).

III.   Virus:Cell Fusion

A.   Cell Surface Events

Enveloped viruses, such as HIV, enter cells after fusion with the cell membrane. The mechanism for this process in HIV infection is not known. In early studies, computer analysis of the amino-terminal external portion of the gp41 of the HIV envelope demonstrated its similarity to fusion domains on paramyxoviruses, such as the Sendai and Newcastle disease viruses (826, 909) (for a review, see reference 2871) (Figure 3.4). This observation suggests that HIV entry might involve viral gp120:CD4 receptor and coreceptor attachments and then fusion via gp41 with another cell surface molecule (Color Plate 2, following p. 188) (Sections II.C and VI). The role of gp41 in fusion has been supported by studies showing induction of syncytium formation by gp41 when expressed by both CD4$^+$ and CD4$^-$ cells (2074). The fusion step could follow a conformational change in CD4 as well as dissociation of the envelope gp120, perhaps following cleavage of the V3 loop (Figure 3.2) (Sections II.A and II.B). This fusion process can be measured by membrane fluorescence dequenching (2512). As noted above, some studies have detected a gp41 cell surface receptor that could be involved (1052, 2167, 2875).

The kinetics of this fusion reaction suggest continued attachment of the virus to CD4 while fusion takes place (637). Thus, complete gp120 shedding most prob-

Figure 3.4   Model of the gp41 (TM) protein of HIV-1. A linear sequence of gp41 is shown in a planar projection of the proposed structure derived from computer modeling and based on the influenza virus HA2 scaffold. The α helices are depicted as modified helical nets alternating three and four amino acids per turn connected by single lines. Hydrophobic amino acids are indicated as solid circles, charged amino acids as open circles, and neutral amino acids as partly filled circles. Nonhelical regions are shown as loosely coiled extended chains; strong turns are indicated by a T, the proposed intramolecular disulfide bond by a double line. Specific functional regions are noted. Figure courtesy of R. Garry. Modified from reference 826a with permission.

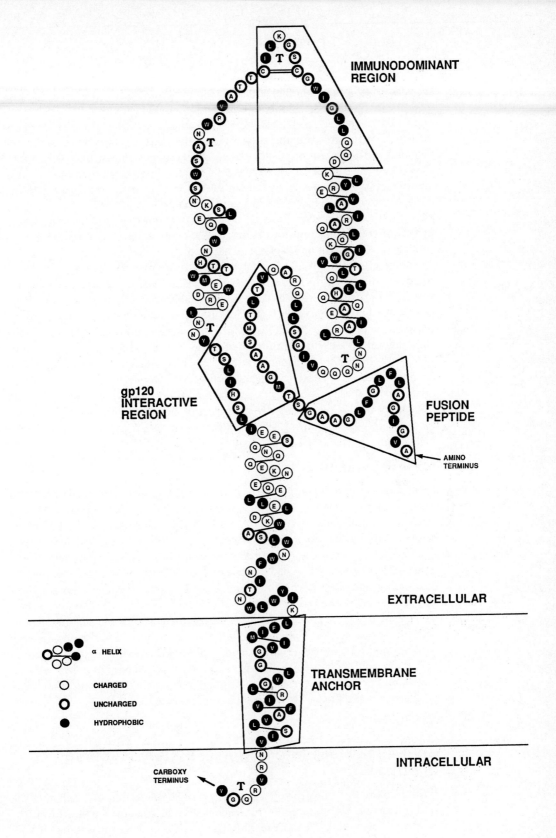

IMMUNODOMINANT REGION

FUSION PEPTIDE

AMINO TERMINUS

gp120 INTERACTIVE REGION

EXTRACELLULAR

α HELIX

CHARGED

UNCHARGED

HYDROPHOBIC

TRANSMEMBRANE ANCHOR

INTRACELLULAR

CARBOXY TERMINUS

ably does not occur, although some displacement, as described in Section II.A, might be involved. The V3 loop, as well as gp41, could be important in this membrane fusion event (179, 182, 2015, 2582). As noted above, the V3 loop may interact with a chemokine receptor, thus bringing the virus envelope closer to the cell membrane to permit fusion (Color Plate 2). Mutational studies with gp41 and with the V3 loop have suggested that cell:cell fusion and infectivity are linked, since in many cases both are affected by the same amino acid changes (see Chapter 6). Infectivity presumably reflects the virus:cell fusion event (182, 589, 792, 795, 945). Nevertheless, the fusogenic property of a virus may not be as important for infectivity as it is for syncytium formation (2582). Thus, virus:cell and cell:cell fusion could involve different processes (see Chapter 6).

Some observations suggest that the CD4 molecule, in addition to binding, could be required for the fusion of the viral envelope with the cell surface. Elimination of the proximal region of CD4 through molecular techniques (e.g., replacement with CD8 regions) reduces viral infection and also eliminates the ability of the cell to fuse with infected cells (2132). Moreover, some monoclonal antibodies to the CD4 molecule block cell:cell fusion but not HIV binding, and vice versa (381, 1042, 1217, 2717, 2881). One explanation is that CD4 must undergo movement involving its hinge region (D2-D3) to bring about this fusion. Nevertheless, in all these approaches, whether virus:cell fusion and cell:cell fusion involve the same processes still has not been answered. Finally, the nature of the putative cellular fusion receptor or receptors is unknown (1495) (Figure 3.2).

B.   ## pH-Independent Entry

Experiments examining the mechanism for virus entry into cells have also evaluated the effect of changes in the relative acidity of the cytoplasmic endosomes. Enveloped viruses enter by either a pH-dependent or -independent process. If a low pH is needed, virus fusion most probably occurs in endocytotic vesicles. With retroviruses that have been examined and many other enveloped viruses, an acidic environment in the cell is generally not needed for virus entry (639, 880, 2871). In the case of HIV, chloroquine and NH_4Cl, which raise the pH in cellular components, do not affect virus infection (1709, 2586). Thus, HIV entry is pH independent. This observation has suggested that the HIV envelope, after attachment and subsequent interactions with the cell surface, can fuse directly with the cell membrane and not necessarily within endocytotic vesicles (Figure 3.2 and Color Plate 2 [following p. 188]). However, the possible entry of HIV through endosomes as well has not been ruled out. Moreover, because HIV can enter by fusing directly with the plasma membrane, phagocytosis may also lead to infection in some cells (915, 2053).

IV.   ## HIV:Cell Surface Interactions Possibly Involved in Virus Entry

The possibility that other factors are involved in HIV infection of a cell, after the viral interaction with a receptor, has been suggested by some studies. Investigators have shown that after attachment to CD4, a delay in viral entry at the cell surface can influence the spread of HIV and the extent of virus production (1292). Different rates and efficiencies of entry are most probably linked to variations in the envelope protein (750, 2485) (see Chapter 7). Other studies suggest that the cytoplasmic domain of gp41 might be partly involved in entry through a role in virus uncoating or penetration (816). Finally, nonprotein components (possibly glycolipids) could play a role in the envelope:CD4-mediated fusion needed for virus entry (662).

The phenomenon of delayed entry has been associated in some studies with the absence of the D3 and D4 regions of the CD4 molecule (2132) and probably reflects inefficient conformational changes in the CD4 molecule associated with fusion (see Chapter 6). These observations suggest that the CD4 protein could be involved not only in the binding but also in the fusion and perhaps penetration of the virion from the cell surface into the cytoplasm of the cell. For a time, the virus might remain attached to CD4 without release of its viral core into the cytoplasm. Alternatively (although this hypothesis is highly conjectural), the core might be kept beneath the cell membrane bilayer without entry into the cytoplasm. Only after penetration and uncoating of the viral core would reverse transcription and the steps leading to viral production take place.

Several reports suggest that attachment and fusion are not the only processes needed for entry of the viral nucleocapsid into the cytoplasm. When certain HIV-1 and SIV strains are used to infect a variety of $CD4^+$ or $CD4^-$ cells, attachment (measured by CD4 binding) and fusion (detected by fluorescence dequenching) may take place, but the presence of the viral core protein in the cell or the production of infectious virus cannot be detected (2568). Studies on infection of alveolar macrophages by HIV-1 have suggested a similar block to infection after virus:cell fusion (2129). These observations suggest that while fusion of the viral membrane to the cell surface might occur, a third major process brings the viral nucleocapsid into the cytoplasm (Figure 3.5) (1495).

The mechanism for the third step, nucleocapsid entry, is not known. One hypothesis is that the binding of the gp41 fusion domain to a fusion receptor on the cell surface brings about an intermixing of the outer lipid membranes of the virus and the cell (i.e., hemi-fusion). However, unless the inner lipid membranes meet, nucleocapsid entry cannot take place (Color Plate 3, following p. 188). The mixing of inner membranes may require other cellular or viral proteins that are yet to be defined. Another explanation could be the need for a particular process for core entry. A Gag protein might be involved in this third step, since this viral protein (e.g., MA) plays an important role in the budding and release of HIV progeny at the end of the replicative cycle (2545, 2948). This possibility has been supported by recent SIV/HIV recombinant studies showing restricted replication of HIV-1 in rhesus macaque cells, in which a region encompassing the *gag* gene appears to be involved (389, 1071).

V.   Down-Modulation of the CD4 Protein

Another early observation made with HIV-1 replication in human T cells was the concomitant disappearance of the CD4 protein from the cell surface (1113, 1311, 2598). The extent and time of the down-modulation depend on the level of virus

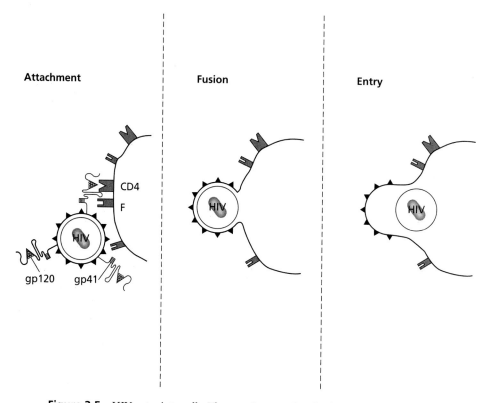

Attachment   Fusion   Entry

CD4
F

gp120   gp41

Figure 3.5 HIV entry into cells. Three major steps involved in virus infection are depicted based on observations in cell culture (2129, 2566). Adapted from reference 1491 with permission.

production (2132, 2598, 2950, 2958). Generally, a loss in CD4 expression in vitro is detected several days after HIV infection of cells, when sufficient progeny virions are produced. Thus, a reduction in chronic HIV-1 production in a T-cell line, as was achieved with a Tat antagonist, restores CD4 expression (2457).

The mechanism involved in the altered expression of this cell surface receptor is still not clear (Table 3.5). The CD4 receptor does not necessarily internalize with HIV during infection, and CD4-related signal transduction events are not needed for virus entry (1991). Moreover, with some HIV strains (HIV-1$_{SF162}$, HIV-2$_{UC-1}$),

Table 3.5 Factors involved in down-modulation of CD4 protein expression

1. Complexing of CD4 with envelope gp160 within the cell (540, 541, 1174, 1334)
2. Vpu dissociation of the CD4:gp160 complex with degradation of CD4 (2884)
3. Down-modulation by Nef (845, 973, 1669)
4. Block in transcription of CD4 mRNA (2344, 2598)
5. Arrest in translation of the CD4 protein (1113, 2950)
6. Masking of viral receptor by gp120 (53, 1719, 2363)
7. Removal of CD4 from cell surface by replicating virions (1028, 1746)

infection with high levels of virus production does not affect CD4 expression (see Chapter 7). Differences in specific regions of the envelope gp120 could be involved. By using interviral recombinants of two HIV-1 strains differing in this biologic property, CD4 down-modulation was linked to the envelope region (2943). Some studies suggest a role of the complexing of envelope gp160 with CD4 in the endoplasmic reticulum of the cell (540, 541, 1174, 1334). Vpu is considered to be involved in this process since this viral protein dissociates the gp160/CD4 complex (540) by inducing the degradation of CD4 (2884). This function could be important in permitting gp160 incorporation into virions and could certainly affect CD4 expression.

In other studies, the Nef protein has been implicated in down-modulation of the CD4 molecule (845, 973, 1669). The mechanism has been linked to an endocytotoxic process in which Nef is degraded in lysosomes (2714). Viruses that lack this activity could have a truncated Nef protein. With both Vpu and Nef, the cytoplasmic portion of the CD4 molecule is the major domain involved (70, 1476). In recent studies of this process, Vpu, Env, and Nef were all shown to play a role in CD4 down-modulation. Nef down-modulated CD4 rapidly during the early steps in HIV infection; Env and Vpu functioned late in infection (414). In general, a combination of all three proteins was the most efficient in reducing CD4 expression.

Other reports indicate that down-modulation of CD4 reflects an arrest of transcription of the CD4 mRNA (2344, 2598) or of translation of the CD4 mRNA (1113, 2950). A few studies have suggested that masking of the CD4 binding site by the envelope gp120 (or gp120 antibody complexes) attached to the cell surface is involved (53, 1719, 2363). The latter phenomenon can be demonstrated by using an antibody to a different region of the CD4 molecule located outside the gp120 binding site. With a monoclonal antibody such as OKT4 (not OKT4A or Leu 3a), the continual presence of the CD4 protein on presumably infected CD4$^-$ cells can be evaluated. In addition, some investigators suggest that the CD4 molecule is removed by budding virions (1028, 1746) (Table 3.5). The relative effect of each of these processes on CD4 protein expression most probably depends on the virus and the cells infected. The relevance to pathogenesis is unclear since some viruses do not modulate the expression of CD4 (432, 721) (see Chapter 7). The removal of this HIV binding site on the CD4 molecule, however, does prevent superinfection of the cells by other HIV-1 strains (see Chapter 4). Finally, HIV infection may induce down-regulation of other T-cell surface molecules, including MHC (1273, 2390, 2598). The effect on MHC class I expression could be mediated by the Tat (1112) or Nef (2428) proteins (see Chapter 11).

VI.   Infection of Cells Lacking CD4 Expression

A.   General Observations

Many CD4$^-$ cells can be infected by HIV (Table 3.6), including human skin fibroblasts, dental pulp fibroblasts, muscle and bone-derived fibroblastoid cell lines, human trophoblast cells, follicular dendritic cells, brain-derived glial cells, brain capillary endothelial cells, cervical epithelial cells, fetal adrenal cells, natural killer cells, and human liver carcinoma cell lines (see Chapter 4) (133, 271, 355, 427, 459, 893,

Table 3.6   CD4⁻ human cells susceptible to HIV infection[a]

In vitro
Fetal astrocytes
Neuroblastoma cell lines (e.g., SK-N-Mc)
Brain-derived capillary endothelial cells
Brain microglia
NK cells
Osteosarcoma cell line (HOS)
Rhabdomyosarcoma cell line (RD)
Primary skin fibroblast cells
Fetal adrenal cells
Follicular dendritic cells
Hepatic carcinoma cell line
Hepatic sinusoidal endothelial cells
Bowel adenocarcinoma cell lines
Trophoblast cell lines
Cervix-derived epithelial cell lines
In vivo
Bowel epithelium
Renal epithelium
Hepatocytes
Dental pulp fibroblasts
Brain astrocytes; oligodendrocytes

[a] In vitro studies involve cell culture with virus replication detected by reverse transcriptase, p24 antigen, and PCR assay procedures. In vivo studies include immunohistochemical and in situ hybridization methods. (See the text for references.)

1012, 1532, 1750, 2049, 2435, 2565, 2638, 2648, 2952). Evidence for the absence of a role of the CD4 receptor in virus entry of these cells comes from a variety of studies, including those involving monoclonal antibodies to CD4, incubation of virus with sCD4, and lack of detectable CD4 mRNA in the cells (Table 3.7).

The extent of virus replication in CD4⁻ cells is generally low, but where evaluated, HIV enters the cells in a pH-independent manner (2648), as it does in CD4⁺ cells. The limited extent of virus production is due in part to inefficient viral entry and subsequent spread; usually less than 1% of cells initially become infected (271, 1750). Intracellular events can also limit steps leading to productive infection (see Chapter 5). Transfection experiments with DNA molecular clones of HIV suggest that once infection is established, substantial virus replication can occur in many of these cell types (1506). To detect HIV production in several CD4⁻ cell types, cocul-

Table 3.7   Evidence for lack of CD4 protein expression in cells

1. CD4 protein is not detected on the cell surface by monoclonal antibodies to the molecule.
2. CD4 protein is not noted in the cells by serologic and immunohistochemical procedures.
3. CD4 mRNA is not detected in cells by Northern blot and PCR procedures.
4. HIV infection is not blocked by pretreating cells with antibodies to the CD4 molecule, e.g., Leu-3a.
5. Infection of the cells is not inhibited by mixing HIV with a soluble CD4 protein.

tivation of the cells with other sensitive target cells, such as PBMC, has been required (2648). Some studies suggest that cytokines produced by PBMC can enhance HIV production in CD4$^-$ cells, particularly those of brain origin (2622, 2691).

The cell surface molecule or molecules responsible for viral entry into CD4$^-$ cells are not known, but conceivably they could be fusion receptors (2648) or secondary binding sites for HIV (e.g., the CXCR-4 receptor) (702) (Section II.C). A portion of the viral envelope that is different from that used for CD4$^+$ cell entry seems to be involved, since antibodies to HIV differ in their ability to neutralize HIV infection of lymphocytes and CD4$^-$ fibroblasts (2648). This route of entry, however, is quite limited compared with the process mediated by CD4. One conclusion could be that for CD4$^+$ cells, the attachment to CD4 enhances the interaction of the viral envelope with a cellular coreceptor (see Section II.C) or a fusion receptor (see below). CD4$^-$ cells would use the same means of entry (a universal one involving fusion), but it would be much less efficient. Likewise, if the coreceptor or cell fusion receptor is absent, infection of CD4$^+$ cells might not occur, as observed with some T-cell lines (1288). Finally, as discussed above, perhaps the third step of virus entry into the cell, the entry of the nucleocapsid (Figure 3.5; Color Plate 2, following p. 188), is blocked in CD4$^-$ cells because of the lack of an appropriate cellular factor or a necessary viral protein:cell factor interaction.

B.   ## Galactosyl Ceramide Receptor

A virus receptor on CD4$^-$ brain-derived cells was identified by using rabbit polyclonal antibodies to galactosyl ceramide (GalC) and galactosyl sulfur (1010). This cell surface product, a glycolipid (204), binds to a different domain on gp120 (the V3 loop) than that for CD4 (203, 204). Like a possible cellular fusion domain for paramyxoviruses (1673, 2871), a glycolipid could be involved in HIV infection of some CD4$^-$ cells. The GalC receptor has also been linked to infection of bowel-derived cells (2926) and of vaginal epithelial cells (814) (Table 3.8). The interaction

Table 3.8   *HIV:cell surface binding interactions*

Major cellular receptors
CD4 (Section I)
GalC (Section VI)
Fc[a] (Section X)
Complement[a] (Section X)
Coreceptors (Section II) (Table 3.3)
CCR-5—macrophage-tropic strains
CXCR-4—T-cell-line-tropic strains
CCR-3
CCR-2b
Other possible cellular binding proteins on HIV (Section VII)
MHC (89, 348, 2319)
LFA-1 (1003, 1068, 2742)
ICAM-1 (2241)
CD44 (673)
Mannose-binding protein (549, 728)

[a] When virus is complexed with antibody.

appears to involve regions, such as the V3 loop and the V4 and V5 domains, that are different from those that interact with CD4 (814, 1011, 2927). Recently, the chemokine receptor CXCR-4 has been identified as a possible coreceptor for HIV-1 entry into CD4$^-$ GalC$^+$ intestinal epithelial cells (615).

The identification of GalC as a means of entry into both brain and bowel cells might explain the reports of gastrointestinal disorders that accompany neurologic signs of HIV infection (722); similar viral strains might use this cellular receptor. Whether the GalC mechanism for HIV entry of CD4$^-$ cells is common is not known, but not all brain cells express this glycolipid. Human fetal astrocytes appear to utilize a different receptor, which has not yet been identified (1618). Moreover, a receptor of approximately 180 kDa distinct from GalC has been demonstrated on CD4$^-$ glioma cells. Binding of recombinant gp120 to this protein receptor appears to induce tyrosine-specific protein kinase activity in the cells (2403). Furthermore, antibodies to GalC do not block HIV infection of CD4$^-$ fibroblasts and fetal adrenal cells (133a).

VII.   Other Possible HIV:Cell Surface Interactions

The incorporation of MHC-related molecules onto the viral envelope might also help in binding of HIV to the cell surface (89, 1115, 2319) via a secondary receptor (Table 3.8). This acquisition of cellular molecules appears to be determined by the viral strain and the infected cells (349), and it has been associated with increased viral infectivity (348). Nevertheless, viruses grown in nonhuman cells are still highly infectious for human cells (1506). Work demonstrating that the lymphocyte function antigen type 1 (LFA-1) adhesion molecule can be a participant in HIV infection offers another alternative mechanism for viral attachment, although its primary contribution appears to be in cell-cell fusion (1003, 1068, 1226, 2030, 2742) (see Chapter 6). Intercellular adhesion molecule type 1 (ICAM-1) on HIV-1 virions has increased the virus infectivity for PBMC by two- to sevenfold (2241). Perhaps adhesion molecules are important in the cell-to-cell transfer of virus. A possible role of the transmembrane receptor for hyaluronan, CD44, in productive infection by macrophage-tropic strains has been suggested (673). The retention of function of the CD44 associated with the viral envelope has been demonstrated (967). In addition, with the high mannose content in the HIV-1 envelope (1003), the macrophage mannose receptor (728) might provide an alternative entry site for infection of macrophages by the virus. This possibility should be explored, particularly since the β-chemokine receptors may not always be involved (Section II.C). Finally, a gp120 binding protein that is a membrane-associated mannose binding lectin on CD4$^-$ placental cells could be a prototype of another receptor for HIV (549).

VIII.   Overview of Early Steps in HIV Infection

A key concept regarding the early events in HIV interaction with a cell (Table 3.9) is that attachment of HIV to the CD4 molecule most probably leads to some conformational changes in both gp120 and CD4. The initial attachment appears to be at two sites on the CDR2 domain of CD4 (Figure 3.1) and probably involves non-

Table 3.9 Steps involved in HIV infection of a cell[a]

1. Attachment of viral envelope gp120 to cell surface receptor (e.g., CD4) or alternative receptor
2. Conformational change in gp120 and perhaps CD4 (i.e., the cell receptor) following attachment
3. Binding of another gp120 region to a coreceptor
4. Displacement of gp120[b]
5. Proteolytic cleavage of the V3 loop or its envelope counterpart (i.e., for HIV-2)[b]
6. Interaction of the fusion domain of HIV (e.g., gp41) with a fusion receptor on the cell surface (conceivably a glycolipid)
7. Virus:cell fusion in a pH-independent fashion
8. Entry of viral RNA associated with the core into the cytoplasm
9. Initiation of reverse transcription
10. Production of viral DNA copy (cDNA) from viral RNA and its duplication into a double-stranded DNA structure; generation of covalently bound circles and non-covalently bound circular forms
11. Transport of cDNA to the nucleus, where integration of the non-covalently bound circular forms into chromosomal DNA takes place
12. Production of viral mRNA and viral genomic RNA from the integrated proviral DNA (extent of production depends on relative expression of HIV regulatory genes [e.g., *tat, rev, nef*] [see Chapter 5])
13. Production of viral proteins from full-length and spliced mRNA
14. Incorporation of viral genomic RNA into the capsid forming at the cell membrane (and in intracellular compartments)
15. Processing of Gag and Gag-Pol polyproteins at the cell surface or in budding virions
16. Budding of the viral capsid through the cell membrane with incorporation of the processed viral envelope glycoproteins present on the cell surface (can depend on viral *vif* gene product)

[a] Summarized from discussions in the text (Section VIII).

[b] May or may not take place.

linear epitopes of gp120 that come into contact with the CD4 receptor site through a specific conformational structure. Subsequent displacement of gp120 and/or cleavage of the envelope protein (e.g., in the V3 loop) by cellular enzymes (Figure 3.2) causes another alteration in the viral envelope. This alteration results in the conformational changes in gp120 and CD4 that give the viral envelope additional binding sites with the cell surface, such as through CXCR-4, CXCR-5, or other coreceptors. This interaction will depend on the viral strain involved. A role for envelope cleavage (Figures 3.2 and 3.3), which does not seem to occur with macrophage-tropic strains, remains to be substantiated. A subsequent process could involve the gp41 fusion domain (Color Plate 2, following p. 188) and the target cell membrane (possibly via another cell surface receptor) (Figures 3.4 and 3.5). Virus:cell fusion, which is pH independent, then takes place (2364) (Figure 3.2; Color Plates 2 and 3, following p. 188) (Section III). The viral core subsequently enters the cell (Figure 3.5; Color Plate 2). Conformational changes in the CD4 molecule following gp120 binding may enhance virus entry (110). Other regions on CD4 and on gp120 (e.g., the V3 loop) could be involved in these processes.

Three major steps—attachment, fusion, and nucleocapsid entry—are thus part of HIV entry (Figure 3.5). Most probably, the virus:cell fusion mediated by gp41 and the nucleoid entry (perhaps mediated by the Gag protein) represent other biologic steps in early HIV infection that need to be elucidated. Conceivably, specific viral and cellular factors are involved. All these findings indicate the promiscuity of HIV in its interaction with the cell surface and the probability that several therapeutic approaches are needed to block infection at entry.

Without CD4 attachment or efficient binding of gp120 to the cell surface, interaction of viral gp41 with the cell membrane (possibly via a specific receptor) might take place but would be highly inefficient. This pH-independent process could explain the limited infection of CD4$^-$ cells. In some cells, the cell fusion receptor could be GalC (1010). Moreover, the gp41-associated cell membrane protein (1052, 2167) or other cell surface molecules interacting with gp120 could be involved. Certainly, the overall conformation of the viral envelope, which differs among strains, influences the infection process (see Chapter 8).

Following virus entry, subsequent intracellular events (e.g., nucleocapsid uncoating and reverse transcription) can determine the extent of virus replication in the acutely infected cell (see Chapter 5). Expression of the CD4 molecule is generally reduced once substantial virus replication occurs (Table 3.5), but exceptions have been observed with some HIV strains (see Chapter 7). Finally, the spread of HIV in the host results from production of infectious progeny and probably also by cell-to-cell transfer of virus (see below) (Table 3.9).

IX.   Cell-to-Cell Transfer of HIV

Besides entering a cell as a free infectious particle, HIV can be passed during cell-to-cell contact (Color Plate 4, following p. 188). In this process, multinucleated cells might result from syncytium formation (Figure 3.6), or cell-to-cell contact could

Figure 3.6 Multinucleated cell formation in PBMC infected by HIV-1. Magnification, ×65.

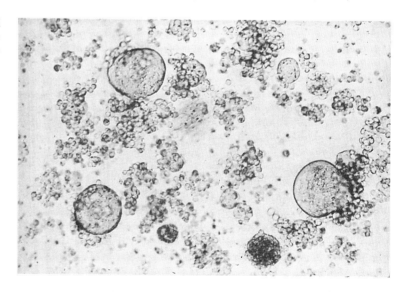

take place by adherence without fusion of cell membranes (Figures 2.4 and 2.6). The cell-to-cell mechanism of HIV transfer has been estimated to be up to 100 times more efficient than infection by free virus particles (2361). Macrophage-to-lymphocyte transfer of virus, presumably involving fusion, has been shown in the presence of neutralizing antibodies (968). In some studies, evidence has been presented that HIV can spread rapidly from one cell to another without formation of fully formed particles (2361). Conceivably, viral nucleocapsids are transferred to a new cell during cell:cell fusion, with subsequent de novo reverse transcription (1534).

In cell culture studies involving cell-to-cell contact without cell fusion, HIV was shown to be transmitted from monocytes or lymphocytes to epithelial cells in the presence of neutralizing antibodies (2055, 2090, 2638). In these experiments, electron micrographs revealed the transfer of complete virus particles that were present at the site of cell:cell adherence without cell fusion (Figures 2.4 and 2.6). In one report, time-lapse photography showed a migrating infected lymphocyte transferring virus particles to several different epithelial cells during short intervals of contact (2055). In other studies with the electron microscope, virus was associated with pseudopods projecting from macrophages, suggesting another means of HIV transfer (2077) (Figure 3.7). Thus, HIV spread in the host could result from cell-to-cell transfer (via cores or virions) as well as from circulating free virus. During cell:cell contact, syncytium formation or cell adherence could be involved, and neutralizing antibodies would not be effective in preventing the infection.

Figure 3.7 (A) Scanning electron micrograph of an HIV-infected (strain P1-2), activated monocyte. The surface of most of the monocyte is characterized by irregular microvilli. However, the pseudopod of the monocyte (top) is covered with small spherical structures, which appear to be HIV virions. The bulges at the tips of these microvilli may be the budding HIV virions. (From reference 2077 with permission.) *(Figure continues next page.)*

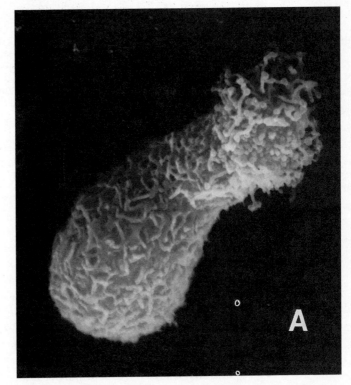

Figure 3.7 *(continued)* (B) Transmission electron micrograph of an activated monocyte showing a pseudopod with budding (strain O/S) virus (top of figure).

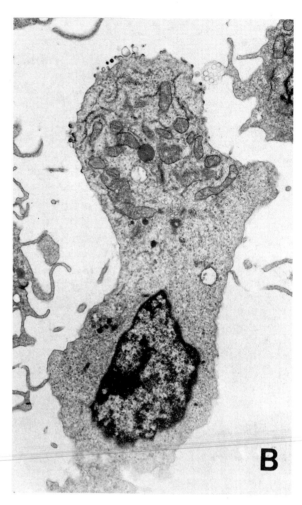

B

X.   Additional Mechanisms Involved in Virus Entry

A.   Fc and Complement Receptors

Besides entering cells via direct interaction of the virus envelope with cell surface receptors, HIV can infect cells by other mechanisms (Tables 3.3 and 3.8). For example, during the course of studies on the humoral response to HIV-1 infection, the phenomenon of antibody-dependent enhancement (ADE) of HIV infection was discovered. Presumably, ADE involves the binding of the Fab portion of nonneutralizing antibodies to the surface of the virion and the transfer of virus into a cell through the complement or Fc receptor (Figure 3.8) (1103, 1446, 2213, 2257, 2633, 2702). Complement-mediated ADE has been demonstrated with fresh serum or plasma from infected individuals and by the addition of complement to heat-inactivated serum (2256, 2257). The assays work best in the MT-2 cell line, which has high-level expression of the complement receptors (1819). Fc-mediated ADE has

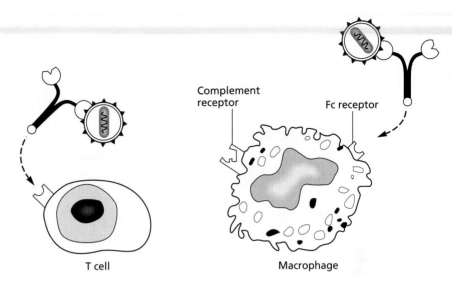

Figure 3.8   Mechanism of ADE of HIV infection. The antiviral antibody binds to the viral envelope glycoprotein. This virus-antibody complex can then enter cells (T cells and macrophages shown here) through an interaction of the Fc portion of the antibody with either the cellular Fc receptor or the complement receptor (after complexing with complement). Adapted from reference 1490 with permission.

been observed with heated (56°C, for 30 min), decomplemented HIV-1-seropositive serum (1103, 1104, 2633) (see Chapter 10).

In some T-cell and monocyte lines and in one study with primary macrophages, the CD4 molecule was reported to participate in viral entry via Fc or complement receptors (2076, 2257, 2632). One proposed process is that these alternative cellular receptors bring the virus closer to the CD4 molecule for subsequent entry. However, from other studies with peripheral blood macrophages, T lymphocytes, human trophoblast cells, and CD4⁻ human fibroblasts, the CD4 protein did not appear to be required for entry (1052, 1103, 1733, 2695). Thus, the complement and Fc receptors could serve as alternative sites for virus infection, although the mechanisms of entry are still not defined.

ADE by HIV highlights the potential role of herpesviruses as cofactors in HIV infection. These viruses can induce both complement and Fc receptors on the surface of infected cells (152, 1742, 2177) that could serve as potential target cells for HIV. Studies with cytomegalovirus (CMV) infection of CD4⁻ fibroblasts have demonstrated the appearance of Fc receptors on the cell surface. Subsequently, the CMV-infected cells were susceptible to HIV infection through antibody:virus complexes (1733). Thus, this study demonstrated the lack of participation by CD4 in HIV infection via the Fc receptor. Fc receptors have also been detected on rectal mucosal cells (1144). Conceivably, infection could take place in the anal canal via antibody:virus complexes in seminal fluid (see Chapter 2).

Finally, other experiments have suggested that HIV alone can enter cells via the complement receptor (CR-2) after activation and binding to the C1 component (i.e., as opsonized particles) (268, 269, 683, 936). This mechanism, involving gp41,

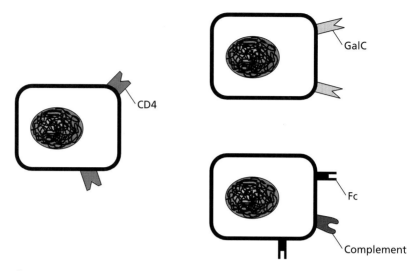

Figure 3.9   Four major cellular receptors that can be utilized by HIV to enter cells.

can lead to enhanced infection of cells by small amounts of virus (2671) and has also been suggested as the mechanism for the attachment of HIV-1 to follicular dendritic cells (see Chapter 9, Section I.H). In summary, at least four major cellular receptors could be involved in HIV infection (Figure 3.9), and several coreceptors can play an important role in the infection process (Table 3.3).

B.   Phenotypic Mixing: Pseudotype Virion Formation

Another mechanism for HIV entry into cells is phenotypic mixing (239, 1126). By this process, a viral genome can be placed in the envelope of a different virus and thus acquire the host range of that virus (Figure 3.10). Phenotypic mixing between HIV-1 and HIV-2 strains has been described (1464). Moreover, cells coinfected by HIV and murine retroviruses have demonstrated pseudotype virion formation in which the HIV genome can be found within the envelope of various mouse retroviruses (345, 434, 1613, 2546). Subsequently, HIV could infect a wide variety of cells susceptible to these animal retroviruses (Figure 3.11).

Figure 3.10   Phenotypic mixing. When two viruses of different types enter the same cell, the progeny produced will consist of the initial viruses and also viruses that have exchanged their outside coat. These new viruses then have the host range of the virus from which they derived their envelope. (From reference 1503 with permission.)

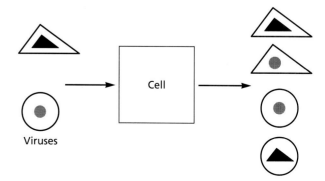

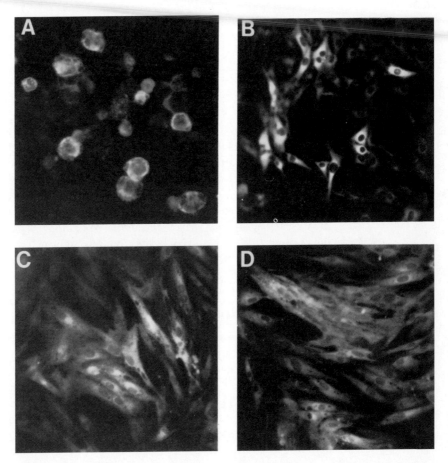

Figure 3.11   Coinfection of a human T-lymphocyte line with HIV-1 and the murine xenotropic retrovirus led to virus preparations that contained phenotypically mixed particles. Thus, the HIV genome enveloped in a xenotropic virus coat could infect a wide variety of animal cell lines previously resistant to HIV infection. (A) HUT 78 human T cells; (B) mink lung cells; (C) horse dermis cells; (D) goat esophagus cells. (All magnifications, ×40). Reprinted from reference 345 with permission.

HIV pseudotypes have also been produced in vitro with herpesviruses and rhabdoviruses (e.g., vesicular stomatitis virus [VSV]) (2846, 2986). The VSV pseudotypes have been helpful in defining the cellular restrictions to HIV entry (2846, 2847). Cells exposed to a virus containing the VSV genome within the HIV envelope show VSV-induced lysis only if they are susceptible to HIV infection. Finally, in vitro phenotypic mixing among different human retrovirus groups (e.g., HTLV and HIV) has also been described (1412, 1464). In preliminary studies, however, we have not observed phenotypic mixing during coinfection of cells with HIV and the human spumavirus (1505a).

In summary, several viruses have shown the ability to undergo phenotypic mixing with HIV-1, including HIV-2; HTLV-1; murine xenotropic, amphotropic, and polytropic type C retroviruses; VSV; and herpesviruses.

Whether pseudotype virus formation occurs in nature is not known. HIV-infected individuals coinfected with herpesviruses or HTLV-1 could have virus populations representing phenotypic mixtures of the two viruses (1412, 2986), but this possibility has not been reported. Electron microscopic studies of nongenital herpes simplex virus (HSV-1) skin lesions have shown virions suggestive of phenotypically mixed particles (1055). The process may have facilitated HIV infection of the keratinocytes as well as HSV infection of the macrophages in the lesions. The findings, if confirmed, could have relevance to sexual transmission of HIV (see Chapter 2). Moreover, as noted above, infection in vitro by HIV-1 and HIV-2 can, under some circumstances, lead to phenotypic mixing of the two virus subtypes (1464). The consequences of these events could include increased pathogenesis, but no evidence of this phenomenon having clinical relevance has been presented. Investigators using animal models to study HIV infection must also recognize that phenotypic mixing with an endogenous virus in the animal (e.g., mouse) (1227, 1856, 1857, 1904) might compromise the study objectives, but this problem has not been encountered in SCID mice (1855a).

XI.   Recombination

The possibility of recombination between the genomes of two different viruses infecting the same cell during early virus:cell interactions must be considered. This process can take place if heterotypic viruses form (i.e., if the two RNA species within a virion core come from different viruses) (1125). The event could produce new viruses with different biologic and pathogenic properties. Recombination could be detected in an HIV isolate by the appearance of genetic differences in specific regions of the viral genome that are usually the same when found together (e.g., Gag and Env) (see Chapter 8).

The process of homologous recombination could allow two defective viruses to become cytopathic (1305) and could introduce new strains into the population, thereby challenging vaccine approaches (631, 949, 1231, 2250, 2322). Following acute infection of cultured cells with two wild-type viruses, recombinants emerged early in infection and represented more than 20% of the entire proviral population within 2 weeks (1392). The results support the possibility that recombination could play an important part in the evolution of drug-resistant strains and new envelope serotypes (322a). Moreover, a recent experiment involving the inoculation of two poorly replicating mutant SIV strains into a monkey, competent recombinant virus was recovered within 2 weeks (623a). This finding emphasizes the potential for the appearance of new strains, particularly if the CD4 molecule is not down-modulated from the cell surface and superinfection takes place (see Chapter 4).

Recombination between HIV strains appears to occur most often within the *gag* and *env* regions (528, 1231, 2250, 2982), but other sites could also be involved. Recent studies have shown recombination between clade B and C viruses in the *tat* region (2459a). Obviously, the viral recombination event will be recognized only when regions having breakpoints that do not interrupt gene expression are involved. Recombination could occur if a cell is infected simultaneously by more than one virus or if the cell is superinfected before the CD4 molecule is down-modulated and resistance is established. This phenomenon could take place early in the infection process (the first 24 to 72 h), with a latently infected cell (2149, 2813), or with cells infected by viruses that do not reduce CD4 protein expression on the cell surface (1464). The extent of recombination between strains is not known, although some investigators believe the frequency in nature may be very high (2250).

Chapter 3	SALIENT FEATURES

1. The CD4 molecule is a major cellular receptor site for HIV infection. The viral regions binding to CD4 include the fourth conserved portion near the carboxyl-terminal end of the viral gp120, as well as other regions involved in the conformational structure of the envelope. The binding region on the CD4 molecule is located on a protuberant ridge along one face of the D1 domain. The binding site on CD4 appears to overlap with the class II MHC binding site.

2. Following binding to the CD4 molecule, attachment to other cellular receptors is needed for HIV infection. These coreceptors are generally the chemokine receptors, CCR-5 (for macrophage-tropic viruses) and CXCR-4 (for T-cell-line-tropic viruses). The expression of these and other coreceptors can differ on CD4$^+$ cells.

3. Primary virus isolates, particularly those that are macrophage tropic, appear to be resistant to inactivation by sCD4. This resistance reflects the conformational structure of the envelope, particularly within the V3 region. Shedding of gp120, lack of envelope cleavage, and perhaps the avidity of the macrophage-tropic strain for cell surface CD4 receptors rather than sCD4 could determine this process.

4. Binding of HIV to a cell may involve displacement of gp120, either completely or partially. Subsequently, cleavage of gp120 may take place (with T-cell-line-tropic viruses), probably by a cellular protease. These two steps could permit the interaction of the fusion domain of HIV (in gp41) with a fusion domain on the cell surface.

5. Virus:cell fusion may take place as a separate step involving gp41 and a fusion domain on the cell.

6. Entry of the viral core into a cell is pH independent. This process may also represent a separate step involving different viral and cellular proteins.

7. Viruses can down-modulate CD4 expression through the function of Vpu, Nef, and the envelope proteins.

8. Galactosyl ceramide (GalC) can serve as a receptor for infection of cells in the bowel, brain, and vagina.

9. Cell-to-cell transfer of HIV appears to be a more rapid mechanism for infection of a cell than direct infection by free virus.

10. After the virus interacts with antibodies, Fc and complement receptors can serve as alternative mechanisms for HIV entry into a cell. Enhancement of virus infection can take place.

11. Phenotypic mixing with pseudotype virion formation could lead to further transfer of the HIV genome inside the envelope of a variety of other RNA and DNA viruses.

12. A recombinant virus can form between viral strains that coinfect a cell. The extent of this process in nature is not known.

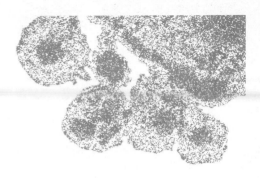

Acute HIV Infection and Cells Susceptible to HIV Infection

THE PRECEDING CHAPTERS DEALT WITH THE IDENTIFICATION OF HIV, the mechanisms involved in its transmission, and the early steps characterizing the interaction of HIV with its target cells. This chapter covers the events surrounding acute HIV infection of the host following transmission and discusses the large variety of cells in the body that are susceptible to HIV infection. The first cellular targets in HIV infection have not been well defined. In one study, the earliest infected cells detected within 24 h after intravaginal inoculation of SIV were dendritic cells in the stratified squamous mucosa or in the endocervical epithelium (2554). When presented at the mucosa, virus can be transmitted by direct infection of mucosal cells (see Chapter 2), transfer via M cells (57), or transcytosis. Transcytosis is a process by which proteins are transferred rapidly from the apical to the basolateral layer of an epithelial cell (246).

I. Acute HIV Infection

A. Clinical Manifestations

Clinical manifestations of initial HIV entry into the body might be expected, since they commonly accompany acute infections

by other viruses. Very early in the studies of AIDS, clinical features of acute HIV infection were described in a number of articles, particularly by Cooper and coworkers (514, 2677, 2679; for a review, see reference 1937) (Table 4.1). A newly infected
individual can present within 1 to 4 weeks with a virus-like illness. Symptoms consist of headache, retro-orbital pain, muscle aches, sore throat, low-grade or high-
grade fever, swollen lymph nodes, and a nonpruritic macular erythematous rash involving the trunk and, later, the extremities (Table 4.1; Color Plate 5, following p.
188) (514, 1739). In some cases, oral candidiasis and ulcerations in the esophagus
or anal canal occur (513a, 2168), and central nervous system (CNS) disorders (e.g.,
encephalitis) can be seen in patients (362, 1084). In other acutely infected individuals, pneumonitis as well as diarrhea and other gastrointestinal complaints have
been reported (653, 2679). These symptoms usually last from 1 to 3 weeks, although
lymphadenopathy, lethargy, and malaise can persist for many months. In general,
primary HIV-1 infection is followed by an asymptomatic period of many months to
years. The presence of the previous virus-like illness can then be elicited only by taking a complete history.

At least 50% and in some series up to 90% of individuals infected by HIV will report a history of this acute mononucleosis-like illness (784, 2382, 2677, 2679). The
rash is a valuable diagnostic sign since it can distinguish primary HIV infection from
other types of infections, but it can be difficult to diagnose. The cause of the rash is unknown, but it could be due to antigen-antibody complexes in the skin (1739). Usually
the clinical findings appear before seroconversion (513a). Some studies suggest that
the occurrence and persistence of symptoms (particularly fever) during primary HIV
infection are associated with a faster disease progression (653, 1260, 2058, 2515, 2770).
Fever and other symptoms observed during acute infection may reflect a hyperresponding immune system with production of cytokines which give rise to the clinical

Table 4.1   Characteristics of primary HIV infection

Clinical[a]
1. Headache, retro-orbital pain, muscle aches, sore throat, low-grade or high-grade fever,
   swollen lymph nodes
2. Nonpruritic macular erythematous rash
3. Oral candidiasis and ulcerations of the esophagus or anal canal
4. Acute CNS disorders (e.g., encephalitis)
5. Pneumonitis
6. Diarrhea and other gastrointestinal complaints

Course
1. Symptoms last from 1 to 3 weeks
2. Lymphadenopathy, lethargy, and malaise can persist for many months
3. Symptoms are generally followed by an asymptomatic period of months to years

Laboratory findings
1. First week, lymphopenia and thrombocytopenia
2. Second week, lymphocyte number rises secondary to an increase in number of $CD8^+$
   cells; $CD4^+/CD8^+$ cell ratio decreases
3. Second week, atypical lymphocytes appear in the blood (generally <50%)
4. HIV antigenemia and viremia detected before seroconversion
5. Virus might be present in CSF and in seminal fluid
6. Anti-HIV antibodies first detected usually within 14 days
7. Alterations in T-cell repertoire presentation
8. Cytokine levels (e.g., IL-1β, TNF-α, and IFN-γ) in plasma can be increased

[a] Some or all of these findings may be present.

signs. The more rapid progression to disease in symptomatic people may then reflect this immune activation that could enhance HIV spread and increase apoptosis. In one report, symptomatic primary infection was found to be associated more frequently with sexual transmission than with intravenous drug use (2515), but when it occurs in an intravenous drug user, it also appears to be associated with a poor prognosis (653). These observations require further evaluation. The use of therapy during primary infection is reviewed in Chapter 14.

B.   Laboratory Findings

Laboratory studies conducted on infected individuals during the first week following HIV infection can show lymphopenia and thrombocytopenia (Table 4.1). In the second week, the number of lymphocytes increases, resulting primarily from a rise in the number of $CD8^+$ cells; the number of $CD4^+$ cells is reduced. Thus, during this period, the $CD4^+/CD8^+$ cell ratio becomes inverted. Moreover, atypical lymphocytes (i.e., $CD8^+$ cells) can appear in the blood (515, 1098), but usually at a smaller number in primary HIV infection than in Epstein-Barr virus (EBV), cytomegalovirus (CMV), or other infections that elicit this response (513a). Within months following primary infection, the quantity of $CD8^+$ cells returns to a baseline or slightly higher level. This amount remains greater than that of $CD4^+$ cells, which increases somewhat; therefore, the inverted $CD4^+/CD8^+$ cell ratio is maintained (2677).

In some studies, the expansion in the number of $CD8^+$ T cells has shown T-cell receptor Vβ gene patterns that might predict the eventual clinical course (991, 2034). A limited diversity of the T cells containing Vβ genes carries a poor prognosis (2033) (see also Chapter 11). The increased $CD8^+$ cells appear to have cytotoxic activity, suggesting a primary immune response to HIV (2033, 2034). In one study, antiviral cytotoxic T-lymphocyte (CTL) activity after seroconversion was noted only in those individuals who showed clinical symptoms of primary infection (1411). Importantly, the levels of viremia were reduced with both an oligoclonal and a polyclonal T-cell response, but the long-term follow-up suggested that the

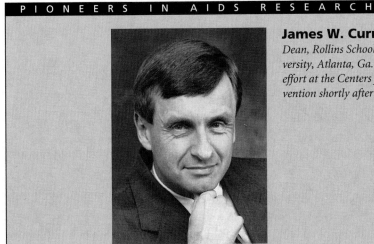

PIONEERS IN AIDS RESEARCH

James W. Curran
Dean, Rollins School of Public Health, Emory University, Atlanta, Ga. Dr. Curran directed the AIDS effort at the Centers for Disease Control and Prevention shortly after the recognition of AIDS.

polyclonal response predicted a better clinical course (2033). Thus, the pattern of immune response early in infection may be a more valuable surrogate marker of a long-term asymptomatic infection than the initial levels of viremia (932, 2033).

During the acute period of infection, levels of certain cytokines associated with immune activation, such as interleukin-1β (IL-1β), soluble CD30, tumor necrosis factor alpha (TNF-α), TNF receptors, and gamma interferon (IFN-γ), have also been found to be increased in the blood (2058, 2239, 2515). These findings could explain some of the symptoms described.

The levels of TH1 and TH2 cytokines detected during acute infection have indicated that peripheral blood mononuclear cells (PBMC) express very low levels of both IL-2 and IL-4, although substantial levels of IL-2 were noted in lymph node cells (937). Production of IL-10 and TNF-α was consistently observed in all subjects, and the levels either were stable or increased over time (937). Likewise, IFN-γ expression was found in all seroconverters, and the levels peaked early in primary infection along with the increase in CD8$^+$ cell numbers, probably induced by these cytokines (937). The results indicate that high levels of proinflammatory cytokines are expressed with primary infection. This response, depending on the cytokine profile, could influence the extent of CD8$^+$ cell expansion (see Chapters 9 and 11).

Finally, during acute infection, certain other laboratory markers, such as persistent low CD4$^+$ cell counts, high immunoglobulin levels, and high CD8$^+$ cell counts (function not specified), have been found to be associated with rapid progression to AIDS (2385) (see Chapter 13). These observations, which need further confirmation, could reflect a lack of early immunologic control of HIV.

C.   Characteristics of the Transmitted Virus

During acute HIV infection, the individual becomes antigenemic and viremic, with very high levels of viral DNA (10^5 to 10^7 virions/ml) present in plasma (Table 2.3). High levels of infectious virus can be detected in the peripheral blood (461, 557, 821, 2092, 2794) (see Chapter 2). How soon virus can be detected in the blood after acute infection has not been fully evaluated in adults. In one study of newborns, HIV RNA was found in the first 10 days of life in about 25% of the infected infants. After 3 months, all of them showed evidence of infection (613a). The early plasma virus is relatively homogeneous in sequence (1383, 2976), probably indicating replication of a dominant strain. In one detailed report, virus was detected in lymphoid tissue before seroconversion (747). Soon after seroconversion, a fairly rapid production of viral variants takes place, as determined by PCR analysis (2027). This heterogeneity of HIV (see Chapter 7) most probably reflects the emergence of virus variants in the face of a host immune response.

In acute infection, both non-syncytium-inducing (NSI) and syncytium-inducing (SI) strains can be isolated initially. In some cases at seroconversion, infection by different strains of HIV-1 has been documented (2985), but this would appear to be rare. During the early period when there is an absence of immune response, the transmitted virus replicates and spreads, with selection of isolates that have increased growth potential (507, 747). In several studies, but not all, the noncytopathic (often macrophage-tropic) strains were found predominantly in the acutely infected individual. This observation has led some researchers to conclude that in adults these NSI strains are the most transmissible (2983), perhaps via macrophages in the genital fluid. Moreover, macrophages or dendritic cells in the vagina, endo-

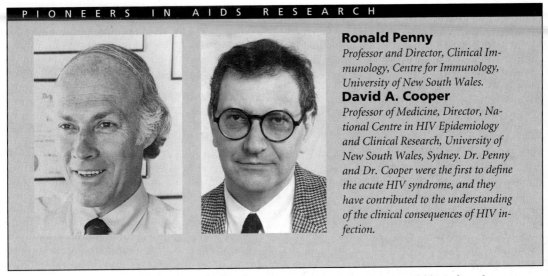

Ronald Penny
Professor and Director, Clinical Immunology, Centre for Immunology, University of New South Wales.
David A. Cooper
Professor of Medicine, Director, National Centre in HIV Epidemiology and Clinical Research, University of New South Wales, Sydney. Dr. Penny and Dr. Cooper were the first to define the acute HIV syndrome, and they have contributed to the understanding of the clinical consequences of HIV infection.

cervix (2554), uterus, bowel mucosa, or penile urethra could be infected most commonly by these strains (Section I.D) (see Chapter 2).

In other studies of transmission by sexual contact (homosexual and heterosexual), about one-third of the subjects had SI viruses after primary infection (755). Several other reports have shown that seroconverters can harbor SI viruses (461, 1931, 2274, 2377). In a review of viruses evaluated during acute infection by different transmission routes, about an equal number of NSI and SI viruses was found (919). In some cases, the initial growth of an SI virus was replaced at seroconversion by an NSI variant (530, 1437, 2140). These findings, together with the fact that most SI viruses can probably infect macrophages (755, 1505a), suggest that these T-cell-line-tropic viruses are not restricted in their ability to infect individuals through sexual contact. The data, viewed together, indicate that there is no apparent block to transmission of the SI virus variants during the sexual route or during transfer of virus from mother to child. Moreover, recent evidence indicates that dendritic cells can express mRNA for the chemokine recpeptors CCR-3 and CCR-5 as well as CXCR-4 (641a). The latter observation suggests that SI viruses could also gain entry into a host through infection of dendritic cells in the mucosal lining. However, intracellular factors could influence the extent of transcription of SI viruses (Chapter 5). Because of their efficient growth in macrophages and dendritic cells, NSI viruses probably have some advantage during transmission. Nevertheless, whether an NSI virus is found much more frequently in the infected individual at the time of seroconversion needs further study.

Quantitative heteroduplex tracking assays on transmission pairs have supported the existence of various genomic complexities during acute infection. In chronically infected transmitters, HIV variants were detected in genital secretions that differed from those in the blood; the sequences of cell-associated virus also differed from those of free virus in the plasma. These findings indicate the heterogeneity of viruses found in asymptomatic subjects as well as the compartmentalization of the virus in different body sites (2984). In contrast to the transmitters, the seroconverters showed relatively homogeneous virus populations, suggesting transmission of a limited number of variants. Furthermore, the virus present in the seroconverter represented only a minor species found in the semen of the transmitting partner. These results provide further evidence of selective transmission during sexual contact.

Virus has been isolated as well from the cerebrospinal fluid (CSF) (1084) and semen (2681) of individuals during the acute phase of HIV infection (Table 4.1). The finding of virus in semen indicates the risk of transmission of the virus through sexual contact during this period.

D.   Selective Transmission of HIV Isolates

As noted above, certain studies have emphasized that during HIV transmission, a selected variant in the large number of viral species present in blood or genital fluid gets transmitted. With homosexual transmission, some reports have suggested the predominance of a macrophage-tropic NSI isolate, based on studies of virus in recipients and in seminal fluids collected from the transmitting partner (2983). Nevertheless, other studies of acute infection (see below) suggest that both SI and NSI isolates can be found and that selection for one specific virus phenotype may not occur (919). In this regard, selective transmission has been studied by using chimeric simian/human immunodeficiency viruses (SHIV) that express the envelope gene from either a macrophage-tropic or T-cell-line-tropic virus. In one case, the dual-tropic $SHIV_{89.6}$ was transmitted by vaginal inoculation to rhesus macaques whereas a T-cell-line-tropic virus was not (1591). In another study, $SHIV_{33}$, a T-cell-line-tropic virus, was more easily transmitted by this route than was $SHIV_{162}$, a macrophage-tropic strain (1597a).

The concept of transfer of predominantly macrophage-tropic NSI strains comes from the idea that Langerhans cells in the vagina or dendritic cells in the rectum are most susceptible to NSI virus in genital fluids. Recent studies have reported that Langerhans cells found in the vaginal canal but not found in the bowel mucosa are more susceptible to some strains of HIV-1 (e.g., clade E) than to others (e.g., clade B) (2539). Thus, the high prevalence of clade E infection by heterosexual contact in Thailand (1386) could be explained. Countering these conclusions are the observations that clade B viruses, which may not grow as well in cultured Langerhans cells (2539), are responsible for high-level heterosexual transmission in parts of Latin America, particularly Brazil, as well as in the United States (1660) (see Chapter 2). Importantly, recent studies have demonstrated that selective infection of Langerhans cells or dendritic cells (DC) does not appear to be associated with certain clades (641a, 2120a).

Mother-child transmission also appears to reflect the selection of a particular viral species, since genetic analysis of virus in the newborn and in the mother often show a variant that is representative of a very low level of virus in the mother's blood (see Chapter 2, Section VI.D). Biologic studies suggest that this variant is resistant to maternal neutralizing antibodies or enhanced by these antibodies (1322). Moreover, as seen by PCR analysis, a dominant single maternal variant is transferred in some cases (1319a, 2910). In other cases, the heterogeneous sequences in the virus recovered from the child suggest multiple viral infections or transmission events (280).

If there is no selection at transmission, the recipient, whether a sexual partner or a child, may encounter a variety of viruses, one of which infects most efficiently and dominates in that individual. In this situation, isolation and culture techniques might detect not the first virus that enters, or a variety that enter at the same time, but the one virus that is able to spread and establish infection in the host. Infection could then be by chance, with both SI and NSI viruses being transmitted (33, 919) but one dominating, depending on certain conditions in the host.

Two noteworthy cases of accidental transmission of HIV provide some insights. In these cases, nonmucosal transmissions were involved. The result of an intravenous inoculation of a small quantity of blood containing predominantly SI virus was compared with the effects of an intramuscular inoculation of a large quantity of blood containing predominantly NSI virus. Inoculation of the blood containing predominantly SI virus gave rise to persistent SI virus replication and rapid loss of CD4$^+$ T cells. The receipt of predominantly NSI virus resulted initially in a selective amplification of SI viruses before seroconversion. Then, at seroconversion, NSI viruses emerged and CD4$^+$ T-cell numbers decreased. Thus, despite the control of the SI viruses, immune deficiency still developed (530). Similar findings on the pathogenicity of NSI viruses have been reported (see Chapter 7). The replacement of an SI virus with a predominant NSI virus has also been observed by others (1437, 2140) and in one case was associated with the presence of host neutralizing antibodies against the SI but not the NSI virus (1437). Although the phenomenon of phenotypic switching during primary isolation appears to be rare (755), it does reflect how the host can modify this virus infection.

E.   Initial Host Responses during Acute Infection

As noted in Chapter 2, within weeks after primary infection, the viremia usually is markedly reduced (Figure 4.1). This phenomenon probably results from an active antiviral cellular immune response in the host (see Chapter 11). Studies of human and animal lentiviruses have shown that efficient control of virus replication soon after primary infection is the best predictor of a long-term asymptomatic course (1260, 1751, 2078, 2208) (see Chapter 13). In certain studies of proliferative responses, HIV peptide-specific T-helper cells have been detected shortly after acute infection, before seroconversion takes place (483). We have documented CD8$^+$ cell anti-HIV noncytotoxic activity associated with a decrease in viremia in infected in-

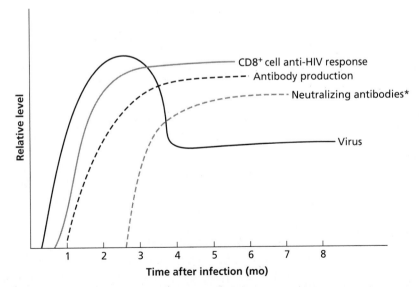

Figure 4.1   Estimated time course for host immune response to acute HIV infection. *, neutralizing antibodies are often directed at the virus that was present earlier, not the virus present in the blood at that time in the individual.

dividuals before seroconversion (1637) (see Chapter 11) (Figure 4.1). Moreover, cytotoxic CD8$^+$ lymphocytes have been detected during acute HIV (253, 747, 1357) and SIV (2934) infection, but usually after seroconversion. Thus, cellular immunity must be a primary mechanism for control of HIV replication soon after infection (Section I.B). Importantly, in one case, CD8$^+$ cell activation and the CTL response were not detected in lymphoid tissue at the time of infection, when a high viral load was present (747). The finding probably reflects the absence of a prompt CD8$^+$ cell response to the infection. Moreover, recent observations suggest that HIV-1 variants that escape CTL activity may be selected during acute infection (2143) (see also Chapter 11).

F.   Production of Antiviral Antibodies

In most cases, the acute viral syndrome occurs before seroconversion (513a), suggesting that the symptoms come from a dominant cell-mediated immune response (Section I.B). Antibodies to HIV generally appear in 2 to 4 weeks, but seroconversion can sometimes occur within days after infection (2679, 2682) (Figure 4.1). In studies performed by Cooper and others, antiviral antibodies were first detected in some subjects as early as 6 days after infection by measuring the IgM response (514). Others have also used IgM measurements to detect infection (822). IgM antibodies have been best detected by an antigen-conjugate enzyme-linked immunosorbent assay (ELISA) rather than the conventional antibody-conjugate assay (828). IgG levels can be demonstrated by ELISA, indirect immunofluorescence, or immunoblot assays (for a review, see reference 142). Present ELISAs can detect antibodies within 2 to 4 weeks in most infected people. Generally, neutralizing antibodies appear several weeks after anti-HIV antibodies are detected (Figure 4.1) (1357, 1637), but in one well-documented case, they were present within 20 days after virus transmission (1437). During acute infection, neutralizing antibodies may be responsible for the emergence of NSI viruses following the initial SI replication (530, 1437). In a recent extensive study, neutralizing antibodies against autologous strains were not noted following initial seroconversion. When identified, the neutralization response was usually evident against viruses present during an earlier phase of HIV infection (1825) (see Chapter 10).

Whether an infected individual can be antibody negative for longer than 3 months is still controversial. Before the development of the current ELISA kits, the "window" period before seroconversion had been estimated to have a median of about 2 months, with more than 90% of infected individuals developing antibodies within 6 months (1107). In one recent case report of infection by needlestick injury, antibodies did not appear until after 8 months (1771). This long delay is rare and could reflect the delivery of a low virus inoculum by the percutaneous route. In another unusual case, a patient developed AIDS without the presence of detectable antibody. The reason is not known (2208a). In nearly all cases presenting today, the period before seroconversion is short (2 to 4 weeks).

Finally, a strategy for estimating the time of infection of an individual has been derived by evaluating serum samples for antibodies using both a less sensitive ("detuned") and a sensitive ELISA procedure. The former involves an increased serum dilution and decreased incubation time. An antibody test negative by the detuned assay but positive by the more sensitive ELISA procedure would indicate that an infection had occurred within the past 100 days (1186a).

II. Cells and Tissues Infected by HIV

Having appreciated the clinical, virologic, and immunologic events that take place during acute HIV infection, it is important to recognize the cellular host range of this virus. In Chapter 3, the studies demonstrating the CD4$^+$ cells as a major target for HIV infection were reviewed. While initially considered a T-lymphotropic virus, HIV has since been shown to infect a wide variety of cells in different tissues of the body. The first cells to be infected may be present in the mucosa, in the blood, or in lymphoid tissue, depending on the route of transmission. After acute infection, the cellular host range of HIV can be extensive and is reviewed below.

A. Cellular Host Range

HIV has been found in several tissues, albeit at a very low level in some (Table 4.2), and can infect many different human cells in culture. These latter observations reflect the polytropic nature of this virus. HIV infection has been detected by recently improved techniques in cell culture, in situ hybridization, immunohistochemistry,

Table 4.2   Human cells susceptible to HIV[a]

Hematopoietic	Other
T lymphocytes	Myocardium
B lymphocytes	Renal tubular cells
Macrophages	Synovial membrane
NK cells	Hepatocytes
Megakaryocytes	Hepatic sinusoid endothelium
Eosinophils	Hepatic carcinoma cells
Dendritic cells	Kupffer cells
Promyelocytes	Dental pulp fibroblasts
Stem cells	Oral mucosal cells
Thymocytes	Pulmonary fibroblasts
Thymic epithelium	Fetal adrenal cells
Follicular dendritic cells	Adrenal carcinoma cells
Bone marrow endothelial cells	Mammary epithelial cells
Bone marrow stromal fibroblasts	Retina
Brain	Uterus-derived epithelial cells
Capillary endothelial cells	Cervix-derived epithelial cells
Astrocytes	Vagina-derived epithelial cells
Macrophages (microglia)	Cervix (epithelium?)
Oligodendrocytes	Prostate
Choroid plexus	Testes
Ganglia cells	Urethra
Neuroblastoma cells	Osteosarcoma cells
Glioma cell lines	Myocytes
Neurons (?)	Rhabdomyosarcoma cells
Bowel	Fetal chorionic villi
Columnar and goblet cells	Trophoblast cells
Enterochromaffin cells	
Colon carcinoma cells	
Skin	
Langerhans cells	
Fibroblasts	

[a] Susceptibility to HIV was determined by in vitro or in vivo studies. See text for details and references.

electron microscopy, and PCR with extracted tissues and individual cells (in situ PCR hybridization) (116, 117, 122, 695, 696, 1954, 1956, 2048). Cell culture studies have shown that a wide variety of human cells are susceptible to HIV, but the extent of infection varies and can depend on the particular virus strain used. In general, $CD4^+$ cells replicate HIV to the highest titers. The in vitro studies indicate that successful virus infection is determined both by the efficiency of viral entry into the cell and by post-entry processes influenced by the intracellular milieu (see Chapters 3 and 5). Clinically, direct infection of the brain, bowel, heart, lungs, kidney, joints, and perhaps other tissues could be responsible for some of the pathologic findings observed in HIV-infected individuals (see Chapter 9).

B. Hematopoietic Cells

1. CD4$^+$ LYMPHOCYTES AND MACROPHAGES

Studies conducted soon after the initial recovery of HIV demonstrated that $CD4^+$ T-helper (TH) lymphocytes were the major target of HIV infection (1310). These observations were soon confirmed by several investigators (see Chapter 3). Recent data suggest that subsets of $CD4^+$ cells may differ in their sensitivity to HIV-1 infection. TH1 cells were found to be less susceptible to productive infection than were TH0 and TH2 cells (468, 1644, 2797) (see Chapters 9 and 11 for a discussion of $CD4^+$ cell subsets, and see Table 11.1). Similarly, preferential infection of $CD4^+$ memory cells (2263, 2405, 2553, 2914) has been reported (see also Chapter 9). The relation of these findings to HIV pathogenesis is under study (see Chapter 13). Many other cells have shown susceptibility to the virus, particularly macrophages (853, 1083, 1512, 1521, 1924), the target cells for other lentiviruses (980). Often, in macrophage infection there is only low-level production of virus, and HIV is found sequestered in intracellular vacuoles (863). Nevertheless, some highly replicating cytopathic macrophage-tropic strains have been identified (177, 2842a).

Macrophage-derived colony-stimulating factor produced by infected cells can increase the susceptibility of macrophages to HIV infection (864, 954). In both $CD4^+$ lymphocytes and macrophages, differences in sensitivity to virus replication, related to both the HIV isolates and the particular cellular target, can be observed (see Chapter 2).

2. DENDRITIC CELLS

Dendritic cells (DC) share a stem cell precursor origin with macrophages. DC are widely distributed in the body (except in the brain) and are called Langerhans cells in the skin, digitary cells in the lymph nodes, DC in the thymus, interstitial DC in the heart, lungs, and intestine, and blood-derived DC in peripheral circulation (Figure 4.2). Their presence in genital mucosa (1145) identifies them as potentially the

Figure 4.2. Dendritic cells uninfected and infected with HIV-1. (A) Purified DC were obtained from PBMC cultured for 6 days in GM-CSF and TNF-α. Magnification, ×9,000. (B) $CD4^+$ cord blood cells were cultured with GM-CSF, TNF-α, and stem cell factor. After 7 days, the derived cells were infected with HIV-1$_{BAL}$, washed, and cultured for a further 8 days. A mature DC with a very indented nucleus and HIV on the surface (arrowhead) is shown. Magnification, ×4,500. (C) Further magnification of the dendritic cell in panel B, showing HIV-1$_{BAL}$ particles on the cell surface. Magnification, ×60,000. All panels provided by N.R. English and S. Knight.

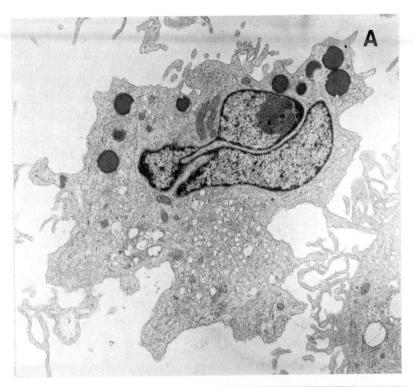

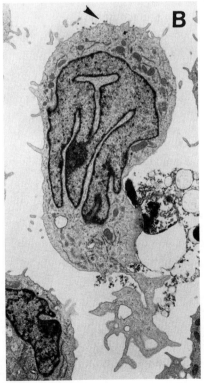

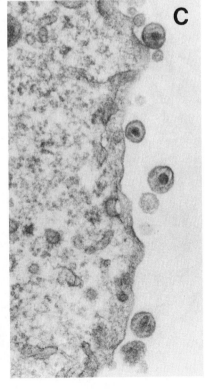

first cell infected by HIV. DC generally take up antigen and then express it—a process foreign to most other immune cells. DC appear to be the major cells for stimulating resting T cells efficiently. They have the unique property of aggregating naive resting T cells as well as memory cells nonspecifically and stimulating primary T-cell responses (1327). In contrast, macrophages and other tissue cells bearing major histocompatibility complex (MHC) molecules cluster only memory cells. The whole balance of the immune system may be regulated by signals provided initially by DC to both T cells and B cells, perhaps in lymphoid tissue through collaboration via signaling with follicular dendritic cells (FDC) (1327). The DC, derived from peripheral blood monocytes by using cytokines (1971, 2630), vary in their phenotype and function, and thus their exact relationship to other DC is not yet clear (for a review, see reference 1326).

Certain of these related cells appear to be susceptible to HIV infection (for reviews, see references 342 and 1326). DC derived from CD34$^+$ progenitor cells in the bone marrow and blood have been shown to produce high levels of the virus after infection in vitro (1425). Other cell culture studies have demonstrated infection of both monocyte-derived DC and DC obtained directly from blood (2049, 2724). Most evidence suggests that DC are productively infected only as they mature (1326, 2851). Infection of the cells appears to depend on CD4, although CD4-independent infection has also been described (411). Nevertheless, some studies suggest that DC are not infected but that they transfer bound virus particles to T lymphocytes in the blood and lymphoid tissue (343). Both processes are most probably involved.

Apparently, only one subpopulation of DC in the peripheral blood is susceptible to HIV infection in vitro (2850). Thus, the controversy over the infectability of these cells may be related to the particular cell subtype examined. In addition, several studies have demonstrated that macrophage-tropic viruses preferentially infect DC (1326, 2539). However, recent observations with DC and monocytes derived from the same population of CD34$^+$ progenitor cells suggest that T-cell-line-tropic viruses replicate best in DC (2824). These observations require further investigation but could explain how SI viruses can also be transmitted during sexual intercourse (see Chapter 3). While perhaps only small numbers of DC in various tissues of the body show infection, reports of infected cells in lymph node, blood, and myocardium (2260; for a review, see reference 1326) suggest that these cells can be infected in vivo, as demonstrated for some of these cell types in vitro.

3. B CELLS AND CD8$^+$ CELLS

B cells and B-cell lines can be infected with HIV in cell culture but appear most susceptible if EBV is also present (561, 1051, 1810, 1813). CD8$^+$ cells can be infected in vitro, after previous infection with HTLV-1 (2811a), and perhaps through the initial expression of CD4 on dual-positive precursor T cells (2722). CD8$^+$ cell infection has also been reported during contact with infected CD4$^+$ cells in culture (593), possibly reflecting contamination with free virus. Some researchers have suggested that infected CD8$^+$ T lymphocytes can be detected in seropositive individuals (1571, 2447). In most cases, as noted above, the infection appears to be due to the presence of the CD4 molecule on the cell surface (i.e., CD4$^+$ CD8$^+$ precursor cells) (2447), as has been observed with SIV infection of CD8$^+$ cells (606). In other studies, a possible contamination of the cells with free virus should be considered, since only late-stage AIDS patients with high virus loads had evidence of HIV infection of CD8$^+$ cells (1571). By PCR assay, we have not detected HIV infection of CD8$^+$ cells recovered in vivo (2022a).

4. BONE MARROW

Stromal fibroblasts (2374) and, recently, endothelial cells from the stroma of the bone marrow (1854) have also been shown to be infected by HIV. The endothelial cell could be an important reservoir of the virus, and HIV infection might influence the level of hematopoiesis in the bone marrow through disturbances in cytokine production (see Chapter 9). In this regard, after HIV infection the BS-1 human stromal cell line did not support the proliferation and differentiation of cultured hematopoietic cells (2589). Some CD34$^+$ bone marrow cells have been found to be infected in certain seropositive individuals (2573) and at times have been susceptible to HIV-1 infection in vitro (i.e., when they express CD4) (413). Nevertheless, conclusive evidence for a major infection of CD34$^+$ stem cells is lacking (576, 591, 1663).

5. SUMMARY

The hematopoietic cells now known to be infectable, at least in cell culture, range from CD34$^+$ stem cells to monocytes, macrophages, B lymphocytes, megakaryocytes, natural killer (NK) cells, eosinophils, thymic epithelial cells, thymocytes, and DC (Table 4.2) (372, 410, 796, 1038, 1391, 1952, 2049, 2330, 2435, 3001). Nevertheless, infection of B cells, CD8$^+$ cells, NK cells, and DC in vivo has not been consistently demonstrated (576, 591, 1806, 2199, 2200, 2792). Moreover, infection of NK cells in vitro is nonproductive (2435) and thus, if infection occurs in vivo, it may not be clinically relevant. Furthermore, the loss of CD34$^+$ hematopoietic progenitor cells has been linked to apoptosis and not to direct infection (2200).

There is still controversy about whether DC are directly infected by the virus or play a role in pathogenesis by carrying adherent virus in vivo to activated CD4$^+$ lymphocytes (342, 343, 2851). Certain studies suggest that mature DC in the blood circulate in association with T cells (1326, 2851). Definitive data on the role of DC in replicating HIV and contributing to pathogenesis await further investigation.

Thus, within the hematopoietic system, CD4$^+$ lymphocytes are the most visibly infected cell type, since they can replicate high levels of virus. Macrophages are infectable, but these HIV-infected cells are not found frequently in the blood or in the lymph nodes, where CD4$^+$ lymphocytes are the predominant cell type infected (122, 696, 2048). Alveolar macrophages also do not appear to be a major source of HIV-1 (1842). Nevertheless, infection of macrophages may go undetected because of low virus production (see Chapter 7). Moreover, these cells may be the first ones infected because they exist in an activated state in lymphoid tissues (see Chapter 13). In the spleen, large numbers of infected macrophages can be detected (981); this organ could be the primary source of tissue macrophages replicating HIV.

C.   Lymphoid Tissue

Virus infection of the lymph node has recently received special attention. The presence of HIV in this tissue was initially described in a series of papers by Racz and associates (2176, 2652). Several subsequent studies showed HIV DNA in lymphoid tissues (783, 2035, 2477). Most virus infection in these tissues is in CD4$^+$ (OPD$^+$) lymphocytes (696). Histologic and electron microscopic examinations have indicated that in the early periods of HIV infection, viral particles can be visualized in the villous processes of FDC, in close contact with lymphocytes (for reviews, see references 2037 and 2038) (see Chapter 9). Some groups have not detected productive HIV infection of the FDC (695, 2037, 2210, 2398, 2726), while other investigators have reported that an average of 20% of these CD21$^+$ cells show HIV DNA (2550). Moreover, some investigators have reported in vitro infection of FDC, probably by a CD4-independent mechanism (2565). Most evidence indicates, however, that these cells, of mesenchymal origin (not from bone marrow), are not directly infected (1326). Lymphoid interdigitary DC can be infected, but probably at a low level compared to other cells in these tissues (1727). Most of the viruses found on FDC are associated with antibody complexes. Certain studies suggest that this antibody:virus interaction is infectious even when neutralizing antibodies are involved. These antibodies do not affect the transfer of virus to CD4$^+$ cells (1043, 2550).

The findings with lymphoid tissues led one group to conclude that HIV is trapped in the lymph node through the FDC network (perhaps complexed with antibody) and therefore that the virus load as reflected in the peripheral blood appears to be reduced in the early stages of disease (for reviews, see references 738 and 2037). By quantitative image analysis and in situ hybridization techniques, it was estimated that the amount of viral RNA in the FDC was 100- to 10,000-fold greater than that in the blood (981). FDC were the largest source of virus in lymphoid tissue, since many of the infected lymphoid cells were not producing virus (981). At first, the virus associated with FDC did not appear to be affected by antiviral therapy (981). However, recent studies with potent triple anti-HIV drug combinations have shown in 6 months a several-log decrease in levels of FDC-associated virus (379) (see Chapter 14). With advancement to disease, the lymph node atrophies, and virus and infected CD4$^+$ cells are released into the peripheral blood. The events responsible for this depletion of cells in the lymphoid tissues and for the destruction of FDC are not well defined (see Chapter 13).

PCR and in situ PCR techniques have confirmed the widespread presence of HIV infection in lymphoid tissue even in healthy individuals. It was estimated that in some asymptomatic individuals HIV infection was up to 100 times more prevalent in lymph nodes than in peripheral blood (226, 1954, 2036, 2038). Similar observations have been made in healthy HIV-1-infected chimpanzees (2334). The important finding is that the high viral infection in lymph nodes (estimated to be 25% of white cells, or 200 billion CD4$^+$ cells in some cases) represents mostly latent infection (Color Plate 6, following p. 188) (695, 696, 981, 1954, 2284b). In asymptomatic individuals, for example, only 1:100 to 1:1,000 infected CD4$^+$ lymphoid cells appear to actively produce HIV-1 (695, 696, 2284b). The actual number of virus-infected cells in lymphoid tissue has recently been reestimated (450) but remains to be defined further (see below). In one study, the number of CD4$^+$ T cells carrying replication-competent HIV-1 was approximately 40 times higher in tonsillar tissue than in peripheral blood (2284b). The finding of HIV latency in vivo has also been made in peripheral blood cells (120, 695, 2048, 2508). The mechanisms involved are considered in Chapter 5.

It is noteworthy that recent quantification of HIV reservoirs in lymphoid tissue has indicated a much smaller number of cells that could potentially release infectious virus (450) than previously estimated (696). In these recent studies of lymph nodes, about 0.5% of the resting $CD4^+$ cells contained HIV DNA, but only 1/10 of these cells carried integrated provirus. Thus, many of these cells seemed to have an abortive infection characterized by a full-length linear unintegrated DNA (313, 2642, 2954). Moreover, only 10% of these latter cells were capable of releasing HIV virions. Thus, in a total of 10^9 $CD4^+$ "resting" lymphocytes containing HIV, 10^7 of these had latent provirus and 10^6 had the potential to produce infectious virus. When activated cells were included, a two- to threefold greater number of infected cells could be detected (450). These studies suggested that a large number of infected cells (up to 10-fold) in the lymph node contain a defective provirus that is unable to produce infectious virions. Furthermore, the frequency of resting $CD4^+$ cells with unintegrated DNA was not different in blood and lymph nodes, suggesting that blood is an accurate mirror of lymphoid tissue.

When the number of infected macrophages in lymphoid tissue was determined in these studies, integrated DNA was found at a very low number (1 per 20,000 cells) (450). Thus, a great deal of the viral DNA detected by standard PCR represents unintegrated virus, perhaps in an arrested state that cannot be replicated. As noted above, these observations counter the quantitative studies on viral load in lymphoid tissue reported earlier (696), but the quantity of infected cells in lymph nodes may be much greater than these most recent findings suggest (979a). The issue remains to be resolved. In any case, the number of cells in the lymphoid compartment that can carry infectious virus still presents a major challenge to antiviral therapies (Chapter 14).

HIV infection of the thymus is another important area of study. All thymic cell subsets, immature and mature, are targets for HIV infection by a CD4-dependent mechanism (for a review, see reference 856). Both lymphocytes and epithelial cells in this organ have been found to be susceptible to HIV (1038, 1952, 2744), but the extent of infection of epithelial cells and DC in vivo requires further study. Most infected cells detected in tissues are of the early precursor type (979a, 2744). Cell death in the thymus occurs by direct cell killing by HIV and by the induction of apoptosis (856). The importance of the thymus in the immune response is discussed in Chapter 11.

D.   Brain

In the brain, resident macrophages and microglia have been the major cells showing the presence of virus (289, 1331, 1766, 1915, 2156, 2467, 2878; for reviews, see references 1777 and 2145). However, the hypothesis that microglia are targets for HIV has been challenged (see also Chapter 9). Peudenier and coworkers (2088) were unable to infect microglia from the fetal brain, and evidence suggests that microglia can be confused with peripheral blood macrophages infiltrating the brain. However, these two cell types can be distinguished by specific antigens (289, 2078, 2088). Reports of other infected brain-derived cell types, including astrocytes, oligodendrocytes, capillary endothelial cells, and perhaps neurons, have appeared in the literature (Table 4.2) (976, 1507, 1766, 1957, 2156, 2878). With the recent use of in situ PCR hybridization procedures, many infected astrocytes and some neurons were detected in patients with dementia (1957). Whether neurons can be infected is controversial. Infection of astrocytes, oligodendrocytes, and brain-derived endothelial cells has also been demonstrated in cell culture (39, 427, 1852) (see Chapter 9). The coexpression of TNF-α mRNA in some cells in the brain suggests a role of this cytokine in the pathology of the CNS (1957) (see Chapter 9). It is noteworthy that, in contrast to brain-derived endothelial cells, endothelial cells from umbilical or saphenous veins do not appear to be susceptible to HIV (1402, 1852). The consistency of these findings on infected cells in the brain and the prevalence of cells infected needs further evaluation.

E.   Gastrointestinal System

In the bowel, the presence of HIV in mucosal cells has been detected by cell culture, in situ hybridization, and PCR studies of all regions of the gastrointestinal tract (882, 1047, 1356, 1696, 1916) (Color Plate 7, following p. 188). The bowel cell types considered infectable include goblet and columnar epithelial cells and enterochromaffin cells (1047, 1516, 1916). The enterochromaffin cells are hormone-producing cells that regulate cell motility and digestion (2110). Macrophages and, presumably, CD4$^+$ lymphocytes in the lamina propria of intestinal tissues are also frequently infected by HIV (767, 782, 1356, 1916) (see also Chapter 9). Moreover, the virus can infect cultured bowel explants and transformed bowel carcinoma cell lines (13, 97, 141, 151, 730, 731, 767, 1870). The in vitro infection can cause impaired function in human colon epithelial cells (730). The in vivo findings on cells infected in the bowel require confirmation (20) and await reports from in situ PCR hybridization studies.

In the liver, infection of cultured CD4$^+$ endothelial cells from human liver sinusoids has been reported (2432, 2580). Other observations suggest that Kupffer cells and hepatocytes can be infected by HIV-1 in vivo (352, 1110, 1134, 2397) and in vitro (2397). Infection of hepatic cells can cause selective impairment in function (1401). The above results showing infection of liver parenchymal cells lacking CD4 expression are supported by the finding that CD4$^-$ cell lines derived from hepatocellular carcinomas are susceptible to HIV (355).

F.   Other Tissues

HIV has also been detected in the synovial membrane in the joints of AIDS patients (716, 1138). In the skin, fibroblasts and possibly Langerhans cells can be infected by the virus, as shown by in situ hybridization, immunohistochemistry, PCR analysis, and cell culture studies (456, 459, 1153, 1750, 2188, 2336, 2600, 2648, 2721, 2961). Evidence of widespread infection of Langerhans cells by HIV in vivo, however, is lacking. Some studies have not detected infection of these cells in the tissues examined (1225, 1236). Certainly, epidemiologic studies do not support the idea of infected skin as a means of HIV transmission (195, 799, 873, 2266). Fibroblasts in dental pulp removed from HIV-positive patients have also been found to contain virus (Table 2.6) (893). Many of the above-cited cell types lack CD4 expression and emphasize the use of other receptors by HIV for infection (see Chapter 3).

Finally, in vivo or in vitro infection of other cells and tissues from organs such as the kidney, heart, lung, muscle, eye, placenta, cervix, vagina, uterus, fallopian tube, prostate, testes, mammary epithelial cells, oral mucosal cells, and adrenal glands has been reported (Table 4.2) (133, 350, 396, 408, 459, 492, 554, 645, 814, 938, 948, 1112a, 1457, 1562, 1701, 1750, 1956, 2103, 2118, 2119, 2152, 2166, 2339, 2688) and could be clinically relevant (see Chapters 2 and 9). In patients with myopathy, HIV antigen and viral nucleic acid have been detected in muscle macrophages and myocytes (390, 2440). These findings suggest that the virus could be involved in the clinical disease. Infection of placenta and fetal tissues is discussed in Chapter 2.

In all these tissues studied, the cells infected could either lack or express the CD4 molecule (see Chapter 3). In several instances, confirmation of the infection is needed (132). Nevertheless, the studies of HIV infection of human cells consistently indicate that this agent is polytropic and not solely T lymphotropic.

III.   # Number of CD4$^+$ Lymphocytes Infected by HIV

In the early period of research on the AIDS virus, in situ hybridization data suggested that only 1 in 10,000 or 1 in 100,000 peripheral leukocytes was infected by HIV (1015). The major target cell was the CD4$^+$ lymphocyte (see Chapter 3). These results raised questions about the viral pathogenic pathway, since the destruction of CD4$^+$ cells, which is characteristic of AIDS, could not be easily explained by direct viral infection.

Subsequently, using quantitative competitive PCR, the number of virus-infected CD4$^+$ cells in the blood was reported to be as frequent as 1 in 10 in some AIDS patients and up to 1 in 1,000 in some asymptomatic individuals (285, 1117, 2149, 2404, 2407). Most recently, in situ PCR hybridization findings have demonstrated infection of as many as 1 in 10 PBMC in symptomatic patients (117, 2048) (Table 2.1). This quantity greatly increases the target cell number considered infected by the virus and might explain the loss of CD4$^+$ cells in this infection (see Chapters 6 and 13). Nevertheless, the number of cells actively replicating the virus (as revealed by in situ hybridization studies measuring viral RNA) could be quite small—only 10% of all PBMC containing the HIV genome (2048, 2507). This observation most probably explains the long incubation period often observed in this infection. It would not support the idea of productive infection by HIV as a major cause of CD4$^+$ cell destruction (see Chapter 6).

Furthermore, as discussed in Section II.C, PCR studies have indicated potentially high levels of HIV predominantly in CD4$^+$ lymphocytes in the lymph nodes of infected individuals (696, 1954, 2036, 2284b). With about 500 billion to 1 trillion leukocytes in the body, some estimate that in asymptomatic infected individuals, 20 to 30% of these cells (mostly CD4$^+$ lymphocytes) could be infected by HIV (696, 979a, 1954, 2284b). Nevertheless, most of these cells are not producing virus when transcription of viral RNA is measured. Only 1 in 300 to 400 infected cells in the lymph nodes of asymptomatic individuals appeared to be releasing virus (Color

Plate 6, following p. 188) (696, 979a, 1954). These findings on viral latency in the lymphoid tissue resemble those noted above for peripheral blood lymphocytes (2048, 2507) and could reflect the antiviral activity of CD8$^+$ cells, both in the blood and in the lymphoid tissues (226) (see Chapter 11). Nevertheless, conclusions about relative levels of infected CD4$^+$ cells in lymph nodes and blood and the number of cells capable of releasing infectious virus still cannot be drawn. As noted above, a recent paper challenged the early estimates and concluded that a much smaller number of cells in lymphoid tissues is infected by HIV (450).

It is important to remember that the CD4$^+$ cell population includes macrophages, which are not readily killed by HIV (863). However, many studies suggest that, aside from the spleen, relatively few infected macrophages are found in the host (122, 2048). This issue needs further elucidation. Moreover, the relation of infected CD4$^+$ cells in the blood to the number of cells carrying HIV in the body (e.g., in lymphoid tissue) is not clear. As noted above, results from some groups suggest that virus in the blood may be a poor reflection of virus content in the host (738, 981, 2037), particularly during the asymptomatic period.

Since the PBMC represent only 1 to 3% of total lymphocytes (2865) in the body, the number of infected CD4$^+$ cells and the virus levels in blood could certainly be misleading. For 1 to 3 years, we have monitored individuals with very low CD4$^+$ cell numbers ($<$150 CD4$^+$ cells/ml) who remain relatively asymptomatic (1497). Several of these people can have good performance status and survive longer than 2 years (76). They could have many more functioning CD4$^+$ cells in their lymph nodes, as suggested in some studies with the HIV and SIV systems (2035, 2176, 2283, 2284), or they could have alternative means for maintaining immune function, such as through NK cell or DC function (2501). These individuals represent an interesting group for further investigation (see Chapter 13). In SIV studies, it was observed that when the number of CD4$^+$ cells in the lymph nodes decreased, simian AIDS quickly developed (2281). Nevertheless, in most cases thus far evaluated, PBMC appear to provide a reasonable indication of the viral state in the individual (i.e., productive versus relatively quiescent) and the extent of HIV infection (see Chapters 5, 11, and 13).

IV.   Interference and Superinfection

A.   Cellular Level

After the initial infection with most retroviruses, the cell becomes resistant to superinfection by a similar virus (Table 4.3). The mechanism for this interference appears to be the elimination or covering of the cell surface receptor needed for viral entry (2579, 2784). This process is observed in the HIV system, in which superinfection cannot occur if the CD4 molecule is down-modulated or blocked by antibody (435, 1023, 1289, 1464) (see Chapter 3). Yet the previously infected cells can replicate a different HIV-1 strain if its DNA molecular clone is transfected into the already infected cells (1464). The block to superinfection is primarily at the cell surface and not intracellular. In some studies, however, superinfection was shown to occur in certain chronically infected cells (e.g., HUT 78). In these examples, replication of the superinfecting virus was blocked at a point in reverse transcription (2626). A similar mechanism for resistance to superinfection has been observed in some infected human cells before CD4 is down-modulated (2787). Further experiments using PCR techniques should determine the universality of these findings. In this regard, the potential role of the complementarity-determining region 3 (CDR3) domain of the CD4 molecule in superinfection has been suggested. Infection of cells has been reported if CDR3 is still expressed after the initial infection when the major CD4 receptor epitope for HIV-1 (e.g., OKT4A) is absent (1975).

The lack of viral interference has been proposed as one cause for cytopathology by HIV strains. Before cells down-modulate CD4, continual infection of these cells by the progeny HIV can take place. This superinfection can lead to an accumulation of unintegrated viral DNA that is associated with cell death (see Chapter 6) (199, 2052, 2252, 2958). However, cells infected by the relatively noncytopathic HIV-2$_{UC1}$ strain continually express CD4, produce high titers of virus, and remain viable (145, 721, 1464). Whether these cells lack an accumulation of extrachromosomal viral DNA copies is not known.

These observations suggest that the relatively slow decrease or lack of elimination of the major viral receptor could lead to superinfection of cells by the same or related HIV strains. Superinfection appears to be possible in vivo, since CD4$^+$ cells infected with HIV but not producing the virus have been recovered from separated PBMC of infected individuals (2149, 2813). Conceivably, these represent nonactivated cells that carry virus for a short time (see Chapter 5) or have virus in a latent state. These cells might be superinfected before the initial virus infection is aborted. The resulting progeny virions might consist of phenotypically mixed particles and even recombinant viruses (see Chapter 3). Nevertheless, in limited studies of individuals dually infected with HIV-1 and HIV-2, one cell that produces both viruses has not been detected (722). Finally, some in vitro studies (190) suggest that noninfectious HIV-1 virions can block HIV replication. An interfering effect on virus spread appears to be involved and could play a role in preventing de novo infection in the host.

Table 4.3 Factors involved in resistance to virus superinfection

The cell
1. Loss of cell surface receptors (e.g., CD4) (1464)
2. Arrest in reverse transcription (2626, 2787)
3. Block by noninfectious HIV particles (190)

The host
1. Different sensitivity to virus strains
2. Differences in viral input levels
3. Down-modulation of virus receptors in sensitive cells (1464)
4. Neutralizing antibody or ADCC (2703)
5. Cell-mediated immune response (e.g., CD8$^+$ cell anti-HIV noncytotoxic response) (137, 1239)

B.   Within the Host

Superinfection is a term also used to denote infection of an individual by more than one HIV strain. Individuals infected with both HIV-1 and HIV-2 have been documented (722, 1480, 2195), but the time at which the infection occurred (i.e., simultaneously or sequentially) is an important question. In a concurrently transfused infant, two distinct HIV-1 strains as well as recombinants were identified (631). However, in a dually exposed adult, only one HIV-1 type was detected (631). The reason could be the relative viral load or differences in sensitivity of the host for infection by particular viral strains (see Chapters 2 and 3). Chimpanzees can be infected by more than one HIV-1 strain (373, 810), but these results reflect a limited spread of the initial virus in the animals and subsequent challenge with high doses of a second HIV strain and infected cells. Recently, resistance to challenge by heterologous virus strains in chimpanzees has been observed (2480). Moreover, recovery of two distinct viral strains from the same cell from a chimpanzee has not been reported. Finally, in some cases, infection of individuals by HIV-2 has been linked to resistance to subsequent HIV-1 infection (2701), but this finding is controversial (82). In one noteworthy report, superinfection of macaques with SIV reactivated the HIV-2 initially used to infect the animals (2087). Both HIV-2 and SIV were present, but the animals were protected from the pathogenic course. We have made a similar observation with baboons infected with different strains of HIV-2 (1577).

The prevalence of infection by more than one strain of HIV-1 in vivo is unknown but is most probably rare (85). Some molecular studies suggest that multiple infections are possible (1231, 2336, 2634, 2985), perhaps even with up to three different HIV-1 clades (2634). However, the time at which the event takes place and the clinical importance of a second or third strain are the key questions. One HIV-1 type usually dominates and must influence the pathogenic course; generally, in both early and late stages of infection of the same individual, the viruses studied by PCR procedures seem related to a dominant strain (1383, 1740). Even if the initial infection potentially involved several viral isolates (e.g., recipients of many Factor VIII units or multiple blood transfusions), a predominant HIV-1 strain seems to emerge and play an important role in pathogenesis. Other strains, if present, are presumably suppressed or eliminated by the dominant strain and/or the host immune response (1502) (see Chapter 11). At most, a different strain might remain as a minor component of the viral load, particularly in lymph nodes. The mechanism for emergence of a predominant strain has not been elucidated but could reflect less efficient recognition by the antiviral immune response or death of cells infected by some viral strains without sufficient spread of this virus type to additional cells.

Other evidence supporting the concept of a predominant strain in the infected host is that the number of incoming virus particles would be quite small compared to the amount of virus already present in the blood and lymph nodes of the individual (1502) (see Chapter 2). Thus, the chance of establishing an infection with another strain would seem unlikely. Moreover, to some extent, down-modulation of CD4 on the surface of infected cells would block the extent of superinfection (1464) (see above). In addition, an active immune system should be capable of eliminating or suppressing virus superinfection through neutralizing antibodies, by antibody-dependent cellular cytotoxicity (ADCC), and particularly by antiviral CD8$^+$ cells (see Chapter 11). As shown in cell culture studies with PBMC, antiviral antibodies produced in the host might prevent superinfection (2703). Importantly, CD8$^+$ cells can establish a state of resistance in the PBMC so that superinfection of the host is limited (137, 1239). In recent in vitro studies, HIV-1 and HIV-2 superinfection of PBMC from asymptomatic infected individuals was found to be blocked by CD8$^+$ cells at the level of virus transcription (137) (see Chapter 11).

Chapter 4   **SALIENT FEATURES**

1. Acute virus infection is characterized by a clinical state that involves a flu-like illness and often a macular-papular rash. This clinical syndrome occurs in 50 to 90% of infected people and generally predicts a more rapid clinical course.

2. During acute infection, CD4$^+$ cell numbers are reduced and CD8$^+$ cell numbers are increased. Subsequently, the CD4$^+$ cell number may return to a near-normal level but remain reduced in relation to the CD8$^+$ cell number.

3. High viral replication during the acute syndrome is subsequently reduced, most probably reflecting the activity of cell-mediated immune activities. A polyclonal CD8$^+$ cell response reflected by the T-cell repertoire is associated with a better prognostic course.

4. HIV is a polytropic virus and can infect many cells in the body. CD4$^+$ lymphocytes produce the highest levels of the virus.

5. Infected macrophages can remain as reservoirs of HIV, continually producing virus, although some cytopathic strains destroy these cells.

6. Dendritic cells in some tissues may be infected, but the extent of this infection in various tissues remains to be elucidated.

7. Cells (primarily differentiated macrophages) in lymphoid tissues may be the first site of virus replication. Virus is found associated with follicular dendritic cells (most probably not infected) and can be passed by these cells to activated CD4$^+$ cells present in lymphoid tissue.

8. In the brain, the major cells infected are the macrophages and microglia, but astrocytes, oligodendrocytes, and capillary endothelial cells can also be infected at various frequencies.

9. In the bowel, a variety of mucosal cells can be infected, but they may be detected at a low level in comparison to the infected CD4$^+$ lymphocytes and macrophages within the gastrointestinal tract.

10. The number of CD4$^+$ lymphocytes infected by HIV can vary from 1 in several million in asymptomatic and long-term survivors to 1 in 10 in symptomatic individuals. Most infected cells in the blood and lymph nodes are in a latent state that eventually can be activated to release virus.

11. A virus-infected cell is usually resistant to superinfection once the CD4 molecule is down-modulated. The establishment of this interference state may take 2 to 3 days.

12. In the host, resistance to superinfection appears to occur once the immune system has responded. Coinfection of individuals with two HIV-1 strains, or with HIV-1 and HIV-2, appears to be an uncommon event. The timing of these dual infections needs to be elucidated. The immune response, particularly by CD8$^+$ cells, most probably controls the inability to have more than one dominant strain within an infected host.

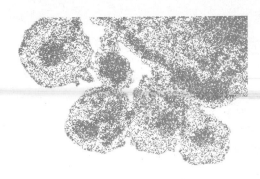

Intracellular Control of HIV Replication

THE DISCUSSION THUS FAR HAS FOCUSED ON EARLY EVENTS INVOLVED in HIV interaction with the cell. This interaction can be influenced by the specific virus involved (see Chapter 7), the cellular receptors expressed (see Chapter 3), and the nature of the cells infected (see Chapter 4). Once virus entry takes place, various functions of the virus determine its ability to replicate. The infectious cycle is influenced by intracellular proteins that may vary for different cell types. Thus, virus entry alone does not necessarily signify productive infection. In this chapter, the virus : cell interactions that take place within the intracellular compartment will be considered. Details on the molecular events involved can be obtained from recent reviews (2003, 2081).

I.   Early Intracellular Events in HIV Infection

Once the virus has entered the cell as a ribonucleocapsid, several intracellular events take place that lead to the integration of a proviral form into the cell chromosome (Figure 5.1). The HIV RNA, enclosed in the viral capsid, exits with the help of the capsid protein, p24, in association with cyclophilins (1596). This process is sensitive to cyclosporine A (2616, 2663). Still associated with

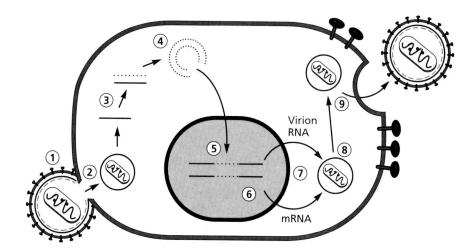

Figure 5.1   The HIV infection cycle. Steps: 1, attachment; 2, uncoating; 3, reverse transcription; 4, circularization; 5, integration; 6, transcription; 7, translation; 8, core particle assembly; 9, final assembly and budding. In steps 3 to 5, some viral core proteins are associated with the viral genome (——, RNA; ⋯⋯, DNA). Double-stranded circular forms can be found both covalently and noncovalently bound. The latter are the forms that integrate into the cell chromosome. Antiviral therapies can be directed against each step and can potentially interrupt virus replication and spread. Adapted from a figure provided by H. Kessler.

core proteins (primarily MA), the viral RNA undergoes reverse transcription by using its RNA-dependent DNA polymerase and RNase H activities and eventually forms a double-stranded DNA copy of its genome (cDNA) (for reviews, see references 2003 and 2081). For efficient transcription, the nucleocapsid protein p7 appears to act like a chaperone protein (744, 1595a). It increases the proportion of long cDNA transcripts produced by reverse transcription (645, 744) and plays a role later in the replicative cycle in efficient packaging of genomic RNA (184a, 1595a). This nucleocapsid protein contains two retroviral zinc fingers that are essential for its function (665). The cDNA is part of a preintegration complex containing the viral MA, Vpr, and integrase proteins (312, 1046). This complex is transported to the nucleus where, as a circular but noncovalently bound molecule, it integrates into the cell chromosome. Recent studies suggest that Tat may also be carried in with the virus particle and help in the internal transcription process (856a). This karyophilic transport depends on an interaction of MA and Vpr with a cellular karyopherin complex (829). The integration of the HIV provirus appears to be random and is essential for the cells to produce progeny virions. As noted above, the cellular protein cyclophilin A, found within the virion, is involved early in the replicative cycle of HIV-1. It binds to the Gag protein and apparently is important in steps occurring before reverse transcription. This function, however, does not seem to be required, since the Gag proteins of other retroviruses, including HIV-2, SIV, and HIV-1 clade O isolates, do not bind to cyclophilin A (788, 2663).

Whether infectious HIV can be produced without integration of the provirus into the cell chromosome is still not certain. This phenomenon has been described for the visna lentivirus (1021). In several studies, HIV integration was found to be necessary for efficient virus expression (703, 2331). In one study with SIV *int/nef* mutants, SIV replication was greatly reduced (2781), although some expression of viral antigen took place. Currently, integration is considered necessary for HIV protein expression and progeny production.

Recent findings on the early events in viral infection have revealed noteworthy features of HIV replication. With peripheral blood T lymphocytes arrested in cell division, virus infection is abortive, whereas in nondividing macrophages or epithelial cells, progeny virus production can take place (Section IV). In permissive activated T cells, HIV undergoes integration and replication within 24 h (1292). In macrophages, the process is similar, but progeny production may take 36 to 48 h (1876). The latter result could reflect the slower incorporation of nucleotide precursors in these nondividing cells (1968). However, under conditions of stimulation with macrophage colony-stimulating factor (M-CSF), replication in macrophages is more rapid and very efficient (1045).

Following virus integration, the earliest mRNA species made in the infected cell are doubly spliced transcripts encoding the major regulatory genes, particularly *tat*, *rev*, and *nef* (942, 1290, 2003). It appears that *nef* mRNA represents the majority (80%) of these species (2246), although it is not known which viral protein is made first. Because of its ability to transactivate promoters influencing transcription, it would appear that Tat is the one most likely to be made at basal levels in unactivated cells. It may function early since it could be carried in by the infecting virion (856a). The interactions of these regulatory genes have been discussed (for reviews, see references 2003 and 2081). Presumably, the predominance of one of these viral gene products determines whether HIV infection will lead to a productive or latent state. High-level expression of Tat will activate substantial virus production (582, 761). Nef has a pleiotropic role and in some cells may induce a latent state (1598) (Section V).

The Rev protein appears to provide a balance in the expression of regulatory and structural proteins of HIV. Rev encourages the production of large, unspliced

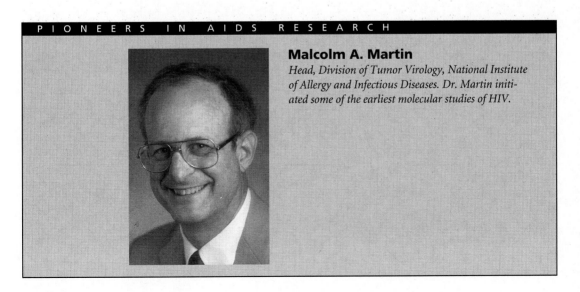

PIONEERS IN AIDS RESEARCH

Malcolm A. Martin

Head, Division of Tumor Virology, National Institute of Allergy and Infectious Diseases. Dr. Martin initiated some of the earliest molecular studies of HIV.

mRNA species responsible for the viral gene products that give rise to infectious viruses (739, 2530, 2531) (for review, see references 2003 and 2081). In the late stages of the virus replicative cycle (Figure 5.1), Rev could down-regulate its own production and cause decreased progeny virus formation and perhaps latency. In cells not fully permissive to HIV replication, the relative expression of the regulatory proteins can differ, leading to abortive infection, low persistence, or a latent state (111, 2120) (Section V).

Viral assembly takes place at the cell membrane, where viral RNA is incorporated into capsids that bud from the cell surface, taking up the viral envelope protein. Final maturation of the virion proteins, mediated by protease, takes place within the budding particle. Cyclophilins can play an important role in the assembly process through their association with the capsid protein (1595a).

II.   Differences in Virus Production: Role of Intracellular Factors

A.   Biologic Studies

How the state of T-cell activation and monocyte differentiation can influence the extent of viral expression has been briefly discussed. These observations emphasize the role of intracellular factors in the HIV replicative cycle. Although the HIV long

Figure 5.2 Variation in HIV replication in PBMC (PMC). The cells from 11 different donors of Asian (bars A to D), African-American (bars E, F, and G), and Caucasian (bars H to K) backgrounds were infected with three different strains of HIV-1 (panel A, SF2; panel B, SF247; panel C, SF170). Reproducible differences in level of replication and time of maximum virus release (number above bar) were observed. Modified from reference 720 with permission.

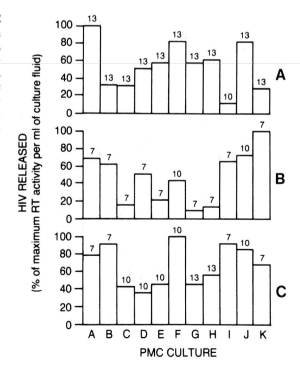

terminal repeat (LTR) alone can be its own promoter, early mRNA transcription appears to rely primarily on binding to the LTR by cellular transcription factors such as nuclear factor kappa B (NF-κB), NFAT, AP-1, SP-1, and the Tat binding proteins (for a review, see reference 2003). Thus, the intracellular milieu can determine the relative dominance of viral regulatory proteins in an infected cell (Section II.B).

Further evidence of this intracellular control is provided by biologic studies showing variations in replication of HIV strains in different cell lines and peripheral blood mononuclear cells (PBMC) from various donors (Figure 5.2) (371, 372, 486, 720, 1521, 2788). Variations in the infectability of macrophages from different sites in the body have also been reported (1977). Viral binding and entry can be similar, but the postentry events differ so that titers of the progeny viruses produced vary widely. The data with HIV infection of PBMC are most dramatic, and the various viral and intracellular factors responsible could influence virus spread and pathogenesis in the host (see Chapter 13) (1490).

These differences in intracellular replication of HIV can be studied after virus entry by transfecting molecular cDNA clones of HIV-1 into cells. The results again show variations depending on cell type. In general, human cells replicate HIV to the highest levels, compared with cells of other animal species, particularly the mouse (1506). Similar observations are made with phenotypically mixed particles that introduce the HIV genome into heterologous cells via a different viral envelope (345) (see Chapter 3). After undergoing reverse transcription from their own RNA genome, the respective viruses replicate to various degrees in cells. Intracellular control of virus replication has also been observed with other retroviruses (1505). These observations suggest either the presence of a cellular inhibitory factor or the relative lack of a cellular product needed for viral replication.

Some studies with human : animal cell hybrids have suggested the dominance of the permissive state for virus replication. Thus, the absence of a particular cellular protein appears to limit viral production. Human:hamster and human:mouse cell hybrids have implicated human chromosome 12 in coding for a permissivity factor that enhances Tat activity (51, 1024, 1922). Several candidate cellular proteins participating in Tat activity have been considered (51, 623, 1064, 1913, 2481). An 83-kDa transactivating response (TAR) RNA loop binding protein has been identified (1025).

Cellular proteins involved with Tat activity could increase Tat binding to the TAR region (51) or to promoters, such as AP-1, upstream from TAR (1064). Thus, two interactions of Tat with the viral LTR could be required to up-regulate HIV replication. Other experiments also suggest that two related cellular Tat binding proteins (TBP) might compete to up-regulate (e.g., MSSI) or down-regulate (e.g., TBP-1) Tat activity and thereby affect HIV production (1913, 2481). The mechanisms need further elucidation.

Some experiments have demonstrated that resistance of a cell to HIV infection can be dominant, and a factor in murine cells that acts against the *rev* gene has been described (2715). These inhibitors of Tat and Rev activities in murine cells act by independent mechanisms (2896) and could be considered in potential approaches to antiviral therapy.

B.   Molecular Studies

In T cells, activation is important for HIV replication and involves the interaction of intracellular factors with regions in the viral LTR (790, 1212, 1252, 1895) (for a review, see reference 2003). This activation is part of a signal transduction process by which the binding of mitogens or antigens within the major histocompatibility complex (MHC) molecules to the surface T-cell receptor (CD3), coupled with co-stimulation via the interaction of CD28 with B7 molecules, affects gene expression within the cell (for reviews, see references 1558 and 2211) (see below). LTA-3 inter-action with CD2 can also activate lymphocytes in a costimulatory manner (2044). The activation is mirrored by an increase in the concentration of intracellular free calcium and depends on the activation of calcium-dependent protein kinase C and other phosphorylation events (Figure 5.3) (1159, 1299, 2003, 2687, 2841).

During these steps in T-cell stimulation, transcriptional factors are activated. For example, NF-κB is normally associated with its inhibitor, IκB (for a review, see reference 140). However, phosphorylation of IκB by protein kinase C dissociates IκB from NF-κB and allows the translocation of NF-κB into the nucleus, where it binds the LTR sequence of the HIV provirus (1941). The interaction of these cellu-lar transcriptional factors with viral LTR regions can up-regulate viral replication (2003) or repress it (e.g., YYI) (1668). With some T-cell-line-tropic virus mutants, a loss in expression of NF-κB DNA binding proteins was shown to be associated with a reduction in HIV infection (2162). Nevertheless, one HIV-1 isolate and an SIV mutant lacking the LTR NF-κB site have been shown to replicate in PBMC (2974), and even to induce AIDS in monkeys (1156). Identification of all the cellu-lar factors involved is an ongoing endeavor (for a review, see reference 2003). Cer-tain cytokines and hormones, as well as transactivating proteins from other viruses, can also increase HIV production via these intracellular events (876, 1299, 1914) (Section III).

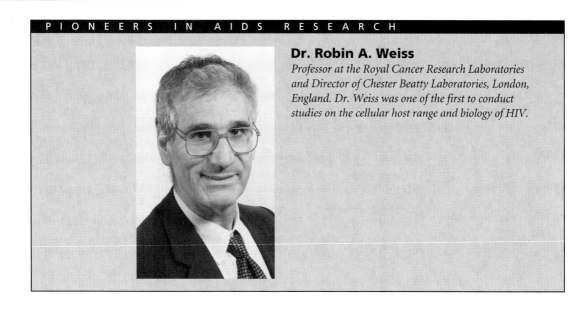

PIONEERS IN AIDS RESEARCH

Dr. Robin A. Weiss
Professor at the Royal Cancer Research Laboratories and Director of Chester Beatty Laboratories, London, England. Dr. Weiss was one of the first to conduct studies on the cellular host range and biology of HIV.

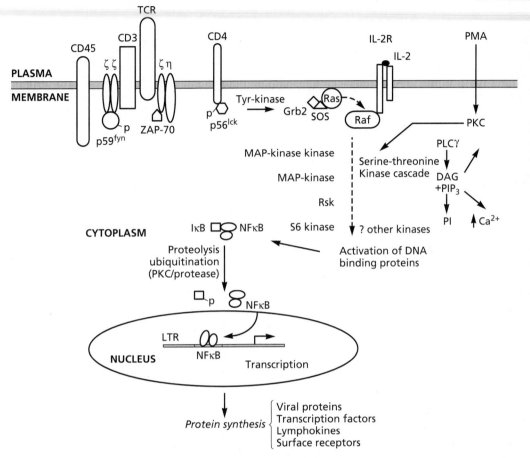

Figure 5.3   Schematic diagram of intracellular signaling events that occur during T-cell activation. The activation process begins with the generation of a signal at the plasma membrane (top) mediated by receptor:ligand interactions, e.g., IL-2 receptor (IL-2R)-and-IL-2 interaction, a receptor-linking T-cell receptor (TCR)-and-CD4 interaction, or passage of membrane-permeating molecules (e.g., phorbol myristate acetate [PMA]) across the membrane. In the case of the T-cell receptor, stimulation results in the activation of tyrosine kinases (top left), such as Fyn (p59^{fyn}), ZAP-70, and Lck (p56^{lck}). This action is probably regulated by tyrosine phosphatases such as CD45. The activated tyrosine kinases phosphorylate a number of different cytoplasmic substrates that initiate a chain of signaling events. These steps usually involve the association of intermediate signaling molecules. As an example, Ras (top middle) can be activated upon binding to Grb2 and SOS. This action results in the activation of cytoplasmic serine kinases such as Raf, which initates a cascade of serine-threonine kinases (e.g., mitogen-activated protein [MAP]-kinase kinase, MAP-kinase, Rsk, and S6 kinase), thereby propagating the activation signal. The serine-threonine kinase cascade results in the activation of DNA binding proteins and transcription factors which regulate gene expression. Phosphorylation and/or proteolysis of IκB in the cytoplasm (bottom left) dissociates it from NF-κB and permits the translocation of NF-κB across the nuclear membrane so that it can bind to DNA and activate transcription and protein synthesis. This signal transduction process can also be initiated by the stimulation of protein kinase C (PKC) by phorbol esters (e.g., PMA) (top right). Activated PKC stimulates phospholipase Cγ to generate the secondary messengers diacyl glycerol (DAG) and phosphoinositol trisphosphate (PIP$_3$), a process which results in the mobilization of intracellular calcium (Ca^{2+}) and liberation of phosphoinositol (PI). Figure and legend courtesy of E. Sawai.

Table 5.1   Level of arrest of virus replication in different cell types

Cell	Virus	Level of block	Possible mechanism	Reference(s)
Macrophages	T-cell-line tropic	Envelope processing	Intracellular factors	2593b
		Reverse transcription	Intracellular factors	1131, 1844, 2393, 2417
Monocytes[a]	Macrophage tropic	Entry	Cell surface receptor	2538
T-cell line	Macrophage tropic	Reverse transcription	Intracellular factors	1131

[a] Undifferentiated macrophages.

With HIV infection, displacement of the Src-family tyrosine kinase, p56^{lck}, from the CD4 molecule could be involved with subsequent activation of protein kinase C, thereby leading to increased virus production (Figure 5.3) (2003, 2687). Since p56^{lck} appears to have a variety of intracellular targets such as the interleukin-2 (IL-2) receptor (1032), it could either directly or indirectly affect the activity of cellular factors binding to the HIV LTR. In some reports, attachment of native gp120 to CD4 alone has activated the CD4$^+$ lymphocytes, as measured by an increase in intracellular levels of inositol triphosphate and calcium, as well as induction of expression of the IL-2 receptor (752, 1353). This observation, however, has not been confirmed by others, who have reported no effect of HIV binding on cellular or CD4 phosphorylation patterns, CD4-associated p56^{lck} kinase activity, or calcium influx (1990, 2799). Furthermore, the calcium channel inhibitor verapamil has shown no effect on HIV entry (1990). Thus, a role for calcium influx in the initial events in HIV infection of T cells is not established. Nevertheless, as discussed in Chapter 9, gp120 can induce calcium influx in certain neural cell lines by a mechanism blocked by verapamil; yet this process does not involve the CD4 protein (664). In brief, signaling via CD4 does not seem to be important in HIV production.

By molecular studies, a selective intracellular block in replication of certain HIV-1 strains can be demonstrated (Table 5.1). For example, by PCR techniques, non-macrophage-tropic strains have been shown to enter macrophages but to undergo only limited reverse transcription (1131, 1844, 2393, 2417). In monocytes, differentiation into macrophages rather than activation is most important for susceptibility to HIV infection (2538) (Section IV.B). Since the ability of HIV to replicate in macrophages has been linked to the envelope region (see Chapter 8), susceptibility could reflect a novel mechanism of envelope-associated signal transduction; a selective induction of cytokines required for completion of the replication cycle may be involved. Alternatively, the viral envelope might not be processed appropriately (2593b). A similar finding of an arrest in the reverse transcription process was reported with infection of a T-cell line by a macrophage-tropic HIV-1 strain (1131). The questions of whether this observation can be made with other viruses and cell lines and whether the viral envelope also plays a role in limiting this infection require further study.

Cytokines, particularly tumor necrosis factor alpha (TNF-α), and other external stimuli have been shown to affect HIV expression differently. Their influence depends on their effect on intracellular transactivating factors within the viral LTR, particularly NF-κB (see Chapter 11) (378, 671, 1007, 1299, 1368, 1994, 2115, 2572,

2746; for reviews, see references 1697, 2114, and 2284). For example, TNF-α can substantially increase HIV production (1697). Moreover, some viruses, such as cytomegalovirus (CMV) and herpes simplex virus, can enhance HIV production through activation of the viral LTR, a process that, in some cases, is mediated by a cytokine (1851, 2084) (Section III).

Finally, intracellular factors are involved with Tat function. This viral protein, after interacting with certain cellular factors, binds to the TAR element of the viral LTR in conjunction with cellular RNA binding proteins (1064, 1229, 2686, 2739, 2918) that may be phosphorylated (1000). Viral expression is subsequently up-regulated, probably following interactions of cellular proteins with other regions of the LTR (1064). The induction of TNF-α production in T cells by HIV Tat could also increase virus production (315, 2194). A role for cellular factors in augmenting subsequent Tat function is under consideration. The Nef protein could also affect virus replication by interacting with cellular factors that may be involved in cellular activation (156, 2368). All these observations reflect how both viral and cellular factors, working together, can affect HIV replication (see Chapter 8).

III. Effect of Other Viruses on HIV Replication

As noted above, some viruses, as shown in cell culture, have the capacity to enhance HIV production by induction of cytokines. Coinfection of cells with certain viruses, including herpesviruses, papovaviruses, hepatitis viruses, and retroviruses, can increase the expression and production of HIV-1 by another mechanism. Generally, these studies have demonstrated that transactivating factors produced by the infecting virus, usually early gene products, interact directly or via intracellular factors with the HIV LTR, usually in the NF-κB region. As examples, CMV, human herpesvirus 6 (HHV-6), and Epstein-Barr virus (EBV) have been shown to activate the HIV LTR, as measured in cell culture by the choramphenicol acetyltransferase

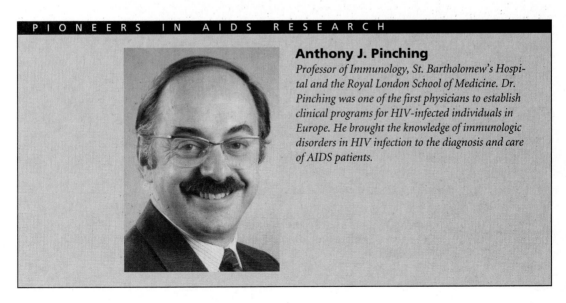

PIONEERS IN AIDS RESEARCH

Anthony J. Pinching
Professor of Immunology, St. Bartholomew's Hospital and the Royal London School of Medicine. Dr. Pinching was one of the first physicians to establish clinical programs for HIV-infected individuals in Europe. He brought the knowledge of immunologic disorders in HIV infection to the diagnosis and care of AIDS patients.

(CAT) assay (38, 580, 865, 884, 1108, 1238, 1266, 2182, 2496, 2779; for reviews, see references 1440 and 1914) (see Chapter 13). Some studies, however, indicate that the activation of HIV replication by DNA viruses can involve regions of the viral LTR that are independent of the normal cellular activation pathways (1896, 2003).

These molecular studies, showing effects on the HIV LTR by other viruses, have been supported by some observations in vitro with dually infected cells, in which HIV production is increased (370, 899, 1051, 1610, 2520). However, in other studies with coinfected cells, CMV, HHV-6, and EBV inhibited HIV replication (365, 1190, 1364, 1513). The differences observed probably reflect the various cell types (1190) or viral strains used.

Some biologic assays have demonstrated an increased production of HIV after coinfection with HTLV-1 or other animal retroviruses (345, 1008). Similarly, some B-cell lines transformed by EBV appear to replicate HIV best, perhaps because of a postinfection process (560, 1810, 1812). Even mouse fibroblasts chronically infected with murine retroviruses replicate HIV to higher levels after transfection of an infectious DNA molecular clone than do transfected uninfected mouse cells (2133a). The mechanism(s) for this enhanced expression of HIV in coinfected cells is unknown but, again, could reflect a cross-reaction with the HIV LTR by induced cellular factors (for further discussion of this topic, see Chapter 13, Section I).

IV.   Virus Infection of Quiescent Cells

A.   CD4$^+$ Lymphocytes

The steps leading to productive viral infection and the consequences of that infection have been discussed. What happens when HIV encounters a "resting" lymphocyte is another important question. The initial experiments with HIV infection of lymphocytes indicated that virus replication occurred best with antigen- or mitogen-induced activation (146, 1667). When established T-cell lines were arrested in growth by drug treatment, HIV replication was blocked in some cells (2643) but unaffected in others (1531). These systems, however, did not reflect what may occur under normal conditions with peripheral blood CD4$^+$ lymphocytes (77).

1. PERIPHERAL BLOOD CD4$^+$ CELLS: IN VITRO STUDIES
Studies with nondividing peripheral blood CD4$^+$ T cells have provided valuable information on the initial events involved in efficient virus infection and progeny pro-

Table 5.2 Studies of quiescent cells[a]

1. Virus replication is blocked at virus entry (928, 2642).
2. Virus enters but is blocked in reverse transcription (2954).
3. Virus enters and is reverse transcribed but is blocked at viral integration (2597).
4. Virus enters and integrates into a resting cell (e.g., epithelial cell) with subsequent virus replication (1526).

[a] In examples 2 and 3, HIV can be produced after activation of the cell. See the text for discussion.

duction. The results indicate that the level of cell activation (expression of HLA-DR and CD25) can influence the extent of viral reverse transcription and release of infectious virus from the cell (2179, 2642) (Table 5.2).

Cells completely blocked in DNA synthesis and kept nonactivated (at the G_0-G_1 stage) (e.g., no HLA-DR and low CD25 expression) cannot be productively infected by HIV (928, 2642). Despite the expression of CD4, these cells show no evidence of viral infection when subjected to subsequent cell activation procedures that can induce infectious virus production in culture. Molecular studies have shown that the virus enters the cell but only short transcripts of viral DNA are made; reverse transcription is not completed and cannot be induced after virus entry (2642). Thus, the infection is abortive.

In contrast to the above observations on nondividing cells, some investigators have reported that "resting" CD4$^+$ lymphocytes can be infected in vitro and that virus replication is arrested but can be induced. Unintegrated viral cDNA forms can be detected by PCR in T cells from a few days to 2 weeks after the initial infection (2597, 2642, 2954). Upon activation, these cells can be induced to release infectious progeny viruses. These studies have suggested that HIV enters the "quiescent" cells but that only limited transcription of the viral gene takes place (2953, 2954). The virus is not integrated, and no viral proteins are produced. In certain cases, if these cells are not fully activated within 3 to 5 days, the infection is aborted (2954). In other situations, long cDNA viral forms may be made in the cell, and this unproductive viral infection can persist for 2 to 4 weeks (2597, 2642). In this type of infection, the preintegration complex remains in the cytoplasmic compartment until activation leads to its rapid transport to the nucleus by a process requiring ATP and not cell division (313). Upon activation, full-length viral DNA is formed (2616) and integrated, and then virus is produced. Recently, quiescent cells lacking CD25 expression have been found to be resistant to HIV infection, most probably at the stage of entry, since no viral transcripts were detected (445). If they were cultured with CD4$^+$ CD25$^+$ cells, however, a nonproductive infection of the resting CD25 cells took place, similar to those described above (2597, 2954). Some factors produced by CD25$^+$ cells (e.g., interleukin-2 [IL-2]) must influence this process to place the target cells in a more responsive state.

In other recent experiments, purified CD45RA$^+$ or CD45RO$^+$ CD4$^+$ cells were exposed to a T-cell-line-tropic virus. Whereas virus entry appeared to take place to an equal extent, initially only the CD45RO$^+$ CD4$^+$ (memory) cell cultures produced virus over time (2914). The authors suggest that virus enters the CD45RA$^+$ naive cell, but unless the cell is activated, the infection is aborted, most likely because the preintegration complex is not transported to the nucleus (see below). Thus, activation determines the extent of HIV replication, as observed in the other studies described above. The data confirm and help explain previous work suggesting preferential infection of memory cells by HIV-1 (2263, 2405, 2553) (see Chapter 4).

2. QUIESCENT CD4$^+$ CELLS: IN VIVO STUDIES
The observations in vitro with purified quiescent CD4$^+$ cells have also been applied to clinical specimens. Purified CD4$^+$ cells from asymptomatic individuals consisted of a large percentage of resting cells that contained primarily unintegrated viral

DNA forms (314). These cells were reported to lack HLA-DR expression, but a low level of DR$^+$ cells (0.3%) was present in the cell population (314). In our studies, this percentage of contaminating DR$^+$ cells is sufficient to give a permissive state to HIV infection in vitro (2642) In individuals with AIDS, the recovered CD4$^+$ cells were primarily DR$^+$ and had integrated HIV with expression of viral RNA (314). These in vivo observations mirror in part those already described from PCR analysis on PBMC specimens; cells from asymptomatic individuals show very little expression of viral RNA (2048, 2507) (see Chapter 4). Moreover, viral mRNA expression in peripheral blood cells has demonstrated latent infection in HIV-infected chimpanzees (2334) and in human subjects (2335). In the human study, the presence of increased levels of viral mRNA in cells predicted progression to disease, most probably because the data reflected infected cells that were no longer in a latent state.

The findings on resting cells support the conclusion that in many CD4$^+$ cells of asymptomatic individuals, HIV can be present in an unintegrated noninfectious form after entry for perhaps many more days than suggested by studies in cell culture. Other cells in the blood, as discussed in Chapter 4, can be present with integrated but nonexpressed virus (2048, 2507). It will be important to determine whether the CD8$^+$ cell factor that suppresses virus replication and prevents virus superinfection (137, 1239) could contribute to this arrest in viral replication in quiescent cells in vivo (see Chapter 11). Conceivably, the free virus in the plasma (see Chapter 2) could be the source of repeated infection of quiescent cells that, unless activated, eventually lose the viral cDNA forms. If virus replication does not take place, CD4 expression could remain intact and reinfection (or superinfection) would be possible (see Chapter 4). Thus, cycles of fluctuation in virus infection and loss could characterize a dynamic situation within an infected individual (Figure 5.4). Under these conditions, there is a chance of recombination (see Chapter 3, Section X.I).

3. INTRACELLULAR MECHANISM

The intracellular factors that might influence the extent of virus production also are not yet identified. They must involve DNA binding (e.g., NF-κB) and RNA binding cellular proteins (Section I). Moreover, as noted above, recent results with macrophage-tropic and non-macrophage-tropic HIV-1 strains, showing a block in reverse transcription in activated T-cell lines (1131) and in macrophages (2393) (Section IV.B) (Table 5.1), respectively, suggest that a similar or other intracellular mechanism could be involved.

Some of the in vitro and in vivo observations on limited reverse transcription of HIV in quiescent cells could have other explanations. For example, heterogeneous viral DNA species, resulting from partial reverse transcription within the virus particles, have been found in HIV virions (1585, 2713, 2972). This DNA might be responsible for the low-level DNA detected by PCR in the experiments with resting cells (2954). The partial reverse transcripts in the cells could be those associated with viruses bound to the cell and not internalized or those failing to continue their replicative cycle. This possibility, however, does not seem feasible because of the control cultures used in the experiments in which the infection of resting cells was evaluated.

Figure 5.4 HIV can infect a resting CD4$^+$ cell that expresses the CD4 molecule (step 1). If that cell is not activated, virus replication cannot take place. Because the CD4 molecule is still expressed on a resting cell, superinfection by another virus can occur (step 2). With no activation of the resting cell after infection, an abortive infection takes place (step 3). With activation, active virus replication takes place (step 4). Similarly, activation of the superinfected cell (step 5) can lead to production of both type viruses, or recombinants might be found. Following activation and virus production (step 5), the CD4 molecule is down-modulated, so that superinfection cannot occur.

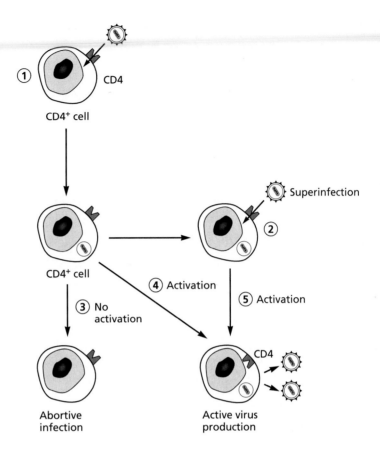

4. CONCLUSIONS

The difficulty in resolving the various findings on resting cells revolves around the definition of quiescence. Most immunologists would insist that such cells should lack CD25 expression (2179). We would emphasize an absence of DR expression as well. If a small number of DR$^+$ cells is present in the inoculated cell population in vitro, they would be permissive to HIV infection and could misleadingly suggest, by the PCR analysis used, successful infection of all cells. In our experiments, this possibility was ruled out by the elimination of all DR$^+$ cells (2642). Moreover, in experiments by others (2597, 2954), macrophages and CD4$^+$ CD25$^+$ cells were not rigorously removed. These cells can be infected or can affect the susceptibility to HIV infection of the other CD4$^+$ cells (445). Nevertheless, full virus replication was not achieved, even in the relatively pure quiescent cells described in these studies. Thus, the findings do suggest that virus entry and expression can be influenced by the state of cell activation. The length of time a cell could carry the unintegrated viral DNA must also reflect the level of its activation (314, 2597, 2954).

How quiescent CD4$^+$ cells lacking HLA-DR expression are infected in vivo is also unknown (314). Whether a DR$^+$ CD4$^+$ lymphocyte can, after infection, return to a quiescent nonproductive DR$^-$ state needs to be determined. Preliminary evidence in our laboratory suggests that this is possible (2644), but other studies suggest that it is a rare phenomenon (452). Alternatively, as noted above, the few quiescent CD4$^+$ cells found infected in vivo (314) could be those few DR$^+$ cells that are present in the resting-cell population (0.3%). Finally, the clinical relevance of these studies on resting T cells needs to be considered. Most CD4$^+$ cells in vivo are in a relatively quiescent state but are still susceptible to productive virus infection. It seems more important, therefore, to focus on activation events that establish the infection in these cells.

B.   Monocytes

Studies of peripheral blood monocytes also suggest that intracellular events are needed to permit productive infection. Monocytes found in the blood are not very susceptible to HIV infection, despite >90% expression of DR (2224, 2420, 2538, 2641, 2643, 2644, 2743). Uncultured, freshly isolated blood monocytes show no evidence of reverse transcription after inoculation with HIV-1. In contrast, cells cultured for at least 24 h show reverse transcripts as well as evidence of virus integration (2538). These observations provide molecular evidence that blood monocytes do not appear to be permissive to viral entry and thus are not susceptible to infection in vivo unless differentiation has taken place. It is noteworthy that nondifferentiated monocytes have more CD4 expression than do differentiated macrophages (502, 1256). Perhaps other specific cell surface receptors are involved, but recent studies suggest that differentiation also affects susceptibility by inducing NF-κB components with transcriptionally active heterodimers (1524).

These findings place further emphasis on differentiated tissue macrophages as a primary initial site of virus infection. These cells could certainly be a source of virus replication in the spleen (979a) (Chapter 4). In some studies, PCR techniques have shown that monocytes in the blood are infected (1215), but this observation has also only been reported in a few cases and in a small number of cells (122, 1722). By in situ PCR procedures, most infected monocyte/macrophages in the blood were shown not to be producing virus (120).

Although in one report, proliferation of the macrophages was found necessary for infection (2420), most studies indicate that HIV can infect a nondividing differentiated macrophage (2538, 2644, 2838). Integration probably takes place (697, 2538). In one study, cultured infected macrophages showed reduced virus production after activation by lipopolysaccharide (LPS) (191). This finding may reflect a differential expression of cytokines. In addition, terminally differentiated macrophages, cultured for a long time, are also not very susceptible to HIV infection (2743); the reason has not been elucidated.

Following acute HIV infection, tissue macrophages in turn could pass the virus to T cells, but only after the lymphocytes are activated. Resting CD4$^+$ cells in the G_0G_1 phase and lacking DR expression cannot be infected when cocultured with virus-releasing macrophages (2642). Moreover, direct cell:cell interactions appear to be necessary for efficient cell transfer to take place (633, 2414). Similarly, the induction of monocyte-to-macrophage differentiation that increases HIV replication depends on CD4$^+$ cell:monocyte contact (633). These findings suggest that macrophages in tissues, particularly lymphoid organs, can be a major reservoir for production and spread of HIV in the host. This concept, however, does not explain why in situ PCR studies thus far do not show many infected macrophages in lymphoid tissue (696, 1954).

Finally, as noted above (Section II.B), experiments with non-macrophage-tropic strains suggest that intracellular events requiring reverse transcription are blocked in differentiated macrophages after infection (1844, 2129, 2393, 2417) (Table 5.1). The explanation for these findings could have relevance to the intracellular events occurring in quiescent T cells and undifferentiated monocytes.

C.   Other Cells

Emerman and colleagues (1526) demonstrated that nondividing human epithelial cells expressing the human CD4 molecule can be infected by HIV; virus integration into the cell chromosome takes place (Table 5.2). The murine type C retroviruses that can infect human cells do not show this biologic activity, and infection does not occur. The reason for the productive infection of these nondividing epithelial cells by HIV is not known, but it does not appear to involve any of the regulatory or accessory genes. Some studies suggest that it could depend on the MA (p17) and Vpr proteins (1046) that direct the preintegration complex to the nucleus (312, 829). The larger preintegration complexes of other retroviruses may not be able to enter the intact nucleus of resting cells via nuclear pores (312). This event, for HIV, appears to not require mitosis (1527), but instead involves a tyrosine phosphorylization of MA (830) by a MAP kinase carried within the virion (2594a); it also involves integrase (828a) and an interaction of the preintegration complex with cellular karyopherins (829). The findings offer some direction for obtaining vectors that might be useful in gene therapy of resting human stem cells. Such an approach has recently been evaluated and shows the increased ability of an HIV vector to transfer genes into human skin fibroblasts arrested at the G_0G_1 stage and into unstimulated $CD34^+$ cells (2212). Nevertheless, the observations on resting T cells cited above suggest that productive infection of quiescent cells could be cell type specific (Table 5.2).

V.   Latency

A.   Cellular Latency

The preceding discussion on HIV infection indicated that some nonactivated cells can harbor the HIV genome in an unintegrated state for several days without evidence of virus replication. This type of silent infection in cells differs from the classic state of viral latency in which the full viral genome is in the cell but expression is suppressed. In the case of retroviruses, very little, if any, viral RNA or protein would be made from the integrated provirus in the cell chromosome (547, 770, 1496). Subsequently, conditions occurring within the cell would alter its state so that HIV replication and spread and cell death would follow. The induction of retroviruses from a latent state has been studied in many different systems, and a variety of approaches can be used (1505) (Table 5.3).

Table 5.3 Induction of retroviruses from a latent state

1. Halogenated pyrimidines (e.g., iododeoxyuridine, bromodeoxyuridine)
2. Nucleic acid analogs (e.g., 5-azacytidine)
3. Protein inhibitors (e.g., cycloheximide)
4. B-cell mitogens (e.g., lipopolysaccharides)
5. T-cell mitogens (e.g., phytohemagglutinin, concanavalin A)
6. Amino acid analogs (e.g., L-canavanine)
7. Cytokines (e.g., TNF-α, granulocyte colony-stimulating factor [G-CSF])
8. Graft-versus-host reaction
9. UV irradiation
10. Heat shock
11. Infection by other viruses (e.g., herpesvirus, retrovirus)

The presence of cellular latency for HIV has been supported by biologic and molecular studies (for a review, see reference 1711). Some groups have observed that virus-producing established cell lines can gradually decrease virus production over time (1230, 1536, 2535). Recently, in both CD4$^+$ lymphocytes and established CD4$^+$ T-cell lines, temporal changes in the steady-state levels of viral mRNA were associated with a shutdown of HIV transcription, and there was enhanced production of spliced mRNAs (1536). The viral genes responsible for the arrest in a T-cell line were mapped primarily to the 3′ LTR, but *tat/rev* and *vpu* also seemed to be involved in the process (2535). The mechanism controlling these temporal changes has not been fully clarified (see below).

In other studies of cells in vivo, the presence of HIV DNA but not RNA has been noted in PBMC, as well as in lymphoid tissue (452, 695, 696, 1954, 2048) (see Chapter 4). Moreover, CD4$^+$ lymphocytes carrying HIV-1 DNA can be recovered from the PBMC of infected individuals, and these cells express the CD4 molecule, conceivably because they are not producing progeny virus (2407, 2813). This state is reflected as well by an excess of multiply spliced or singly spliced viral RNA compared to unspliced RNA in infected cells recovered in vivo (2048, 2453, 2507) (Section I). High levels of viral mRNA species in peripheral blood cells have predicted progression to disease (2335), presumably reflecting the onset of virus replication.

In one of the first in vitro studies of cellular latency by HIV in vivo, Hoxie et al. (1116) reported a long-term culture of naturally infected human CD4$^+$ lymphocytes that did not express much virus until several weeks after the start of the culture. Then high levels of HIV were spontaneously produced, and this was followed by cell death. These observations were subsequently confirmed by using purified resting CD4$^+$ T cells from infected individuals (452). Moreover, clones of CD4$^+$ lymphocytes isolated from seronegative donors have been shown to harbor virus in a latent state after infection with HIV-1 in vitro (402). Thus, a state of postintegration latency appears possible in some cells in vivo.

Some researchers have used established cell lines such as the infected U-1 and ACH-2 cell lines to study cellular latency; these cells produce very low levels of HIV (769, 772, 2115). The lines were derived from established monocyte (U-1) or T-cell (ACH-2) lines chronically infected with HIV-1$_{LAI}$ and generally show only 2-kb mRNA (1774, 2120). Thus, they appear to lack production of Rev (2280, 2531, 2739). A possible effect of low Tat expression should also be considered. When the cell lines are activated by treatment with a variety of cytokines (e.g., TNF-α, IL-1, phorbol esters, and granulocyte colony-stimulating factor [G-CSF]), viral RNA and infectious virus production are markedly increased and are often associated with activation of the cellular NF-κB protein that binds to the viral LTR (671, 770, 771, 1007, 1895, 1896, 1994, 2115, 2284; for a review, see reference 2003). During this activation process, a shift in mRNA patterns occurs, with a reduction in spliced mRNA levels and an increase in unspliced mRNA levels (1774). Thus, expression of Rev does appear to be involved. Similarly, a block in Rev function has been linked to restricted HIV-1 production by human astrocytoma cells (1917).

Moreover, silent infection of monocytes has been reported with mutant HIV-1 strains lacking *vpu* or *vpr* functions (2866). Virus can be recovered from these cells by cocultivation with uninfected PBMC. A similar observation on the amplification of HIV release by adding PBMC to the cultures has been made with established T-cell and monocyte lines, as well as HIV-infected macrophages (720, 770, 2413) and fibroblasts (2648). Thus, the "latent" state in monocytes and other cells could reflect an arrest in virus release rather than earlier events. Nevertheless, the role of cytokines or cell:cell activation should be considered; the mechanism has not yet been elucidated.

In other studies, halogenated pyrimidines, UV rays, and heat shock have led to virus activation (378, 1507, 2572, 2585), perhaps secondary to DNA damage (2746) (Figure 5.5). As noted above, other viral infections can reactivate a latent HIV infection in vitro, most probably via effects on the viral LTR (1851) (Sections I and II). Again, the molecular events in this process are not well characterized.

A cell line has been described that oscillates between a latent CD4$^+$ state and a

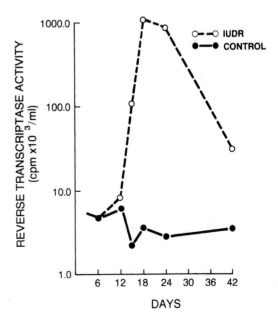

Figure 5.5 Latent HIV infection of an established T-cell line. The HIV-1$_{SF247}$ strain, obtained from a patient of E. Koenig from the Dominican Republic, was used to infect the Jurkat T-cell line. After 6 days in culture, very little virus replication was detected by the reverse transcription assay. After the addition on day 6 of iodo-deoxyuridine (IUDR) (50 μg/ml), HIV-1 was released to high levels, as measured by particle-associated reverse transcriptase activity. Within 2 weeks, virus replication decreased to almost a latent state. Reproduced from reference 1507 with permission.

virus-productive CD4$^-$ state (327). Derived from the HL60 promonocytic cell line, this model of latency seems more typical of classical viral latency; little if any viral RNA and protein are made unless virus activation is induced. TNF-α predominantly influences the state of virus expression in this cell line.

Persistent nonproductive HIV infection of EBV-transformed B lymphocytes has also been described (561). Clones from these cells, however, showed many intracytoplasmic viral particles. This result indicated that although the virus seemed to be latent, the state reflected the effect of cellular and not viral factors: HIV was not released by the particular B-cell clone. Once produced, it replicated like the parental virus in PBMC. Finally, in one report, latency in the U937 monocyte cell lines was associated with methylation of high levels of extrachromosomal viral DNA copies (2513).

It is important to recognize that nearly all these in vitro studies of cellular latency have used established cell lines with integrated HIV genomes and not infected normal lymphocytes which would be more relevant to the in vivo situation (402). Moreover, whether observations on cells that produce low levels of virus (e.g., U-1 and ACH-2 cells) mirror conditions within cells in a completely latent state (in which relatively no viral RNA is produced) is still not known.

B. Mechanism of Cellular Latency

1. POSSIBLE PROCESSES

Several hypotheses have been presented to explain the mechanism of cellular latency with HIV (Table 5.4) (for reviews, see references 770, 1711, and 2594a). Each may relate to certain processes within a specific cell type and to particular viral strains (668). The latency could be caused by methylation of certain portions of the integrated viral LTR needed for induction of the replicative process (160) or, as cited above, by methylation of extrachromosomal viral DNA sequences (2513). It could result from chromatin interaction with the HIV-1 promoter (2752) or from inactivation of the *tat* or *rev* gene (17, 95, 666, 746, 770, 1024, 2120, 2429, 2715) or a TAR mutation (699). Alternatively, the specific site of proviral integration (2895) and/or histone suppression of gene expression could be involved (1439).

Table 5.4 Possible mechanisms of HIV latency^a

1. Methylation of viral DNA (160, 2513)
2. Lack of sufficient viral Tat expression (746, 1024)
3. Expression of viral Nef protein (422, 1598)
4. Lack of expression of Rev (2120, 2715)
5. Lack of viral Vpu and Vpr expression (2866)
6. Inhibition of intracellular factors that interact with the NF-κB protein or other regions on the viral LTR (1895, 2003)
7. Inhibition of virus expression by CD8$^+$ cell antiviral factor (2811)
8. Site of virus integration (2895)
9. Histone suppression of viral gene expression (1439)

^{a} See the text for other references and discussion.

Early studies suggested that the virus itself produces a protein, such as Nef, that interacts with cellular factors and establishes the silent infection (27, 422, 1598, 1930). Suppression of *vpu* or *vpr* function could be responsible (1488, 2866). However, more recent studies have suggested that Nef and Vpr carried within the virion play a role in activating cells, thus making them susceptible to HIV replication (546, 1488, 2025, 2054). For example, when Vpr was added to non-virus-producing cell lines (U-1 and ACH-2), HIV replication was induced (1488). Moreover, Vpr is found in the serum, suggesting that it may play a role in activating HIV replication. Countering these observations is the evidence that Vpr arrests cells in the G_2 phase of the cell cycle (150). This viral protein may therefore play a role in blocking the efficiency of virus replication (1040, 1487, 2198). Thus, as may be true for other viral proteins, the relative effect of Vpr on activating or suppressing virus replication must depend on its interaction with a particular cell and could be a determinant of HIV pathogenesis.

Likewise, the finding of Nef within virions (2025), its association with protein kinase activity (2368, 2369), and its potential function in activating $CD4^+$ lymphocytes (see below) suggest that it plays a role in inducing a permissive state for virus replication early in infection. Nef appears to associate with a 65-kDa protein that is serologically and functionally related to the p21-activated kinases that are involved in signal transduction (1953). In all these processes, certain cellular proteins appear to be involved (1252). Finally, cellular latency could be induced by $CD8^+$ cell anti-HIV-suppressing activity, perhaps via a novel cytokine (1239, 1515, 1635, 2811) (see Chapter 11).

2. THE Nef PROTEIN

The role of the *nef* gene in latency was initially proposed because deletion of this viral gene from the molecular clone of the HIV-1$_{SF2}$ strain produced a variant that replicated to high titer and was more cytopathic than the original SF2 isolate (1598). Work with other HIV isolates and with SIV supported the conclusion that the *nef* gene can down-regulate virus replication in T cells and monocytes (27, 212, 1929, 1930, 2661, 2725).

Other findings suggested an association of *nef* with latency. The HIV-1$_{SF2}$ *nef* gene (linked to the viral LTR or the simian virus 40 [SV40] promoter) transfected in T-cell lines suppressed virus replication (422). Most noteworthy was the observation that highly cytopathic strains (e.g., HIV-1$_{SF33}$ or strains recovered from individuals with disease) replicated in the Nef-expressing T cells without any visible effect of the viral protein on HIV production (422). The results suggested that HIV virulence in the host could depend on the sensitivity of the particular virus to the effects of the viral Nef protein (see Chapter 7). The observations on viral heterogeneity were provided as one explanation for why some investigators did not find a silencing effect of Nef on HIV expression (998, 1291). More important, however, appear to be the target cells used to study Nef. Different results on its activity are obtained when normal $CD4^+$ lymphocytes are used instead of transfected T-cell lines (see below).

HIV-infected human astrocyte cell lines have also demonstrated a correlation between an arrest in virus replication and high-level Nef expression (271, 2690). One latently infected astrocyte cell line contained as much as a 10-fold-greater amount of multiply spliced mRNA species than of unspliced mRNA species, concomitant with a high expression of the Nef protein. Similarly, biopsy specimens from brains of children and adults have shown high expression of Nef in non-virus-producing cells (2329, 2692). Down-modulation of HIV LTR activity by a portion of the *nef* gene has been detected (1601) (see also below). Thus, Nef might play an inhibitory role in certain cells.

An alternative explanation for a role of Nef in latent infection of astrocytes is that the intracellular milieu of these cells may affect virus expression differently from that of T cells. Some studies do indicate that Tat can transactivate the viral LTR in astrocyte cell lines in the absence of the TAR region. The results suggest that an element upstream from TAR participates in viral gene expression in these cells (2650). Some studies suggest that a restricted expression of Rev is involved (1917). Thus, cellular factors interacting with certain viral genes could be directly involved in the latent infection in these brain-derived cells.

Most studies indicate that the function of Nef can be pleiotropic (Table 5.5). The sequences in the Nef region are highly heterogeneous (614), and, as noted above, differences in activity can be found among various alleles and in different cell types (e.g., T-cell lines versus CD4$^+$ lymphocytes) (2313). For example, the Nef protein of certain viruses down-modulates CD4 in some T cells (845, 973, 1669), but the Nef protein of other viruses does not (422). Moreover, Nef expression can affect IL-2, gamma interferon (IFN-γ), and IL-10 production in some cells (284, 499, 1608). Thus, an effect on the levels of these cytokines could be important in HIV infection (see Chapter 11). In addition, studies in our laboratory have demonstrated that Nef proteins from some viruses have no influence on replication kinetics or can even enhance it (420). Others have shown that some viruses with *nef* mutations can replicate better in macrophages than in T-cell lines (2662). Some studies suggest that the *nef* allele of some strains is associated with acceleration in virus replication in CD4$^+$ lymphocytes and T-cell lines (595, 2968, 2969). Nevertheless, a

---

Table 5.5   Reported activities of HIV Nef

1. Enhances HIV replication (i.e., PBMC and particularly nonstimulated CD4$^+$ lymphocytes)[a] (447, 595, 1793, 2427, 2550, 2968, 2969)
2. Decreases virus replication (astrocytes, T-cell lines) (27, 271, 422, 1598, 2661)
3. Induces activation in association with serine kinase activity (156, 2368, 2369)
4. Down-modulates CD4 expression (845, 973, 1669)
5. Down-modulates MHC expression (2428)
6. Decreases expression of IL-2 (1608)
7. Decreases IFN-γ production (499)
8. Induction of IL-10 production (284)
9. Suppresses viral LTR expression (27, 1601, 1650, 1845, 2945)
10. Inhibits NF-κB induction and AP-1 DNA binding proteins (1927, 1928)
11. Cytotoxic for CD4$^+$ cells (802, 803)
12. Determines pathogenesis in rhesus macaques (1281)

[a] Affects early steps in virus entry and/or reverse transcription.

mutant from another strain (HIV-1_{SF2}) that does not express Nef replicates faster and to higher levels in PBMC than the parental wild-type virus (1505a, 1598).

Recent reports suggest that the importance of Nef for high-level virus production is secondary to its influence on early steps in virus entry of cells and/or reverse transcription (447, 1793, 2427, 2550). This difference becomes most evident in non-stimulated CD4$^+$ lymphocytes (1793, 2550, 2552). In these cells, most *nef*-deleted viruses that grow efficiently in activated CD4$^+$ lymphocytes do not replicate substantially. In studies in our laboratory, however, the *nef*-deleted mutant of HIV-1_{SF2} replicated as well as or better than the wild-type virus in resting CD4$^+$ cells (1518a). Conceivably, reduction in CD4 expression, attributed in part to Nef (845, 973), helps virus replication by preventing cell death by fusion or other CD4-mediated events (Chapter 6). In this regard, studies have demonstrated that the down-modulation of CD4 by Nef can be separated from its enhancing effects on virus replication (902).

How Nef could suppress HIV replication is not known. Some investigators initially proposed that the viral LTR is affected (27, 974, 1650, 1845, 2945). Other data suggested alternative conclusions (111, 998). An inhibition by Nef of NF-κB induction in T cells and of AP-1 DNA binding proteins was reported (1927, 1928). Our studies with T-cell lines showed that sensitive HIV strains infecting Nef-expressing T-cell lines made little viral protein and only small spliced mRNA species (e.g., 2 and 4 kb) (1514), suggestive of *rev*-deleted mutant viruses (2280, 2531). Moreover, experiments with interviral recombinants resistant to Nef mapped this property to a region encompassing the second exon of Rev (1514). Observations on the effect of Rev on Nef expression also support these conclusions (26). However, these findings need further clarification, particularly since they were made in established T-cell lines.

Animal experiments also do not support a virus-suppressing role of Nef. In rhesus macaques, the *nef*-deleted mutant virus was less pathogenic than its wild-type counterpart (1281). The requirement for Nef in pathogenicity was also inferred from studies in the SCID mouse system, in which *nef*-deleted mutants of HIV-1 strains had attenuated growth properties and did not induce depletion of human CD4$^+$ cells in the animals (965, 1185). Recently, a deletion in the *nef* gene was found in some HIV-1 isolates from long-term survivors (1028, 1303, 2025, 2855) and in viruses recovered from transfusion recipients who did not progress to disease (1773). These studies suggest that Nef could play a role in delaying disease progression in some cases. However, several other studies characterizing *nef* sequences in long-term survivors and progressors with HIV infection have shown that deletions or functions of the *nef* gene do not correlate with the rate of disease progression (1127, 1773). One potential mechanism for its role in attenuation is that a *nef*-deleted mutant virus might express its proteins more efficiently in vivo so that the host immune system can recognize them more readily and suppress viral growth. Nef has been shown to reduce cellular expression of MHC molecules (2428), so that the immune system might better recognize a *nef* mutant. This possibility requires further study.

In summary, Nef proteins most probably function through an interaction with cellular proteins, probably via phosphorylation events yet to be fully defined (973, 974, 1448, 1953, 2133, 2368, 2369, 2903). The effect on HIV depends on the particular *nef* allele, the cell type infected, and perhaps the location of Nef in the cell. Also, conceivably, specific domains in the *nef* gene differ in their biologic function. The potential effect of Nef on T-cell activation (156, 2521) and its association with serine kinase activity (2368, 2369) also suggest that its influence on HIV replication is linked to signal transduction (Figure 5.3). Thus, how Nef affects the intracellular milieu could determine its ultimate effect on the replication in a cell by a particular HIV isolate. Most investigators currently consider that the function of this viral protein carried within the virion (2855) is to induce activation rather than suppress virus replication (for a review, see reference 546). Nevertheless, the exceptions noted above do suggest a potential role of Nef in latency, along with certain other viral proteins.

3. CONCLUSION

The mechanisms involved in the induction of a state of latency with HIV have not yet been fully defined (Table 5.4), and the reason that certain viral strains can enter latency more readily than others is unexplained (Chapter 7). Moreover, whether the in vitro studies of viral latency have relevance in vivo has yet to be determined (Section V.C). Nevertheless, the HIV regulatory proteins, Tat, Rev, and Nef, and intracellular factors certainly could be involved either positively or negatively in inducing this biologic process. The potential role of Nef in latency appeared to be a plausible function and was responsible for its name as negative factor. However, more recent studies with $CD4^+$ lymphocytes have strongly suggested that the major role of Nef is in activating $CD4^+$ cells, making them more susceptible to HIV replication. Nevertheless, the studies of *nef*-deleted mutant viruses in T-cell lines may yet uncover a mechanism by which this viral protein could play a role in both a positive and negative regulation of HIV regulation. In this regard, the Vpr gene product, also present in virions, appears to play dual roles in HIV infection and replication (see above).

C.   Clinical Latency

The interval between infection and clinical disease in an individual has often been called latency. This state is quite different from the latent state within the cell. The factors influencing this clinical condition not only are cellular but also, most importantly, involve the immunologic response of the host against the virus (discussed in Chapters 10 and 11). Evidence today indicates that clinical latency, defined as an absence of symptoms, can be present at the same time that virus replication is active in the host (see Chapter 3). Thus, the interrelationship and differences between biologic and clinical latency need to be appreciated.

A clinical reflection of cellular latency in the host was suspected when antibody-negative, viremia-negative healthy individuals whose blood contained non-virus-producing HIV-infected cells were identified by PCR and other analyses (734, 1157, 1194, 2001, 2185, 2909). In some cases, the PBMC from these individuals were induced to produce anti-HIV antibodies in vitro (1195, 2765), but this observation needs confirmation. The existence of this HIV cellular latency in the host for a long period is now controversial and probably occurs rarely, if at all. Most studies point to a short seronegative interval in HIV-infected individuals (735, 878, 1107, 1543,

1670, 2023). In the infected person, the virus is continually being expressed in some cells (see Chapter 3). Therefore, a seronegative status in infected individuals most probably reflects a delay in the response of the immune system rather than the presence of a completely latent cellular state in vivo.

In essence, many non-virus-producing HIV-infected cells are present in tissues in the host throughout the course of infection, but virus continues to be produced by some cells, as shown by in situ PCR techniques (Section II) (see Chapters 4 and 9). With low virus expression, individuals can remain clinically asymptomatic. Thus, they are often considered to be in a clinically latent state. Rarely, newborn infants infected in utero become seronegative after elimination of maternal antibodies (684), but they show clinical signs of productive virus infection. A similar finding has been made in SIV-infected newborn monkeys which progress to disease and show no production of antibodies (1679a), probably as a result of their infection in a naive immune state. Moreover, in rare cases, adults will be infected by HIV and develop AIDS without production of detectable antibodies (1772). The mechanism has not been defined but most probably reflects a greatly compromised immune system. Finally, the early reports of seroreversion of HIV-1 antibody status (734), suggesting elimination of HIV infection, have not been substantiated (2298). The few cases of virus elimination from newborn children (see Chapter 2) appear to be rare, and the mechanism is not known.

Chapter 5 SALIENT FEATURES

1. The replicative cycle of HIV involves the intracellular interaction of a variety of viral, structural, and regulatory gene products with cellular genes. Some regulatory genes (e.g., *tat*) up-regulate virus replication, and others may suppress virus expression.

2. Differences in virus production can be noted in PBMC and appear to be related to intracellular differences. In the productive infection of cells, intracellular factors as well as coreceptors on the cell surface and the particular virus involved need to be considered.

3. Activation is important for HIV replication and involves several intracellular factors that interact with regions of the viral LTR. Intracellular blocks may be responsible for lack of replication of some SI viruses in macrophages and NSI viruses in T-cell lines.

4. Other viruses coinfecting a cell can enhance transcription of HIV.

5. Quiescent $CD4^+$ cells are resistant to productive infection by HIV. Either limited transcripts of the viral RNA are made, or virus entry is completely blocked. Unless the cells are activated, the virus infection can be aborted.

6. Differentiated macrophages are most susceptible to virus replication. The reason may be the up-regulation of NF-κB transcriptionally active proteins.

7. Nondividing macrophages, as well as certain other human cells, can be infected by HIV, with integration of virus into the cell chromosome. This process, different from that of other retroviruses, depends on the MA and Vpr proteins that direct the preintegration complex to the nucleus.

8. A state of cellular latency has been found in HIV infection in which $CD4^+$ cells or other cells can contain unexpressed HIV that can be activated under certain conditions.

9. Cellular latency may be explained by an inactivation of certain viral genes (e.g., *tat* and *rev*). In some cases, the Nef protein appears to bring about suppression of virus expression.

10. The Nef protein is pleiotropic and, in general, carried in the virion, functions to activate cells during virus infection. The *nef*-deleted mutant viruses appear to be less pathogenic in animal experiments. Nef may have various functions, depending on the cellular proteins with which it interacts and the particular alleles of the virus.

11. The state of clinical latency defines an individual who has not developed disease. These individuals may have complete control of virus replication, although most evidence suggests that low-level virus replication takes place continually. Low virus expression in infected individuals correlates with a long-term asymptomatic clinical course.

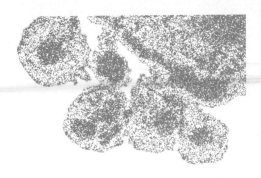

Cytopathic Properties of HIV

AN IMPORTANT PART OF OUR UNDERSTANDING OF THE PATHOGENESIS of HIV in the host should come from studying the cytopathic effects of the virus or its proteins on individual cells. As reviewed in Chapter 7, certain HIV-1 isolates, particularly those recovered when the infected individual is advancing to disease, have a greater capacity for killing infected cells in culture than do strains isolated in the clinically asymptomatic period. Cell death appears to result from formation of multinucleated cells, necrosis, and apoptosis. This chapter reviews various processes involved in the cytopathic effects of HIV (Table 6.1).

I. HIV Induction of Cell Fusion

An important biologic feature of HIV infection is the formation of multinucleated cells (syncytia) in culture (and perhaps in the host) as a result of the fusion of infected cells with uninfected CD4$^+$ cells (Figures 3.6 and 6.1; see Chapter 7, Figure 7.4) (1544, 1548). Syncytium formation is often the first sign of HIV infection of peripheral blood mononuclear cells (PBMC) in culture and can appear in these cells within 2 to 3 days; accompanying this cytopathic effect is balloon degeneration of the cells, most probably resulting from changes in membrane permeability (Section III) (Figure 6.1). In

121

Table 6.1 Possible mechanisms of cytotoxicity by HIV or its proteins[a]

1. Syncytium formation
2. Accumulation of unintegrated viral DNA
3. Virus release causing changes in membrane integrity
4. Virus alteration of plasma membrane permeability to cations
5. Decrease in synthesis of membrane lipids
6. Decrease in "second-messenger" (diacylglycerol) activity
7. Interference with cellular heteronuclear RNA processing
8. Degradation of cellular mRNA and reduction in cellular protein synthesis
9. Induction of apoptosis[b]
10. Release of toxic cytokines by infected cells and/or uninfected cells
11. Destruction by immunologic responses (ADCC, CTL)[c]
12. Competitive inhibition by HIV of normal growth factors (e.g., in the brain)

[a] The viral proteins gp120, gp41, Tat, Nef, and Vif have been considered potentially responsible for cell death (see Chapters 7 and 8).
[b] Cytokines might be involved as well as superantigens.
[c] Abbreviations: ADCC, antibody-dependent cellular cytotoxicity; CTL, cytotoxic T lymphocytes.

culture, cell fusion can be observed within 2 h (2641) and is monitored by redistribution of fluorescent dyes (Color Plate 8, following p. 188) (636, 2842). HIV isolates can be distinguished by their ability to induce cell fusion (or syncytia) in established T-cell lines (e.g., MT-2 cells) (1347, 2649). Viruses that are syncytia-inducing (SI) are found more frequently in individuals advancing to disease than the non-syncytia-inducing (NSI) type (see Chapter 7).

This cell:cell fusion is temperature dependent (798) and does not require cellular DNA, RNA, or protein synthesis (1004, 2641); it appears to involve cell surface carbohydrates (1004, 1700, 2641) and glycolipids (662) (Table 6.2). Some studies suggest that a certain number of gp120:CD4 complexes are required for the process, which most probably involves multiple envelope:CD4 molecule interactions (798).

Whether syncytium formation is directly related to virus:cell fusion is not clear. The cell fusion event, as shown by specific antibodies, also involves the CD4 molecule and both the HIV gp120 and gp41 envelope proteins (72, 762, 792, 1004, 1544, 1546, 1548, 1700, 2522, 2530, 2595) (Figures 3.6 and 6.1; Table 6.2). Conformational changes in gp120/gp41 occur after binding to CD4 and appear to be important in rapid fusion (900) (Color Plate 2, following p. 188). Shedding of HIV-1 gp120 has been observed but is probably not necessary for cell fusion (801). Moreover, cell fusion can be influenced by the pattern of viral envelope glycosylation (741, 1700), as well as by the extent of proteolytic cleavage of gp160 within the cell (257) (Table 6.2).

Regions of CD4 and gp120 different from those used for viral attachment can play a role in the cell:cell fusion (72, 339, 1547, 2132). As discussed in Chapter 3, certain monoclonal antibodies to CD4 will not block virus binding but will prevent cell:cell fusion and HIV infection (100, 381, 1042, 2717). Results with interviral recombinants have indicated that syncytium formation can be linked to specific regions of gp120 (see Chapter 8) (426, 2566, 2943).

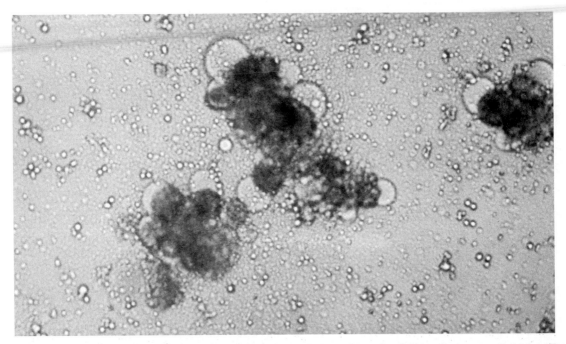

Figure 6.1 Multinucleated giant cells formed by cell:cell fusion during acute infection of PBMC by HIV-1. Balloon degeneration of the cells is also evident. Phase microscopy; magnification, ×80.

In other studies with HIV-1 and HIV-2, gp41 was noted to contain an important determinant for the fusion process (Section III) (762, 792, 794, 2074, 2522, 2582). Whether gp41 alone can mediate this process, however, has not yet been determined (1665). Moreover, it is still not clear which viral epitopes are directly involved in cell fusion and which only influence this biologic event. For example, certain coreceptors for HIV entry that were discovered by using cell fusion assays (see Chapter 3) are not directly involved in the virus:cell membrane fusion (Color Plate 2).

The possible role of cellular membrane proteins such as the integrin lymphocyte functional antigen 1 (LFA-1) (1068) or the CD7 glycoprotein (2360) in cell:cell fusion has been considered (see Chapter 3). Monoclonal antibodies to these cell surface proteins block cell aggregation and/or syncytium formation. Those directed against LFA-1 do not prevent virus infection (2030), but anti-CD7 antibodies do (2360). These findings underline possible differences between cell:cell fusion and virus:cell fusion. In addition, the absence of fusogenic activity when murine cells that express the human CD4 molecule are mixed with HIV-infected cells appears to reflect the lack of a human cell factor (291, 660, 2660). In one study, this factor appeared to be a glycolipid (662). A similar observation has been made with certain human-human cell heterokaryons (659). These observations have been partially explained by the absence of certain viral coreceptors (see Chapter 3). Moreover, the relation of these findings to a fusion domain for gp41 (Figure 3.4), which has been proposed as a necessary part of HIV entry (826, 2522), needs to be determined. Im-

Table 6.2   Factors influencing cell:cell fusion in HIV infection

Cell
    Does not require DNA, RNA, or protein synthesis (1004, 2641)
    Temperature dependent (798)
    Surface glycolipids (662)
    Surface adhesion molecules (LFA-1 and CD7 glycoprotein)
Virus
    Envelope proteins (1544, 1545, 1792, 2074)
    Pattern of gp120 glycosylation (741, 1700)
    Extent of proteolytic cleavage of gp160 within the cell (257)

portantly, events involved in cell:cell fusion may be distinguishable from those mediating virus:cell fusion. Nevertheless, in vitro cell fusion assays have supported a correlation between the fusogenic capacity of a virus envelope and the infectivity of cells by that virus (e.g., macrophage tropism and T-cell-line tropism) (290). These studies provided the basis for the discovery of the CXCR-4 (formerly called fusin) coreceptor for T-cell-line-tropic viruses (743) (see Chapter 3).

   The process of cell membrane fusion has been linked to viral cytopathicity and cell death (351, 1544). Some investigators believe that cell fusion is important in the depletion of CD4$^+$ cells resulting from single-cell lysis and perhaps multinucleated-cell formation (351, 1044; for review, see references 850 and 1030). Evidence for multinucleated cells in vivo is lacking except in the brain (2026, 2460, 2461). Moreover, in other retroviral systems, multinucleated cells can remain viable for long periods (1505). Recent studies suggest that necrosis can be the mechanism involved in single-cell lysis (351). In addition, rapid cell lysis could result from the contact of normal CD4$^+$ cells with HIV-1-infected cells in the absence of syncytium formation (1044).

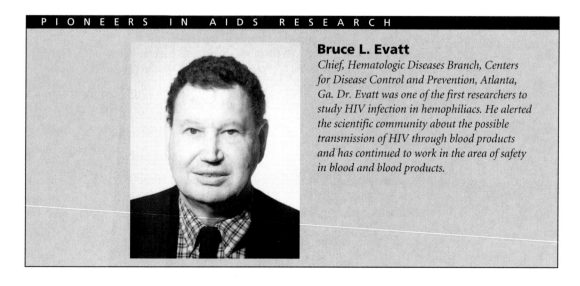

P I O N E E R S   I N   A I D S   R E S E A R C H

Bruce L. Evatt

Chief, Hematologic Diseases Branch, Centers for Disease Control and Prevention, Atlanta, Ga. Dr. Evatt was one of the first researchers to study HIV infection in hemophiliacs. He alerted the scientific community about the possible transmission of HIV through blood products and has continued to work in the area of safety in blood and blood products.

II.   Accumulation of Extrachromosomal Viral DNA and Cell Death

Besides cell:cell fusion, the cytopathology and cell death that occur during acute HIV infection in vitro can be associated with an accumulation of viral cDNA in the cytoplasm of the cells (1512, 2466). Whether this process occurs during virus infection in vivo is not known. Neurologic damage has been found to be associated with large amounts of unintegrated HIV DNA in cells in the brain (2026). The possible role of superinfection in this process is discussed in Chapter 4. Similar observations have been made with infected T cells arrested in division (2643). In this case, continued production of the unintegrated cDNA could be the cause of cell death, since viral progeny are not produced. The same phenomenon linked to cytopathology has been previously reported with in vitro infection of cells by the avian spleen necrosis virus (1277).

These observations support the conclusion that high levels of intracellular DNA can be toxic to the cell and could contribute to the initial cell killing observed in the early stages of infection (1512, 2466). Nevertheless, single-cell killing is not always associated with the accumulation of viral DNA in the cytoplasm (181, 2534) (see Chapter 9). Moreover, accumulation of extrachromosomal viral DNA sequences during a noncytopathic latent HIV infection of a monocyte cell line has been reported, although in that case, the DNA was methylated (2513).

III.   Toxicity of the Virus and Viral Proteins

Several observations link cell death with direct toxicity of the virus or viral envelope proteins (for reviews, see references 850 and 982) (Table 6.3). The mechanism of cell death is not always specified in the studies reported but can involve a disturbance of cell membrane integrity (Section I; see below) and/or apoptosis (Section IV). The relative quantities of the viral envelope protein produced by the cell (1366, 1545, 2190, 2530, 2596), as well as the extent of glycosylation of the viral envelope (1821, 2595), can determine cytopathicity. Presumably, the cytopathic effect of irradiated HIV (2190) also results from the viral envelope proteins.

In interviral recombinants, cytopathicity, including cell fusion, has been mapped to regions in gp120 (72, 426, 589, 2943) (see Chapter 8). Moreover, the cell:cell fusion that often leads to cell death can be induced directly by gp120 (430, 1545, 1546, 2530). In one study, just a doubling in the production of gp120 following HIV infection gave rise to cytopathology and cell death (2596). In another, two changes in the N-linked glycosylation sequences of gp120 produced a cytopathic strain (2595). In another report, the accumulation of gp160 without secretion of the processed envelope proteins (gp120, gp41) led to single-cell death (1333), linked to apoptosis (Section IV) (1594). Moreover, adding gp120 to PBMC or cultured brain cells caused cell killing in a dose-dependent manner (276, 664, 1221). Finally, some studies suggest that gp120 on the surface of $CD4^+$ cells (uninfected or infected) can activate complement components, leading to cell death (2617).

Gp41 can also be toxic to cells, most probably through alterations in membrane permeability (1791, 1792). Mutations in the viral gp41 (762) have modified the ex-

Table 6.3   Viral proteins that are cytotoxic for CD4+ cells[a]

gp120 (664, 1544, 1545)
gp41 (1791, 1792, 2074)
Nef (802, 803, 2861)
Tat (1529, 2320)
Vpu, Vpr (1040, 1408, 2198)

[a] Other references can be found in Section III.

tent of cytopathicity or produced cytopathic variants. Gp41 alone can induce the cell fusion that accompanies cell death (2074, 2522). Finally, the *vif* gene has been linked to cytopathology, probably by increasing replication of infectious virus (2333).

The mechanisms for the induction of cell death by the viral envelope proteins are not yet defined. Disturbances in membrane integrity could be involved, as reflected by the balloon degeneration of cells in vitro (Figure 6.1). HIV binding to and entry into cells have shown membrane discontinuities and pores in association with ballooning (749). For example, cells producing cytopathic HIV are unable to control the influx of monovalent and divalent cations that accumulate in the cell along with water (485, 850, 971, 1616, 2796) (Figure 6.2). The resulting loss in intracellular ionic strength not only leads to cell death (visualized by balloon cells) when carried to its extreme (Figure 6.1) but also, at relatively noncytopathic levels, could change the electrical potential of the cell, thereby compromising normal cell function.

The phenomenon of direct damage to the cell membrane has been demonstrated with cultured brain cells exposed to HIV gp120 (see Chapter 9). There was a

Figure 6.2   Membrane permeability changes resulting from HIV infection. PBMC were infected with HIV strains with different cytopathic properties, and the influx of radioactive potassium (K^+) was measured by standard procedures. A correlation of cytopathology with a greater ingress of K^+ was noted. UC1 is from a relatively noncytopathic HIV-1 strain (721). Experiments conducted with R. Garry.

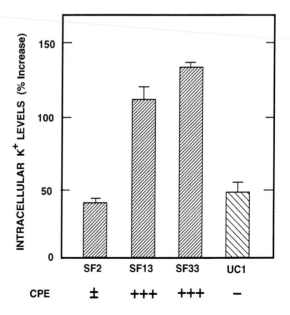

high influx of calcium concomitant with a disturbance in membrane integrity and cell function (664). The toxic effect of the viral envelope was reversed by the calcium channel antagonist nimoptene (664). This observation sparked therapeutic trials with nimoptene to reverse neurologic abnormalities during HIV infection (1563); the results have not yet been reported. Conceivably, the glycosylated HIV protein expressed on the surface of the infected cell disturbs membrane permeability in some manner, leading to cell death. Alternatively, the viral envelope could induce N-methyl-D-aspartate (NMDA) receptor-mediated neurotoxicity (1564). As noted in Section IV, gp120 can also be involved in the induction of cell death by apoptosis.

Other viral proteins can be involved in cell toxicity. Changes in cell membrane potential have been demonstrated after exposure to the Nef protein, which contains a small region with some sequence homology to scorpion toxin (2861). Soluble Nef can be cytotoxic for human $CD4^+$ T cells (803). This viral protein, expressed on the cell surface, could cause the death of normal uninfected $CD4^+$ cells by cell contact (802). Domains on other viral proteins (e.g., Tat and gp41) have also shown similarities to a neurotoxin (851). Moreover, the Tat protein causes the death of neuronal cells in culture (2320) and can cause apoptosis of $CD4^+$ cells (1529) (Section IV). In addition, Vpu and Vpr could affect processes affecting cell viability through their ion channel activities (for a review, see reference 1408).

The cytopathic effects of HIV also have been linked to a cellular activation process involving gp41 and CD4 in which tyrosine phosphorylation of a newly recognized 30-kDa protein was detected (493). Inhibition of this phosphorylation led to reduced syncytium formation, apparently related to a block in cell mitosis (2674). This mechanism resembles the effect of HIV envelope and Vpr on $CD4^+$ cells, in which a block in cell replication at the G_2 phase can result in apoptosis (1040, 1341, 2198) (Section IV). The question whether modifying specific intracellular signals would decrease $CD4^+$ cell loss via this process merits further study. Moreover, some evidence suggests that cellular protein synthesis is reduced during HIV infection of cells; a degradation of cellular mRNA may be involved (25).

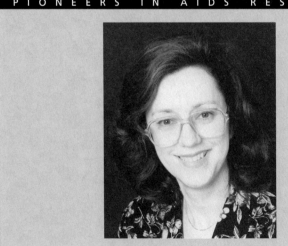

Margaret A. Fischl

Professor of Medicine, University of Miami, Miami, Fla. Dr. Fischl was one of the first physicians to devote clinical programs to the diagnosis and care of AIDS patients, particularly women and Haitians.

IV.   Apoptosis

A.   General Observations

Apoptosis is an alternative general mechanism for cell death besides necrosis (Figure 6.3) and has received increased attention in recent years. The phenomenon is a normal physiological response during embryogenesis, thymocyte maturation, and other differentiation processes and can be elicited in cells by a variety of stimuli, including virus infection (495, 872, 1274, 1275; for reviews, see references 2674 and 2675). Apoptosis requires cell activation, protein synthesis, and the function of a Ca^{2+}-dependent endogenous endonuclease that fragments the cellular DNA into small, measurable nucleotide units (Figure 6.4). It may involve cells sensitized by interleukin-2 (IL-2) to antigen recognition (2197). The process can be blocked by the administration of IL-2, which appears to suppress the down-modulation of *bcl*-2 expression (14).

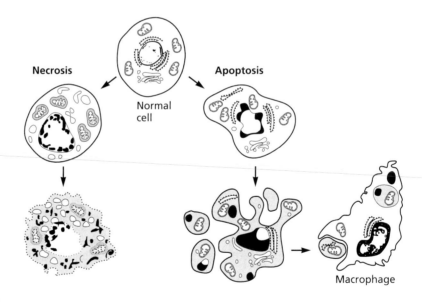

Figure 6.3 Processes of cell death. The sequential ultrastructural changes occurring in apoptosis and necrosis are shown. In apoptosis (right), a normal cell undergoes compaction and segregation of chromatin into sharply delineated masses that lie against the nuclear envelope. Condensation of the cytoplasm and convolution of the nuclear and cellular outlines occur. Rapid progression of the process is associated within minutes with nuclear fragmentation, marked convolution of the cellular surface, and the development of pedunculative protuberances. The protuberances then separate to produce membrane-bound apoptotic bodies, which are phagocytosed and digested by macrophages. In necrosis (left), chromatin is clumped into ill-defined masses and gross-volume organelles, and folliculin densities appear in the matrix. Membranes break down, and the cell disintegrates at the late stages. Figure modified from reference 1274 with permission.

B. ## Mechanisms

Accelerated T-cell apoptosis in HIV infection can be related to a variety of mechanisms (922) (for a review, see reference 2675). These include induction by specific viral proteins (e.g., Tat), interaction of the HIV envelope protein with the CD4 molecule (cross-linking), and interactions of cytokines with their receptors (particularly the Fas and Fas-ligand [Fas L] system) (Table 6.4). In addition, disorders in antigen-presenting cells (e.g., macrophages and dendritic cells) leading to defects in T-cell activity as well as superantigen activity (Section V) can be involved. In general, whether in the peripheral blood or lymph nodes, apoptosis is increased in immune cells (B and T lymphocytes) during HIV infection, concomitant with a state of immune activation (925, 1880). Some studies suggest that enhanced apoptosis is related to a high sensitivity to stimulation by Fas (718, 2506).

In this connection, most studies indicate that cell proliferation alone, as occurs with exposure to phytohemagglutinin, does not lead to apoptosis of CD4$^+$ cells from HIV-infected individuals; cell activation is needed. In support of this conclusion, cross-linking CD4 or stimulation with major histocompatibility complex (MHC)-restricted class II recall antigens (e.g., tetanus toxin) or pokeweed mitogen can cause up to 40% cell death by apoptosis in CD4$^+$ cells from asymptomatic HIV-infected subjects (130, 953, 2009).

C. ## Role of Virus Replication and Cytokine Production

Both CD4$^+$ and CD8$^+$ lymphocytes of HIV-infected individuals can undergo apoptosis, but the process appears to be most evident in CD4$^+$ cells (922, 923, 953, 1449, 1764). Apoptosis has been linked to active HIV-1 replication (1449, 1681, 2655) and disease progression (925, 2024), but whether the infected cells or the uninfected cells (or both) are the major targets of this process is not yet known. Some studies strongly suggest that apoptosis occurs primarily in uninfected cells (478, 753). As noted above, apoptosis has been reported in T cells during other viral infections (e.g., Epstein-Barr virus [EBV], and lymphocytic choriomeningitis virus) (2197, 2734). Apoptosis has been observed in feline CD4$^+$ cells with certain strains of the feline leukemia retrovirus (2269). Furthermore, enhanced CD8$^+$ cell apoptosis has been noted in HIV-infected children in whom EBV is reactivated (1438).

Table 6.4 Causes of apoptosis in HIV infection[a]

1. Immune activation (925, 1880); stimulation with recall antigens or mitogens (953, 2009)
2. Interaction of HIV envelope protein with the CD4 molecule (cross-linking) (130)
3. Exposure to viral proteins (e.g., Env, Tat, and Vpr) (1040, 1450, 1529, 1706, 2655)
4. Exposure to cytokines (e.g., TGF-β) (478, 1655)
5. Interaction of cytokines with specific receptors (Fas and Fas ligand) (8)
6. High sensitivity of cells to Fas stimulation (718, 2506)
7. Superantigen activity (Section V)

[a] For other citations, see the text and references 922 and 2675.

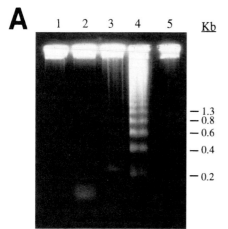

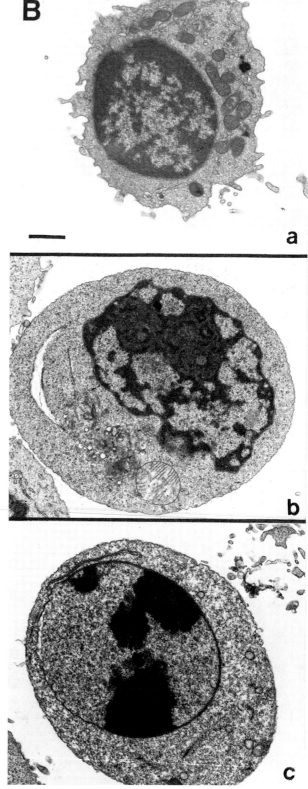

Figure 6.4. Activation-induced apoptosis in human CD4$^+$ peripheral blood T lymphocytes following CD4 ligation by anti-CD4 antibody or by anti-gp120. (A) Agarose gel electrophoresis of total DNA after treatment of cells with anti-TCR (lane 2), with gp120 cross-linked with polyclonal anti-gp120 antibody and then incubated with anti-TCR (lane 3), with 500 rads of gamma radiation (lane 4), and with gp120 cross-linked with polyclonal anti-gp120 (lane 5). Lane 1 shows untreated cells. The typical ladder pattern of DNA digestion associated with apoptosis is observed only after gamma irradiation and the cross-linking experiments conducted with anti-gp120 and anti-TCR antibodies. (B) Ultrastructural morphology of apoptotic T cells induced by ligation of TCR after gp120-CD4 interaction. (a) Untreated CD4$^+$ cells. (b and c) CD4$^+$ T cells treated with the recombinant chimeric protein gp120 plus antibody to gp120 and then incubated with anti-TCR. No apoptotic cells were seen in the control sample (a). Apoptosis in its early (b) and late (c) stages was observed in the treated samples. Bar, 1 μm. Figures courtesy of T. Finkel. Reproduced in part from reference 130 with permission.

The apoptotic process involving CD4$^+$ cells is related in part to alterations in cytokines. Some cytokines (e.g., IL-4) can increase apoptosis in macrophages by countering the protective effects of other cytokines (e.g., tumor necrosis factor alpha [TNF-α], and gamma interferon [IFN-γ]) (1655). In some studies, IL-1α and IL-2 used together (but not alone) prevented apoptosis of CD4$^+$ cells from HIV-infected individuals (922). As reviewed in Chapter 9, CD4$^+$ cells can be separated into TH1 and TH2 (T helper) cell subsets, depending on the cytokines they produce. TH1 cells make IL-2 and IFN-γ, whereas TH2 cells produce IL-4 and IL-10. These cells and their cytokines are also referred to as type 1 and type 2, respectively. In some studies, selective rescue from glucocorticoid-induced apoptosis has been observed with the different CD4$^+$ cell subsets: IL-4 protects TH2 cells, whereas IL-2 protects TH1 cells (3000). Such interactions may be involved in the normal immune response.

In related studies, removal of IL-2 has caused apoptosis in murine cytotoxic effector cells (672). Moreover, with CD4$^+$ cells, some results suggest that type 1 cytokines (e.g., IL-2 and IFN-γ) prevent apoptosis whereas type 2 cytokines (e.g., IL-4 and IL-10) can accelerate this process (479, 718) (see Chapter 9, Section I.G, and Chapter 11, Section II). It is therefore somewhat surprising that type 1 CD4$^+$ cells appear to be more susceptible to HIV gp120-sensitized apoptosis than are type 2 cells (8) (Table 11.1). For example, enhanced expression of the Fas ligand by HIV-infected macrophages could increase apoptosis of uninfected CD4$^+$ T lymphocytes (113a). Differences in expression of Fas (CD95) or the Fas ligand might be involved. Apoptosis can be inhibited by anti-CD95 neutralizing antibodies or antibodies to the CD95 ligand. Type 1 cells, but not type 2 cells, appear to express cell-associated and soluble CD95L. The resistance of type 2 cells, therefore, may be due to a relatively reduced production of CD95L (8). Alternatively, this resistance could reflect a difference in distribution of receptors for the type 1 and type 2 cytokines on the CD4$^+$ cells. These possibilities need further study. Transforming growth factor β (TGF-β) has also been identified as another cytokine that can mediate antigen-stimulated CD4$^+$ cell apoptosis (478).

In other studies of CD4$^+$ cell subsets, the memory T cells were found to be more susceptible to the cytopathic effects of a T-cell-line-tropic virus (451) whereas both naive and memory cells could be infected similarly. Cell death appeared to result in part from apoptosis, but the mechanism was not determined. It could be mediated by a particular viral envelope (see above). The role of this enhanced killing of memory CD4$^+$ cells by SI strains in HIV pathogenesis remains to be determined.

D.   Effect of Viral Proteins

The viral protein Tat has been shown to induce apoptosis in normal, uninfected CD4$^+$ lymphocytes in association with an activation of cyclin-dependent kinases (1529). Tat also enhanced the apoptosis of T cells exposed to antibodies to CD3, Fas, and TNF-α (1706). In contrast, Tat-expressing cells appeared to be resistant to the cytopathic effect of Tat as well as to other inducers of apoptosis (1706). Conceivably, by activating uninfected cells, Tat makes them sensitive to processes leading to cell death (e.g., Fas:Fas ligand interaction and antigen recognition). In this regard, $CD4^+$ cells, activated by immobilized CD3 monoclonal antibodies and exposed to soluble Tat, underwent apoptosis (2965). In the Tat-expressing (and, conceivably, virus-infected) cells, this process was prevented. This observation could explain the absence of apoptosis in the HIV-infected cells found in lymphoid tissue and in the brain (see above). The extent of HIV-1 replication and perhaps the virus strain can influence this process (1681).

In certain studies, the Tat protein has been found to protect human T cells and epithelial cells, as well as rat neuronal cells, from apoptosis (2966). Thus, a possible role of this viral protein in the cell proliferation preceding B-cell transformation and, perhaps, the induction of Kaposi's sarcoma has been considered (2966) (see Chapter 12). Nevertheless, it is perplexing how Tat can suppress cell function (2775) and induce cytotoxicity (2320) and apoptosis (1529) (see above) in some cases and prevent cell death in others.

Another viral protein, gp120, can elicit apoptosis alone, through virus:antibody complexes (2655), or by a gp120:gp41:CD4 interaction (1450). Cross-linking of the gp120 bound to human $CD4^+$ lymphocytes followed by T-cell activation by anti-CD3 antibodies has caused apoptosis of these cells (Figure 6.4) (130). The importance in this process of monocytes expressing FasL has been reported (2007). Other studies suggest that this process requires the cytoplasmic tail of CD4 and is most efficient when p56 on the CD4 molecule is intact (522). Thus, apoptosis can result from a signal transduction type of response. This rapid induction of apoptosis by the interaction of the viral envelope with CD4 can be demonstrated as well in the cell:cell transmission of HIV (1652). Finally, as noted previously, the HIV envelope and Vpr can cause apoptosis of $CD4^+$ cells by blocking their replication at the G2 stage of the cell cycle (1040, 1341).

Apparently, $CD4^+$ cells from HIV-1-infected chimpanzees or SIV-infected African green monkeys do not undergo apoptosis (922, 924, 2421), even after expo-

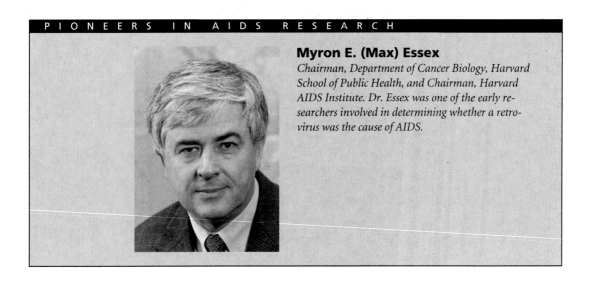

PIONEERS IN AIDS RESEARCH

Myron E. (Max) Essex
Chairman, Department of Cancer Biology, Harvard School of Public Health, and Chairman, Harvard AIDS Institute. Dr. Essex was one of the early researchers involved in determining whether a retrovirus was the cause of AIDS.

sure to Tat (688). These animals do not generally develop disease. In contrast, apoptosis was observed in CD4$^+$ cells from SIV-infected macaques that can advance to AIDS (922). This distinction was most evident when CD4$^+$ cells and not CD8$^+$ cells were compared (717), even under conditions of activation (924). Thus, the lack of a pathogenic course in some animals could be explained by the absence of the apoptotic pathway or could be related to the extent of immune system activation. Levels of expression of activation markers on CD4$^+$ and CD8$^+$ cells are not increased in HIV-1-infected chimpanzees compared to uninfected animals (924). We have also noted apoptosis in CD4$^+$ cells from HIV-2-infected baboons (134b). These animals show a loss of CD4$^+$ cells with time; the finding of apoptosis in their cells may presage the development of disease.

E.   Conclusions

Considering all these features of apoptosis, it is not known if this process plays an important role in HIV pathogenesis. Because the studies thus far have used different techniques and different cell populations, consistent results are not always available. For example, unstimulated CD4$^+$ cells removed from infected individuals do not undergo apoptosis (1764), but PBMC do (2009). A role of gp120 in this process, whether cross-linked or not or whether the cells are activated or not, has not been confirmed in all studies (1681). This viral protein does, however, seem to be involved. Thus, the potential factors influencing apoptosis (Table 6.4), and the extent of this process in vivo (from activation), are not yet fully defined. HIV-1 strains cytopathic for macrophages appear to induce the death of these cells by necrosis (177). Nevertheless, in attempts to find alternative reasons for a loss of CD4$^+$ lymphocytes, apoptosis provides a provocative area of study (see Chapter 13). Importantly, approaches to prevent apoptosis in CD4$^+$ cells (e.g., via *bcl-2* expression) (75, 2353) could sustain the viability of uninfected CD4$^+$ cells and might allow immune control of virus production by infected cells. Perhaps normal function could return to the infected cells in which virus has been sufficiently suppressed (Chapters 11 and 13).

V.   Role of Superantigens

HIV may have a peptide that acts like a superantigen that can attach to CD4$^+$ lymphocytes by one portion of the MHC class II molecule (e.g., the alpha but not the beta chain) and the beta-chain region on the T-cell receptor (TCR) (Color Plate 9, following p. 188) (see Chapter 11 and Color Plate 12 [following p. 188] for a description of viral antigen interaction with the TCR). This phenomenon could induce cell death by the process of apoptosis just described (491, 922; for reviews, see references 531 and 2864). Importantly, it could lead to an imbalance in the T-cell repertoire by expansions and deletions with "gaps" that may compromise the robustness of the immune response (see Chapter 11). Some support for this concept comes from the observation that individuals with AIDS show a disproportionate loss of T-cells that have certain T-cell receptor beta chains (566, 1090, 1158, 1444, 2202). Furthermore, in many HIV-1-infected individuals, a Vβ-specific (e.g., Vβ8) anergy has been found in both CD4$^+$ and CD8$^+$ lymphocytes (558). One report suggests that HIV replicates more efficiently in CD4$^+$ cells that express certain Vβ genes (e.g., Vβ12), presumably because they are influenced by a superantigen-like activity (643).

Superantigens have been considered responsible for the loss of T cells in other retrovirus infections, such as those with the murine mammary tumor virus and the murine model of AIDS (491, 1139, 2913). The nucleocapsid of the rabies virus has also been reported to be a possible superantigen (1400).

Despite these findings in other systems, the changes in T-cell repertoire observed are not the same for each cohort of subjects examined and can be influenced by environmental and other external factors (for reviews, see references 531 and 2864). Considering this fact, some studies do not support a role of superantigens in Vβ deletion and loss of CD4$^+$ cells in HIV infection (418, 532, 1936, 2127). Moreover, whether the alterations in the PBMC reflect changes in the lymphoid tissue needs to be examined (531). Thus, the phenomenon needs further evaluation. If there is a superantigen-induced loss of T cells in HIV infection, the particular antigen involved has also not been determined. Conceivably, it might come from other organisms or foreign proteins present during HIV infection.

A reduction in the number of B cells expressing the immunoglobulin V$_H$3 gene product has also been described. This subpopulation of normal B cells was found to bind to HIV gp120 by a membrane IgM. This interaction induced immunoglobulin secretion, suggesting functional activation (175). A portion of gp120 identified recently as a discontinuous epitope spanning the V4 domain and the amino-terminal region flanking the C4 domain appears to serve as a superantigen for V$_H$3 B cells (1248). This viral protein could induce some of the B-cell responses observed in HIV infection (Chapter 10).

Chapter 6 SALIENT FEATURES

1. HIV induces cell fusion by an interaction of its envelope gp120 with CD4. Co-receptors on the cell surface may help in enabling this virus envelope:cell membrane fusion, which can result in cell death.

2. Accumulation of viral extrachromosomal DNA can be responsible for cell death.

3. HIV envelope proteins can induce cell death through changes in cell membrane integrity, permitting an influx of monovalent and divalent cations with water, leading to balloon degeneration.

4. HIV infection can be associated with apoptosis, resulting from the direct action of viral proteins (e.g., Tat), gp120 binding to the CD4 molecule, disorders in antigen-presenting cells, and superantigens. Immune system activation is needed to induce apoptosis.

5. Apoptosis may be more common in uninfected than infected CD4$^+$ cells. The process can be observed in other cells, including CD8$^+$ T lymphocytes, B lymphocytes, and neuronal cells.

6. Apoptosis is influenced by cytokine alterations. Type 1 cytokines can prevent apoptosis, whereas type 2 cytokines can enhance the process. TGF-β can also mediate antigen-stimulated CD4$^+$ cell apoptosis.

7. The Tat protein is associated with the induction of apoptosis but can protect human T cells, epithelial cells, and neuronal cells from this process. The role of this protein appears to be pleiotropic, as demonstrated by its ability to suppress cell function and to prevent cell death, as well as to induce cytopathicity and apoptosis.

8. HIV gp120 and Vpr can cause apoptosis of CD4$^+$ cells by blocking viral replication at the G2 stage of the cell cycle.

9. Some macrophage-tropic HIV strains induce the death of macrophages by necrosis.

10. Superantigens can play a role in up-regulating cell replication and inducing cell activation associated with apoptosis. A portion of gp120 can also serve as a superantigen for V_H3 B cells and thus could induce some of the B-cell responses observed in HIV infection.

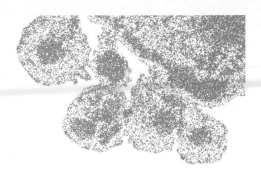

Heterogeneity of HIV and Its Relation to Pathogenesis

7

TWO MAJOR TYPES OF AIDS VIRUSES, HIV-1 AND HIV-2, CAN BE distinguished. Several studies that were conducted after many HIV strains had been isolated indicated quite early that these viruses are highly heterogeneous and exist as subtypes with a variety of biologic, serologic, and molecular features. These include

- cellular tropism
- replication kinetics
- level of virus production
- modulation of CD4 expression
- cytopathicity
- plaque- or syncytium-forming ability
- latency and inducibility
- genetic structure
- sensitivity to neutralizing or enhancing antibodies

These characteristics of HIV strains and how they could influence disease are discussed in this chapter. Other distinguishing features defined by laboratory studies include sensitivity to soluble CD4 (sCD4) inactivation, sensitivity of the viral envelope to proteolytic cleavage, and stability of the gp120-gp41 complex. These properties are discussed in Chapters 3 and 8. The features of viral diversity, discussed in this chapter, relate to HIV-2 as well as HIV-1. Some specific findings with HIV-2 are covered in the first section.

I. HIV-2

A. Discovery and Characteristics

Shortly after the identification of HIV-1, a second AIDS virus was recovered in Portugal from AIDS patients from West Africa, particularly the Cape Verde Islands and Senegal (462). This virus, after cloning and sequence analysis, differed by more than 55% from the previous HIV-1 strains isolated and was antigenically distinct. Thus, it was designated a new type of HIV (462, 489, 975) (Figure 1.3). Other HIV-2 strains were subsequently isolated from individuals from Guinea Bissau, The Gambia, and Ivory Coast (32, 371, 722, 1345, 1381, 2424). The major serologic difference between HIV-2 and HIV-1 resides in the envelope glycoproteins (Figure 7.1). Antibodies to HIV-2 will generally cross-react with the Gag and Pol proteins of HIV-1 but might not detect HIV-1 envelope proteins and vice versa (463, 894). For this reason, blood banks are now required to use enzyme-linked immunoasorbent assays (ELISAs) consisting of both HIV-1 and HIV-2 proteins (1961). Sera from some individuals from Africa have reacted with both HIV-1 and HIV-2 proteins, suggesting cross-reactivity or dual infection. In certain cases, infection by both types of virus has been documented, but the prevalence of this event is not known (722, 869, 2062, 2195).

HIV-2 glycoproteins appear to cross-react serologically with envelope proteins from strains of SIV (463) (Figure 7.1), a complex group of primate lentiviruses.

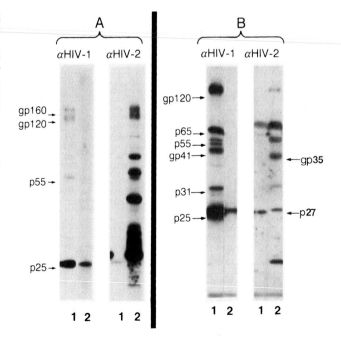

Figure 7.1 Immunoblot analyses showing antibody reactions with HIV-1, HIV-2, and SIV proteins. (A) Serum from an African patient with HIV-1 and HIV-2 infections was tested for reactivity against electrophoretically separated cell lysates containing HIV-1 (lane 1) and SIV$_{mac}$ (lane 2). Note the differential detection of the envelope gp160 and gp120 proteins. (B) Proteins from purified HIV-1 (lane 1) and HIV-2 (lane 2) isolates were reacted with serum from an HIV-1- or HIV-2-infected individual. Reprinted from reference 721 with permission.

Some SIV isolates can give rise to an AIDS-like disease in certain primate species (rhesus macaque) but are relatively nonpathogenic in their species of origin (e.g., SIV_{agm} in African green monkeys) (for reviews, see references 847 and 1504). Since antibodies to SIV and HIV-2 cross-react and their sequences are similar, some investigators believe that HIV-2 was derived from SIV sometime in the near distant past (see Chapter 1) (694, 1076, 1685).

B.   Epidemiology of HIV-2 Infection

HIV-2 strains have been recovered from patients in several parts of Africa, primarily in the western region. They have been detected in individuals in Europe, the United States, and South America (1961, 2848). Most recently, HIV-2 infections have been increasing rapidly in India (1660). In the United States, as of June 30, 1997, 73 HIV-2-infected individuals had been reported to the Centers for Disease Control and Prevention, of whom 49 were of West African origin (1763). The spread of HIV-2 throughout the world, therefore, has not been as extensive as that of HIV-1.

Some investigators believe that the transmissibility and pathogenic potential of HIV-2 strains are lower than those of HIV-1 (66, 1237, 2071, 2134). For example, some data have suggested a five- to ninefold difference in infectivity of HIV-2 compared with HIV-1 per sexual act. Observations on mother-child transmission have shown that HIV-2 transmission is 15- to 20-fold less than that of HIV-1 (74). In a study of mother-child transmission in the Ivory Coast, perinatal transmission of HIV-1 (24.7%) was significantly higher than that of HIV-2 (1.2%) (21). In Burkina Faso, however, HIV-2 appears to be transmitted as readily as HIV-1 from mother to child (27.8 and 29.5%, respectively) (2141).

In terms of levels of disease, individuals infected solely by HIV-2 have developed AIDS, but some reports indicate that people infected with HIV-2 survive longer than those infected with HIV-1 (2872, 2873). In one study of femate commercial sex workers in Senegal, the HIV-2-infected women showed a markedly reduced rate in loss of $CD4^+$ lymphocytes compared to HIV-1-infected women (649a).

The reasons for these potential differences in HIV-2 transmissibility and pathology are not clear (Table 7.1). The epidemiologic observations could reflect a low viral load in HIV-2-infected individuals (585, 2510). In support of the decreased replicative ability of HIV-2 (and perhaps, therefore, a reduction in emergence of pathogenic variants) is the observation that for HIV-2 infection, the intra-patient nucleotide variability rate in the *env* gene was 0.6% for healthy individuals and 2% for those with clinical AIDS. For HIV-1-infected patients, the V3 sequence heterogeneity was as high as 6.1% (2355; for a review, see reference 1674). These findings cannot yet be explained but might result from a strong host immune re-

Table 7.1 Features of HIV-2 that may explain a slow pathogenic course and reduction in transmission

1. Low virus load (585, 2510)
2. Neutralizing antibodies (221)
3. Cellular immune response
4. Reduced cytopathicity (721, 1015)
5. Lack of modulation of CD4 protein on the cell surface (721)

sponse that limits the replication of HIV-2. For example, autologous neutralizing antibodies have been found more frequently in HIV-2-infected than in HIV-1-infected subjects (221). Studies on cell-mediated immune responses have not been reported.

Another potentially relevant observation with some HIV-2 strains has been their reduced cytopathic properties in cell culture and lack of modulation of the CD4 antigen on the cell surface (371, 721, 1345, 1385). These findings could indicate the presence of relatively noncytopathic strains of HIV-2 in certain populations (721). Those observations could explain the reduced pathogenic course suggested by the epidemiologic studies cited above. An HIV-1 strain with noncytotoxic features has yet to be reported, although non-syncytium-inducing (NSI) isolates and *nef*-deleted mutant viruses may be less pathogenic in the host (see Section IV).

Another study of Senegalese women has suggested that infection with HIV-2 could protect the individual against subsequent infection by HIV-1 (2701). The HIV-2-infected women had a lower incidence of HIV-1 infection compared to the overall prevalence of HIV-1 in the women studied. In contrast, in preliminary short-term longitudinal studies, HIV-1 infection did not appear to protect against HIV-2 infection (2701). These findings on protection by HIV-2 have been questioned (82) and require further evaluation.

C. HIV-2 Genome: Molecular Features

The genetic sequences of individual HIV-2 strains can differ substantially, and, like HIV-1, HIV-2 can be separated into sequence subtypes according to genetic relationships (Figure 7.2) (145, 1890). The genome of HIV-2 is very similar to that of HIV-1 except for the absence of *vpu* and the presence of *vpx* (Figure 1.3); *vpx* appears to be a duplication of *vpr* (2709). Five distinct sequence subtypes of HIV-2 (A to E) have been identified (837). Subtype A is the most commonly isolated subtype thus far. Most recently a new subtype, designated F and having very divergent

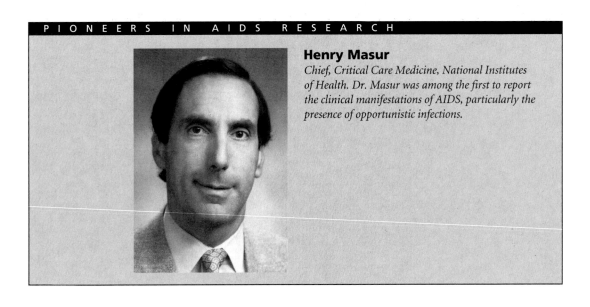

Henry Masur
Chief, Critical Care Medicine, National Institutes of Health. Dr. Masur was among the first to report the clinical manifestations of AIDS, particularly the presence of opportunistic infections.

Figure 7.2 A neighbor-joining tree showing the phylogenetic relations between HIV-2 and SIV *gag* gene sequences. The subtype classification of the HIV-2 sequences was proposed by Gao et al. (837). The SIV sequences are classified according to their natural host. It can be seen that the different subtypes of HIV-2 and SIV are approximately equidistant, suggesting that they may have arisen around the same time. Figure courtesy of C. Kuiken.

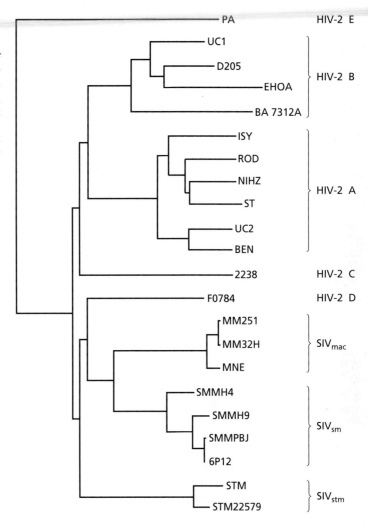

transmembrane envelope sequences, has been identified in an infected person in Sierra Leone (416a). Subtype D appears to be particularly closely related to SIV strains, leading some researchers to conclude that the SIV from sooty mangabeys has entered humans on more than one occasion (837) (see Chapter 1).

II. Differences in Cellular Host Range among HIV-1 Strains

A. General Observations

In Chapter 4, we reviewed the variety of cells and cell lines susceptible to HIV-1 infection in vitro. Ongoing studies continually demonstrate the wide and varied cellular host range of both HIV-1 and HIV-2 strains (Table 4.2). When HIV-1 was initially recovered, the virus was grown in mitogen-stimulated normal peripheral blood mononuclear cells (PBMC) (146). Because with time the cells died, fresh PBMC had to be added on a regular basis. After a few months of study, however, the virus was shown to infect and grow persistently in established lines of T and B cells that were not killed by the virus. These lines were useful in growing large quantities of HIV-1 through cell culture procedures (1510, 1521, 1813, 2122). Established cell lines soon became the source of screening tests used for detecting antibodies to HIV (163, 1230).

One early observation on HIV diversity, however, was that many HIV-1 strains could not be propagated in established human T-cell lines (96, 720, 1507). Subsequent studies with several independent HIV-1 isolates have since demonstrated that some can grow in certain established human T, B, and monocyte cell lines and others cannot (96, 372, 486, 746, 1521, 2332, 2429). Nevertheless, nearly all the isolates can replicate in peripheral blood CD4$^+$ lymphocytes, except for cells lacking CCR-5 expression (e.g., NSI strains) (see Chapter 3). Certain strains replicate well in primary macrophages, whereas others grow efficiently only in peripheral blood CD4$^+$ T cells (see below) (372, 863, 864, 2429, 2788).

These early findings led to the subsequent demonstration that T-cell-line-tropic viruses are those that readily induce cell syncytia in T-cell lines. The macrophage-tropic viruses are generally NSI when assayed in T-cell lines. This feature is not surprising since they cannot grow well in these cells (1347). These differences have now been explained in part by the specific coreceptor used by NSI and SI strains (Tables 3.3 and 7.2). Several NSI strains, however, can induce cytopathology and syncytia in CD4$^+$ lymphocytes (2947). Moreover, some syncytium-inducing (SI) HIV-1 strains are both macrophage and T-cell-line tropic (429), and some NSI viruses do not replicate well in macrophages (see below). Thus, the SI viruses are distinguished biologically from the NSI viruses primarily by their growth and cytopathic properties in T-cell lines, particularly MT-2 cells (1347). They also differ generally in other features discussed in the book, particularly in the coreceptor used for virus entry into cells (see Chapter 3) (Table 7.2).

In recent studies with T-cell clones, SI isolates have shown a more consistent ability to infect CD4$^+$ lymphocytes than have NSI isolates (780). This finding could have relevance to the extent of CD4$^+$ cell loss by people infected with SI viruses and also to the relative sensitivity of different PBMC to infection (Figure 5.2). In other studies, however, macrophage-tropic NSI strains appeared to infect all types of CD4$^+$ lymphocytes, whereas T-cell-line-tropic HIV isolates grew primarily in TH2-type cells (2640) (see Chapter 11). The results could explain the dominance of NSI strains early in infection and the loss of TH1-type cells as a person advances to disease (see Chapter 13). NSI strains can be associated with a loss of CD4$^+$ cells (1859) and the development of AIDS (see Chapter 13). Furthermore, when unstimulated PBMC are used, some investigators have found that human cord blood mononuclear cells are more susceptible to macrophage-tropic NSI isolates than to SI strains (2209). With unstimulated adult PBMC, the opposite observations were made (2209). All these results need to be reanalyzed in light of further knowledge about the relative expression of different coreceptors for HIV on the cell surface (see Chapter 3).

Some HIV-1 (usually SI) strains can infect B-cell lines and even B lymphocytes in culture, particularly if Epstein-Barr virus (EBV) is present (560, 1051, 1813).

Table 7.2 Characteristics of NSI and SI isolates of HIV[a]

Characteristic	Associated with:	
	NSI	SI
Growth in macrophages	+ +	±
Growth in T-cell lines	−	+ +
Cytopathicity[b]	−	+ +
Sensitivity to sCD4	−	+ +
Use of CD4 receptor	+ +	+ +
Chemokine coreceptor usage	CCR-5	CXCR-4
Associated with substantial loss of CD4$^+$ cells	−	+ +
Associated with CNS disease	+ +	−

[a] Further differences have been reported but need confirmation (Section II).
[b] Usually defined by induction of CPE in MT-2 cells. Some NSI viruses can cause CPE in PBMC.

Likewise, viruses can be distinguished by their ability to grow in bowel- and brain-derived cell lines as well as in primary cells from fetal and adult organs (see Chapter 4) (432, 746, 2332, 2429; for a review, see reference 372).

Even in the highly sensitive target cell for all HIV strains, the CD4$^+$ lymphocyte, variations in virus production can be observed. An HIV-1 or HIV-2 strain might grow to high titers in the PBMC of only certain individuals (Figure 5.2) (371, 486, 720). In some cases, up to 1,000-fold differences in virus replication can be demonstrated (486). No HIV strain has been found that grows well in PBMC from all individuals; likewise, PBMC from one individual have not shown an equal susceptibility to infection by all HIV isolates. In certain rare cases, as noted above, the PBMC (both CD4$^+$ lymphocytes and macrophages) are very resistant to infection by NSI strains, since the cells lack the required CCR-5 coreceptor (see Chapter 3) (508, 1568, 2181).

Similar differences in HIV-1 infection of peripheral blood macrophages can be demonstrated (543, 2740) (see below). Thus, it is conceivable that one virus infecting two individuals could induce different pathogenic pathways, depending on its ability to grow and spread in the peripheral lymphocytes of each person. The susceptibility to virus replication appears to be determined by the genetic makeup of the host cell (e.g., cell surface molecules and intracellular factors) (Table 7.1) (see Chapter 5).

B.   Macrophage Tropism

In reference to growth in macrophages, there is no evidence for a purely macrophage-tropic virus. Low-level virus replication in these infected cells can be detected with HIV-1 strains considered to be non-macrophage tropic (2741) (Table 7.2). The mechanism has been related with some viruses to coreceptor usage (see Chapter 3) but also can involve a block in reverse transcription (see Chapter 5) (see below). It is noteworthy that after cocultivation with CD4$^+$ lymphocytes, virus can be readily recovered from the inoculated macrophages, supporting a role for cellular factors in controlling virus replication (2413).

In general, all HIV strains grow well in CD4$^+$ lymphocytes, although there are some exceptions (see above). HIV-1 isolates that preferentially infect T-cell lines can be identified (Section II.C), and are called T-cell-line-tropic viruses. Macrophage-tropic viruses replicate well in both peripheral blood macrophages and CD4$^+$ lymphocytes (863). In both cell types, the CD4 protein on the cell surface is the major receptor for entry (502, 543). Some investigators reported that HIV-1 strains that were initially isolated from macrophages of infected individuals would grow primarily or only in macrophages (1413, 2121, 2419). In these cases, the ability of these viruses to infect CD4$^+$ T lymphocytes was not well documented. After cocultivation of infected macrophages with T cells, a virus with a dual host range has been demonstrated (2394). In other studies, fresh isolates from PBMC that were initially macrophage-tropic were found, after growth in cell culture, to change into non-macrophage-tropic strains that retained their ability to replicate in CD4$^+$ lymphocytes. In this case, selection of a biologic variant most probably occurred in culture. Other investigators have reported that some HIV-1 strains grow better in macrophages than in CD4$^+$ lymphocytes (863, 864, 2419), but these findings have not been substantiated (1505a).

While macrophage-tropic strains have been characterized as noncytotoxic (see Chapter 4) (Table 7.2), several can induce cytopathic effect (CPE) in PBMC (1505a, 2947). Moreover, some HIV-1 strains grow to high titers in macrophages and can be cytopathic in these cells (177, 429, 1924). Usually, differentiation of monocytes to macrophages is needed for efficient infection (2224, 2420, 2743) (see also Chapter 5). However, these cells are much less susceptible to HIV once terminal differentiation has occurred (1505a, 2743). In addition, HIV-1 strains can differ in their ability to replicate in macrophages from different tissues (e.g., lungs) (2129). Macrophages from neonates appear to have an increased susceptibility to HIV-1 infection compared to macrophages from adults (2548).

Another suggested characteristic of macrophage-tropic strains is resistance to sCD4 inactivation (1833), but this feature can be separated from tropism (see Chap-

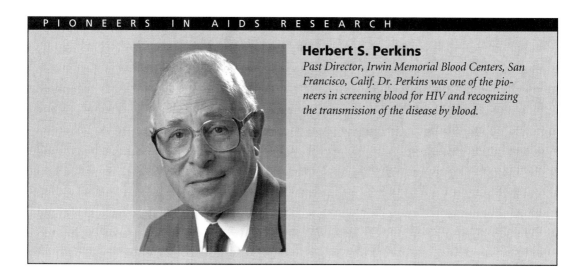

PIONEERS IN AIDS RESEARCH

Herbert S. Perkins
Past Director, Irwin Memorial Blood Centers, San Francisco, Calif. Dr. Perkins was one of the pioneers in screening blood for HIV and recognizing the transmission of the disease by blood.

ters 3 and 8) (2570). Moreover, resistance of the V3 loop to cleavage during infection has been considered a common feature of macrophage-tropic NSI strains (962, 2859) (Table 7.2). This characteristic would not seem to be a determinant for infection of macrophages, since exceptions can be found (see Chapter 8) (962, 2015, 2570).

C. T-Cell-Line Tropism

When T-cell lines are used in studies of cellular host range, differences among strains can be appreciated. As noted above, nearly all HIV strains can grow to different levels in CD4$^+$ lymphocytes from PBMC, but viruses can differ substantially in their ability to replicate in T-cell lines (720, 2657, 2660). The T-cell-line-tropic viruses are generally associated with SI HIV-1 strains recovered from infected individuals late in the course of infection (Section IX). As noted previously, they generally use the CXCR-4 coreceptor for entry into cells (Table 7.2). T-cell-line and macrophage tropisms are not often found as properties of the same strain, although viruses with this dual tropism and the SI phenotype have been reported (429, 652) (see Chapter 3). Likewise, HIV-1 strains that grow only in PBMC and not T-cell lines or macrophages have been recovered from the blood of infected people (674, 1150, 1322). The relevance of these observations to diversity in the viral envelope and pathogenesis is under study (Chapter 8).

D. Other Considerations of Cellular Host Range

Most HIV-1 strains can infect both peripheral blood CD4$^+$ T cells and macrophages but with great differences in efficiency in virus production, particularly in the case of macrophages. For instance, all of the non-macrophage-tropic strains in our laboratory can be detected in macrophages after inoculation, if PCR procedures or cocultivation of the cells with PBMC are conducted (1505a). Others have made similar observations with both HIV-1 and HIV-2 isolates (2740). The number of cells infected, reflecting the efficiency of virus entry, may be a determinant. As discussed in Chapter 5, however, some studies suggest that virus strains that are poorly tropic for macrophages enter the cells but undergo limited steps in reverse transcription and thus have greatly reduced progeny production (1844, 2393, 2417). The reason for this observation is not known but could involve a variety of factors including intracellular events determined by the viral envelope and cytokine production (Table 7.3) (see Chapters 5 and 8). Moreover, as noted above, some isolates grow only in PBMC and not in macrophages or T-cell lines. Variations in the ability of T-cell-line-tropic viruses to productively infect certain established human T-cell lines are also commonly observed (372). These differences could reflect relative affinities of the viral envelope for CD4 (2104) and for a particular viral coreceptor (see Chapter 3) (Table 7.3). In terms of clinical relevance, conceivably, an evolution of HIV-1 takes place from CD4$^+$ lymphocyte tropism to a virus that can also grow well in macrophages, then to a dual-tropic virus (macrophage and T-cell-line-tropic), and finally a T-cell-line-tropic virus (Section IX).

As with HIV-1, the biologic phenotypes of HIV-2 can be distinguished by their ability to form syncytia and to grow rapidly to high titer or slowly to low titer (34).

Table 7.3 Factors influencing HIV infection and replication: host range

1. Presence of cellular receptor(s) for virus
2. Virus envelope (structure, conformation, charge)
3. Extent of viral envelope glycosylation
4. Number of envelope spikes—extent of gp120 shedding
5. Cellular proteases
6. Interaction of intracellular factors with the viral LTR and with viral proteins (e.g., Tat, Rev, Nef)
7. Extent of expression of viral regulatory and accessory genes (e.g., *tat, rev, nef, vif, vpu, vpx,* and *vpr*)

The relation of these host range differences to HIV pathogenesis is discussed in Section IX.

Some fresh (primary) isolates, particularly from plasma, might not readily infect cultured PBMC, perhaps because of a reduced affinity for the $CD4^+$ lymphocyte in culture or the use of a specific coreceptor (see Chapter 3). For these reasons, some investigators warn about artifacts introduced by in vitro techniques that can affect the biologic characterization of HIV-1 (1392, 1767). Furthermore, prolonged growth in vitro of virus from an individual could select for a more rapidly growing SI variant (1603) when both NSI and SI are present (2350). Nevertheless, studies using the same approaches for isolation, short-term culture, and comparison among strains should help control for these variables. Moreover, evaluation of viral strains directly in tissues and PBMC (e.g., by PCR) carries the risk of studying defective virions (2349). Most measurements indicate the presence of up to 1,000-fold more noninfectious than infectious viruses in HIV preparations (1294), and up to 100,000-fold more noninfectious than infectious particles in the plasma of seropositive individuals (1451, 2092). In this regard, some studies indicate that limited cell culture procedures for isolation of HIV-1 (7 to 10 days) can provide a good indication of the major infectious virus variant present in the specimen studied (2322).

These differences in cellular host range among HIV-1 strains appear to be determined primarily by the initial steps involved in virus entry (see Chapter 3), because they are influenced by the diversity of the HIV envelope (for a review, see reference 1729) and the polymorphism in the coreceptor. Subsequently, intracellular factors can affect the extent of virus production (see Chapter 5) (Table 7.3). These replicative properties of HIV-1 strains have been used by some investigators to classify viruses into subgroups (96, 746, 2788) or to designate their degree of virulence (Tables 7.2 and 7.4) (Section IX) (96, 429, 746, 1494, 2657, 2659). Most recently, a classification of HIV-1 based on coreceptor usage has been proposed (177b). By this system, the NSI, macrophage-tropic viruses would be known as R5, the SI viruses as X4, and the dual-tropic viruses as R5X4 viruses.

E.   Influence of Glycosylation on Cellular Host Range

Two reports (428, 2057) demonstrated that HIV-1 strains, passed through a variety of cell types, were modified in their host range properties. Although selection of a variant could be involved, posttranscriptional modification of the infecting virus strain should be considered. For example, some HIV-1 isolates grown in the HUT

Table 7.4 Classification of HIV strains by host range and replicative properties

Subtypes

1. Virulent versus nonvirulent strains (429)
2. SI versus NSI strains (2649, 2659)
3. Rapid/high versus slow/low strains (746)
4. Groups a to d (for lymphocytes) or α to γ (for macrophages)[a] (2788)

Phenotype considered

1. Host range is defined by replication in macrophages versus established human T-cell lines. Some differences in growth in $CD4^+$ lymphocytes and established B-cell and monocyte lines have been used.
2. Replication is defined by how soon virus is released from the cell (kinetics, e.g., rapid versus slow) and to what levels it is produced at peak virus replication (titer, e.g., high versus low).
3. Cytopathology is defined by cell killing as well as induction of syncytia via cell:cell fusion.

[a] Kinetics not a parameter.

78 T-cell line, in contrast to PBMC, take on biologic features permitting infection of a variety of other established T-cell and macrophage lines. When the virus is passed back in PBMC, this expanded host range disappears. The only viral proteins that appear to be changed during this transfer of HIV-1 are the envelope glycoproteins. On exposure to tunicamycin, the nonglycosylated envelope proteins for all the viruses studied have the same size (428); it is the extent of glycosylation that differs.

This intracellular modification of an HIV-1 strain was observed as well with an infectious molecular clone of HIV-1$_{SF2}$. When it was passed through different cell lines or the PBMC of different individuals, variations in replicating ability in PBMC and established T-cell lines were noted (428). The results strongly suggest that the glycosylation pattern of the envelope protein determined by events within the cell (741) can affect the host range of the progeny virions. One hypothesis considers that carbohydrate binding proteins on the cell surface or a macrophage endocytosis receptor (728) can interact with oligosaccharides on HIV-1 and affect its infectivity and cellular host range (741). Other studies suggest that only some N-linked glycosylation sites might be important for infectivity (1462). Nevertheless, this posttranscriptional alteration is another example of the influence that intracellular factors could have on HIV infection and spread (Table 7.3). Therefore, glycosylation differences could be added to the general features of HIV that might determine pathogenesis in individuals infected by the same HIV strain (Section IX). Glycosylation could also affect the sensitivity of certain HIV strains to antiviral antibodies (167) (see Chapter 10).

F. Kinetics and Level of Virus Replication

The difference in ability of HIV strains to infect cells is reflected not only in virus entry, as discussed above, but also in the rate of virus replication (kinetics) and the extent of viral progeny production (titer) in various cell types. In part, the virus titer over short periods can reflect the extent to which a strain of HIV-1 can spread among the cells inoculated. The relative ability to replicate in cells, as measured by kinetics and titer, has been used by some investigators to categorize HIV into "rapid/high" and "slow/low" strains (96, 746) (Table 7.4; Figure 7.3). The rapid/high strains are associated with disease in infected individuals (Section IX). In general, these distinctions in kinetics and titer fit most isolates; however, some low-titer viruses have been found to replicate rapidly, and certain slowly replicating viruses can eventually grow to high titers after a prolonged period in culture (1505a, 2788). Moreover, in some studies, slow infection kinetics was found to reflect a low production and spread of infectious virus rather than a long replication time (638).

Differences in replication among viruses can also result from external stimuli (e.g., cytokines) acting on intracellular factors that influence the expression of particular HIV strains (see Chapter 5). For example, tumor necrosis factor alpha (TNF-α) and interleukin-1 (IL-1), via protein kinase C activation, appear to induce the attachment of the NF-κB protein to a promoter region of the viral long terminal repeat (LTR) and enhance virus replication (Figure 5.3) (671, 1299, 1368, 1697, 1994, 2798). These cytokines are produced by activated macrophages and T cells and by HIV-infected cells (see Chapter 9). Moreover, a particular *tat* gene could influence the extent of virus replication (see Chapter 8). Following transfection with a *tat* gene, certain CD4$^+$ T-cell lines become susceptible to high-level replication of HIV strains that previously did not grow well in these cells (746). Since high expression of Tat induced in other cells does not change the phenotype of slow/low viruses, cellular factors in addition to this HIV regulatory protein must be involved in these differences in virus production (1352). As discussed in Chapter 5, certain cellular factors may be needed to interact with Tat to increase virus replication. Furthermore, infection of cells by other viruses can result in enhanced HIV replication that can differ among viral isolates.

All these findings, as well as those on virus entry and the intracellular modifications, emphasize again how both external and internal cellular factors, interacting with different viral gene products, can influence the extent of infection and replication by individual HIV strains (Table 7.3).

Figure 7.3 Replication of two strains of HIV-1 recovered from the same individual over time. HIV-1$_{SF2}$ (○), isolated early in the course of infection, replicates slowly and to low titer in the established HUT 78 T-cell line. In contrast, HIV-1$_{SF13}$ (△), recovered when the patient had AIDS, grows rapidly and to high titer in the same cells. These and other biologic differences among HIV isolates have been used to distinguish viruses in culture as nonvirulent and virulent strains as well as slow/low and rapid/high strains (Tables 7.4 and 7.8; Figure 7.14).

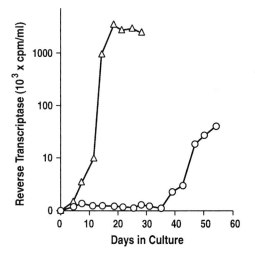

III.   Modulation of CD4 Protein Expression

In early studies of HIV-1, infection of CD4$^+$ cells was associated with elimination of CD4 protein expression on the cell surface (see Chapter 3). In subsequent evaluations of HIV-1 and HIV-2 strains, some viruses were found that did not down-modulate the CD4 receptor. One HIV-2 strain (UC1) (721), which is also generally noncytopathic, replicates to high titer in CD4$^+$ lymphocytes without disturbing the expression or intensity of the CD4 molecule on the cell surface. This observation was made with both CD4$^+$ lymphocytes and established T-cell lines. Another HIV-2 strain (ST) (1385) has also been shown to have minimal effects on CD4 protein expression. This variation in extent of CD4 modulation can be seen as well with diverse HIV-1 strains (1507) and is one notable property of viruses recovered from the brain (432) (Section IX) (see Chapter 9). Whether this feature, which varies among viral strains, plays any role in the pathogenic pathway is still unknown. The mechanism for this process is discussed in Chapter 3, and the potential viral determinants of this process are reviewed in Chapter 8.

IV.   Cytopathology

In addition to the relative ability of HIV strains to infect and replicate in cells, and to modulate CD4 protein expression, the extent of cytopathology produced by a variety of HIV-1 and HIV-2 strains can differ substantially (see Chapter 6) (65, 429, 1347, 2595, 2649). The mechanisms for cell death involve several processes discussed in Chapter 6. As mentioned above, some HIV-2 strains have been recovered that replicate to high titer in PBMC but do not induce any cytopathology, as defined by syncytium formation and reduction in cell viability (722, 1345). Some HIV-1 strains also have limited cytopathic properties in PBMC, but thus far, all those described cause some cell:cell fusion. With cytopathic HIV-1 and HIV-2 strains, however, the relative extent of cell killing can vary dramatically (371, 721, 2649). By using T-cell lines as noted above, SI and NSI strains have been described (2657) and differences in the plaque-forming ability of HIV-1 strains have been reported (1008, 2649).

The highly cytopathic SI strains replicate well in T-cell lines and produce plaques in MT-4 T-cell-line monolayers, reflecting syncytium formation and cell death (Figure 7.4) (2649). Most noteworthy are the variations in the induction of CPE and syncytium formation observed with viral isolates recovered from the same infected individual over time. The later viruses, isolated when the person is symptomatic, are the most cytopathic (429) (Section IX). This observation on heterogeneity in cytopathicity measured by syncytium formation has been standardized in the MT-2 cell line (1347), which is used by many investigators to group virus isolates into SI and NSI strains (2657, 2659) (Table 7.2). As noted previously, the host range, replicative abilities, and cytopathic properties of HIV-1 strains have helped to classify viruses into separate biologic subgroups (Table 7.4).

Figure 7.4 Plaques formed in the MT-4 cell line by a cytopathic strain of HIV-1. (A) Cytopathology induced in PBMC by HIV-1$_{SF33}$. Magnification, ×65. (B) HIV-1$_{SF33}$-induced foci of syncytia and cell death detected by staining as plaques in the MT-4 cell monolayer. Magnification, ×40. Photograph courtesy of C. Cheng-Mayer.

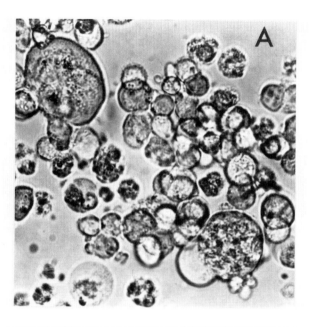

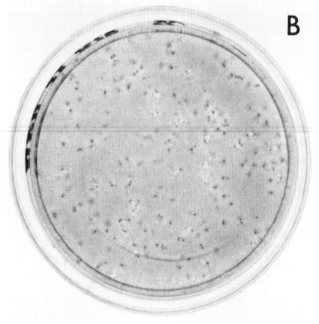

V.   Latency

Just as other virologic properties show heterogeneity, so does the induction of latent infection in cultured cells (see Chapter 5). Some HIV isolates enter into a latent or silent state in vitro much more rapidly than others. Again, this biologic feature depends on the cell type as well as the viral strain. For example, the HIV-1$_{SF247}$ strain induces a latent state in the established Jurkat T-cell line but replicates well in PBMC (1507) (Figure 5.5). Sometimes, the early isolates from an asymptomatic individual will enter a latent state in established T-cell lines whereas later isolates from the same person, when symptomatic, will replicate efficiently in the cells (424a). Certain HIV-1 strains studied in our laboratory (e.g., HIV-1$_{SF33}$) have never induced a latent infection in T cells in vitro. If the definition of latency is expanded to include low-level virus production (i.e., viral persistence), similar variations among HIV strains in different cell types (e.g., macrophages versus T cells) can be appreciated (327, 770). The observations on latency therefore emphasize the dependence of this state both on genetic differences in viral genes (e.g., *tat*, *rev*, and *nef*) and on their various interactions with intracellular factors. The mechanisms are probably diverse and require continued study (see Chapter 5).

VI. Molecular Features of HIV Strains

A. General Observations

The extensive biologic and serologic heterogeneity of HIV strains (Section VII) is mirrored in the genetic sequences of the viruses (Figure 1.3). How these diverse strains of HIV arise is not clear, but the viral reverse transcriptase (RT) is very error prone and thus appears to give rise readily to changes in the genome (2142, 2248, 2636). Fidelity has been found to be severalfold higher with RNA than with DNA, suggesting that most mutations occur with the DNA template-DNA primer (266). It has been estimated that up to 10 base changes in the HIV genome occur per replicative cycle. Molecular techniques have helped to define the variations in the viral genome associated with HIV heterogeneity (see Chapter 8).

B. Genome Sensitivity to Restriction Enzymes

One of the first differences recognized among HIV-1 strains was the variation in sensitivity of the cloned, proviral genome to digestion by restriction enzymes. When the restriction enzyme patterns of two prototype isolates, HTLV-III and LAV, were examined, they were virtually identical (44, 986), but that of a third, ARV-2 (HIV-1$_{SF2}$), showed marked differences (305, 1599). The latter observation became the rule as highly divergent strains were recognized by their different restriction enzyme patterns.

Viruses recovered from one individual appear to conserve several restriction enzyme sites and thus can be identified as coming from the same person (169, 429, 987). Similarly, HIV-1 isolates from a mother and child, individuals receiving a blood transfusion or clotting factor from the same donor, or two sexual partners could show a close relationship among the viruses by similar restriction enzyme patterns.

C.   Genetic Sequence Differences

When complete genetic sequence data were available on the initial HIV-1 strains, it again became evident that HTLV-IIIB and LAV were the same strain (HIV-1$_{LAI}$) whereas SF2 and subsequently other HIV-1 strains could be differentiated by their viral genomic sequence (1871, 2193, 2351, 2804). At least 6 to 10% of the total viral genome can differ among strains from different individuals. Some isolates vary widely in both synonymous sequence changes (mutations that do not affect amino acid representation) and nonsynonymous sequence changes (mutations that affect the amino acid expressed). The greatest nonsynonymous sequence heterogeneity is observed in the genes of the regulatory and envelope proteins (1683, 1767, 1892); with some strains, nearly 40% differences in amino acid sequences in some viral genes can be appreciated (Figure 7.5) (1887, 1892). Currently, a major focus of research has been centered on correlating these sequence differences with functional variations among HIV strains (see Chapter 8).

D.   Sequence Subtypes (Clades)

The amplification of parts of the viral genome by PCR followed by DNA sequencing has been particularly helpful in conducting rapid comparisons of different sequences among HIV-1 and HIV-2 strains (1224, 1394, 1587, 1683, 1714, 1715, 2001), particularly in the V3 region. By amino acid analyses, this procedure has shown extreme envelope diversity as well as certain similarities among strains. Thus far, based on the viral C2-V3 envelope sequences, 11 sequence subtypes (or clades) of HIV-1 (A to J and O) have been identified in the world (Figure 7.6) (1889, 1891) (for a review, see reference 1211). Each clade differs from the others in amino acid composition by at least 20% in the envelope region and 15% in the Gag region. Within each clade, the differences in Env can be up to 10% and those in Gag can be up to 8% (1889). Their interrelationship has been established by either phylogenetic trees (Figure 7.7), stars (Figure 7.8), or bushes (Figure 7.9). Subtype A is found primarily in Central Africa, subtype B in North America and Europe, subtype C in South Africa and India, subtype D in Central Africa, and subtype E in Thailand; subtype F includes a few isolates from Brazil (2131) and all of the viruses thus far characterized from children in Romania (674) (Figure 7.6).

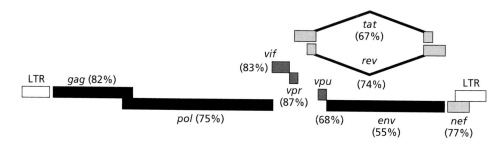

Figure 7.5   Estimated similarities in amino acids for the different HIV-1 gene products. Figure compiled from data analyzing several HIV-1 strains worldwide in reference 1887 and provided by C. Kuiken.

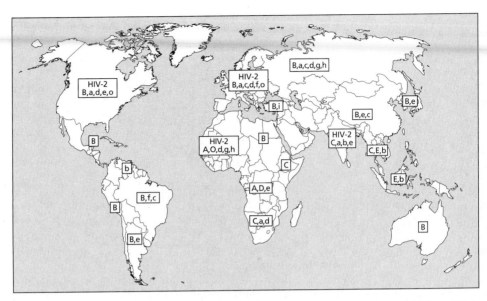

Figure 7.6   HIV-1 is the predominant HIV type distributed throughout the world, but HIV-2, which is less common, has still been found in West Africa and most recently in India at an increasing rate. The distribution of the various genotypes (clades) of HIV-1 is indicated by the letters A through I. Clades of HIV-2 are not shown separated. Source, UNAIDS, 1996.

The other sequence subtypes include viruses from Russia (G) (237), Africa and Taiwan (H) (1890), Cyprus (I) (1354), and Africa (clade J). Some isolates appear to be genetically outside the other clades in this interrelationship. These viruses (e.g., ANT70), originally identified in Cameroon, have been placed in the sequence subtype O for "outlier" (1890). They have since been found at low frequency in other African countries (2063). The other clades have been grouped under the category of M, for "major" (or "main") genotype. All of the clades identified can be found in Africa (1186b, 1586). The distribution of clades in other countries varies but most probably reflects the number of viruses recovered as well as epidemiologic spread (Figure 7.6). In servicemen returning to the United States, viruses from three group M clades aside from type B (i.e., types A, D, and E) have been detected (293). Most recently, clades G and O were found in AIDS patients who had come to the United States from Africa (2614a).

About 10% of isolates from Cameroon are of the clade O genotype (1939). Most people infected with this genotype are detected by using the antibody-based assays for the other HIV-1 strains. Nevertheless, up to 20% of individuals infected with clade O may not be detected by these assays (2381). This finding has raised concerns about the safety of blood donations. A clade O isolate has been recovered from a West Central African woman living in the United States (2196). Thus far, however, the screening procedures and the relative rarity of clade O in other parts of the world have not made contamination of blood a major issue.

A biologic difference involving the capsid (CA) protein has been described between the HIV-1 group M and group O viruses. The O viruses do not appear to be very sensitive to cyclosporine in culture, suggesting that the interaction of cy-

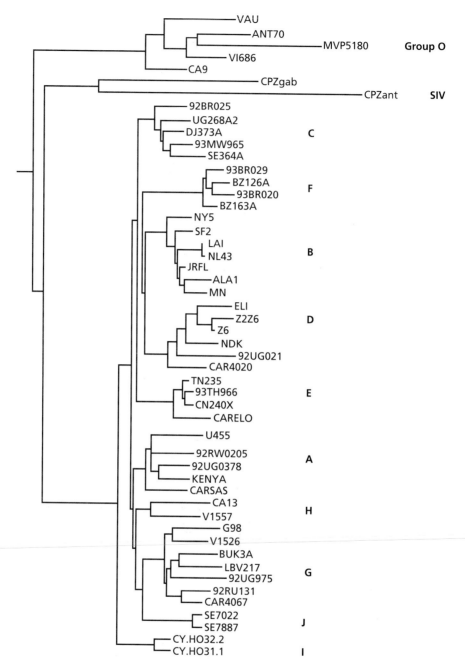

Figure 7.7 A neighbor-joining tree, based on C2-V3 sequences (the only region available for subtypes I and J), showing the interrelations between the HIV-1 major group M (main, clades A to J) and the O (outlier) group. The two groups are separated by two rather distinct SIV sequences isolated from chimpanzees (CPZ), which suggests that M and O could be the result of two separate cross-species transmissions. The origin of the subtypes is still completely unknown. The distribution of the subtypes partly follows geographical lines (Figure 7.6). Subtype A is found mainly in Africa and India; subtype B is mostly a "Western" virus and is the major type in Western Europe, most of the Americas, and Australia, but is also present in the Far East and Russia; subtype C is the most common subtype in East and South Africa, India, and China; subtype D is mostly African; subtype E is found in the Far East (Thailand) and also in central Africa; subtype F is common in Brazil and Eastern Europe (particularly Romania) and is also found in Africa; subtypes G and H are both mainly African, but G has migrated to Eastern Europe; subtype I so far has been found only in two related infections in Cyprus; and subtype J was isolated from two Zaireans living in Sweden. Figure courtesy of C. Kuiken.

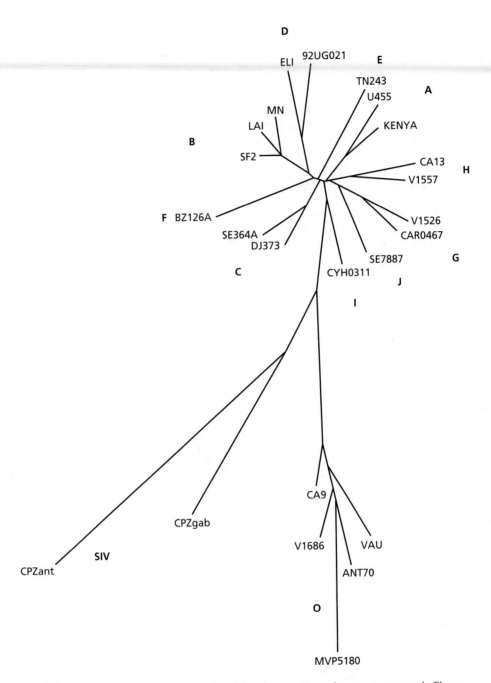

Figure 7.8   A neighbor-joining tree involving the same Env subtype sequences as in Figure 7.7. While this analysis is equivalent to that in Figure 7.7, the presentation makes clear the equidistance; this evolutionary pattern is known as a "star" phylogeny. Figure courtesy of C. Kuiken.

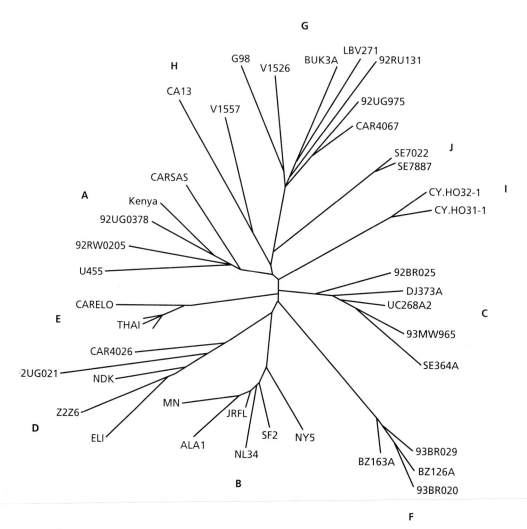

Figure 7.9 A phylogenetic tree in "bush" format, showing the 10 clades in the M group of HIV-1. Only the length of the branches and the location of their connection to the tree are significant, not their orientation. Within HIV-1, these genetic subtypes appear to be more or less equidistant, suggesting that they must have arisen around the same time. The tree is a neighbor-joining tree based on genetic distances estimated by using Kimura's two-parameter method. Figure courtesy of C. Kuiken.

clophilins with this Gag protein is not required for group O virus replication (270) (see Chapter 5).

Another technique involving DNA heteroduplex mobility on an agarose gel has been used to detect HIV-1 quasi-species diversity when evaluating different genetic regions (617). This approach is a rapid procedure for studying genetic differences among HIV strains and the evolution of genetic variants over time (617).

It seems apparent that several regions within a virus need to be considered when the final classification of HIV-1 strains takes place. Nevertheless, the distribution of virus subtype according to sequence should focus on the genetic structure of the envelope region, which is most important for vaccine development. How the clade classification relates to antigenic subtypes is an important, unresolved area of study (Section VII).

The process by which these clades evolved remains a mystery (see also Chapter 1). The earliest evidence for infection by HIV came from studies of three Norwegian people (a couple and their daughter) who died in 1976 after 10 years of clinical evidence of immune deficiency (1553). Recent data indicate that HIV-1 was present in these individuals and it was clade O type (1211). These results indicate that this recently recognized clade of HIV-1 existed long before the onset of the present epidemic. The reason for the emergence of this subgroup and its limited spread remains to be determined.

It would seem that viruses maintained and spread in one habitat could, after several transmissions and selection in different hosts, emerge with sufficient mutations to be classified as a separate clade. However, the distribution of clades worldwide has remained relatively constant. For instance, the lack of a large number of people infected with clades other than B in North America raises questions about the singular emergence of certain virus subtypes in other countries. The dominance of clades in some parts of the world, such as Romania (F), Cyprus (I), and Russia (G), reflects this occurrence. In some instances, recombination among clades in certain genetic domains has taken place. Some of these recombinants at first appeared to be new clades until their genetic sequences were more fully determined. Thus, whether some of the recently recognized viruses will qualify as distinct clades (e.g., clades I and J) requires further evaluation (1211). Recombinant A/E (*gag/env*) and A/I strains have been identified in Thailand and Cyprus, respectively (985a, 2250) (see below). Moreover, the viruses in clade F from Brazil have GPGR in their crowns, whereas the clade F isolates from Romania have GPGQ (1889). Similarly, the clade B virus in Thailand differs from clade B viruses in North America by the animo acids in its V3 loop (GPGQ or GPGH versus GPGR) (1889). The meaning of these findings to the biologic heterogeneity of HIV-1 strains within a specific clade and the potential for intergenetic recombinant virus formation in vivo merit further evaluation.

In this regard, when similarities in proteins were compared among various M clades, some convergence in the V3 loop protein sequences was identified. Clades A and C have similar genetic sequences; in contrast, clade D has very divergent V3 loop sequences (1351). These and other data suggest that the extent of replication influences the interpatient variation that develops during the spread of virus subtypes through populations in the world. Some researchers have estimated that the level of variability among viruses within a clade in a country can predict how long that virus has been present in the country (Figure 7.10) (2857). Similarities in clades obtained from various countries would indicate a recent introduction of the virus into these countries. Great diversity would suggest a longer period that these viruses have existed, spread, and diversified in the population.

Finally, molecular approaches used on uncultured PBMC have suggested HIV-1 diversity in infected hosts that is not appreciated after isolation of virus in vitro (1392, 1767). Whether selection in culture influences conclusions made about HIV heterogeneity and pathogenesis remains to be determined. As noted above, short-

Figure 7.10 Relationship between the degree of genetic diversity of a genotype and the duration of the epidemic in a region. Each curve represents the expected distribution of intrasubtype nucleotide substitution frequencies, expressed as a percentage, among all possible pairs of a typical sample of sequences from a country or area. Examples named reflect the most recently reported genetic divergence. The width of each curve represents the approximate range of these frequencies, and the height represents the relative proportion of pairs with that frequency of substitution. Genetic divergence is believed to increase at a rate of approximately 0.5 to 1% per year. Reprinted from reference 2857 with permission.

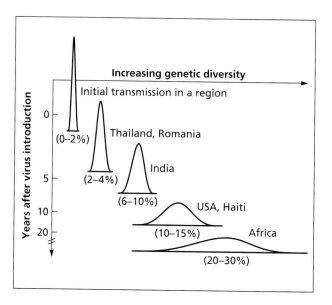

term culture of virus appears to identify the major infectious HIV strain present in the specimens being evaluated from infected individuals (2322) (Section II.B).

E.   Identification of Viruses Involved in Transmission

The distribution of HIV-1 clades in Thailand has suggested that one genotype may be transmitted more readily by sexual contact (clade E) and another genotype by intravenous drug use (clade B) (2002). Whether these conclusions will hold true over time (1714) remains to be seen. Some investigators have reported that clade E viruses replicate better in Langerhans cells than do clade B viruses (2539). Since Langerhans cells are found in the vaginal canal but not in the anal canal, this in vitro observation may explain the high prevalence of clade E in Thai women, whose risk is from heterosexual contact. This possibility needs further study but seems unlikely, since clade B isolates have been associated with extensive spread by heterosexual activity in other parts of the world (see Chapter 2). The findings have raised concern about possible increased spread of HIV-1 by heterosexual contact in the United States, since small numbers of clade E viruses (as well as other clades) have been detected in this country (84, 293). Recent studies, however, have not confirmed a specific tropism of the clade E viruses for Langerhans cells or dendritic cells (641a, 2120a).

Phylogenetic and molecular analyses of common (signature) sequences in the viral envelope (particularly the V3 loop) by PCR have also been useful in demonstrating transmission of one HIV-1 strain to other individuals in the recent past (321, 1741, 2907) and from mothers to infants (1409, 1410, 2910). In most cases, a selected transfer of one or a limited number of HIV-1 variants was shown (1410, 2907, 2910). In recipients of the same clotting-factor preparation, some data from PCR sequencing revealed a lack of substantial change in the virus isolated from different individuals (455, 1314). In another study of recipients of blood components from one HIV-infected donation, the degree of viral diversity correlated with the individual's different genetic background (630a) The results most probably reflect the influence of the host's immune system on the evolution of virus. In this regard, a blood transfusion to monozygotic triplets showed a similar evolution of viral genotypes (2367). The PCR procedure was also helpful in demonstrating that a dentist infected five of his patients during surgical procedures (2000).

VII. Serologic Properties of HIV Strains

Differences among HIV strains can also be demonstrated by the reactivity of the host immune system to the virus. Antibodies measured in peptide ELISAs, antibody-dependent cellular cytotoxicity (ADCC) assays, and neutralization/enhancement assays can distinguish virus isolates. sCD4 inactivation procedures also show variations in virus sensitivity (see Chapter 4). This section reviews observations on differences in sensitivity of virus to antibodies. Other information on the humoral immune response to HIV, particularly reactions with selected viral proteins and antigens, is reviewed in Chapter 10.

A. Sensitivity to Antibodies Mediating Neutralization

1. METHODS FOR MEASURING NEUTRALIZING ANTIBODIES

For many of the early studies on neutralization, laboratory strains and T-cell lines were used with serum from infected subjects. It is now recognized that neutralizing antibodies used as an in vitro correlate for immune response should be measured optimally by procedures utilizing autologous primary virus isolates and normal PBMC. These components of the assay come closest to being the potential targets for neutralizing antibodies and the potential cells for HIV infection in vivo. Some investigators recommend using unstimulated PBMC for the assays, since cells in vivo would not be activated (2995). The value of this procedure needs further study (2981), particularly since unactivated cells may express different viral coreceptors (see Chapter 3) (234). A definition of a primary isolate has not been formally made, but it conventionally represents a virus that has been replicated only in cultured PBMC and only for a short period after the initial recovery (<2 months).

2. VIRAL REGIONS MEDIATING SENSITIVITY TO NEUTRALIZATION

The viral envelope gp120 appears to contain the major regions susceptible to neutralization by specific antibodies (see also Chapter 10; Table 10.1 and Figure 10.1). These regions include the CD4 binding domain (2095, 2584, 2615) and the V3 loop (945, 1191, 1192, 1433, 3003). The latter immunodominant region is important in postbinding events needed for virus entry (for a review, see reference 1835). Other portions of gp120 (1079, 2712) and gp41 (400, 1885) and perhaps p17 (2358) could also be sensitive to neutralization antibodies.

Polyclonal and monoclonal antibodies to the V3 loop are type specific but have been found to react with several strains (188, 553, 910, 990, 1191, 2996). This response is observed because the cysteine-bound V3 region has a central portion with certain amino acid sequences (e.g., GPGRAF), now termed the principal neutralizing domain (PND), that are shared by many HIV-1 isolates (e.g., HIV-1$_{SF2}$), particularly those found in the United States and Europe (Figure 7.11) (1191, 1433). Unrelated virus strains with different sequences in the PND are resistant to neutralization by the same monoclonal antibody (553). Broadly reactive anti-V3 loop antibodies have been found (910, 1191) that probably reflect a reaction with a nonlinear conformational V3 epitope (see Chapter 10). Antibodies to the CD4 binding site on gp120 are often cross-reacting, since they are conformational (2584). Nevertheless, several anti-HIV monoclonal antibodies are type specific (553), most probably because they interact only with part of the CD4 binding site on gp120. The domains on this viral envelope protein are discontinuous, so that multiple monoclonal antibodies may be needed for virus neutralization (see Chapter 3).

3. NEUTRALIZATION OF SIMILAR AND DIVERSE GENETIC SUBGROUPS

Differences in the susceptibility of various HIV strains to serum neutralization have been demonstrated. Initially, evidence for neutralizing antibodies against HIV was limited, most probably because of the viral assays used. Subsequently, a number of laboratories demonstrated that sera from HIV-infected individuals from many parts of the world could neutralize HIV-1 and HIV-2 strains to different extents (373, 423, 1085, 1699, 2846, 2847). Some viruses, such as HIV-1$_{SF2}$, are easily neutralized by many sera, particularly from the United States. High titers of serum-neutralizing antibodies can often be detected with this isolate (421, 1104, 2846). One explanation for these observations is that this virus is a member of the North American sequence subtype, clade B (Section VI) (Figure 7.7), and shares envelope properties with many HIV-1 isolates. The HIV-1$_{MN}$ strain is a similar antigenic type (1192, 1433). Another possibility is that the high sensitivity of these strains to neutralization could reflect the increased release of their envelope gp120 from the virion and/or the reduced number of gp120-bearing knobs on the virion surface (1728). These properties could have resulted from culturing the virus for a long time in the laboratory.

In early studies of neutralization, HIV-1 isolates could be placed into at least four subgroups depending on their sensitivity to neutralization by three different sera (Table 7.5) (421). Viruses recovered from the brain, in contrast to those from

Figure 7.11   Comparison of the amino acid sequence of the V3 regions of the HIV-1$_{SF2}$ and HIV-1$_{SF162}$ strains. The complete V3 sequence of a molecular clone of HIV-1$_{SF2}$ is shown, and the five amino acid residues that differ in HIV-1$_{SF162}$ are designated. The positions of amino acid residues are relative to the HIV-1$_{SF2}$ genome referenced in the Los Alamos AIDS and Human Retroviruses database. Reprinted from reference 2485 with permission.

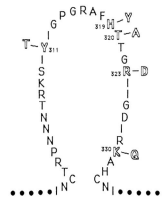

Table 7.5   Neutralization of HIV-1 infectivity by anti-HIV-1 sera[a]

Proposed subtype	HIV-1$_{SF}$	Source	Serum		
			1	2	3
A	2	PBMC	≥1,000	100	10
	4	PBMC	≥1,000	100	100
	13	PBMC	≥1,000	100	10
	33	PBMC	≥1,000	100	10
	66	PBMC	≥1,000	100	10
	113	PBMC	≥1,000	100	100
	117	PBMC	≥1,000	100	10
	301A	CNS	≥1,000	100	100
	315	PBMC	100	10	10
B	97	PBMC	80	20	−
	171	PBMC	20	10	−
C	98	CNS	20	−	−
	128A	CNS	20	−	−
	161B	CNS	100	−	−
	162	CNS	100	−	−
	178	CNS	20	−	−
	185	CNS	20	−	−
	153	PBMC	20	−	−
	247	PBMC	100	−	−
D	170[b]	PBMC	−	−	−

[a] Tenfold and twofold dilutions of anti-HIV-1 sera (1, 2, and 3) were tested for their ability to neutralize infectivity of PBMC by 20 different HIV-1 isolates from individuals in the United States, the Dominican Republic (SF247), and Africa (SF170 and SF171). Numbers represent the reciprocal of the highest serum dilution causing a reduction greater than or equal to 67% in RT activity in the culture fluid. A minus sign (−) indicates no virus neutralization at a 1 : 10 serum dilution. Reprinted from reference 421 with permission.
[b] Rarely neutralized by sera from individuals outside Africa.

the blood, were not very sensitive to neutralization, a characteristic of brain-derived strains (Section IX) (432). Also noteworthy is the fact that an isolate from Africa (SF170) was resistant to neutralization by these sera as well as many other North American sera but could be neutralized by African sera.

Several more recent studies with sera from individuals infected with different HIV-1 strains have indicated that cross-neutralization of a variety of HIV genomic subtypes (including clades A to F and O) can be achieved (1688, 1829, 2832), even with some human monoclonal antibodies (2711). Nevertheless, certain clade-specific reactivity has been noted (438, 674, 1150, 1319a, 1687, 1829). In extensive neutralization studies with diverse HIV-1 isolates and sera from people infected with either group M (A to H) or group O HIV-1 strains, cross-neutralization was found among the M group of clades and some clade O isolates (1958, 1959). In contrast, antibodies from individuals infected with HIV-1 group O showed a reduced ability to neutralize primary isolates from the group M genotypes (1958). What controls the breadth of this immune response (e.g., host or antigenicity of the virus) remains to be determined. The potential sharing of conserved neutralizing epitopes among group M and group O viruses offers some encouragement for vaccine development.

Variations in sensitivity to neutralizing antibodies have also been found with viruses recovered over time from the same individual. Generally, the sera from infected individuals do not neutralize the homologous virus (the strain replicating in the person at the time of serum collection) as effectively as they neutralize previous autologous strains or other heterologous HIV-1 strains, especially those grown in the laboratory (1102, 2789). This finding, particularly noted in individuals after primary infection and those leading to disease, suggests that the virus changes to "escape" the immune antiviral responses in the host (31, 80, 1732, 1825, 2214, 2720) (see below). The observation further emphasizes the serologic diversity of isolates even within the same individual. Most importantly, the results raise concern about evidence of neutralizing antibodies in subjects when *laboratory* strains and T-cell lines are used in the assay instead of PBMC (1005, 1102).

With HIV-2 isolates, specific neutralizing domains of the viral envelope, such as a PND, have not been conclusively identified, although such a region has been suggested by some reports (220, 238, 604). Neutralization studies, however, have also demonstrated heterogeneity in antibody responses against HIV-2 isolates (371, 2847). Furthermore, cross-neutralization of HIV-1 and HIV-2 strains has been described with HIV-1 sera but not HIV-2 sera (2847). In general, however, the neutralizing capacity against HIV-2 isolates is low (1959), reflecting important serologic or antigenic differences between these two virus types.

4. NEUTRALIZATION-RESISTANT VIRUS ISOLATES

The generation of viruses that have "escaped" neutralization by serum antibodies has been demonstrated and studied by cell culture studies. HIV-1 strains grown in the presence of neutralizing monoclonal antibodies mutate to become resistant to neutralization (1732, 2214, 2247). In these studies, an alteration within (1309, 1321, 1732) or outside (2664, 2889, 2892) the epitope identified by the monoclonal antibody brings about this resistance. Such a modification, for example, was found in gp41 (1309, 2214, 2664, 2887, 2889). A change from alanine to threonine at position 582 in gp41 conferred resistance to neutralization by antibodies to the CD4 binding site on gp120 (2664). A single amino acid substitution at position 281 in the conserved region of gp120 conferred virus resistance to a broadly reactive antiserum (2828). This change apparently affected several regions of the envelope that were involved in antibody neutralization. A single amino acid change within the V2 domain can be responsible for escape from neutralization by an anti-V2 region monoclonal antibody (911, 2944). Changes in the V3 region can affect the neutralization sensitivity (1321; for a review, see reference 1829). On another note, mutations in gp41 also conferred a neutralization-sensitive phenotype to HIV-1 by affecting the interactions of antibodies with gp120 (112).

These observations on sensitivity to antibody-mediated neutralization emphasize the influence of other envelope domains on the overall conformation of the viral envelope that can determine effective antibody binding. This conclusion has also been reached by studies of fractionated antibody preparations (2584) and monoclonal antibodies (681, 1321, 1827, 1828, 2570) (see Chapters 8 and 10). Thus, viral escape from anti-HIV responses most probably occurs by multiple mechanisms, including conformational changes in the envelope. Development of successful envelope-based vaccines, therefore, may require the identification of conserved regions

Table 7.6   Factors influencing virus sensitivity to neutralization[a]

Genetic
1. Linear epitope on viral envelope protein
2. Conformational epitope on viral envelope protein

Nongenetic
1. Glycosylation differences
2. Virus envelope stability
3. Cellular proteins on the virion surface (e.g., HLA, blood group antigens)
4. Age of virus preparation

[a] See Section VII.

in the viral envelope that are critical for function, so that any alteration within them would render the virus inactive (2828).

5. OTHER FACTORS INFLUENCING VIRUS SENSITIVITY TO NEUTRALIZATION

Besides linear and conformational epitopes on the virus envelope, other, nongenetic factors can also affect serologic responses to HIV-1 strains (Table 7.6). Viruses cultivated in one cell line in a laboratory, for example, can yield progeny that become more or less sensitive to neutralization by specific sera (see below) (2888). In some instances, the serologic effect could be due to reactivity with cell surface proteins (e.g., human leukocyte antigen [HLA]) on the virions (89, 168, 1115) (see Chapter 3), carbohydrate moieties (1001), or differences in viral envelope stability. In the last case, studies of virus sensitivity to sCD4 inactivation have suggested that the resistance of primary isolates reflects the density and stability of the envelope gp120 (see Chapters 4 and 8). However, recent studies suggest that those factors are not involved in this resistance (1243). Antibody to the histo-blood group A antigen has been reported to neutralize HIV-1 produced only by lymphocytes from blood group A donors (81).

Antibodies to the human major histocompatibility complex (MHC) class II molecules protected monkeys from infection by SIV grown in human but not monkey cells (88). In other cases, glycosylation patterns differed and affected antibody binding (577, 741, 855, 1001, 2888). Thus, some researchers have noted a difference in sensitivity to neutralizing antibodies between viruses grown in PBMC and those grown in macrophages or T-cell lines (2371, 2888; for a review, see reference 1831). The possible mechanisms for these differences could be selection in the target cells of different subpopulations within a virus preparation, cellular posttranslational modifications of the virus (e.g., glycosylation and envelope stability), genetic mutation during passaging in culture, or incorporation of different host cell proteins on the virion surface (see Chapter 3, Table 3.8).

In addition, the age of the virus preparation can affect antibody sensitivity. With time in culture, the envelope region of the virion becomes less stable and detaches early; neutralization becomes more effective (1452, 1728). Thus, it has been recommended that viruses, for serologic study, should preferably come from the individual being evaluated and that culture fluids 2 days old or less be used. Moreover, as noted above, for the most clinically relevant results, the immunologic assays should be performed in PBMC and not in established T-cell lines.

B. Sensitivity to ADCC

Anti-envelope antibodies mediating ADCC (reviewed in Chapter 10) also reflect the serologic heterogeneity of HIV strains. In some cases, they can be distinguished from neutralizing antibodies (259, 2791). The relative binding of the antibodies to the viral antigenic determinant on the surface of cells infected by a variety of isolates can differ depending on the specific gp120 and gp41 proteins expressed (1359, 1572). Thus, certain viruses can be distinguished by their sensitivity to ADCC following infection of target cells.

C. Sensitivity to Enhancing Antibodies

Enhancing antibodies were recognized during the evaluation of sera for neutralizing activity against HIV. Two types of antibody-dependent enhancement (ADE) were detected: complement mediated and Fc mediated. The mechanisms are discussed in Chapters 3 and 10 (Figure 3.8). Robinson et al. (2256) noted that HIV-1 seropositive sera in the presence of complement could enhance the infection of the MT-2 T cell line by certain HIV-1 strains. Homsy et al. (1104), in studies of guinea pigs immunized with various HIV-1 strains, noted that instead of inducing a neutralizing antibody, the immunization produced sera that enhanced HIV infection. This reaction took place in the absence of complement. Some sera from chimpanzees infected with HIV and from HIV-infected individuals showed similar results. Depending on the viral strain used and the serum selected, virus infection was neutralized or enhanced (1104). Others reported comparable results for decomplemented sera (2633). Most notable have been the observations that a viral strain within the same individual can change over time from sensitivity to serum neutral-

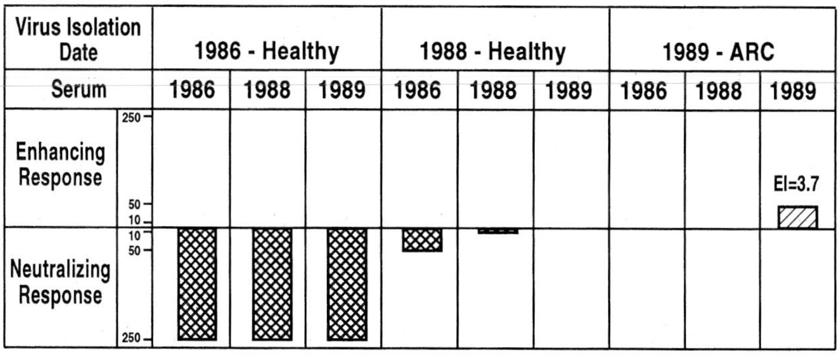

Virus Isolation Date	1986 - Healthy			1988 - Healthy			1989 - ARC		
Serum	1986	1988	1989	1986	1988	1989	1986	1988	1989
Enhancing Response									EI=3.7
Neutralizing Response									

Figure 7.12 Neutralization or enhancement of infection by sequential autologous HIV-1 isolates. HIV-1 strains recovered from the same individual were tested for enhancement or neutralization by the corresponding sera obtained early or late in the infection. The sera were evaluated at fivefold dilutions (1:10 to 1:1,250; reciprocal titer shown). Normal control serum was used at similar dilutions. The clinical status of the individual at the different time points is indicated (ARC, AIDS-related complex). The extent of neutralization is shown below the bar; the enhancement index (EI) is shown above the bar and is defined as the ratio of the viral RT activity in supernatants of cultures receiving virus preincubated with autologous serum compared to the RT activity in supernatants of cultures receiving virus preincubated with control serum. Modified from reference 1102.

ization to sensitivity to enhancement (1102) (Figure 7.12). Generally, this modification in HIV is associated with progression to disease (Section IX.D). Recent studies suggest that very few amino acid substitutions in the V3 loop can bring about this alteration in the serologic sensitivity of the virus (1321) (see Chapter 10).

In the laboratory, certain HIV-1 strains can be grown that are more sensitive to serum neutralization than others (e.g., SF2). Likewise, other strains are found to be most susceptible to enhancing antibodies (e.g., SF128A, a brain isolate, or SF170, an isolate from an AIDS patient from Rwanda) (1104). The reason for these differences is not known, but they appear to be related to specific regions in the viral envelope (1321). The variation could also result from distribution of the viral gp120 on the virion surface and its stability. The relative binding affinity of the gp120 to the antibodies can also be involved (1321) (see Chapter 10). Enhancement of infection by some HIV-2 strains has also been noted with certain sera (374a). Thus, this immunologic phenomenon, which also reflects viral heterogeneity, could have relevance for pathogenesis by either HIV type.

VIII.   Sensitivity to Cell-Mediated Immune Responses

Another property that could differ among HIV strains is their recognition by the cellular immune system, with subsequent killing of the infected cells or suppression of virus replication in the cell (see Chapter 11). In one study with PBMC cultures, PCR procedures detected viral genomes from HIV-1 strains that were not eliminated by antigen-specific CD8$^+$ cytotoxic T lymphocytes (CTL), but no consistent strain of virus could be identified (1768). In another report, the escape in vivo of a specific virus strain from the effect of CD8$^+$ CTL was described (2091). That finding supports in vitro studies showing that a single amino acid mutation in the viral gp41 can eliminate killing of the infected cell by CD8$^+$ CTL (562). These observations have been confirmed in some studies (see Chapter 11) but not others (419, 1768). Thus, the importance of CTL escape mutants in HIV pathogenesis needs further evaluation (see Chapter 11, Section V).

Work in our laboratory has suggested that slower, less virulent HIV-1 strains are somewhat more sensitive to the inhibition of virus replication shown by antiviral CD8$^+$ lymphocytes (1629, 2814) (see Chapter 11). This difference most probably reflects the relative extent of virus replication and spread rather than the specific recognition of an HIV strain resistant to suppression by the cell-mediated response.

IX.   Relation of HIV Heterogeneity to Pathogenesis

Several studies have been initiated to determine if certain HIV-1 subgroups distinguished by specific biologic and serologic features are associated with pathology in certain tissues. HIV appears to evolve independently in different tissues of the body. This in vivo compartmentalization can be noted by the presence of biologic and genetic differences (see also Chapters 4 and 8) (2912). The three major tissues with potential subgroups are reviewed below, but others could eventually include the heart, lungs (1169), kidneys, and endocrine organs.

Table 7.7   Characteristics of HIV-1 strains recovered from different tissues[a]

Characteristics	Source of virus		
	Peripheral blood[b]	Brain	Bowel
Growth in CD4+ lymphocytes	+ +	+ +	+ +
Growth in established human cell lines	+ + (or −)	−	±
Growth in macrophages	± (or + +)	+ +	+
Modulation of CD4 antigen expression	+ +	−	+
Cytopathicity	+ (or + +)	−	+
Serum neutralization	+ +	±	+

[a] Summary representative of several viral isolates. Relative extent noted by number of + signs; −, not evident. Modified from reference 1490 with permission.
[b] Can be NSI or SI.

A. ## Brain Isolates

Studies in our laboratory have demonstrated that HIV-1 strains recovered from the brain or cerebrospinal fluid of patients with neurologic symptoms can be distinguished from viruses recovered from the blood of individuals who are asymptomatic or who have a marked reduction in CD4+ cell number (Table 7.7) (423, 424, 432). In general, the brain-derived isolates, although growing to high titer in CD4+ lymphocytes, are not cytopathic for these cells and do not down-modulate the CD4 protein on the cell surface. These characteristics could explain in part the finding of central nervous system (CNS) disease in some individuals with near-normal CD4+ cell numbers (1507, 1908). Brain-derived isolates grow to higher titer in macrophages than do many blood-derived isolates (423, 1331, 1367). Moreover, the CNS isolates can rarely be propagated in established lines of T cells, B cells, or monocytes (e.g., U937) (432). Thus, they have the features of NSI viruses (Section II) (see Chapters 3 and 4) (Table 7.2). Finally, brain-derived strains are not as sensitive to serum neutralization as are the blood isolates (432). In one report, certain strains from the brain appeared to be more sensitive to cerebrospinal fluid antibodies than to serum antibodies (2536), but this finding has not been confirmed (2790). These biologic and serologic differences can also be appreciated when comparing brain and blood isolates from the same individual (432).

When the relative ability of the HIV-1 isolates to replicate in brain-derived cell lines was examined, other noteworthy observations were made that could have relevance to neuropathogenesis (see Chapter 9). In one study, the blood-derived isolates (T-cell-line-tropic viruses) grew better in the human glioma cell lines than did the macrophage-tropic, brain-derived isolates (427). Similarly, a non-macrophage-tropic HIV-1 strain recovered from the cerebrospinal fluid (and not a brain-derived macrophage-tropic isolate from the same individual) grew in a glioma explant culture (1367).

Other investigators showed that only the macrophage-tropic HIV-1 strains (characteristic of brain isolates) grew well in adult microglial cells in culture (1213, 2465, 2827). This observation was not unexpected, since brain microglia are supposedly derived from macrophage precursor cells. Nevertheless, as noted previously, Peudenier et al. (2088) have challenged the report of infection of microglia, particularly since these cells most probably lack CD4 protein expression. The infected cells could have been peripheral blood macrophages that reside in the brain. Thus, the issue of cell identity is still not resolved and has relevance to any hypothesis on CNS pathogenesis (see Chapter 9). Finally, the relative ability of HIV strains to infect brain capillary endothelial cells (1852) could determine entry into the CNS and hence selection of a specific strain. In studies completed thus far, macrophage-tropic HIV-1 isolates are not infectious for these cells (1852).

The biologic differences between blood and brain isolates have also mirrored variations in restriction enzyme sensitivities and viral LTR and envelope V3 loop sequences. Although the HIV-1 strains from the brain and blood from the same individual are related, there are certain genetic differences between them (28, 709, 985, 1283, 1537, 2594, 2912). Similar findings have been made with HIV-2 isolates recovered from one individual. The brain virus had a macrophage-tropic NSI phenotype, and the blood virus an SI T-cell-line-tropic phenotype (2354). The observations further indicated that distinct but related viral strains can evolve independently in various tissues in the infected host (Section IX.B) (Figure 7.13) (1329).

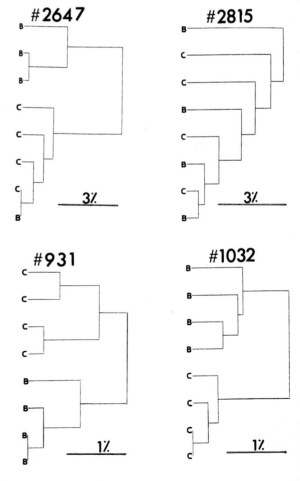

Figure 7.13 Relationship of nucleotide sequences of viruses isolated from the blood (B) or cerebrospinal fluid (C) of the same infected individual. Results with viruses from asymptomatic carriers (#2647 and #2815), one patient with persistent generalized lymphadenopathy (#931), and one patient with AIDS (#1032) are shown. The lines at the bottom of each phylogenetic tree indicate the percentage of sequence differences for comparison. A separation of blood and brain isolates by genome sequence analyses is apparent in the symptomatic patients. Reprinted from reference 1283 with permission.

B.   ## Bowel Isolates

HIV-1 strains have been detected in the bowel mucosa along the gastrointestinal tract from the esophagus to the rectum (141, 882, 1047, 1356, 1916). Studies similar to those described above with brain isolates have indicated some differences between the blood and the bowel isolates (141), but the distinctions were not as great as those defining the brain-derived HIV-1 strains. Nevertheless, the bowel isolates did show substantial macrophage tropism and were less capable of infecting established T- and B-cell lines than were blood isolates. In contrast to brain isolates, however, they were sensitive to serum neutralization and were cytopathic for CD4$^+$ cells in culture. The existence of subgroups of bowel-tropic HIV-1 strains was suggested, particularly by the extent of these differences observed when closely related blood and bowel isolates from the same individual were evaluated (Table 7.7) (141).

Molecular studies on bowel and blood isolates from the same person have not yet been conducted to determine if separate evolutionary pathways have taken place within the host, as suggested for the brain-derived isolates (Section IX.A). Nevertheless, studies with SIV strains recovered from different tissues of a monkey have shown sequence changes in the envelope that suggest specific evolution of the virus in the bowel as well as the brain (1329). One tantalizing possibility is that brain and bowel isolates will show an increased ability to enter cells expressing the GalC molecule since cells from both these tissues have this HIV-1 receptor (1010, 2926). The role of a bowel subgroup of HIV in gastrointestinal disorders is discussed in Chapter 9.

C.   ## Plasma Virus Isolates

Several studies have indicated that most infected individuals have free infectious virus circulating in the blood (512, 1081, 2023) (see Chapter 2). In asymptomatic individuals, it is found in small amounts (1 to 100 infectious particles [IP]/ml); in AIDS patients, it can be detected in larger quantities (100 to 10,000 IP/ml) (Tables 2.2 and 2.3). In most situations, virus has been recovered from both the blood and the cultured PBMC. In others, infectious HIV has been found only in the plasma and not in PBMC (1776). This latter finding may indicate a different source for the plasma virus (e.g., lymph node). Alternatively, the lack of HIV recovery from PBMC could be related to the antiviral activity of CD8$^+$ cells (see Chapter 11).

Studies in our laboratory indicated that some plasma-derived viruses replicate less efficiently in PBMC than do the associated PBMC-derived isolates. Only low-level p24 antigen production and no RT activity was detected in culture fluid (2023). While the results may reflect the presence of less infectious virus, HIV recovered from the plasma of the same individual could have less affinity for the cultured PBMC, since the virus comes from another cellular source. In this regard, one study has demonstrated that at any one time, the predominant plasma virus variant may be antigenically distinct from the virus in the PBMC (2508). Moreover, in another study, only the virus from the plasma, and not viruses obtained from the lymph nodes of the same individual, was sensitive to serum neutralization (2637). In addition, genetic analyses of HIV-1 isolates grown for a short time in cultured PBMC have revealed some differences between plasma and PBMC isolates (2322).

These findings may relate to the "escape" mutants detected by neutralization assays in individuals over time (see above and Chapter 10). Finally, during zidovudine (AZT) treatment, plasma virus could be distinguished from viruses represented in cellular proviral DNA (2979) and from viruses (viral sequences) in the lymph node (1396). All these observations suggest that the plasma virus might better represent the actively replicating virus in the host and be a more reliable predictor of clinical state than are isolates from cultured PBMC. In the same way, the infectious virus in genital fluids may better reflect the agent transmitted by sexual contact (see Chapter 2).

D.

HIV and Virulence: Changes in Biologic and Serologic Properties of HIV over Time in the Host

One of the first observations linking biologic heterogeneity to disease was the finding that HIV-1 strains isolated from AIDS patients differed in biologic properties from those recovered from asymptomatic individuals (96, 429, 746, 2657, 2659) (Table 7.8). Similarly, viruses obtained from the PBMC of an individual in the early asymptomatic period were remarkably different from HIV-1 strains isolated from the same person at later times, when disease had developed (429, 2658). The earlier virus replicated in a limited number of cell types, grew to a relatively low level, and showed slower virus replication than did the later strain associated with disease in the host (429) (Figure 7.3). Moreover, the early virus or the strain in asymptomatic individuals, in contrast to the later one, was not very cytopathic for PBMC (Figure 7.14). Other distinctions of HIV-1 strains probably linked to virulence in the host include lack of induction of latency in established cell lines (424a), resistance to the suppressing effect of Nef as determined in T-cell lines (422), and sensitivity to enhancing and not neutralizing antibodies (1102) (Table 7.8).

Other studies demonstrated by molecular techniques that viruses from the same individual are highly related by restriction enzyme sensitivities and sequence homology (429, 2317). However, at any time, a large number of genetic variants (related but distinguishable) can coexist in an individual (760, 2317). This variation

Table 7.8 Characteristics associated with HIV virulence in the host

1. Expanded cellular host range
2. Rapid kinetics of replication
3. High titers of virus production
4. Disruption or alteration of cell membrane permeability
5. High level of syncytium induction (SI phenotype)
6. Increased cell killing (cytopathicity)
7. Failure to enter a latent state in vitro
8. Lack of sensitivity to suppression by the Nef protein[a]
9. Sensitivity to antibody-mediated enhancement of infection

[a] As assayed with the HIV-1$_{SF2}$ *nef* gene product in T-cell lines (422).

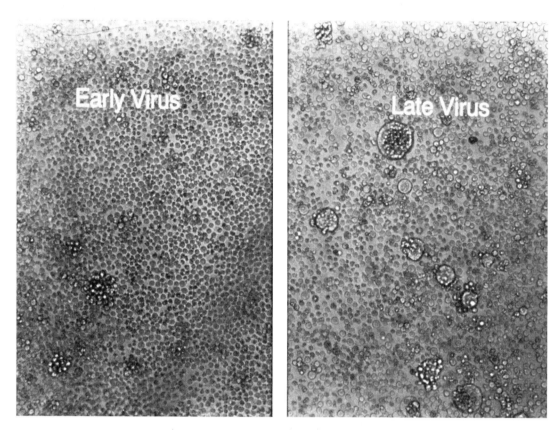

Figure 7.14 HIV-1$_{SF2}$ recovered early during infection from a relatively healthy individual shows very little CPE when inoculated onto normal PBMC. In contrast, HIV-1$_{SF13}$ isolated later from the same individual when he had AIDS shows the syncytium formation and balloon degeneration characteristic of "virulent" strains (Table 7.8). Reprinted from reference 1490 with permission.

appears to be generated more rapidly in vivo than in vitro (2317), most probably reflecting the selective effect of the immune response on HIV replication. The differences are noted particularly in certain sequences in the envelope region (see below) (429, 430, 760, 1099) (see Chapter 8). Specific genetic changes have correlated with changes in host range, enhanced cytopathicity, and "escape" from the immune response (430, 454, 1382, 2566, 2908) (see Chapters 8, 10, and 11).

Many studies have indicated that during acute infection, a homogeneous population of viruses is recovered from the individual. These relatively similar variants are replaced by viruses with varying genetic differences (as noted above), reflected by high complexity. They have been called quasi-species (1767) because they represent variants of the same virus. Finally, during AIDS, a more homogeneous population of viruses is again observed (616). Thus, the initial dominant HIV strain(s), after infection, appears to change over time, probably reflecting responses to the antiviral activity of the immune system. This possibility is supported by the finding of greater diversity in HIV isolates in individuals who have been infected and re-

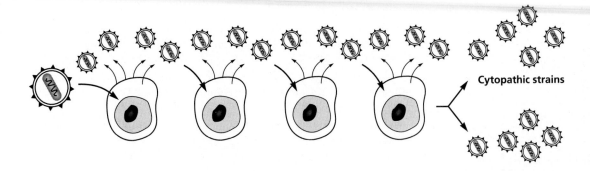

Cytopathic strains

Neuropathic strains

Figure 7.15 HIV replication permits genetic mutations to the virus. HIV, when replicating through different cells, mutates toward a strain that replicates rapidly, is more cytopathic, and can adapt to grow in various tissues such as the brain. Each replicative cycle can lead to up to 10 mutations (most of them lethal), but the surviving virions generally have a rapid kinetics of replication and a high level of virus production (see Section IX.D).

main asymptomatic for the longest period (616, 1604). Evidently associated with a demise in the immune system, the viruses acquire properties of virulence in the host (Table 7.8) (429, 2659). The possible evolution of those strains by multiple cycles of replication is illustrated in Figure 7.15. At that time, a dominant strain again emerges, and the earlier virus population, made up of quasi-species, again becomes homogeneous. The genetic bases for these differences are reviewed in Chapter 8. In some studies, this transition in virus phenotype over time seemed evident in the infected individuals, since virus clones with different biologic properties could be found in the blood at the same time (951, 2418). These results mirror those cited above for variation in genetic sequences among viral species in one individual. The relevant quantity of each type could influence pathogenesis or be a consequence of immune deficiency.

The association of disease with viruses with more "virulent" SI features, as defined in cell culture, is suggestive of causation. For example, SI variants appearing 2 years earlier in the blood can predict progression to AIDS (1346). Moreover, individuals with SI viruses in primary infection have been reported to advance more rapidly to disease (1931, 2274). Several reports suggest that the SI phenotype of HIV leads to a more rapid decline in $CD4^+$ cell counts, which is a predictor of disease progression. Furthermore, studies of sequential primary isolates of HIV from individuals progressing to disease have shown not only a switch from an NSI to SI phenotype but also an expansion in coreceptor usage. The switch to the SI phenotype is associated with the use of CXCR-4 for virus entry (509, 1187). In some cases, the initial virus isolated over time has shown an increased diversity in its coreceptor use to include not only CCR-5 but also CCR-3, CCR-2b, and CXCR-4 (509) (see Chapter 3). Most often, an SI phenotype develops and uses the CXCR-4 coreceptor. The results suggest that the evolution of HIV during infection includes an expanding cellular host range involving the use of several coreceptors. Nevertheless, as noted previously (Chapter 4), some studies have not always shown a direct correlation of SI isolates with progression to AIDS (1242). Adults or children infected with NSI viruses can reach the same CD4$^+$ cell level over time and progress to AIDS (919, 2229, 2547, 2551). Thus, the virus phenotype does not always correlate directly with induction of AIDS. More importantly, it may be the cytopathicity for CD4$^+$ cells that is a common property of NSI strains associated with AIDS (2683, 2947). Whether these observations reflect an etiologic role for the virus or the result of an already compromised immune system is not known. Less immune control of HIV replication could permit mutations leading to the SI strain (see Chapter 13).

How these biologic changes relate to pathogenesis are best evaluated in animal models. In cats, the induction of immune deficiency by the feline leukemia virus has been linked to its envelope region and its ability to cause cytopathic effects in an established feline T-cell line (2004). Work in the SIV system has indicated that other portions of the viral genome (e.g., *nef*) could be responsible for its pathogenic characteristics in vivo (1281, 1679). Moreover, studies with SCID-hu mice reconstituted with human PBMC have shown that macrophage tropism and not cytopathicity by an HIV strain correlates best with CD4$^+$ cell loss (1859). The reason for this observation is not known but might involve the relative levels of cytokines produced and their influence on apoptosis (see Chapters 6, 8, and 13). The possible predominant expression of a particular coreceptor on the target CD4$^+$ cells may need to be considered (see Chapter 3). A reduction in IL-1 production by HIV-infected macrophages and/or an increased expression of Fas ligand (113a) could cause CD4$^+$ cell death by apoptosis (Figure 7.16) (495) (Chapter 6). Apoptosis could also be responsible for the loss of thymocytes following HIV infection of fetal liver and thymus implants in SCID-hu mice (248). In this latter animal model system, in contrast to the SCID-PBMC-hu mouse system (1859), SI viruses are the most destructive (338). Thus, both biologic phenotypes can play a role in CD4$^+$ cell loss (see Chapter 13).

In summary, noncytopathic strains (NSI variants) have been associated with development of AIDS in some patients (648, 1242, 2229), particularly children (2547). Thus, as is true of many conclusions on HIV infection, exceptions to general observations could provide further insights into the true pathogenic pathway.

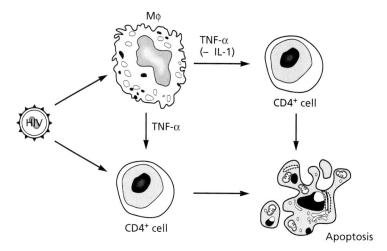

Figure 7.16 Cell killing by noncytopathic HIV-1 strains. A proposed mechanism for indirect loss of CD4$^+$ cells is shown. HIV-1 infection of macrophages can lead to the production of cytokines (e.g., TNF-α) that can induce apoptosis of CD4$^+$ cells (infected or uninfected) (495). Moreover, the loss of IL-1 production by infected macrophages (704, 2299) can cause apoptosis of CD4$^+$ cells, particularly in the presence of antigen. In some cases, infection of CD4$^+$ cells may increase this process of apoptosis. Reprinted from reference 1491 with permission.

The possible role of the relatively noncytopathic macrophage-tropic strains in the slow but persistent loss of CD4$^+$ cells over time in infected individuals merits further study (see Chapter 13). High virus replication rather than cytopathicity may be the important parameter. Moreover, whether SI strains induce progression to disease or result from this event needs further evaluation (Chapter 13). All these results indicate that no conclusions on HIV pathogenesis can be drawn from in vitro studies alone. The best insights can be made by using animal systems, if available.

An important question under consideration is whether a virus showing "virulence" in one individual will do so upon transmission to another. As described in Chapters 4 and 5, the PBMC of individuals can differ in their sensitivity to virus replication and cytopathicity (Figure 5.2). Thus, the relative growth and spread of HIV in the blood and tissues of an infected subject could be one of the parameters determining the extent of pathogenesis. Moreover, the ability of the individual's immune system to counter virus replication is an important factor. A fast-replicating SI virus may be more readily recognized by the host than an NSI virus. Some reports indicate the suppression of SI strains after acute infection and the emergence of NSI variants (530). Neutralizing antibodies could be involved (1437). One concern, however, is that more "virulent" strains of HIV will eventually emerge and pass through the population. While no definitive evidence of this phenomenon has been shown, certain recently infected individuals, whom we are monitoring, have progressed much more rapidly to AIDS than did others first seen 10 years ago. Moreover, some epidemiologic studies have suggested that individuals infected since 1989 have progressed more rapidly to disease than did those infected earlier (2514). This concern about transmission of virulent strains should be given further attention, particularly if the same virus infects individuals with similar genetic backgrounds. How the virulent strains might emerge over time is discussed further in Chapter 13.

Chapter 7   SALIENT FEATURES

1. HIV-1 and HIV-2 can be distinguished by a variety of biologic, serologic, and molecular features, including cell tropism, replication kinetics, levels of virus production, modulation of CD4 protein expression, cytopathicity, latency, genetic structure, and sensitivity to antiviral antibodies.

2. HIV-2 strains appear to be less pathogenic in the host than HIV-1 but are still responsible for induction of AIDS. HIV-2 may be transmitted less efficiently to adults and children.

3. Viruses can be distinguished by their growth in PBMC, macrophages, and T-cell lines. In general, macrophage-tropic viruses are non-syncytium-inducing (NSI) when assayed in T-cell lines, and they do not replicate well in these cells. T-cell-line-tropic viruses are SI and do not replicate well in macrophages. Both types of viruses can be cytopathic in PBMC.

4. Viruses differ in their kinetics and level of replication, which can be influenced by cytokines, concurrent viral infections, and differential expression of the viral regulatory proteins (e.g., Tat).

5. Differences in the molecular structure of HIV can be observed by restriction enzyme analyses and genetic sequencing. Eleven separate sequence genotypes (clades) can now be identified throughout the world, with particular clades dominant in certain countries. An outlier (O) clade that differs substantially from the other major or "main" (M) clades has been recognized.

6. Neutralizing antibodies to HIV-1 and HIV-2 can be demonstrated, and some can cross-neutralize several isolates from all clades, except usually clade O. Resistance to neutralization results from changes within the envelope epitope that are recognized by the antibody or regions outside the epitope that can affect the conformation of the viral envelope.

7. Sensitivity to virus neutralization can be influenced by the cell line in which the isolate is grown, cell surface proteins on the virus, and age of the virus preparations.

8. Virus sensitivity to enhancing antibodies differs; enhancing antibodies are particularly noted in individuals as they advance to disease.

9. Some strains show differences in sensitivity to cell-mediated immune responses, but evidence of resistance is not common.

10. Viral clades can be used to identify transmission of particular viruses among populations and between individuals.

11. HIV heterogeneity can be observed in the host. Virus isolates from the brain, bowel, and plasma can be distinguished from viruses found at other sites.

12. HIV strains appear to become more virulent over time in the host. NSI strains can be replaced by SI strains, which are associated with a greater reduction in $CD4^+$ cell number. The direct relationship of this event to pathogenesis is not yet established.

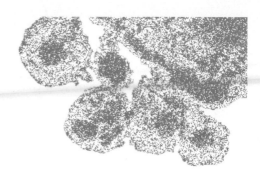

Viral Regions Determining Biologic Features of HIV

INITIAL MOLECULAR STUDIES OF THE HIV GENOME DEFINED IN GENERAL the relative importance of various viral genes for infection and replication. These approaches led to the recognition of several regulatory genes influencing virus production (for reviews, see references 2003 and 2081). Subsequent studies have emphasized the identification of specific genetic regions in the virus responsible for certain biologic and serologic properties, such as cell tropism, kinetics of replication, cytopathicity, CD4 modulation, sensitivity to sCD4, and sensitivity to antiviral antibodies. The findings on most of these features are summarized in this chapter; studies on serologic properties are discussed in Chapter 10. Results from work with both HIV-1 and HIV-2 are considered.

I. Envelope Region and Cell Tropism

A. Genetic Studies

1. GENERAL OBSERVATIONS

Attempts to find limited alterations (perhaps only one amino acid change) associated with a particular viral feature such as cell tropism have focused on the generation of recombinant viral genomes. Advantage is taken of restriction enzyme sites shared among diverse HIV strains or the introduction of such sites by PCR techniques. Selected regions of a virus are removed by the restriction enzymes and reinserted into the backbone of another cloned virus. In some studies, two biologically active molecular clones have been used. In others, a noninfectious molecular clone has been used to donate regions to, or exchange regions with, a biologically active clone. Subsequently, site-directed mutagenesis has been helpful to further define the genetic sequences governing a specific in vitro property of the virus.

Several reports initially demonstrated that the envelope region contains the primary genetic sequences responsible for T-cell-line and macrophage tropism, cytopathology, CD4 protein modulation, and virus neutralization (347, 426, 430, 435, 526, 1148, 1569, 1966, 2484, 2943) (see Chapter 10). In all these studies and others cited in this book, it is important to recognize that differences in the ability of HIV isolates to infect established (transformed) T-cell lines do not indicate variations in tropism for $CD4^+$ lymphocytes. All viral mutants, except those losing infectivity in general, maintain the ability to infect peripheral blood $CD4^+$ cells, assuming that the appropriate coreceptor is present (see Chapter 3). Moreover, most if not all HIV isolates can infect macrophages, but the extent of replication varies. Thus, macrophage tropism refers to viruses that grow to high titer in macrophages. In addition, macrophage tropism does not necessarily indicate an inability to replicate in established T-cell lines. Dual-tropic viruses can be identified. Many viruses grow well only in $CD4^+$ lymphocytes and not in macrophages or T-cell lines (see below and Chapter 3). Finally, tropism for primary macrophages does not correlate with infection of transformed monocytic cell lines. Thus, results from cell culture studies may not have direct relevance in vivo, but the observations do reveal the importance of certain genetic regions and envelope conformation in cell tropism.

Importantly, before the discovery of the coreceptors for macrophage-tropic (CCR-5) and T-cell-line-tropic (CXCR-4) viruses, studies were aimed at identifying the region of the viral envelope that determines infection of different cell types. With the recognition that specific cellular coreceptors are involved, the past findings presented in the following sections are now particularly relevant to understanding the interaction of macrophage-tropic or T-cell-line-tropic viruses with their specific cell surface receptor. For example, for CCR-5 and CXCR-4, the V3 loop appears to be an important determinant (488, 2545a) (see also Chapter 13), as had been previously demonstrated by the early experiments with the interviral recombinants described below. However, the diversity of strains that use this receptor (different clades of HIV-1, HIV-2, and SIV) implies that regions other than this variable envelope domain are involved. Reviewed in this section are data on certain genetic regions and on the conformation of the envelope protein that can determine cellular host range as defined by the virus envelope:cell receptor interactions (see also Chapters 3 and 4) (Table 3.3).

2. MACROPHAGE TROPISM

Certain experiments conducted several years ago examined the cellular host range of HIV and considerably narrowed the region(s) of the virus responsible for macrophage tropism. Studies of two unrelated HIV-1 viruses (the T-cell-line-tropic

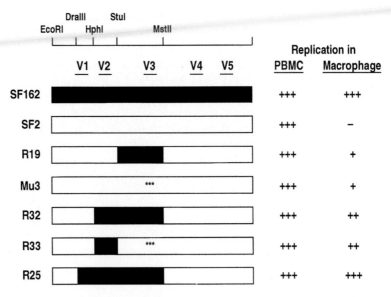

Figure 8.1   Recombinant virus strains were derived from HIV-1$_{SF162}$, a macrophage-tropic virus, and HIV-1$_{SF2}$, a T-cell-line-tropic virus. Previous studies had indicated that only three amino acid changes (stars) in the V3 loop (positions 319, 320, and 323) (Figure 7.11) could convert the SF2 strain (Mu3) into a macrophage-tropic strain (2485). Subsequent studies shown here indicated that both the V1 and V2 regions are important in conferring optimal macrophage tropism on the SF2 strain (R25) (1338). Plus signs indicate the extent of virus replication.

SF2 strain and the macrophage-tropic SF162 strain) initially showed that infection of primary macrophages was associated with a 159-amino-acid region in the 3' portion of the gp120 (2484). A similar finding was made with two other viral strains (1966). Subsequently, the involvement of the V3 loop alone (amino acids ~304 to 324 of gp120) in macrophage tropism was demonstrated (435, 1148, 2485, 2867). As few as three amino acid changes in the V3 domain (positions 311, 319, and 323) were found to confer macrophage tropism on a T-cell-line-tropic strain (2485) (Figure 7.11). Nevertheless, conversion of a T-cell-line-tropic strain such as HIV-1$_{SF2}$ to a macrophage-tropic strain with replicative properties equal to those of HIV-1$_{SF162}$ required the transfer of the V1 and V2 regions as well the V3 loop (1338) (Figure 8.1). Similar observations on the importance of the V1 and V2 regions for efficient replication in cultured macrophages have been made with other virus recombinants (2689).

   In other mutant-virus studies, elimination of two N-linked glycosylation sites in the V2 region of SF2 conferred macrophage tropism and eliminated the T-cell-line tropism of HIV-1$_{SF2}$ (1340). This dramatic finding appeared to reflect the importance of envelope conformation and/or charge on viral entry (see Section B). Finally, recent studies suggest that productive infection of macrophages involves two distinct genetic regions and mechanisms: envelope gene for virus entry, and *vif* and *vpr* for efficient virus replication (1075).

Work with SIV infection of macrophages has uncovered other potential roles of the envelope region in virus replication besides the interaction with cell surface receptors. Envelope recombinant mutants that replicate poorly in macrophages were found to enter with an efficiency similar to that of macrophage-tropic strains, but steps involved in the late stages of reverse transcription were inhibited (1844). The mechanisms responsible could be induction of cytokines, signal transduction (i.e., following viral envelope interaction with the cell membrane), or events involving the processing of Env (see also Chapter 7). In some studies of macrophage-tropic and non-macrophage-tropic strains, the processing of the Env and Gag precursor proteins of an envelope chimeric virus was blocked (1204).

3. T-CELL-LINE TROPISM

For T-cell-line tropism, studies with the SF2 and SF162 strains of HIV-1 indicated initially that the specific sequences associated with infection of these cells were somewhat broader (310 amino acids) than those for macrophages; however, again, no regulatory proteins were involved (2484). Subsequently, the V3 loop was also found to be important for T-cell-line tropism (346, 1148, 2485). The SF2 recombinant virus with the SF162-like V3 domain described above lost its T-cell-line tropism when it gained macrophage tropism (2485). Moreover, substituting the five different amino acids in the V3 loop of HIV-1$_{SF162}$ with the amino acids of HIV-1$_{SF2}$ did not convert the HIV-1$_{SF162}$ recombinant to a T-cell-line-tropic strain. However, in one SF2 mutant (Mu8), a single amino acid change in the V3 loop (position 323, Figure 7.11) eliminated the ability of the SF2 mutant virus to infect one particular T-cell line (MT-4) but not others (2485) (Table 8.1). Noteworthy was the observation that the substitution of three amino acids in the V3 regions of SF2 produced a

Table 8.1 Cellular host range of HIV-1$_{SF2mc}$ and HIV-1$_{SF162mc}$ mutant viruses[a]

HIV-1 strain	V3 region sequence	Virus replication in:[b]			
		PBMC	Macrophages	HUT 78	MT-4
SF2					
wt	iYigpgrafHTtgRiigdirKa	+ + +	−	+ + +	+ + +
Mu1	-T-------YA--D------Q-	+ + +	+	−	−
Mu2	-T-------YA--D--------	+ + +	+	−	−
Mu3	---------YA--D--------	+ + +	+	−	−
Mu8	-------------D--------	+ + +	−	+ + +	−
R19	-T-------YA--D------Q-	+ + +	+	−	−
SF162					
wt	iTigpgrafYAtgDiigdirQa	+ + +	+ +	−	−
Mu10	-Y-------HT--R------K-	+ + +	+	−	−
Mu11	-Y-------HT--R--------	+ + +	+	−	−

[a] Mutant proviral DNAs were generated by site-directed mutagenesis with mutant oligodeoxynucleotides as primers. Mutant viruses were recovered by transfection of mutagenized proviral DNA into human RD4 cells followed by cocultivation with PBMC from seronegative individuals. These viruses were inoculated at 10^6 cpm of reverse transcriptase activity onto PBMC, primary macrophages, and the HUT 78 and MT-4 T-cell lines. Adapted from reference 2485.

[b] The relative extent of virus replication is represented by plus signs. Minus sign indicates no detectable virus production.

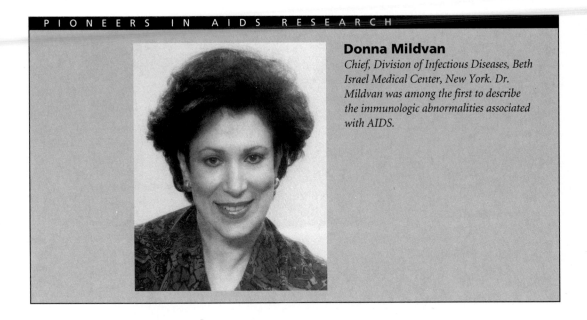

Donna Mildvan

Chief, Division of Infectious Diseases, Beth Israel Medical Center, New York. Dr. Mildvan was among the first to describe the immunologic abnormalities associated with AIDS.

mutant (Mu3) with both macrophage and T-cell-line tropisms, although somewhat reduced in comparison to parental strains (2485) (Table 8.1).

In studies with other HIV-1 T-cell-line-tropic isolates, replacement of the V3 region with that of a non-T-cell-line-tropic virus eliminated that tropism. However, the reciprocal exchange did not confer T-cell-line tropism (368). Thus, the V3 domain is needed for T-cell-line infection, but other regions in the envelope must help to determine the extent of T-cell-line tropism. Some studies suggest that a small region of the C4 domain can be involved (366, 2922). The C4 region is part of the CD4 binding site (see Chapter 3). Others suggest an interaction of the V3 loop with the V1 loop (366). In perhaps unusual cases, the V3 domain of a virus shows dual tropism. In addition, two specific amino acid changes in the V3 domain of the macrophage-tropic strain SF162 (amino acids 307 and 312) have been found to produce a virus with T-cell-line tropism, syncytium-inducing (SI) phenotype, and sensitivity to soluble CD4 (sCD4) neutralization. The reason for the alteration in host range and cytopathicity appears linked to envelope conformation or charge (1022). Finally, as noted above, two changes in the V2 region of SF2 that brought about macrophage tropism eliminated T-cell-line tropism (1340). All these observations emphasize the role of envelope conformation on viral host range (Section I.B), particularly interactions with CD4 and coreceptors (see also Chapter 3).

Other studies examining structure-function relationships have used HIV-1$_{SF2}$ and HIV-1$_{SF13,}$ which are closely related but biologically distinct viral isolates recovered over time from the same individual (423, 430). With these two strains, more direct comparisons of genetic differences are possible since the genomes of these two viral isolates differ by less than 3%. Cytopathicity and tropism for macrophages and certain T-cell lines were found to be associated with 10 or 12 amino acid differences in the envelope gp120 of SF2 compared to SF13 (Figure 8.2).

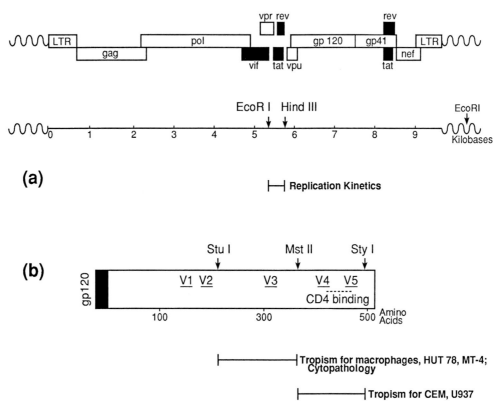

Figure 8.2   Structure-function relationship of HIV-1. The HIV-1~SF2~ and HIV-1~SF13~ related isolates were used. The regions of HIV-1 needed for cell tropism, cytopathology, and CD4 down-modulation are indicated (b). A region in the second exon of *tat* has been found to be associated with the kinetics of virus replication (a). Reprinted from reference 431 with permission.

Most noteworthy in these SF2/SF13 studies was the observation that tropism for certain cell lines and cell types was determined by nonoverlapping regions of the HIV gp120. Infection of macrophages, HUT 78, and the MT-4 cell lines was associated with the envelope domain encompassing the V3 loop. Tropism for CEM and U937 cells was linked to a separate portion of gp120 containing V4, V5, and the CD4 binding domains (Figure 8.2). A similar selective effect of an amino acid change in the CD4 binding region on tropism for U937 cells, but not a T-cell line, was shown by others (526). That separate regions controlled entry into primary macrophages and into the U937 cells further indicated that the U937 line is not an ideal target for examining macrophage tropism. Moreover, these studies confirmed that the V3 loop alone does not determine productive infection of all cell types.

4. THE V3 LOOP
Focusing on the V3 loop, mutations made in the crown (GPGRA) of this HIV envelope region have generally induced a loss of infectivity and changes in the fusogenic potential of the viruses examined (945, 1170, 2015, 2566) without affecting

CD4 binding. Furthermore, in certain experiments (779, 1785, 2485), the envelope charge in the V3 loop (e.g., the presence of a positively charged amino acid at position 11 or 28) was found associated with efficient T-cell-line infection, syncytium formation, and virus replication. In other cases, however, this correlation of SI viruses with specific amino acids in the V3 sequence has not been confirmed (431, 2323). Such discordance has also been reported in 3 to 10% of isolates from children and adults (2377, 2378). Furthermore, differences among HIV-1 clades in terms of concordance with these molecular findings have been noted (2323). With HIV-2, the association of cell tropism with the V3 loop has also been reported (34).

In some experiments with the SF2 and SF13 strains, changes outside the crown but within the V3 loop, as well as in the C2 envelope region, were found to affect spontaneous gp120 shedding and infectivity of peripheral blood mononuclear cells (PBMC) by recombinant viruses (2566) (see Chapter 3). The latter findings may reflect the importance of the C2 region in both the gp120:CD4 interaction and gp120:gp41 attachment (1982, 2570). Finally, as discussed in Chapter 3, other viral regions, including those on gp41 (2522), may have envelope domains needed for postbinding steps involved in virus entry. The latter are presumably linked to virus:cell fusion (see Figures 3.2 and 3.5 and Color Plate 2 [following p. 188]).

5. TROPISM FOR BRAIN-DERIVED CELLS

Studies of infection of CD4$^+$ brain-derived fibroblasts with other isolates of HIV-1 (e.g., the GUN strains) have shown that a single amino acid in the V3 loop (amino acid 311) can affect HIV infection (2635). The results demonstrated that changes in this region of the virus can affect cell tropism and sensitivity to neutralizing antibodies (1737). Moreover, perhaps as expected, using the strains JR-FL (macrophage tropic) and NLY-3 (T-cell-line tropic), the infection of brain-derived microglia was linked to the same envelope region controlling macrophage tropism (2465). In other studies, the pattern of envelope N-linked glycosylation appeared to be important for this infection (1462).

In addition, as noted with T-cell and macrophage tropisms, changes within the crown of the V3 loop were found to be needed for infection of brain-derived cells (e.g., meningiomas) (2483). Moreover, sequences regulating the tropism of HIV-1 for brain capillary endothelial cells were localized to a region encompassing the C1 portion of Env and overlapping reading frames for Vpr, Vpu, Tat, and Rev. This domain does not cosegregate with either macrophage or T-cell-line tropism (1853). Nevertheless, the sensitivity of brain capillary endothelial cells to HIV-1 infection correlated best with T-cell-line tropism and not with macrophage tropism (see Chapter 7). In addition, sequences in either V3 or V4/V5 appear to determine the tropism of some viruses for neural cell lines, in which entry is mediated by galactosyl ceramide (GalC) (1010, 1011). The relevance of these findings to other brain isolates requires further study.

6. INFECTION OF CD4$^-$ CELLS

In investigations of the CD4-independent tropism of HIV-1 and HIV-2, certain regions in the envelope protein were found to be responsible. With HIV-1, as noted above, regions within the V3 loop that interact with GalC on CD4$^-$ brain- and bowel-derived cells have been identified (1010, 1011, 2927). With HIV-2, the sequences including portions of the transmembrane protein and the V3 loop and areas flanking the base of the V4 loop could be involved (702, 2205).

B. ## Role of Envelope Conformation in Cell Tropism

All the results have indicated that generally more than three amino acid changes are required to affect cell tropism, particularly if substantial replication is measured. Nevertheless, in some cases, one modification has affected the infection of a single cell line (526, 2485) (Table 8.1). The findings emphasize the importance for HIV entry of a variety of viral epitopes, determined most probably by the conformation of gp120, particularly in the V3 loop. In support of this conclusion, additional regions of the envelope gp120 outside the V3 loop were found to enhance the extent of virus replication in T-cell lines and macrophages, probably by increasing the efficiency of virus entry via the V3 loop (366, 367, 435, 2484, 2566, 2867). In this connection, certain studies suggest that the V1 and V2 domains, together with the V3 loop, can increase viral infectivity and replication in macrophages (Figure 8.1) (1338). Moreover, conserved regions in gp120 (such as the C4 region) can influence HIV infection of certain cell types; with the help of V1/V2, these additional domains can determine syncytium formation in culture and affect viral tropism (1267). It seems likely that the envelope of each viral strain, depending on the amino acid makeup of the envelope, will have a different conformational structure. Therefore, various envelope regions for specific viruses could influence their ability to enter cells.

These observations strongly suggest that emphasis should be placed on the role in infection of the three-dimensional structure of the viral envelope, and not on individual epitopes. Various viral properties reflect the importance of envelope conformation (Table 8.2). Among these, cell tropism and antibody binding (including serum neutralization) appear to be the best correlates (682, 1839, 2570). Most of the properties do not occur together consistently and thus most probably reflect varia-

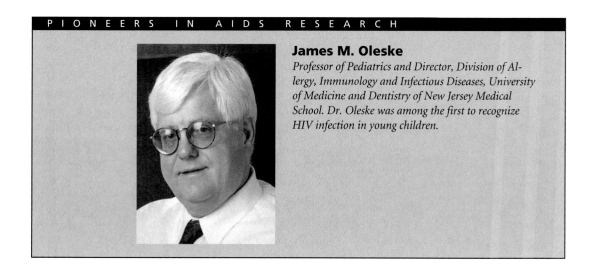

Table 8.2 Viral properties reflecting envelope conformation[a]

1. Host range: macrophage versus T-cell-line tropism
2. Antibody neutralization—conformation-dependent epitopes
3. Antibody binding efficiency
4. Envelope cleavage
5. Virus:cell fusion
6. Soluble CD4 inactivation
7. Virus:CD4[+] cell binding
8. Spontaneous gp120 shedding

[a] Most of the above parameters do not appear together consistently.

tions in envelope conformation but not universal sites responsible for the particular conformation.

This conclusion on the importance of the envelope conformation is supported by studies with the T-cell-line-tropic strain HIV-1$_{SF2}$, the macrophage-tropic strain HIV-1$_{SF162}$, and their V3 loop mutants (Table 8.3; Figure 7.11) (1338, 2485, 2570). The SF2/SF162 mutant virus Mu8, in which only the arginine in the SF2 V3 loop has been replaced by an aspartic acid at position 323, shows an inability to infect the MT-4 cell line but infects other T-cell lines readily, like the parental strain SF2 (Table 8.1). Mu8 demonstrates other SF2 properties, including an inability to productively infect macrophages, but this mutant virus is resistant to gp120 cleavage, like the SF162 strain (Table 8.1). Thus, only one amino acid change modifies two properties of SF2 (Table 8.3). The Mu3 mutant of SF2, with only three amino acid substitutions in the V3 loop, resembling SF162 (Section I.A), shows some characteristics of both T-cell-line and macrophage tropism. Like the SF2 strain, Mu3 undergoes spontaneous shedding of gp120 and envelope cleavage (Table 8.3) and is inactivated by sCD4. Its reaction with monoclonal antibodies shows a dual-tropic response (2570); its envelope binds to both macrophage-tropic and T-cell-line-tropic related monoclonal antibodies (Table 8.3) (2570).

This reaction of HIV-1 strains to specific monoclonal antibodies appears to distinguish macrophage-tropic from T-cell-line-tropic isolates very well (682, 2570). Such antibodies can detect conformational changes in gp120 that occur after virus:receptor binding and that distinguish viruses with different cell tropisms (2567). Observations with the other viral mutants, Mu1 and Mu8 (Table 8.1), also demonstrate that cell tropism correlates with antibody binding but not with the other properties listed in Table 8.3.

Other studies reflecting the role of envelope conformation have shown that certain genetic changes that reduce the infectivity of one HIV strain may not have any effect on the infectivity of another virus if the sequences surrounding the mutated site are different (2015). Moreover, certain amino acid changes in the C2 and V3 loop regions of the SF2/SF13 mutant viruses discussed earlier can increase the extent of gp120 shedding by the viral envelope without affecting binding to the CD4 cell surface protein. In this case, virus infectivity of T-cell lines can be increased, perhaps secondary to enhanced exposure of the gp41 fusion molecule (see Chapter 3)

Table 8.3 Correlation of HIV-1 properties with envelope sequences[a]

Property	SF2	SF162	Mu1	Mu3	Mu8
Host range	T	M	M	M-T	T
Monoclonal antibody binding[b]	T	M	M	M-T	T
gp120 cleavage	+	−	−	+	−
sCD4 inactivation	+	−	−	+	+
Spontaneous gp120 shedding	+ +	−	+	+	
Virus:cell binding[c]	+ +	±	+ +	+ [d]	+

[a] Relative extent of the properties listed is expressed by + and − signs. T, T-cell-line tropic; M, macrophage tropic. Data from references 1322, 1338, and 2570.

[b] Measured with monoclonal antibodies to the V3 loop. Certain monoclonal antibodies show preferential reactivity with T-cell-line- or macrophage-tropic viruses.

[c] Measured with CD4+ HUT 78 cells.

[d] Shows delayed replication in HUT 78 cells.

(Figure 3.2 and Color Plate 2 [following p. 188]). In contrast, some mutant viruses with increased spontaneous gp120 release are less infectious and not very cytopathic (2566). In this case, the affinity of gp41 for its binding region on gp120 (which does not involve the V3 loop) also appears to have been affected by the V3 loop changes, but other alterations must influence infectivity.

This effect of amino acid substitutions in the V3 loop on the virion gp120:gp41 envelope complex has been noted in other studies on cell tropism (2890). In both instances, the modifications in the V3 region most probably changed the conformational structure of the viral envelope and caused the increased displacement of gp120 from the virus envelope. The result alters the biologic properties observed, depending on the particular viral strain. Obviously, gp120 shedding alone is not sufficient to determine a viral biologic phenotype (Table 8.3). Finally, the influence of gp120 glycosylation on cell tropism supports the importance of envelope conformation in cell tropism (1340, 1462)—essentially the ability of certain regions of this viral protein to interact with receptors or coreceptors on the cell surface (Chapter 3).

II.   Regulatory Proteins and Virus Replication

The relative role of HIV regulatory genes in determining the extent of virus replication has also been studied with recombinant viruses. With the interviral SF2/SF13 recombinants, substantial virus replication in PBMC and the HUT 78 cell line was linked to the first exon coding region of *tat* and reflected only two amino acid differences (430, 431) (Figure 8.2). A change in one of these two amino acid differences in Tat$_{SF13}$ reduced the extent of replication of the SF13 strain to that of the SF2 strain (1465). While initially Tat was thought to regulate the kinetics of virus replication, close examination with a mathematical equation showed that the effect was on the level of virus production (638). HIV-1$_{SF13}$ produces nearly twice as many infectious viruses as does HIV-1$_{SF2}$. Thus, the faster kinetics reflected increased number and spread of progeny viruses in culture. The results indicate that for some isolates, limited modifications in the Tat regulatory protein can greatly affect virus replication.

Additional studies using the chloramphenicol acetyltransferase (CAT) assay have supported the effect of HIV-1$_{SF2}$, HIV-1$_{SF13}$, and HIV-1$_{SF33}$ Tat proteins on their respective long terminal repeats (LTR) (1465). The results showed that cell type can influence the effect of Tat and that the LTRs from the high-producer strains (SF13 and SF33) were more sensitive to Tat$_{SF2}$ than was the LTR from SF2 (1465). Moreover, no substantial difference was observed in the extent of transactivation by Tat$_{SF13}$ when using the LTR from the three different viruses. Finally, in the CAT assay the function of the Tat mutant of SF13 described above resembled that of the Tat$_{SF2}$ protein. Thus, these findings further indicated the substantial effect of Tat on the viral LTR and the important role of this interaction in virus replication.

As noted previously, introducing the *tat* gene into Jurkat cells that are relatively nonpermissive for replication of a particular HIV strain can convert them into actively producing cells (95, 746). Furthermore, rodent cells lacking a cellular factor that interacts with the Tat protein are less sensitive to HIV replication (1024) (see Chapter 5). All these observations indicate a major role of the *tat* gene in promoting virus replication but also reflect its important interplay with the viral LTR as well as with cellular proteins. Despite these findings in the laboratory, studies of viruses from individuals with different rates of progression to disease have not revealed a major influence of the TAR and *tat* regions (1304). Other studies of clinical isolates are warranted.

Some reports suggest that small changes in *vif*, as well as *vpr* and *vpu*, can also affect the extent of virus infectivity and replication (2333) (see Chapter 5). Finally, Rev, Nef, and intracellular factors appear to affect HIV production by a variety of mechanisms (2003) (see Chapter 5). In clinical isolates, alterations in these other accessory viral genes, except for Nef, also do not correlate with either a progressive or a long-term asymptomatic course (see Chapter 13).

III.   Envelope Region and Cytopathicity, CD4 Protein Modulation, and sCD4 Neutralization

A.   Cytopathicity

Other observations with interviral recombinants have identified to some extent the specific regions in the viral envelope that determine cytopathicity as measured by syncytium formation and plaque formation in MT-4 cells (426, 2566, 2943). As noted above, this region in the SF2/SF13 recombinants is the same as that associated with tropism for primary macrophages, HUT 78, and MT-4 cells (431) (Figure 8.2) but does not involve the V3 loop (2566). In some mutational studies, the role of the V1, V2, or V3 loop in cytopathicity has been identified, depending on the viruses studied (72, 589, 793-795, 2015, 2614, 2820). The influence of the V3 domain on this biologic property was suggested by earlier work in which cell:cell fusion was blocked by the RP135 (amino acids 307 and 330) peptide of HIV-1 gp120 (2308). In this regard, amino acid substitutions outside the V3 loop can affect syncytium formation (2566).

In evaluating viral cytopathicity, De Jong et al. (588) demonstrated that the introduction of one positively charged amino acid (e.g., arginine) into a specific region of the V3 loop can, in some cases, produce an SI virus. This observation was supported by other investigators examining SI versus non-syncytium-inducing (NSI) viruses. Most of the SI viruses had a positive charge near the crown of the V3 loop (778, 779). Nevertheless, some SI strains, particularly of the HIV-2 type, do not show this characteristic (431, 2323) (see Section I.A).

In addition, the V1 and V2 regions can influence the extent of syncytium formation (950, 2614), perhaps through a functional interaction with the C4 region of gp120 (793). This potential interaction between the V1/V2 domains and C4 has also been suggested by studies with monoclonal antibodies (1734, 1837). The possible role of gp41 in this process has been considered as well (see Chapter 6) (762, 792, 794, 1365, 2074, 2522). Furthermore, only two glycosylation sites in the viral gp120 can determine the extent of cell death resulting from lysis independent of cell fusion (2595). This observation supports the role of glycosylation in cytopathology (1821). The mechanism(s) by which the viral envelope would bring about this cytopathology is discussed in Chapter 6. In other studies of cytopathicity, a more cytopathic HIV-1 isolate was Vpu deficient and on infection led to the accumulation of envelope glycoproteins at the cell surface. This phenomenon suggested that the cellular retention of virions that are usually released with the help of Vpu could be partly responsible for the cytopathic effects of HIV-1 (1173).

Finally, recent studies with SIV mutants showing increased pathogenicity have indicated that the nucleotide changes potentially responsible for disease are present particularly in the envelope region but also in *tat* and the LTR. These observations are noteworthy since they are among the first to relate changes in the viral genome to pathology in vivo (1244). Nevertheless, as noted above, similar findings with *tat* and TAR have not been made with clinical isolates of HIV-1 (1304).

B.   CD4 Protein Modulation

CD4 down-modulation was first mapped to the envelope region of HIV (426, 2943). While a specific domain has not been definitively identified, it is most probably the CD4 binding region of gp120. Nevertheless, the potential role of Nef (844, 974, 2714) and/or Vpu in this process must be appreciated (see Chapter 3, Table 3.5). For example, Vpu causes a release of gp160 from the CD4 envelope complex in the endoplasmic reticulum (2884). This dissociation appears to result from CD4 degradation induced by Vpu. The results suggest that the cytoplasmic domain of CD4 contains one determinant susceptible to this Vpu-induced degradation (1476). This region of CD4 is also a determinant for CD4 down-modulation by Nef (70). Recently, CD4 down-modulation was shown to occur rapidly as a result of Nef, but the later expression of Vpu and the viral envelope gave the optimal reduction in CD4 expression (414). Further studies may indicate the sites in Vpu and Nef that influence these processes that can affect CD4 protein expression.

C.   sCD4 Neutralization

The structural basis for HIV heterogeneity with regard to sensitivity to sCD4 has been examined. In general, macrophage-tropic viruses are resistant to sCD4 and appear to bind this molecule less avidly. Early studies showed that sCD4 resistance and macrophage tropism are associated with the V3 and flanking regions of gp120 (1147). With molecular clones of macrophage-tropic and T-cell-line-tropic strains, sCD4 sensitivity corresponded to a rapid shedding of gp120 after interaction with sCD4. The sCD4 sensitivity is temperature related, since there is increased shedding of gp120 and inactivation of the macrophage-tropic viruses at 4°C, whereas at that temperature the sensitivity to sCD4 is reduced for the T-cell-line-tropic viruses (1967). The number of gp120 molecules on macrophage-tropic viruses appears to be about four times greater than that on the T-cell-line-tropic viruses (1967). Thus, potential posttranslational changes to the virion occurring within a cell can affect not only cell tropism and sensitivity to antibody neutralization but also sensitivity to sCD4 neutralization. The results support previous studies showing that adaptation of macrophage-tropic viruses to T-cell lines increases their binding to sCD4 (1839). Nevertheless, recent studies suggest that gp120 density and stability are not involved in resistance to sCD4 (1243).

IV.   Conclusions

All of the work directed at mapping the genetic determinants of cell tropism was conducted before the identification of the coreceptors for HIV entry of macrophages and T-cell lines. Therefore, the evidence reviewed in this chapter can provide insights into the probable domains on the envelope of HIV isolates that determine their interaction with CCR-5 and CXCR-4. While the V3 loop in many of the genetic studies appears to be required for the virus:cell interaction, the diversity of viral strains interacting with CD4 and coreceptors suggests that other domains are necessary and can be very important. Studies aimed at identifying the regions of the HIV envelope that bind to the coreceptors (2545a) should relate very well to the results obtained over the past years, when virus infection of cultured macrophages versus T-cell lines was measured. Only further work with interviral recombinants performed with HIV strains from a variety of individuals will determine if a common conformational structure or a particular region in a viral envelope correlates with a certain cell tropism or biologic property. Besides studies of T-cells and macrophages, evaluation of genetic regions controlling infection of brain-derived cells and CD4⁻ cells also needs to be continued. Specific virus envelope:cell interactions should be examined, and several mechanisms will most probably be found to be involved. With some HIV isolates, the influence of electrical charge should be considered, but this feature is only one of several that could influence tropism and cytopathicity. In general, the envelope conformation appears to be the major determinant of several biologic properties of HIV, particularly cell tropism (Section I.B) (Table 8.2) (2015, 2566). For analysis of the potential three-dimensional structures, studies with monoclonal antibodies offer promising results (2570). These reagents could eventually provide valuable insight into the three-dimensional form of the HIV envelope until full crystallization is achieved.

Chapter 8	SALIENT FEATURES

1. The cellular host range of HIV is determined to a great extent by linear and conformational epitopes of the viral envelope region. The conformation of the viral envelope appears to be the major determinant for cell tropism.

2. Small differences (as few as two or three amino acids) can determine whether a virus is macrophage tropic or T-cell-line tropic. Both types of viruses have the capacity to infect CD4$^+$ lymphocytes.

3. The V3 loop of the viral envelope is a major determinant for infection of cells, most probably through its role in the interaction with coreceptors on the cell surface (Chapter 3).

4. Tropism for brain-derived cells is also determined by the envelope region but can involve other viral regions, including the HIV regulatory proteins.

5. Infection of CD4$^-$ cells involves in part the V3 loop as well as other regions of the viral envelope.

6. Regulatory proteins (e.g., Tat) are involved in the kinetics of virus replication and level of HIV production.

7. The envelope region is an important determinant of viral cytopathicity, down-modulation of CD4 expression, and sensitivity of HIV isolates to sCD4 neutralization. Nef and Vpu can also affect the expression of CD4 on the cell surface.

8. The heterogeneity of HIV, resulting from its error-prone reverse transcription, can lead to the emergence of viral strains with differing biologic features involving virus:cell interactions, induction of cell death, and modulation in CD4 expression on the cell surface.

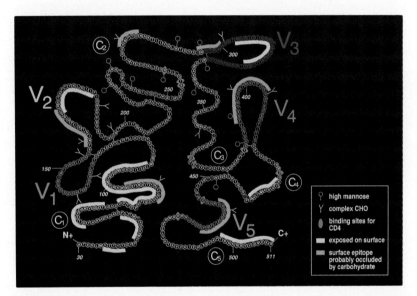

Color Plate 1   Schematic representation of gp120 HIV-1$_{LAI}$, showing disulfide and glycosylation sites. Glycosylation sites containing high-mannose-type and/or hybrid-type oligosaccharides are indicated, as well as the glycosylation sites with complex-type oligosaccharide structures. The variable regions are designated V1 to V5. The conserved regions are designated C1 to C5. Parts of the envelope exposed on the surface and those portions probably occluded by carbohydrates are demonstrated. The CD4 region contains a major attachment site for CD4 (1434). Also noted are other regions on gp120 that, according to studies with amino acid substitutions (1982), appear to be involved in binding to the CD4 molecule (1838). Reprinted from reference 1479 with permission. (See p. 44.)

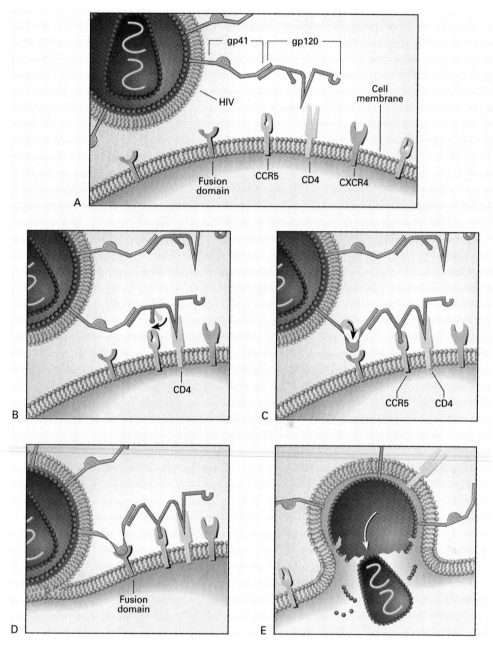

Color Plate 2 Interactions between HIV and the cell surface. (A) HIV interacts with a cell surface receptor, primarily CD4, and through conformational changes becomes more closely associated with the cell through interactions with other cell surface molecules, such as the chemokine receptors CXCR-4 and CCR-5. Alternatively, some viruses, such as certain strains of HIV-2, could attach to CXCR-4 directly. (B to E) The likely steps in HIV infection are as follows. The CD4-binding site on HIV-1 gp120 interacts with the CD4 molecule on the cell surface (B). Conformational changes in both the viral envelope and the CD4 receptor permit the binding of gp120 to another cell surface receptor, such as CCR-5 (C). This second attachment brings the viral envelope closer to the cell surface, allowing interaction between gp41 on the viral envelope and a fusion domain on the cell surface. HIV fuses with the cell (D). Subsequently, the viral nucleoid enters into the cell, most likely by means of other cellular events (E). Once this stage is achieved, the cycle of viral replication begins. (See p. 52.)

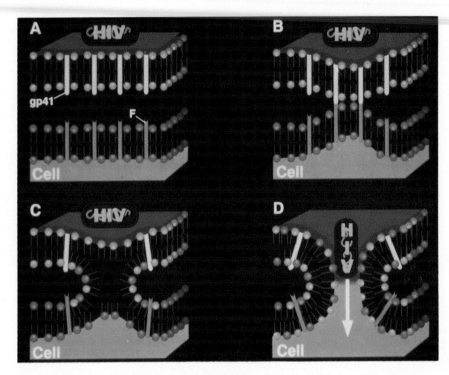

Color Plate 3   HIV:cell fusion. The fusion molecule on the HIV envelope (i.e., gp41) interacts with a fusion receptor (F) on the cell surface (A and B). This process leads to an intermixing of the inner lipid membranes (hemifusion) (C), but unless the outer lipid membranes also undergo intermixing (D), the HIV core cannot enter into the cell cytoplasm. This nucleocapsid entry may also depend on specific viral and cellular factors. Figure derived from a design provided by L. Stamatatos. (See p. 59.)

Color Plate 4   An HIV-infected T lymphocyte (HUT 78 cell), shown by immunofluorescence staining, fuses with an uninfected HUT 78 T cell. This interaction permits virus transfer to the uninfected cell. Magnification, ×65. Photo courtesy of E. Lennette. (See p. 66.)

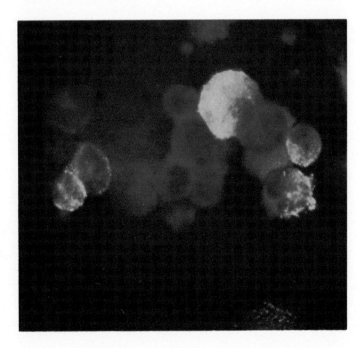

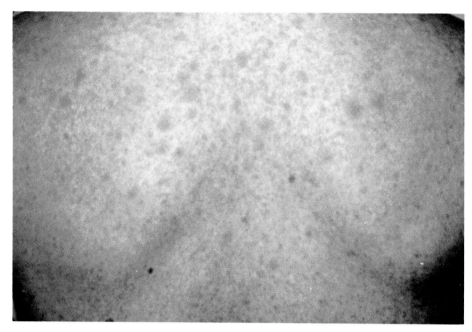

Color Plate 5 Typical macular-papular rash on the surface of the skin occurring within days after acute (primary) HIV infection. Photograph courtesy of R. Hutt and C. Farling. (See p. 76.)

Color Plate 6 HIV infection of lymphoid tissue. By using both in situ DNA and RNA PCR procedures, the presence of HIV infection in cells of the lymph node was evaluated (695). (A) A large number of cells are infected, as demonstrated by in situ DNA PCR procedures. Note the green grains (designating reaction with the HIV probe) over virus-infected cells. (B) In the same lymph node, evaluated by in situ RNA PCR, only two cells replicating virus particles (dark grains indicate viral RNA) can be detected. It has been estimated that 1 in 300 to 1 in 400 infected cells in the lymph node is producing virus (695). Photomicrographs courtesy of A. Haase. (See p. 88.)

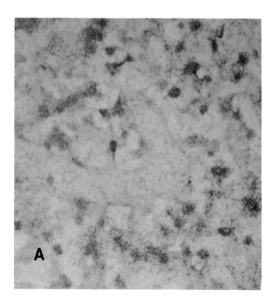

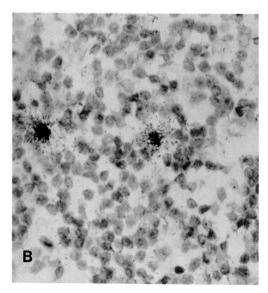

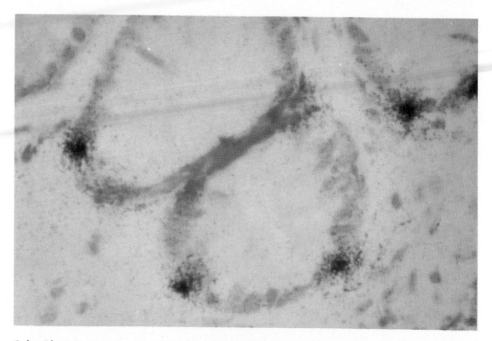

Color Plate 7   Histologic section of a colon biopsy specimen from an HIV-infected individual with a gastrointestinal disorder. In situ hybridization shows the presence of HIV-1-infected cells in the bowel epithelium (see reference 1916). The presence of grains of radioactivity designates reaction of cells with the viral protein. Photomicrograph courtesy of J. Nelson. (See p. 90.)

Color Plate 8   The HUT 78 T-cell line (pretreated with dye) was mixed with Chinese hamster ovary cells expressing the HIV-1$_{LAI}$ envelope glycoprotein. The resulting fusion between these two cells permitted dye transfer from the T lymphocyte into the CHO cells. Photomicrograph courtesy of C. Weiss. (See p. 122.)

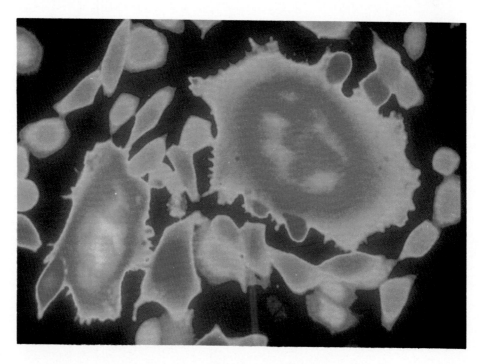

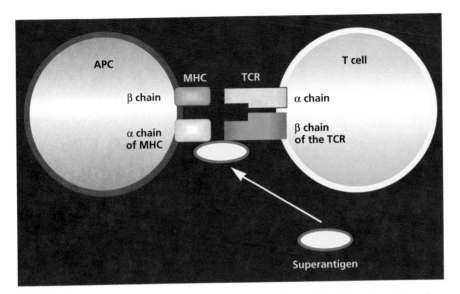

Color Plate 9 A superantigen is not processed by cells but can bind directly to either class II molecules or the Vβ portion of the T-cell receptor (see Color Plate 12). This interaction can lead to a nonspecific activation of T cells. (Adapted from reference 531 with permission.) (See p. 133.)

Color Plate 10 Effect of HIV infection on lymphoid tissue. (A) Early stage. Follicular and paracortical hyperplasia can be seen secondary to an increase in the number of germinal centers associated with B-cell proliferation. Paracortical hyperplasia reflects the increase in the number of CD8+ cells. (B) Follicular lysis stage. In the early advancement to symptomatic infection, germinal centers break down and FDC death occurs. Eventually, an involution of the germinal center takes place. (C) Terminal stage. At this level of infection, lymphoid tissue depletion is noted, with an absence of lymphocytes and a complete disruption of normal lymph node architecture. Photomicrographs courtesy of B. Herndier. (See p. 203.)

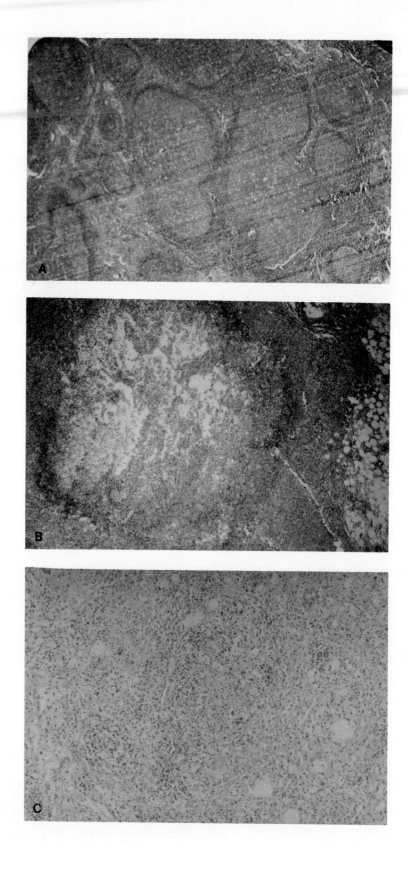

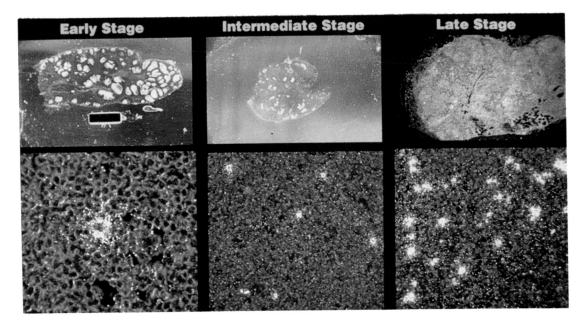

Color Plate 11 Effects of HIV infection on lymphoid tissue. Panels indicate the changes in the lymph node germinal centers as determined by selective staining (top panels) and by the location of virus replication in lymph node tissue (bottom panels). HIV replication was detected by PCR procedures. The events are reflected for the early, intermediate, and late stages of HIV infection. (Data provided by the HIV Information Network; figure derived from reference 2038.) (See p. 203.)

Color Plate 12 (A) Antigen (Ag) presentation to CD4$^+$ T cells. An exogenous antigen with various epitopes is endocytized by an antigen-presenting cell and processed in intracellular vesicles such as acidified endosomes. These vesicles then fuse with other vesicles containing MHC class II molecules, which transport the peptide to the cell surface. The antigen is subsequently presented to the CD4$^+$ cells through an interaction with the TCR (generally the α and β chains) and the CD4 molecule. (Adapted from reference 531 with permission.) *(Figure continues next page.)*

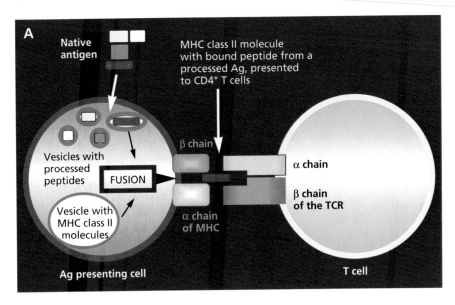

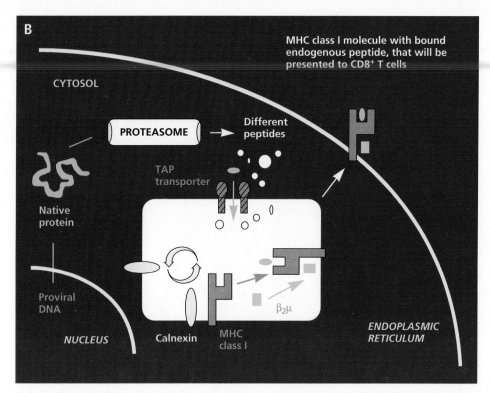

B

MHC class I molecule with bound endogenous peptide, that will be presented to CD8⁺ T cells

CYTOSOL

PROTEASOME → Different peptides

TAP transporter

Native protein

Proviral DNA

NUCLEUS   Calnexin   MHC class I   β₂μ   ENDOPLASMIC RETICULUM

Color Plate 12 (continued) (B) Presentation of antigen to CD8⁺ cells. Endogenous antigens expressed by a cell are first processed by proteosomes into small peptides. These molecules are then transported by specific molecules (the TAP transporters) into the endoplasmic reticulum. In this organelle, MHC class I molecules are bound first to calnexin (Csc), a chaperone protein, and then to peptide antigen. Binding of the peptide to the α chain allows for stable interaction with β₂-microglobulin. The peptide bound to the MHC class I complex is transported through the Golgi complex to the cell surface. From this site, it interacts with the TCR and the CD8 molecule on the CD8⁺ cell surface. (Adapted from reference 531, with permission.) (See p. 256.)

Color Plate 13 Kaposi's sarcoma in a young HIV-infected man. Note the distribution of the lesions, suggesting lymphatic involvement. Photo courtesy of P. Volberding. (See p. 288.)

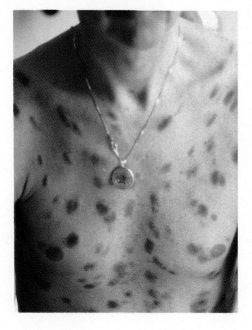

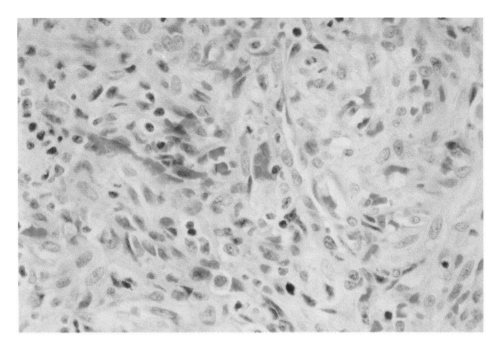

Color Plate 14 Histologic picture of Kaposi's sarcoma. Magnification, ×100. Photomicrograph courtesy of B. Herndier. (See p. 288.)

Color Plate 15 AIN grade 2 lesion observed at analscopy. A 3% acidic solution was applied to the surface of the anal canal. A well-circumscribed lesion that has turned white compared to the normal mucosa ("acetowhite") is visualized through an anal scope at ×160 magnification. The lesion is smooth and has prominent vacuolization. Reprinted from reference 2020 with permission. (See p. 304.)

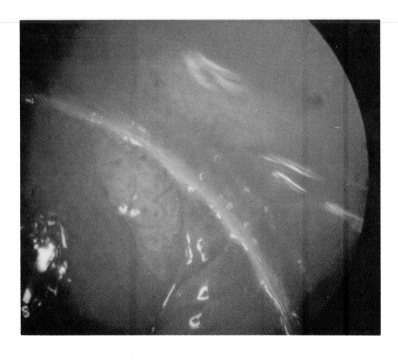

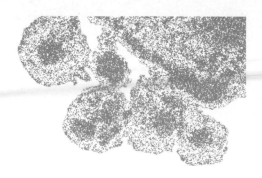

Effect of HIV on Various Tissues and Organ Systems in the Host

9

Hematopoietic System: Immune Function

Central Nervous System

Gastrointestinal System

Other Organ Systems

H IV INFECTION, EITHER DIRECTLY OR INDIRECTLY, CAN AFFECT A wide variety of tissues in the host. This chapter will review the major organ systems that appear to be affected by the virus. Other aspects of this topic are presented in Chapters 10 and 11.

I. Hematopoietic System: Immune Function

HIV replication has been considered pathogenic to bone marrow, as demonstrated by a reduced number of clonal cells growing out in culture and clinical evidence of bone marrow dyscrasias (1663, 2374) (Sections I.A and I.E). Suppression of myeloid activity in the bone marrow, as measured in cell culture, has been attributed partially to the viral Gag p24 protein (2178). The effect appears to result from the induction of soluble factors released by the bone marrow stroma. The findings have clinical relevance, since levels of p24 that can suppress bone marrow activity in vitro can be found circulating in the blood of AIDS patients (2178). Other effects of HIV on hematopoiesis are discussed in Section I.E.

A simplified presentation of the major cells involved in immuno-

Table 9.1 Abnormalities of the immune system in HIV infection

B lymphocytes
  Polyclonal activation
  Hypergammaglobulinemia
  Lack of response to T-cell-independent antigens
  Production of autoantibodies

Macrophages
  Decreased chemotaxis
  Decreased IL-1 production (or production of IL-1 inhibitor)
  Decreased microbicidal activity
  Reduced antigen-presenting activity

NK cells
  Decreased cytotoxic activity

CD4$^+$ lymphocytes[a]
  Loss of CD4$^+$ cell number
  Decreased proliferation to recall antigens, alloantigens, and subsequently to mitogens
  Decreased production of IL-2
  Disturbance in cytokine production
  Disturbance in memory cell number and function

CD8$^+$ lymphocytes
  Decreased antigen-specific proliferation
  Decreased antigen-specific cytotoxic activity
  Decreased redirected cytotoxic activity
  Decreased anti-HIV responses (cytotoxic and suppressing)

Dendritic cells
  Decreased cell number
  Decreased ability to function as antigen-presenting cells
  Decreased ability to stimulate primary T-cell proliferative response
  Decreased ability to increase antibody production
  Decreased cytokine production (e.g., IL-12)

[a] See Table 9.3.

logic activities is provided in Figure 9.1. Precisely how HIV causes disorders in the immune system (Table 9.1) still is not fully understood. Most studies on the effect of HIV on the immune system have concentrated on evaluating specific cell subsets obtained from the blood. Immune abnormalities can be observed in T cells, B cells, and natural killer (NK) cells early in infection, before the loss of CD4$^+$ cells begins (333, 483, 1421, 1781, 2274, 2469) (see Chapter 3) (Section I.E). Moreover, a reduction in the function of polymorphonuclear leukocytes can develop soon after HIV infection (2099). Some studies suggest that interleukin-4 (IL-4) and IL-10 could be involved in this reduced function (2647). The result could explain the serious bacterial infections encountered. More recently, the role of HIV in the destruction of lymphoid tissues (including the thymus) has received renewed attention (Section I.H). Aside from the direct cytotoxic effects of viral proteins and HIV itself, described in Chapters 6 and 8, several other possible causes of HIV-associated immune disorders are discussed in this chapter. The alterations in CD8$^+$ cell subset populations occurring in response to HIV infection are covered in Chapters 11 and 13.

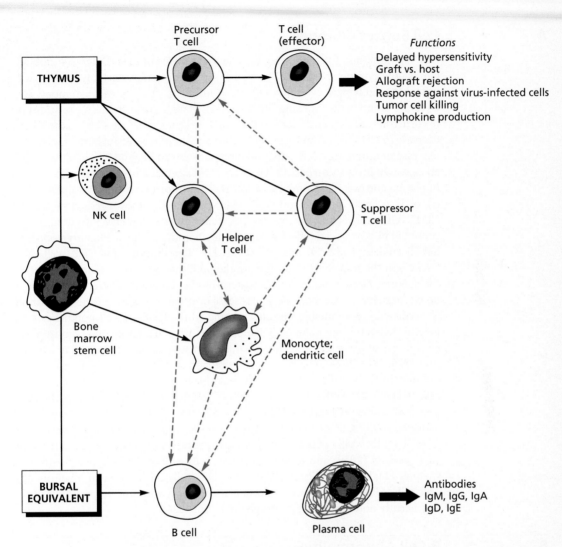

Figure 9.1   A simplified version of the major cells involved in immune function in the host. Bone marrow stem cells circulating through the thymus give rise to T cells that can have helper or suppressor/cytotoxic cell functions. Monocytes or DC (APC) are derived from the bone marrow and interact with T-cell subsets to present antigens to induce an immune response. B cells from bone marrow pass through the bursal equivalent in humans to evolve into B cells that produce antibodies (plasma cells). All these functions entail interactions with several different members of the immune system, particularly APC. The CD4$^+$ helper cells can assist in both cell-mediated and humoral immune responses. Their separation into type 1 or type 2 cells provides some distinction in these cell types (Chapter 11, Table 11.2). The final result is a balance in both arms of the immune system with functions used in defending against incoming organisms. The complex interaction of the cytokines produced by the various immune and other cells in the body is presented in Figure 9.3. Cells derived from a particular precursor cell are designated with a solid-line arrow; the influence of a cell on another cell is designated with a broken-line arrow.

A. Cell Subset Changes

One rapid method for examining the effect of a virus on the cellular immune system is flow cytometry (885, 1414). In measuring this parameter, it is important to note that total lymphocytes and cell subset numbers show diurnal variations. Low levels are found in the morning and high levels at night, with an inverse relationship to corticosteroid concentrations in the blood. Recent studies have also shown that a decrease in $CD4^+$ cell count can occur after 60 min of rest. At night during sleep, a decrease in monocytes, NK cells, and lymphocytes can be found concomitant with an increased production of IL-2. These effects of sleep do not correlate with changes in plasma cortisol. Sleep does not affect IL-1β, tumor necrosis factor alpha (TNF-α), or IL-6 levels in the blood (251, 344a). Besides the known reduction in total $CD4^+$ cell numbers and the rise in $CD8^+$ cell numbers with HIV infection, certain subsets of these cells can reflect abnormalities in immune status. Phenotype changes have been described for B cells, NK cells, $CD4^+$ lymphocytes, and $CD8^+$ cells. Differences in the results are evident from the published studies and appear to reflect the cohorts selected; no definitive pattern has yet emerged. Therefore, the use of flow cytometry for assessing stage of disease or prognosis needs further evaluation. Nevertheless, reproducible findings relating to the $CD8^+$ T-cell populations are helpful. Activation markers on T lymphocytes are consistently observed from the early stages of infection, and changes in certain subpopulations can be noted over time (886, 1414, 2829). For example, progression to AIDS is reflected by an increase not only in the number of $CD8^+$ cells but also in the subpopulations of activated cells ($CD38^+$, HLA-DR$^+$), memory cells ($CD45RO^+$), and cells showing the cytotoxic cell marker ($CD11b^+$ $CD28^-$) (166, 886, 1414, 1416, 2761). The number of activated $CD8^+$ $CD28^+$ cells in AIDS is reduced in comparison to the number of $CD8^+$ $CD11b^+$ cells (1416). These findings appear to correlate with observations on clonogenicity (2039) and functional studies with cultured $CD8^+$ cells (1416) (see Chapter 11). In terms of both $CD4^+$ and $CD8^+$ cells, a loss in the number of naive cells ($CD45RA^+$), which are important for primary immune response, has been consistently noted with disease progression (166, 2263).

B. B-Cell Abnormalities

HIV infection is associated with abnormal activation of B lymphocytes, leading to B-cell dysregulation (62, 439, 1162, 1175, 1421, 2406) (Table 9.1). Evidence from several laboratories indicates that the viral envelope protein, particularly gp41, induces a polyclonal B-cell activation (439, 2017, 2406). Hypergammaglobulinemia develops and is particularly evident in children (59). Whether the antibody response is general or virus specific is still not clear, but most probably both types are involved (54, 2487). This proliferation of B cells may be mediated by the production of IL-6 or IL-10 by monocytes (55); the activation can be shown in cell culture by spontaneous production of antibodies to HIV as well as to other proteins (55). Moreover, the hypergammaglobulinemia observed early in infection correlates with increased amounts of immune complexes in the blood (1421).

The polyclonal B-cell response can be reflected by a persistent generalized lymphadenopathy (1175). Histologically, the adenopathy shows reactive follicular

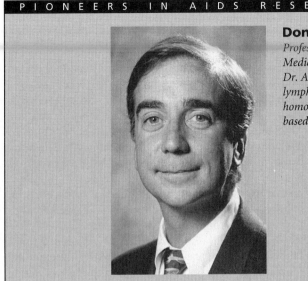

Donald I. Abrams
Professor of Clinical Medicine, Department of Medicine, University of California, San Francisco. Dr. Abrams pioneered the early studies of persistent lymphadenopathy syndrome in HIV-infected homosexual men. He has also initiated community-based trials of antiviral drugs.

hyperplasia of B cells with an increase in the number of secondary germinal centers (323) (Section I.H). Binding of gp120 to B cells expressing the V_H3 immunoglobulin has been associated with the induction of immunoglobulin synthesis by the B cells (175). The role of this interaction in B-cell abnormalities needs further evaluation. The activation of B cells has been linked to a defect in the ability of infected individuals to mount a novel immune response to immunization with new antigens, as well as to an impaired response of individuals to T-cell-independent antigens, such as lipopolysaccharides (62). This presumed anergy to new antigens may be related to a reduced number of naive $CD4^+$ cells or the poor function of the $CD4^+$ helper cell population (483, 1781, 2469) (Section I.E).

C.   Macrophage and NK Cell Abnormalities

Major abnormalities in the function of macrophages have not been conclusively demonstrated in HIV infection (Table 9.1). Many studies do not show a substantial effect on phagocytic activities (131, 1949), but some do (209, 407). For example, certain reports indicate a deficiency in macrophage binding to yeast, but normal ingestion of the organism takes place. Nevertheless, the yeast cells show increased intracellular growth (407). A similar finding was noted with *Cryptococcus neoformans* infection, and the impaired intracellular degradation activity appeared to be related to defects in both oxidative and nonoxidative effector pathways (1021a). Other studies have also suggested that infected macrophages from the peritoneum and the blood but not the lungs (341) have reduced antifungal activity. In some cases, a reduction in phagocytosis activity has been reported in association with the presence of circulating immune complexes (2705).

Most of the evidence on macrophage function suggests reduced antigen-presenting function (e.g., decreased ability to induce lymphocyte proliferation)

(669, 704, 1807, 2459, 2942), reduced response to chemoattractants (2112, 2525), and a disruption in normal cytokine production (2299) (for reviews, see references 863 and 2942) (Chapter 11). Part of the reduced function of macrophages (and other antigen-presenting cells) could be the loss of expression of major histocompatibility complex (MHC) class II (2117a) and of B7 molecules needed for costimulation (669) (Section I.D). In certain studies, the decreased proliferative response of CD4$^+$ cells on contact with HIV-infected macrophages in culture appeared to be mediated by a cytokine released by macrophages (1749). The abnormalities may result directly from HIV infection (341, 2800, 2916) or from an abnormal cross-communication among cytokines produced by other cells (Section I.G). The lack of a consistent and major defect in macrophage activity could reflect the relatively small number of these cells infected by HIV (117, 2048).

NK cell function, as discussed in Chapter 11, is reduced in HIV infection (333, 776) (Table 9.1). The loss of this activity, which is not related to cell number, probably mirrors a reduction in cytotoxic factor production (247), perhaps affected by a decrease in IL-12 synthesis (412). It might result from direct infection of NK cells by HIV (410) or from suppressive effects of the viral envelope (377). In some studies, the reduction in cell function has correlated with alterations in subpopulations of NK cells. The number of cytotoxic CD16$^+$ CD56$^+$ cells is decreased, whereas the number of CD16$^-$ CD56$^-$ cells, with low lytic activity, is increased (1121).

D.   Dendritic Cells

The dendritic cells (DC) found in lymphoid tissue and circulating in the blood, and their counterparts in the skin (Langerhans cells), are very important for antigen presentation, T-cell proliferation, and the normal immune function of both T and B lymphocytes (for reviews, see references 1326, 1327, and 2592). The earliest report on potential involvement of DC in HIV infection showed a reduction in ATPase and MHC class II antigens on Langerhans cells of the skin (165). The DC from several tissues appear to be susceptible to HIV infection (1425, 1619, 1621–1623, 2049), but probably not all DC in the blood are sensitive to the virus (343, 2850; for review, see references 1326). The number of cells infected, however, seems too small to suggest that infection itself causes much dysfunction. These cells could be affected indirectly by certain viral or cellular proteins (Section I.E). In addition, low-level HIV replication in DC can provide a reservoir for transfer of virus to activated CD4$^+$ lymphocytes and subsequent high-titer virus replication (2120b).

The DC number in skin, bone marrow, and peripheral blood mononuclear C cells (PBMC) has been reported to be reduced in individuals with HIV infection (1326, 1621) (Table 9.1). Most importantly, these cells from HIV-infected individuals, as well as cells infected in vitro, have decreased ability to stimulate primary T-cell proliferative responses, to act as antigen-presenting cells (APC), and to increase B-cell antibody production (1326, 1619, 1621–1623). This reduced function could explain the decrease in CD4$^+$ cell numbers (1049). Conceivably, these disorders are caused by HIV infection of the cells, alterations in cytokine production by the DC (874, 1326), or reduced expression of the costimulatory molecule, B7, on their cell surface (669) (Table 9.2). For example, DC produce IL-12, which directs the development of the TH1 cells (1620) and helps the activity of NK cells. DC function can affect CD4$^+$ cell cytokine production (type 1 to type 2) (see Chapter 11, Section III)

Table 9.2 Causes of the loss of APC number and function

1. HIV infection
2. Cytokine dysregulation
3. Decreased expression of costimulatory molecules (e.g., B7)
4. Cytotoxic T-lymphocytes (CTL)

and $CD8^+$ cell antiviral responses (see below). In this regard, measles virus infection of DC induces apoptosis and compromises the production of cytokines, such as IL-12, which are needed in T-cell proliferation and function (for a review, see reference 202a). Finally, the effect of HIV on DC may relate to cytotoxic T-lymphocyte (CTL) antiviral responses. Viral antigen presentation by these APC might elicit cytotoxic effects of CTL that kill the DC (1515) (see Chapters 11 and 13). Thus, the number of DC will be decreased if fresh cells cannot be replenished at an equal rate by $CD34^+$ progenitor cells. A defect in DC renewal appears to be present in HIV infection but needs further substantiation. This possible process of DC destruction is supported by observations with infection by lymphocytic choriomeningitis (LCM) virus in mice. Destruction by CTL of LCM virus-associated DC leads to immune deficiency (252).

E.

$CD4^+$ Lymphocyte Abnormalities

1. DIRECT AND INDIRECT EFFECTS OF HIV INFECTION

The first immunologic disorder recognized in AIDS was a loss of $CD4^+$ lymphocytes of the helper (inducer) cell type (918, 1782, 2562). Whether this loss reflects direct cell destruction by the virus or its proteins (as discussed in Chapter 6) or a secondary effect of the immune system disorder (e.g., anticellular effects of CTL) is still not known. Other studies demonstrated that the function of $CD4^+$ cells, measured by proliferative responses to specific stimuli, can be reduced before a loss in cell number is noted (483, 961, 1420, 1781, 2469, 2754). The latter finding could be related to decreased APC function (see above). In this regard, T-helper (TH) cell subsets can be out of balance (see Chapters 11 and 13).

The earliest abnormality reported in $CD4^+$ cells is a loss of response to recall antigens (see above) followed by a reduced proliferation in response to alloantigens and finally a loss of response to lectins (e.g., phytohemagglutinin) (Figure 9.2; Table

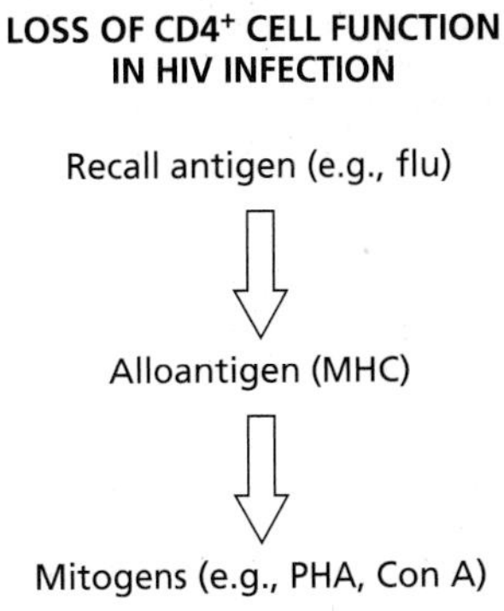

Figure 9.2 The earliest abnormality noted in $CD4^+$ cell function has been the inability to respond to recall antigens (e.g., tetanus and influenza), followed by a reduced proliferation to alloantigens and finally to mitogens (e.g., PHA, concanavalin A [ConA]). This progression in loss of response by $CD4^+$ cells has correlated with a more rapid progression to disease (483, 2469).

LOSS OF $CD4^+$ CELL FUNCTION IN HIV INFECTION

Recall antigen (e.g., flu)

⇩

Alloantigen (MHC)

⇩

Mitogens (e.g., PHA, Con A)

9.1). Thus, CD4$^+$ cells from the healthiest HIV-infected individuals have all three responses $(+/+/+)$, whereas those cells from many AIDS patients show none $(-/-/-)$ (483, 2469). The assays are particularly helpful when examining asymptomatic individuals. Those subjects who show a loss of all three responses progress much more rapidly to disease than do those who have all or some of these immunologic functions. The factors potentially involved in inducing these disorders are covered in Chapter 11.

Other direct effects of HIV-1 replication, besides cell destruction, might contribute to the reduction in CD4$^+$ cell number and their function (Table 9.3). For example, infection of T-cell clones by HIV has led to disorders in cytokine production (1625). Moreover, despite the inability to detect HIV-1 replication in a large number of CD4$^+$ cells, particularly in asymptomatic individuals (see Chapter 4), HIV could be present in a latent or "silent" state and affect the function, long-term viability, and growth of these cells. The presence of this covert cellular state is supported by studies using in situ DNA and RNA PCR methods (695, 696, 1954, 2048) (see Chapter 5). Thus, HIV, even if not replicating to high levels, might alter cytokine production and membrane integrity of CD4$^+$ cells sufficiently that not only is normal function affected (see Chapter 6) but also the sensitivity of these cells to cellular factors (e.g., cytokines) could be increased (Section I.G).

Some investigators believe, based on cell culture studies, that a preferential infection of CD4$^+$ memory T cells (2405, 2553) causes immune dysfunction. In this regard, virus entry appears to be the same in cultured CD45RA$^+$ and CD45RO$^+$ cells but virus replication occurs only in the CD45RO$^+$ cells (2553, 2914), and these memory cells are more susceptible to the cytopathic effects of HIV (451). A loss of memory T cells (CD4$^+$ CD45RO$^+$) has been noted in asymptomatic HIV-infected

Table 9.3 Possible factors involved in HIV-induced loss of CD4$^+$ lymphocyte number and immune function[a]

1. Direct cytopathic effects of HIV and its proteins on CD4$^+$ cells (see Chapter 6)
2. Effect of HIV on cell membrane permeability; enhanced fragility of CD4$^+$ cells
3. Effect of HIV on production of cytokines needed for CD4$^+$ cell function
4. Preferential destruction of CD4$^+$ memory cells
5. Destruction of bone marrow (e.g., stem cells and stromal cells)
6. Destruction of lymphoid tissue (e.g., thymus and FDC)
7. Immunosuppressive effects of immune complexes and viral proteins (e.g., gp120, gp41, Gag, and Tat)
8. Effect of HIV on signal transduction
9. Induction of apoptosis (Chapter 6)
10. Cell destruction via the attachment of circulating envelope to normal CD4$^+$ cells (ADCC and CTL)
11. Anti-CD4$^+$ cell cytotoxic activity (mediated by CD8$^+$ and CD4$^+$ cells)
12. CD8$^+$ cell suppressor factors
13. Anti-CD4$^+$ cell autoantibodies
14. Cytokine cytotoxicity

[a] See Section I.E.

PIONEERS IN AIDS RESEARCH

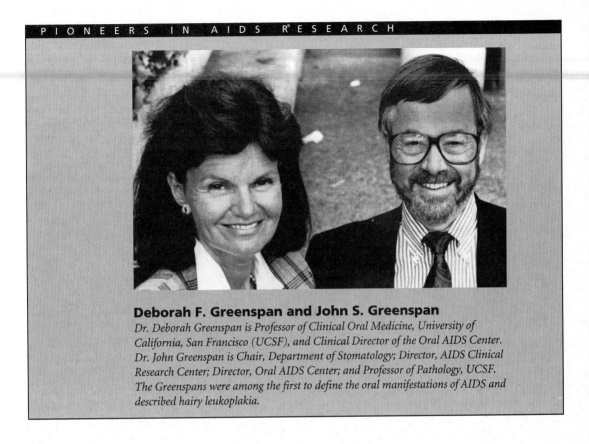

Deborah F. Greenspan and John S. Greenspan
Dr. Deborah Greenspan is Professor of Clinical Oral Medicine, University of California, San Francisco (UCSF), and Clinical Director of the Oral AIDS Center. Dr. John Greenspan is Chair, Department of Stomatology; Director, AIDS Clinical Research Center; Director, Oral AIDS Center; and Professor of Pathology, UCSF. The Greenspans were among the first to define the oral manifestations of AIDS and described hairy leukoplakia.

individuals (2754), and HIV can be detected in these cells in vivo (2405). Importantly, over time the naive T cell ($CD45RA^+$) is found at reduced frequency (2262). Whether selective infection occurs in vivo in the host and has relevance to immune dysfunction needs further study.

The virus could infect or suppress production of the early precursors of $CD4^+$ cells (e.g., stem cells) and reduce the quantity of fresh lymphocytes and DC added regularly from the bone marrow to the peripheral blood. Hematopoiesis is suppressed in vitro in some (591, 647, 1470, 2590) but not all (1806) studies with HIV. Moreover, an inhibitory effect of gp120 and gp160 on in vitro growth of $CD34^+$ progenitor cells has been reported by some investigators (2967) although not confirmed by others (2611). Some investigators (773) have infected early bone marrow progenitor cells in vitro, but most researchers believe that $CD34^+$ cells are not directly infectable. Infected $CD34^+$ cells have been detected in some HIV-infected subjects in vivo (2573) but not in others (576, 1663), and they are probably not usually infected before expression of CD4. Bone marrow endothelial cells appear to be infected by HIV (1854). Thus, an effect on stem cells caused by alterations in cytokine production by the infected established cells could occur (see Chapter 4).

Since the circulation of lymphocytes in the blood represents only 1 to 3% of their total population in the body (2865), the loss of stem cells or early precursor cells would influence the replenishment of the normal $CD4^+$ cells required to maintain a steady state. Nevertheless, as noted above, PCR and other analyses have not confirmed the presence of HIV in early bone marrow progenitor cells in vivo (576, 591, 1663). Some studies emphasize that HIV can directly inhibit hematopoiesis or that the virus (or gp120) could induce tumor necrosis factor alpha (TNF-α), which is toxic to the bone marrow (1627). As noted above, in some studies, p24 levels correlate with suppression of bone marrow myeloid activity (2178).

The potential damage by HIV to precursor cells or stromal cells in the thymus also has been considered (41, 248, 1038, 2574; for a review, see reference 856). Infection of T-lymphocyte precursors in the thymus has been noted (2744). Such an infection could affect the production and release of fresh T lymphocytes, particularly naive cells, that are believed to reside in lymphoid tissue throughout the body. These cells are vital for response to new antigens (Section I.H). Finally, the formation of antibody:virus antigen complexes (1849) could "tie up" the reticuloendothelial system, affect cytokine (e.g., IL-1) production, and influence CD4$^+$ cell function. The interplay of all these processes in reduction in CD4$^+$ cell number and function requires further evaluation.

2. EFFECT OF VIRAL PROTEINS

Several investigators have demonstrated that viral envelope proteins (e.g., glycosylated gp120 and gp41) have immunosuppressive effects on the mitogenic responses of T lymphocytes (401, 630, 1658, 2008, 2017, 2800, 2840). Considering the role of CD4$^+$ cells in B-cell function, gp120 could interfere with normal T-cell helper function via a block in contact-dependent interactions (441). Some cell culture studies suggest that gp120, through its interaction with CD4, inhibits IL-2 production by CD4$^+$ lymphocytes (2008), perhaps by the induction of IL-10 production by monocytes (2410). In addition, gp120 could block T-cell activation and function by interfering with costimulation (440a).

Initial studies with the envelope gp41 placed particular emphasis on portions of this protein that could suppress immune responses (401, 2305, 2306), most probably by inhibition of activation pathways (2306). A related protein in other animal retrovirus systems (i.e., p15 in murine and feline retroviruses) causes depressed immune reactions (453). In addition, gp41 and gp120 can be toxic to CD4$^+$ cells (see Chapter 6).

The HIV Gag protein might also affect normal intracellular activities and function through binding to cellular cyclophilins (1596) (see Chapter 5). Moreover, the HIV *tat* gene, expressed in infected cells, can reduce in vitro the proliferative responses of CD4$^+$ cells to recall antigens (e.g., tetanus) (2775). This potential effect on immune function would be most evident via transfer of extracellular Tat to uninfected CD4$^+$ cells (2775). The above mechanism, if present, could involve CD26 and an interference with a signal necessary for IL-2 production (2609). In this regard, restoration of the recall antigen response can be achieved in vitro by the addition of soluble CD26 (2400). Moreover, Tat and gp120 have been implicated in the induction of apoptosis of CD4$^+$ cells (see Chapter 6). Whether any of these processes affect the major phenotype of immune dysfunction (loss of CD4$^+$ cells) is not known. However, as noted above, they could reduce the ability of the host to provide sufficient fresh CD4$^+$ cells to keep up with loss by a variety of other mechanisms.

3. DISTURBANCE IN SIGNAL TRANSDUCTION

Besides certain indirect effects of HIV and its proteins on CD4$^+$ lymphocytes and their precursor cells, infection of these cells by HIV could interfere with the normal events in signal transduction. This process, as discussed previously (see Chapter 5), involves an extracellular signal that affects the activity of sequence-specific intracellular transcription factors (Figure 5.3). These events lead to an information transfer within the cell involving a protein kinase cascade and protein phosphorylation. It occurs when natural ligands bind to the CD4 antigen or interact with other membrane surface proteins to bring about T-cell activation and effective immune response (for reviews, see references 1241 and 2003).

HIV-1 gp120 has been found to form an intracellular complex with CD4 and p56^{lck} in the endoplasmic reticulum (541). The retention of this tyrosine kinase in the cytoplasm could be toxic to the cell or affect its function. In addition, both HIV and envelope gp120 have been reported to inhibit the early steps of lymphocyte activation (1093, 1555). Thus, the function of these cells could be compromised by HIV even if they are not directly infected. Moreover, induction of the phosphorylation of a 30-kDa protein has been linked to CD4$^+$ cell death by apoptosis (493, 2674), ascribed to a block in mitosis (2674).

Furthermore, in neuropathogenesis, a possible gp120:receptor interaction on CD4$^-$ brain cells with subsequent activation of tyrosine phosphorylation of certain cellular proteins might be involved (2403). Finally, cell death by apoptosis could reflect intracellular disturbances that affect normal cell activity and function (see Chapter 6).

4. BYSTANDER EFFECT

Another indirect mechanism for CD4$^+$ cell loss is the covering of cells carrying the CD4$^+$ molecule with gp120 released by infected cells. In this case, the gp120 peptides would be associated with MHC class II and not class I molecules (380). These uninfected cells are recognized as virus-infected cells by NK effector cells or CTL (1428, 2505, 2839, 2840) and are subsequently destroyed even though they are not infected by the virus. This process, because it involves presentation by class II MHC molecules, appears most evident with CD4$^+$ cytotoxic cells (999). Proof of this hypothesis would require the detection of circulating gp120 in the blood of individuals or on uninfected cells. While some gp120 released from cells has been found in in vitro studies (881, 2401), this phenomenon has not been well documented in vivo.

5. CYTOTOXIC CELLS AND IMMUNE SUPPRESSOR FACTORS

Cytotoxic CD8$^+$ cells recovered from the blood of infected individuals have shown the ability to kill normal CD4$^+$ cells as well as those infected with HIV (205, 2839, 2963). A role for these cells in alveolar disease of the lung has been suggested (106) (see Chapter 11). Some investigators report that CD4$^+$ cells can demonstrate this cytotoxic activity against infected CD4$^+$ cells (1988). This event may not reflect a CTL response but may result from contact of normal CD4$^+$ T cells with HIV-infected cells, in which rapid cell lysis can occur (1044).

In some studies, the induction of immune suppressor factors, several of which block IL-2 activity and reduce cell proliferation, has been described (63, 1053, 1443,

2503), although none has been well characterized. A factor produced by CD8$^+$ cells has been found to reduce the response of CD4$^+$ cells to certain recall antigens (477). This effect could explain the early abnormalities observed in TH cell function (483, 1781, 2469) (Table 9.3). Its relation to a known cytokine awaits further definition.

F.   Antilymphocyte Antibodies

Autoantibodies to lymphocytes could also play a role in immune deficiency (see Chapter 10). In some of the early studies of HIV infection, antibodies to both TH and T-suppressor lymphocytes were detected, and their presence was later confirmed (79, 654, 1325, 1874, 2836). In general, the anti-CD4$^+$ cell antibodies appear first, but autoantibodies to both lymphocyte subsets can be noted as symptoms of disease appear. Even antibodies to B lymphocytes have been detected (1300a). Some of these antibodies could result from anti-MHC responses induced by the HIV proteins (see Chapter 10). Moreover, autoantibodies to the CD4 protein itself (although not to the HIV binding site) have been detected in HIV-infected individuals (392, 2672); these antibodies could be responsible for the death of some CD4$^+$ lymphocytes.

Some studies suggest a link of these anti-lymphocyte autoantibodies to CD4$^+$ helper cell defects (2836) and disease (1308, 1874). However, all the observations suggesting that this humoral immune response could affect the immune system require further study. For instance, plasmapheresis, which eliminates autoantibodies and can result in clinical improvement (e.g., in conditions involving loss of platelets and neutrophils, and in peripheral neuropathy) (1302), does not change the CD4$^+$ cell number (1300a).

G.   Effect of Cytokines on Immune Function and HIV Replication

A great deal of information has been accumulated on the influence of various cytokines on the activity of the immune system (see Chapter 11) (for a review, see reference 1697; for a review of the nomenclature and the biologic roles of cytokines, see reference 1549). Disturbances in cytokine production brought about by HIV infection can affect normal immune function. Macrophages (and DC) produce IL-1, IL-12, and other cytokines that permit CD4$^+$ cells to reach the level of maturation to produce IL-2 (2433). IL-2 is needed for self-replication of the CD4$^+$ cell population and for growth and function of CD8$^+$ cells. IL-12 enhances NK-cell function (2433; for a review, see reference 2707). Certain cytokines can induce the differential production of other cytokines by CD4$^+$ cells. This observation has led to the classification of CD4$^+$ cells into TH1 (or type 1) and TH2 (or type 2) cells, depending on their cytokine production (see Chapter 11 and Table 11.1). For example, IL-12 enhances the development of TH1 cells, which produce IL-2 and gamma interferon (IFN-γ), and IL-4 promotes the emergence of TH2 cells, which produce IL-4 and IL-10 (1861, 1862, 2270; for reviews see references 481, 1862, 2270, and 2602).

Other cytokines, such as IL-6 and IL-10, which enhance B-cell growth and function, and IL-4, which induces T-cell maturation, are also important in maintaining an effective immune response (for reviews, see references 481 and 2270).

Certain studies suggest that type 1 cytokines (e.g., IL-2 and IFN-γ) can protect against apoptosis of $CD4^+$ cells whereas type 2 cytokines (e.g., IL-4 and IL-10) encourage this process (479) (see Chapter 11, Table 11.1). Some cytokines (e.g., IL-4) increase apoptosis by inhibiting the function of other cytokines that prevent this process (e.g., TNF-α and IFN-γ in macrophages) (1655) (see Chapter 6). TNF-α helps maintain a balance in production of several lymphokines but itself can be toxic to T cells and can induce apoptosis. To some investigators, TNF-α is a major cause of HIV pathology (1697). Nevertheless, recent studies of lymphoid tissue have not found any correlation between TNF-α gene expression and the level of HIV-1 production (1534a). These results differ from those obtained with brain cells from patients with dementia (2863); high levels of TNF-α RNA were detected (Section II.C). More studies of cytokine expression in vivo are needed.

HIV infection and viral proteins can affect cytokine production (Table 9.4). For example, production of IL-1 and TNF-α by macrophages infected by HIV or exposed to the viral gp120 has been observed (1758). Moreover, activation of TNF-α, but not IL-1 or IL-6 production, has been reported with Tat expression by HIV-infected T cells (315). TNF-α increases the production of IL-1 and IL-6, and these cytokines can in turn enhance HIV expression (Table 9.5) (see below). In this connection, the reported increased levels of TNF-α in serum in patients with AIDS and not in asymptomatic individuals (105, 1405) merits further study. Moreover, the question of whether these cellular products act as cofactors to influence the destruction of $CD4^+$ cells or compromise their function needs further evaluation. Induction by HIV of IL-6 production by human B lymphocytes has also been described (261). This event can contribute to the polyclonal activation of these cells (Section I.B). Recently, recombinant Nef was shown to induce IL-10 production in PBMC (284). Whether sufficient extracellular Nef is made to affect the immune response via this cytotoxic production remains to be studied.

Despite the above reports, some studies suggest that HIV-infected macrophages, on stimulation, release diminished amounts of cytokines or have no change in production of these cellular factors (1807, 2299). Thus, the relative extent of cytokine expression during HIV infection in vivo is not yet defined.

In addition to their potential effects on immune function, several cytokines, produced by immune cells activated during infection, can affect HIV replication as

Table 9.4 Effect of HIV and HIV proteins on cytokine production[a]

Cell type and viral protein	Cytokine produced	Reference
Cell types		
$CD4^+$ lymphocyte	TNF-α	315
Macrophage	IL-1, TNF-α	1758
B lymphocyte	IL-6	261
Viral proteins		
gp120	IL-1, TNF-α	1758
Tat	TNF-α	315
Nef	IL-10	284

[a] Some of these observations need to be confirmed.

Table 9.5 Effect of cytokines on HIV-1 replication[a]

Cytokine	Major source	Effect on HIV replication in:			
		T-cell line	PBMC	Primary macrophage	CD4$^+$ cells
TNF-α	Macrophage, T cell, B cell, keratinocyte	↑↑	↑↑	↑↑	↓$^+$ or ↑
TNF-β	T cell, B cell	↑↑	↑↑	NT	↕
GM-CSF	Macrophage, T cell	—	↑↑	NT	↕
IL-1	Macrophage, fibroblast, endothelial cell	↑ or —	NT	NT	—
IL-2	T cell	—	↑	NT	—
IL-3	T cell	—	NT	↑↑	—
IL-4	T cell	—	NT	↑↑	↕$^+$ or ↕
IL-5	T cell, mast cell	NT	NT	NT	↑
IL-6	Macrophage, T cell, glia, fibroblast	—	NT	↑↑	↕
IL-7	Bone marrow stromal cell	NT	NT	NT	↕
IL-8	T cell, monocyte, keratinocyte, fibroblast, endothelial cell	NT	NT	NT	↕
IL-9	CD4$^+$ T cell	NT	NT	NT	↑
IL-10	T cell, B cell, mast cell	NT	NT	NT	↕
IL-12	Macrophage, B cell	NT	NT	NT	—
IFN-α	B cell	↓↓	↓↓	↓↓	↓↓
IFN-β	Fibroblast, B cell	↓	↓↓	NT	↓↓
IFN-γ	T cell, NK cell	↓ or —	↑ or —	↑	↑
TGF-β	Platelet, macrophage, T cell	—	↓	↓↓	↓$^+$ or ↑

[a] Data on acute infection of the cells listed by HIV-1 is presented. Results show by the number of arrows an increase (↑) or decrease (↓) in virus production. A line through the arrow indicates a slight effect. In limited studies, M-CSF increased HIV replication in primary macrophages and G-CSF enhanced HIV production in CD4$^+$ cells. IL-13 has been shown to inhibit HIV replication in peripheral blood macrophages but not in CD4$^+$ lymphocytes (1811). Symbols and abbreviations: +, high concentration only; −, no effect; NT, not tested. Adapted from references 1635 and 1697.

observed by in vitro studies (Table 9.5) (1635, 1811; for reviews, see references 1697, 2113, and 2284). In certain cases, virus production is affected in some cells (e.g., decrease in replication in macrophages by IL-10 and IL-12) and not in others (e.g., CD4$^+$ lymphocytes) (Table 9.5) (29, 754, 1348, 1811). In one recent study, the enhancement of HIV replication noted in vitro with granulocyte-macrophage colony-stimulating factor (GM-CSF) (864) was also observed in vivo (1398), but this effect can be blocked by antiviral therapy (2373).

Cytokines could cause cell death via enhanced virus growth or by direct toxicity. For example, TNF-α increases HIV production and can be toxic for cells (see also Chapter 6). In other situations, the relative amounts of cytokines produced can influence the results. For instance, high levels of IL-10 reduce HIV replication in macrophages, probably secondary to a decrease in TNF-α production (2853). Low levels can increase virus production in the presence of other cytokines (2852). Moreover, HIV replication has been inhibited in the SCID-hu mouse by the administration of IL-10 (1342). These observations have led some investigators to examine the use of this cytokine in therapy (see Chapter 14).

Other studies have indicated that levels of TNF-α in plasma, which can be increased during HIV infection, have a detrimental effect on normal sleep patterns; high levels can be related to the fatigue symptoms associated with severe HIV infection (574). This finding is important since sleep patterns can affect immune cell numbers and cytokine production. Sufficient nocturnal sleep has been associated with a low number of cells in the morning but higher levels in the afternoon. It enhances the production of IL-2 but not TNF-α, IL-1β, or IL-6 (251). These observations indicate the need to consider circadian rhythm when assessing immune cell number and function.

β-Chemokines and IL-16 have been reported to suppress HIV replication (127, 487). These cellular factors produced during HIV infection, particularly immune activation, have therefore been considered potential immune antiviral factors affecting pathogenesis (see Chapter 11). These cellular factors are made by a wide variety of cells, including CD8$^+$, CD4$^+$, NK, and B cells. Within the CD4$^+$ lymphocyte subset, β-chemokines appear to be produced primarily by the TH1 or TH0 subtype (2416). If these cytokines have an effect in reducing virus replication, their association with a type 1 response found in asymptomatic individuals may be noteworthy (2416). We have noted that infection of CD4$^+$ cells with NSI viruses leads to an increase in β-chemokine production, whereas infection with SI viruses reduces chemokine production (1630). These effects of HIV infection on chemokine production could influence cytokine production by CD4$^+$ cells (e.g., IFN-γ, IL-4) (1247) (see Chapter 11, Section II.B). A relevance of chemokines to HIV expression in vivo, however, has not been demonstrated (1630). Importantly, the chemokines might be responsible for the inflammatory reactions that are harmful to the host (15, 1985). Their production could cause recruitment of inflammatory cells to tissues and result in cell destruction. They could be responsible in part for the symptoms observed in acute HIV infection and the later course of the infection.

In summary, as cited above and discussed in detail later, cytokines can influence the extent of cell-mediated versus humoral immune responses (see Chapter 11), affect HIV replication (Table 9.5), and induce symptoms in the infected host. The balance in secretion of certain of these cell factors is needed for the normal functioning of the immune system (1597, 2468, 2475). Their interactions are very complex, as illustrated in Figure 9.3. The known importance of cytokines for intercellular activities emphasizes their potential role in modulating or enhancing HIV pathogenesis.

H.   HIV Effects on Lymphoid Tissue

The effects of HIV on the immune system, defined mostly through studies of the peripheral blood, have also been described in the lymph node. Lymphoid tissues may, in fact, be the first sites for virus replication following acute infection (see Chapter 4) (1396). Initially, with primary infection, lymph nodes show reactive hyperplasia and high levels of virus replication (for a review, see reference 497a). The tissue enlarges with particular increases in secondary germinal centers (or follicles) filled with activated B cells (for a review, see reference 322) (Color Plates 10 and 11, following p. 188). This event reflects the polyclonal B-cell activation and hypergammaglobulinemia found early in HIV infection (Section I.B). The paracortical areas

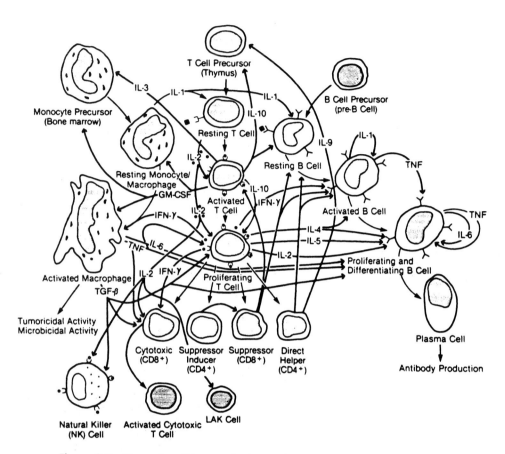

Figure 9.3   Illustration of the complex interactions among cells in the immune system and their secreted cellular factors (cytokines). Each represents a process of checks and balances to ensure a normally functioning immune system. Figure courtesy of A. Fauci.

also become increased in size (Color Plate 10, panel A), with the expanding number of CD8$^+$ cells that is also seen in the peripheral blood (700, 2176). The ingress of CD8$^+$ cells may reflect enhanced production of β-chemokines by resident macrophages (240, 2651). Many appear to be short-lived cells (240). In this acute period, the follicular mantle and paracortical regions can show many infected CD4$^+$ cells (696, 979a).

During the subsequent asymptomatic clinical period, the lymph node may contain a large number of virus-infected CD4$^+$ cells, particularly in the mantle regions (see Chapter 4), but most of these cells are latently infected (696) (see Chapter 5) (Color Plates 6 and 11 [following p.188]). Germinal-center CD4$^+$ T cells are also an important site of HIV infection (1135). Despite this infection, CD4$^+$ T-cell number in lymphoid tissue in asymptomatic HIV-infected individuals may be maintained at normal levels, even when CD4$^+$ T-cell counts are reduced in the peripheral blood (2284b). Virus particles can be best visualized by molecular techniques (PCR procedures) and by electron microscopy in close contact with follicular dendritic cells (FDC) (83, 700, 2210, 2652) (Color Plate 11), but very few, if any, of these cells seem infected (2210). Evidence suggests that these cells, localized to germinal centers, facilitate the infection of CD4$^+$ cells (2550). The virus particles appear bound to the FDC in a complement component C3-dependent manner (1209). Antibodies to the virus can increase this effect of complement. A role of gp41 in the binding of complement to virions has been considered (683) (see Chapter 3, Section IX). Some evidence suggests that neutralizing antibodies are associated with virions on FDC but do not block virus infection of CD4$^+$ cells (1043).

In our studies of lymphoid tissue from HIV-infected individuals at different clinical states, only symptomatic patients showed extensive ongoing virus replication as detected by in situ RNA hybridization techniques (226). Importantly, the number of virus-infected cells was substantially larger (up to 100-fold) in the lymph node mononuclear cells than in PBMC. Moreover, the percentage of cells that contained infectious virus (detected by infectious-center assays after cell activation) ranged from 1 to 10%. Since up to 25% of CD4$^+$ lymphoid cells could contain HIV as detected by DNA PCR (695, 696), probably about half of these infected cells have defective viruses, but the others could have viruses under tight cellular control (see Chapters 4 and 5) (Color Plate 6, following p. 188). CD8$^+$ cells appear to play a role in suppressing HIV replication in the lymphoid tissue (226) (see Chapter 13).

A noteworthy finding is the relatively small number of infected macrophages detected in lymphoid tissue (695, 981), although a large number of these infected cells have been found in the spleen (979a). The relation of these observations to HIV pathogenesis is not known (see Chapter 13).

Over the course of the infection, the lymph node gradually loses its normal architecture owing to the slow but persistent destruction of CD4$^+$ cells, deterioration of the stromal elements (e.g., FDC), and release of virus from intercellular trappings in the FDC or from infected lymphoid cells producing virus (Color Plates 10, panel B, and 11, following p. 188) (738, 2037, 2040, 2210). According to some studies, a loss of CD4$^+$ cells may not be evident in some lymphoid tissues at the time the number of these cells in the blood is reduced (2284b, 2286). The causes of these events are unknown but most probably resemble those suggested for loss of immune cells in the blood (see Chapter 13): an inability to control virus replication and a reduction in CD4$^+$ and CD8$^+$ cell function. As the FDC undergo destruction, immune function falters, mirrored as well by a return to high levels of virus replication (2031) (Color Plate 11).

The end-stage lymph node shows typical atrophy (Color Plate 10, panel C), with marked depletion of CD4$^+$ cells and destruction of FDC, resulting from the virus itself (738, 1954, 2040, 2550), from cytokine production by cells in responding to increased virus replication (700), or conceivably from activated CD8$^+$ cells (1515). In SIV-infected macaques, a possible detrimental role of CD8$^+$ cells in destruction of lymphoid tissue has been considered (2282) (see Chapter 13). At this late stage of infection, a large percentage of the remaining CD4$^+$ cells show active HIV replication (Color Plate 11). A loss of the FDC reduces efficient antigen presentation and the ability of the host to generate strong antiviral immune responses (1624, 2628; for a review, see reference 1326). In some studies, a further increase in the prevalence of CD8$^+$ cells has been described in the late-stage lymphoid tissue (1656), reflecting in part the loss of CD4$^+$ cells. The antiviral function of the CD8$^+$

cells in the lymphoid tissue appears to be markedly decreased (see Chapter 13) (226). Finally, CD4$^+$ lymphocytes producing virus emerge from the lymph node and become a large part of the virus-expressing cells found in the blood.

This disruption of lymphoid tissues has been demonstrated as well by direct HIV-1 infection of the human fetal thymus in SCID-hu mice (41, 248, 2574) and histoculture of human lymphoid tissue (893a). Loss of precursor T cells and destruction of lymphoid tissue structure take place. Whether the changes noted in the thymus transplant occur in infected individuals is not yet clear, but infected precursor cells in the thymus have been detected (979a) and are susceptible to HIV infection (2744) and cell death (2736; for a review, see reference 856). The findings probably have relevance to the capacity of the immune system to replenish T lymphocytes (see Chapter 14).

Whether these histologic and immunologic events occurring in lymphoid tissue directly reflect the functional changes in lymphoid cells described is not known. Nevertheless, the reduction in virus load in the lymph nodes with increased virus expression in the blood is a common finding in end-stage disease or AIDS. The findings suggest a breakdown in the FDC network and release of virus into the blood. Similar alterations appear to occur in Peyer's patches, the lymphoid structures in the bowel (979a). Observations on HIV infection in lymphoid tissue during therapy are described in Chapter 14.

II. Central Nervous System

Lentiviruses are associated with encephalopathies and other brain disorders (980, 1496), and similar conditions are observed with HIV infection (1777, 2086, 2144). HIV has been readily isolated from the central nervous system (CNS) (see Chapter 4) (for reviews, see references 423 and 424). In some cases, CNS disorders may be the only manifestation of HIV infection (1507, 1908), but HIV-induced CNS disease generally is a late feature of the infection (Table 9.6). Encephalopathy can sometimes be the presenting symptom of acute HIV infection (362, 1084). The findings of brain pathology in conjunction with immunologic disease are not surprising when one appreciates the many shared features of these two systems, particularly cell surface markers and cytokines (2591) (Table 9.7). General pathologic conditions include gliosis, reflecting increased numbers of astrocytes (primarily in the white matter) (Figure 9.4), and perivascular infiltration of lymphocytes and macrophages (310, 710, 2145, 2460). The clinical disorders range from acute encephalopathies to the AIDS dementia complex (2145) (also called HIV dementia or

Table 9.6 Common features of neuropathogenesis

1. Multinucleated giant cell encephalitis
2. Vacuolar myelopathy
3. Astrocytosis (gliosis)
4. Macrophage/microglia activation and proliferation
5. Neuron loss
6. Sensory neuropathy

Table 9.7 Interrelationship of the nervous system and the immune system[a]

1. Neural cell adhesion molecule (N-CAM)
2. L1
3. Axonal glycoprotein 1 (TAG-1)
4. Contactin
5. Neuroglican
6. Fasciclins II and III
7. Thy-1
8. CD4
9. Myelin/oligodendrocyte glycoprotein (MOG)

[a] These cell surface molecules are members of the immunoglobulin gene superfamily.

Figure 9.4 Reactive astrocytes in intragyral white matter of the cerebral hemisphere of a 25-month-old boy with AIDS and severe progressive encephalopathy. Astrocytes stain dark in this photograph with the GFAP avidin-biotin immunoperoxidase reaction. Magnification, ×64. Photomicrograph courtesy of L. Sharer. Reprinted from reference 710 with permission.

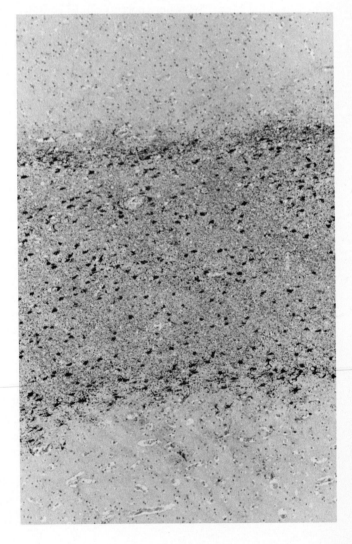

the HIV-associated cognitive/motor complex) (310) (Table 9.6). Dementia has correlated with high levels of β_2-microglobulin and neopterin in the cerebrospinal fluid (CSF) (279) and, most recently, the presence of CD69$^+$ macrophages in the peripheral blood (2153). These cells appear to be responsible for release of products toxic to brain cells (Section II.D).

In animal model systems (e.g., visna/maedi virus and caprine arthritis-encephalitis virus [CAEV]) (Table 1.1), CNS disease usually results from direct infection of the brain parenchyma, particularly glial cells, astrocytes, and possibly microglia (979). Microglia, as noted above, form the macrophage counterpart in the brain compartment. Most observations indicate that these cells enter the CNS only during embryonic development; after birth, peripheral blood macrophages circulate but generally do not take up residence in the CNS (1435, 1556, 2078). The cause of neurologic disease with HIV infection is not yet defined but obviously depends first on HIV entry into the CNS.

Six major concepts can be considered to explain how HIV enters and causes pathology in the CNS (Table 9.8): (i) transfer of free virus or infected cells into the brain directly or through infection of endothelial cells with effects on the blood-brain barrier; (ii) specific HIV neurotropism; (iii) the induction of toxic cellular factors (e.g., cytokines); (iv) the toxic effects of viral proteins; (v) autoimmune and immunologic phenomena; and (vi) potential copathogens (e.g., herpesviruses and papovaviruses). These concepts are considered below.

A.   HIV Entry into the Brain

1. TRANSFER BY INFECTED CELLS

The mechanism(s) by which HIV gains entry into the CNS is not known. Infection, either by free virus or by infected cells, seems to be involved (Table 9.9). Multinucleated giant cells (presumably of microglial origin) are an important component in this infection of the CNS, particularly in children (Figure 9.5) (1766) (for reviews, see references 710 and 2460). These cells are the only specific finding associated with HIV infection of the brain. Moreover, studies with HIV-associated CNS disorders have indicated that the one cell type that readily shows evidence of HIV infection is the macrophage, particularly macrophages found in perivascular areas (1331, 2145, 2878). There are conflicting data on whether these cells resembling macrophages are brain microglia. Some investigators believe that the infected cells in the brain are peripheral blood macrophages (2088, 2827) (see Chapter 4), but infection of both cell types seems to be possible.

Table 9.8   Concepts in HIV neuropathogenesis

1. Effects on blood-brain barrier (endothelial cells, astrocytes)
2. HIV neurotropism: glial cells, microglia, neurons (i.e., membrane permeability changes)
3. Effects of cellular factors produced by macrophages and astrocytes (e.g., TNF-α, quinolinic acid)
4. Effects of viral proteins (gp120, gp41, Tat, Nef)
5. Immune response (autoimmunity, cytotoxicity)
6. Viral cofactors (herpesviruses, papovaviruses)

Table 9.9   HIV entry into the central nervous system (CNS)

Sources
1. Infected CD4$^+$ lymphocytes
2. Infected macrophages
3. Infected endothelial cells
4. Virus passage through fenestrations in brain endothelium
5. Transcytosis of free virus through endothelial cells

Mechanisms
1. Activated infected cells express adhesion molecules (627)
2. Cytokines (e.g., TNF-α, IL-6, and IL-10) up-regulate adhesion molecules in brain endothelial cells (587, 1948, 2079)
3. Tat production up-regulates adhesion molecules on endothelial cells and alters the permeability of the blood-brain barrier (1092, 1403)
4. Cytokines (e.g., TNF-α) produced by infected macrophages or endothelial cells cause endothelial cell leakage (742); passage of virus and virus-infected cells can occur
5. Adhesion molecules on infected cells (and endothelial cells) help in cell attachment and transendothelial migration into the CNS (1067)

Based on these early CNS findings on macrophage infection by HIV, many researchers concluded that peripheral blood macrophages brought the virus into the brain and caused neurologic disease (1331, 2145). Nevertheless, studies in animals have indicated that activated T cells as well as some macrophages continuously circulate in the CNS (1067, 1435, 2078, 2854). Cell activation appears to be a prerequisite for this trafficking in the brain (1067), since cytokines produced by the activated cells (e.g., TNF-α, IL-6, and IL-10) up-regulate adhesion molecules on brain

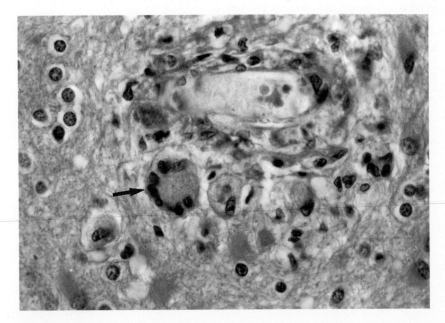

Figure 9.5   Multinucleated giant cell (arrow) and inflammatory cells surrounding a blood vessel in the brain of a 6-year-old boy with AIDS and severe progressive encephalopathy. Hematoxylin and eosin. Magnification, ×555. Photomicrograph courtesy of L. Sharer.

endothelial cells (1066a, 1948, 2079). These adhesion proteins help in cell attachment and migration but are not necessary on the endothelium for cell trafficking. Moreover, HIV infection can elevate levels of adhesion molecules on monocytes (627). The activated cells enter by attachment and diapedesis between endothelial cells (1067) (Figure 9.6). Both types of peripheral blood cells, therefore, could be the initial source of HIV infection, although recent in vitro studies suggest that infected CD4$^+$ lymphocytes preferentially migrate through the endothelium (213).

Some investigators believe that Tat released from infected cells activates endothelial cells and alters the permeability of the blood-brain barrier (1092). Other studies suggest that TNF-α released by infected macrophages can cause endothelial cell leakage (742), as well as an enhanced expression of adhesion molecules (587, 1948). These changes can promote the entry of the infected cells in the CNS. Tat also appears to up-regulate the expression of β_2 integrins, which increase lymphocyte adhesion to endothelial cells. This process can cause destruction to the endothelial cell structures (1403) and affect the integrity of the blood-brain barrier (Sections II.B and II.C).

How HIV establishes infection in the brain is also not known. In acute HIV infection (and in asymptomatic individuals), free virus and mild pleocytosis can be found in the CSF without any signs of neurologic disorder (1084, 1098). In one case report, HIV-1 was isolated from the brain of a man 15 days after accidental transfusion with contaminated PBMC (579). Therefore, conceivably, free virus can readily enter the CSF and brain from the blood via the vascular endothelium. Then, infection of brain cells might be established if a "neurotropic strain" is present (Section II.C).

Figure 9.6 Light microscopic analyses of migration of HIV-1-infected and uninfected monocytes through a blood-brain barrier (BBB) model system involving bone marrow microvascular endothelium (2079). (A) Uninfected control monocytes added to the blood-brain barrier. (B) HIV-infected cells added to the blood-brain barrier; they attach but do not alter the bone marrow microvascular epithelial cells, and the astrocyte portion remains intact. (C and D) Lipopolysaccharide-stimulated uninfected (C) and HIV-infected (D) monocytes modify the morphology of endothelial cells, and the monocytes penetrate the barrier system. Astrocytes are found partially detached from the membrane in sites of active monocyte transmigration. (Reprinted from reference 2079 with permission.)

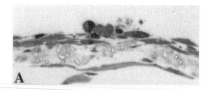

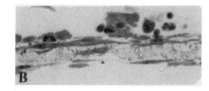

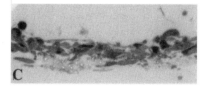

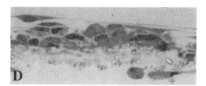

2. INFECTION OF ENDOTHELIAL CELLS AND ASTROCYTES

Both detection of HIV in brain capillary endothelial cells (2878) and the ability of the virus to infect these cells in vitro (1852, 2111) suggest that the endothelium itself could serve as an initial portal of entry for HIV. Subsequently, as observed with cultured glioma (astrocyte) cell lines (Section II.C), HIV could infect the astrocytes associated with the blood-brain barrier. Thus, circulating HIV from the blood might first infect the vascular endothelial lining cells in the brain and then pass from the basolateral surface layer (Figure 9.7) (2005) to astrocytes. Alternatively, the virus could enter via fenestrations in the brain endothelium or pass through endothelial cells by transcytosis without infecting the cells (246). Subsequent mutational changes in the transferred virus could determine its ability to spread from astrocytes and cause disease in the CNS (i.e., as a neurovirulent strain) (Section II.C).

Observations in the SIV system support the conclusion that the virus must penetrate the blood-brain barrier to infect the brain. Lymphocyte-tropic SIV strains cannot replicate in the brain (2462), and certain macrophage-tropic viral isolates cannot induce CNS disease in primates unless the viruses are injected directly into the brain. It is also noteworthy that replication of these macrophage-tropic SIV strains in the blood and other tissues of the animals studied did not induce neurologic disease (e.g., via circulating cytokines) and that infected T cells and macrophages were not found in the CNS (2463). Thus, entry of free virus seems to be the initial step in neuropathogenesis in this animal model. Subsequently, emergence of a "neurotropic" strain would occur. Recent intraviral recombinant studies with SIV have confirmed that macrophage tropism alone is not sufficient for the development of neurologic disease. Portions of the transmembrane envelope protein and/or *nef* conferred neurovirulence (1656a). This evolution of the virus seems to be necessary, since some studies suggest that certain SIV strains can be neuroinvasive but not pathogenic (1205). Moreover, neuropathogenic viruses do not necessarily have the capacity to pass through the blood-brain barrier (1679, 2463). Therefore, the inability of viruses to infect the brain endothelial cells (or to pass through their fenestrations) and their ability to infect certain brain cells (e.g., microglia and astrocytes) could be the important determining factors in neurotropism.

Some studies indicate that passage of macrophage-tropic SIV strains in vivo can select a virus that readily goes from the blood into the brain compartment of the monkeys, causing CNS disease to develop. The virus has been selected to infect endothelial cells (1657). In this regard, neuropathogenesis of a murine leukemia virus is determined by its ability to infect brain capillary endothelial cells (1694).

Since astrocytes help to maintain the integrity of the blood-brain barrier (775), this proposed infection of brain endothelium and subsequently of astrocytes could cause a disturbance within the blood-brain barrier. The infection of endothelial cells could also result in the release of TNF-α, which can induce endothelial cell leakage (742), increase adhesion molecule expression, and permit entry of virus-infected cells. Moreover, other proinflammatory cytokines, such as IL-6 and IL-10, secreted by activated immune cells can contribute to a transendothelial migration of infected or uninfected monocytes (2079). Tat can also increase the permeability of the blood-brain barrier and affect the integrity of this structure (1092, 1403). Toxic products as well as infected cells could enter the brain and might induce the de-

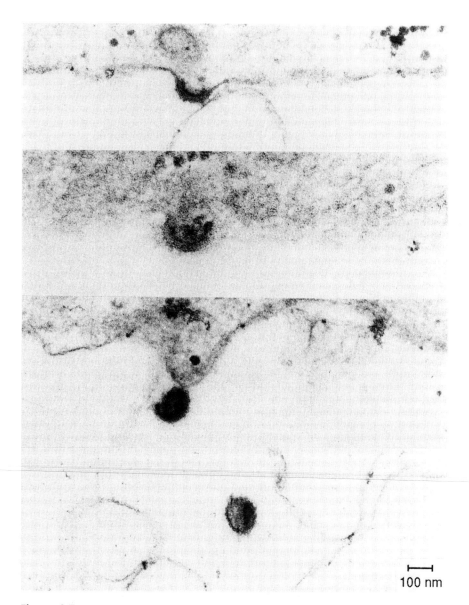

100 nm

Figure 9.7 HIV-1 maturation at basolateral surfaces of polarized epithelial cells. Vero monkey monolayer cells were grown to confluency on Millicel-HA filters and prepared for electron microscopy. All stages of virus assembly were observed from the first signs of budding (top) to the final release of progeny virions (bottom). Reprinted from reference 2005 with permission.

mentia and other neurologic disorders observed. Arguments against this concept include the fact that other viruses, such as cytomegalovirus (CMV), can infect endothelial cells and astrocytes but do not appear to give rise to certain neurologic conditions found in HIV infection, such as vacuolar myelopathy (2086). CMV, however, can cause a virulent encephalitis in AIDS patients.

B.   ## Neurotropism

Once transmitted to the brain compartment by one of the processes described above, a neurotropic HIV strain emerges, as indicated by the consistent recovery from the CNS of HIV with certain biologic properties (see below) (Table 9.10) and detection of virus in glial cells (oligodendrocytes and astrocytes) and perhaps even neurons (119, 1766, 1957, 2156, 2878; for reviews, see references 424 and 2145) (see Chapter 4) (Figure 9.8). Infection could occur via the CD4 molecule that is expressed on neurons and glial cells in the brain (812), but this latter observation still needs confirmation. In addition, cell culture, immunohistochemical techniques, and ultrastructural examination have indicated that brain-derived cells, including astrocytes, oligodendrocytes, and fetal neuronal cells (many lacking CD4 expression), can be directly infected by HIV (39, 289, 427, 708, 976, 1012, 1013, 1039, 1213, 1389, 1766, 2088, 2156, 2329, 2465, 2536, 2692, 2827, 2831, 2874) (Table 9.11). A cellular receptor for HIV-1 other than CD4 (galactosyl ceramide [GalC]) has been found on some brain-derived cells (1010) (see Chapter 3). In a recent study, certain HIV-1 isolates were found that preferentially grew in microglia compared to macrophages (2604). The viruses induced cytopathic effects in microglial cultures and had a V3 loop sequence similar to those isolated from patients with HIV dementia. The findings place further emphasis on the selection for a virus in the CNS and one that is cytopathic. The presence of a microglia-tropic (versus macrophage-tropic) virus merits further study.

The identification of certain HIV-1 isolates that show biologic and serologic properties distinct from those of blood-derived strains (Table 7.7) supports the idea that a neurotropic strain exists (424, 432). A common feature is macrophage tropism, but the ability of this HIV strain to infect brain cells must be considered (see below). Furthermore, as previously noted (see Chapter 7), PCR studies suggest that a viral strain in the same host can evolve independently in the brain and in the blood and can be distinguished by molecular as well as biologic features (Figure 7.13) (709, 1137, 1283, 1329, 1350, 2028, 2137, 2594). Some genetic differences correlate with neurologic disorders (2137). Finally, observations with transgenic mice containing the long terminal repeat (LTR) of either a CNS-derived strain or a T-cell-line-tropic strain of HIV are noteworthy (525). Only animals generated with the CNS-derived LTR showed gene expression in the brain, particularly in neurons. In newborns, this HIV-1 expression was noted in endothelial cells and macrophages as well as in neurons (329). These findings support a differential ability of brain-derived strains to replicate in the CNS and the presence of temporarily regulated cel-

Table 9.10 Recovery of HIV from CSF and brain tissues

Clinical conditions	No. positive/total no. (%)
Neurologic disorder[a]	74/96 (77)
Asymptomatic	36/68 (53)

[a] Meningitis, myelopathy, peripheral neuropathy, encephalopathy, dementia. For a review, see reference 424.

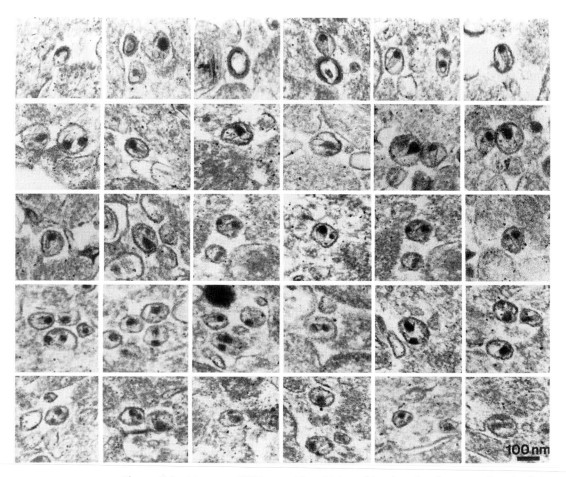

Figure 9.8   Montage of HIV-1 particles within multinucleated and mononucleated cells in the brain of a 6-year-old boy with AIDS and severe progressive encephalopathy (same patient as in Figure 9.5). Several types of virions are present, including immature particles and mature particles. Other particles have an atypical morphology, which suggests that they may be defective. Reprinted from reference 1766 with permission.

lular transcription factors in the CNS. The results also suggest that neurons could be involved in a neuropathic process in infected individuals (725, 1282, 1957).

In further support of this neurotropism is the observation that persistent non-cytopathic low-level infection of glial cells can occur. This infection cannot be detected by in situ hybridization studies but can be demonstrated after exposure of the cells to infected lymphocytes, cytokines, or culture fluids of PBMC (2691) or by in situ PCR procedures (1957). Without killing the cell, such a phenomenon in HIV-infected oligodendrocytes, for example, could reduce myelin production by these cells and thus could affect normal nerve transmission.

The cytopathicity of HIV itself in the brain could be related to its proteins, its effects on the permeability or function of the cell membrane, or the accumulation of unintegrated HIV-1 DNA in brain tissue (2026). Effects similar to those induced in other cells by the virus might be involved (Section I.E) (Chapter 6). In summary,

Table 9.11 Cultured brain-derived cells susceptible to HIV infection[a]

Cells	CD4 expression[b]
Astrocytes (fetal)	±
Microglia	±
Dorsal root ganglia (glia)	−
Choroid plexus	−
Glioma cell lines	±
Medulloblastoma[c]	−
Neuroblastoma	−

[a] Generally low virus replication takes place and is amplified with addition of PBMC.

[b] Symbols: ±, CD4 detected in some cells or cell lines; −, no CD4 expression.

[c] Expresses glial and neuronal cell markers.

transmission and subsequent development of a neurotropic strain in the brain could be a major factor in HIV neuropathogenesis.

C. Toxic Cellular Factors

Once HIV has infected the brain, it could induce a high production of toxic cellular products that could have neuropathic effects (for review see reference 1757). Apoptosis of neurons and astrocytes has been detected in brain tissue of AIDS patients; most of the apoptotic cells were found near HIV-infected cells but did not involve them (2476). These observations, mirroring those noted in lymph nodes (753), provide further support for the role of soluble cellular factors in CNS disorders. Several cytokines are produced by cells in the CNS (1538) (Table 9.12). Moreover, high levels of quinolinic acid have been found in the CSF of HIV-1-infected patients (299, 1065). A direct relationship of this protein to CNS disease has not been shown in adults (2877) but was reported to occur in children (299). Which cells make this excitotoxin, an N-methyl-D-aspartate (NMDA) agonist, is not known, but work with poliovirus suggests that macrophages and microglia are involved (1066).

Many investigators believe that after HIV infection or exposure to viral envelope proteins, the microglia and macrophages within the brain could be induced to produce certain cytokines (e.g., TNF-α, IL-1, and IL-6), including chemokines

Table 9.12 Cytokine production in the brain

Cells	Cytokines
Astrocytes	TNF-α, lymphotoxin, IL-1, IL-6, IFN-α, IFN-β, TGF-β
Microglia (macrophages)	IL-1, TNF-α, TGF-β, IL-6, low-molecular-weight cytotoxins (?), quinolinic acid
T cells	Lymphotoxin (TNF-β), neuroleukin

(1582, 2394), that can be directly toxic to the CNS (344, 833, 1697, 1758, 1759, 2732, 2733, 2863, 2939) (Figure 9.9). Essentially, activated cells (whether infected or not) could produce these toxic products.

TNF-α mRNA, for example, was found in high levels in brain cells from infected patients with dementia (2863) and by in situ PCR techniques in infected astrocytes and microglial cells in the brain (1957). In addition, some studies suggest that stimulated astrocytes (perhaps via HIV infection or exposure to viral envelope proteins) could produce TNF-α, which is toxic to brain cells such as oligodendrocytes (1759, 2242) (Table 9.13). TNF-α might also induce the production of β-chemokines that could have anti-HIV activity in the brain (1582) but most probably cause harmful inflammatory effects.

At high concentrations, TNF-α has been shown to destroy rodent neurons and human fetal neurons (859). TNF-α is toxic for myelin and human brain-derived cell lines (2312, 2444, 2868). Moreover, TNF-α and lymphotoxin have been found to be cytotoxic for bovine oligodendrocytes but not astrocytes (2442). The mechanism of this cell destruction appears to be apoptosis, perhaps by activation of AMPA (α-amino-3-hydroxy-5-methylisoxazole-4-proprionic acid) receptors (859). Whether these cytokines could be damaging to the CNS in vivo is not known. In some reports, relatively low levels of TNF-α have been found in CSF (946, 2732). However, elevated amounts of TNF-α and quinolinic acid have been detected in brain tissue (9). Thus, the toxicity of TNF-α, if important in the CNS, would most probably result from an apocrine secretion process.

IL-1 production has also been linked to CNS disease, although IL-1 mRNA was not detected by in situ PCR techniques in infected cells in the brain (1957). This cytokine, which is secreted by monocytes, microglia, and endothelial cells, can be cytotoxic and can induce proliferation of astrocytes in vitro (1984, 2733), as do TNF-α and IL-6 (2443, 2733). Thus, the role of these cellular factors in the gliosis observed in HIV-associated infection should be considered.

Induction of transforming growth factor β (TGF-β) production by macrophages and astrocytes has also been linked to CNS disorders (2801). Expression of

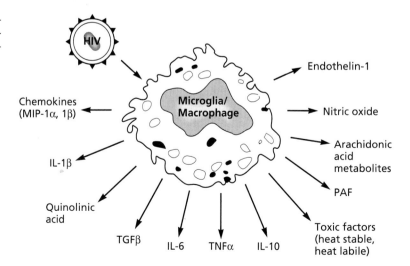

Figure 9.9 Neuropathogenesis. The role of infected microglia/macrophages is illustrated.

Table 9.13 Toxic effects of TNF-α in the CNS

1. Induces IL-1 secretion
2. Enhances monocyte toxicity
3. Can act synergistically with IL-1 and IFN-γ to augment monocyte/macrophage cytotoxicity
4. Can destroy oligodendrocytes and neurons
5. Can cause degeneration of myelin (direct and indirect)

TGF-β was found in the brain, and purified human monocytes infected with HIV were shown to secrete increased levels of this cytokine. Moreover, infected macrophages release substances that induced uninfected cultured astrocytes to secrete TGF-β. Since TGF-β is a very potent chemotactic factor and can augment the production of other cytokines, including TGF-α, its role in CNS disease deserves further attention. Another monocyte-derived cellular factor with potential neuropathic effects is endothelin-1, which has potent vasoconstricting activity in the brain (732). One report shows increased production of this cytokine by monocytes after exposure to gp120 in vitro (687).

In further support of the role of toxic cellular factors in neuropathogenesis is the observation that HIV-infected macrophages, in contrast to uninfected macrophages, release factors (in addition to TGF-α and TGF-β) that are destructive to rodent neuronal cells and to cultured human brain cells (890, 2154) (Figure 9.9). Macrophages recovered from the PBMC of HIV-infected individuals also induce damage in cultured human brain cells (2154). Low-molecular-weight substances produced by infected macrophages appear to mediate the effects. One is heat labile (2152a); the other is heat stable and protease resistant (890, 891). The heat-stable factor can be blocked by antagonists to NMDA receptors and by soluble CD4 (891). Recently, a factor toxic for brain cells that is produced by CD69$^+$ macrophages was detected at high levels in the blood of HIV-infected patients with dementia (2153). Whether this factor is one of the above-described toxic cellular products remains to be determined (2152a).

Certainly, the induction of brain pathology by macrophage-tropic and not T-cell-tropic strains of SIV does suggest a major role for infected macrophages (or the microglial counterparts) in human CNS disorders (Section II.B) (2462). The hypothesis is also supported by studies showing pathology in human neural xenografts only with HIV-infected macrophages (550). Moreover, coculturing HIV-infected macrophages with astrocytes leads to production of high levels of the neurotoxins IL-1 and TNF-α. Arachidonic acid metabolites (eicosinoids) and platelet-activating factor (PAF), produced by activated macrophages, have also been implicated in the observed toxicity to astrocytes and neurons (860, 867, 2868). Moreover, elevated levels of the immunologic isoform of nitric oxide synthase have been noted in the CNS of patients with dementia. Its production appears linked to gp41 expression (see below) (18). All these results, if confirmed, could explain the cell death described in human neural cells after direct contact with infected macrophages (2645).

This overexpression of eicosinoids, PAF, and TGF-α by activated monocytes during HIV infection of the brain can be countered by the function of astrocytes that inactivates these substances in the CNS (1950; for a review, see reference 172)

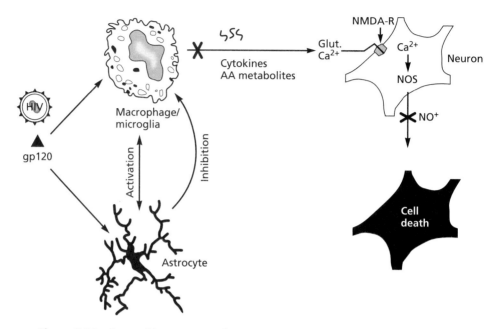

Figure 9.10   Some evidence suggests that astrocytes play an active role in inactivating toxic substances entering the CNS (1950). The cells, by interacting with macrophages and microglia, can inhibit their production of cellular products that are toxic to neurons. This toxicity is mediated via the NMDA receptor (NMDA-R). Thus, a balance is established by which astrocytes can either synthesize neurotoxins or remove them from the CNS (Section II.C).

(Figure 9.10). Thus, a balance seems to be established, with astrocytes either synthesizing neurotoxins or removing them from the CNS. The end result of this activity could determine the pathogenic pathway. Nevertheless, as mentioned above, whether any of these cytokines detected in vitro are produced in the brain in sufficient quantities to cause pathology is not yet known.

D.   Toxic Viral Proteins

Another consequence of macrophage or microglial infection could be the production of high levels of HIV-1 proteins in the CNS (Table 9.8). As noted previously, the envelope protein gp120 has been found to be toxic to cultured brain-derived cells from a variety of animals as well as humans (170, 276, 1564, 2155, 2939) (Table 9.14). Distinct changes in the ultrastructure of the cells, particularly tubular fibrils, can be seen (2155). The toxic effect may reflect gp120 induction of IL-6 and TGF-α (2939), which are known to cause damage in the CNS (Section II.C). HIV infection of primary brain cell cultures induces apoptosis in neurons and astrocytes once virus production is at its peak (2476). Moreover, viral gp120 or other viral proteins could be responsible for the endothelial cell apoptosis observed in the brains of AIDS patients (2476).

HIV gp120 can affect the permeability of the cell membrane and its electrical potential via an effect on ion transport and calcium channels (170, 664, 1221, 1563)

Table 9.14 Potential role of gp120 in HIV neuropathogenesis

1. Kills cultured rodent neuronal cells (276, 1068a)
2. Kills cultured human brain cells (2154)
3. Intracerebral injection induced cell death in rat brain cortical neurons (123, 1068a)
4. Inhibits β-adrenergic regulation of astrocytes and microglial function (1483)
5. Causes alterations in membrane integrity and astrocyte function (e.g., GFAP expression; ion transport) (170, 1221, 1563, 2155)
6. Stimulates monocytes to release neurotoxic factors (891)
7. Induces IL-6 and TNF-α in brain cultures (astrocytes and macrophages) (2939)
8. Stimulates secretion of endothelin-1 (also TNF-α) by macrophages (687)
9. Increases intracellular adhesion molecule 1 (ICAM-1) levels in glial cells (2493)
10. Transgenic expression of gp120 through the GFAP promoter causes astrocytosis and neuron loss (192, 2684)
11. Blocked by anti-gp120 antibodies (664, 1221)
12. Prevented by anti-CD4 antibodies (murine system; not rat retinal cells) (276, 1221)
13. Prevented by calcium channel blockers (nimodipine) (664, 1563)
14. Prevented by antagonists to NMDA receptor (1564)
15. Reversed by neuroleukin (1460)
16. Prevented by vasoactive intestinal polypeptide (VIP) (276, 2080)

(see Chapter 6). The effect can be exacerbated in cultured cells by glucocorticoids or abrogated by estradiols (296a). The relevance of these observations to therapies given during HIV infection merits study. The toxicity from gp120 can involve production of nitric oxide (581) and can act via the NMDA receptor (1564). Quinolinic acid has also been implicated in this process (Section II.C). Thus, NMDA antagonists can reduce the toxic effect of gp120 (1564). Moreover, the HIV envelope could be involved in inducing membrane damage directly (749, 850) or in activating, via a receptor, toxic tyrosine kinase activity in brain cells (2403) (see Chapter 6). Perturbations in astrocyte function induced by gp120 could also affect neurons (2155). A detrimental effect of gp120 on the β-adrenergic regulation of astrocytes and microglia has been suggested from studies of rat cells (1483). Finally, the increased expression of adhesion molecules and changes in signal transduction induced by Tat or gp120 in astrocytes and microglia have been cited as possible pathogenic factors because of enhanced binding of monocytes to these cells (1403, 2493).

The potential toxicity of gp120 on the CNS was demonstrated in studies of transgenic mice expressing the HIV-1 envelope under the control of the glial fibrillary acid protein (GFAP) promoter or neurofilament light gene promoter (192, 2684). Extensive vacuolization of dendrites and a reduction in the number of neurons were found in animals expressing gp120. Furthermore, the brain showed a widespread reactive astrocytosis, particularly in areas of high gp120 mRNA expression. As noted above, this pathologic finding is common to individuals infected with HIV-1 (310). Whether similar results would be observed if gp120 were expressed in cells from the macrophage/microglia lineage merits further study. Intracerebral injection of HIV-1 gp120 also induced cell death in rat brain cortical neurons. The toxicity appeared to be secondary to a relative balance in the expression of nerve growth factor and nitric oxide synthase (123). The possibility also remains that gp120 induced the production of cytokines that caused the neuropathology (see above). In any case, these studies emphasized the potential toxic effects of gp120 in the CNS (Table 9.14).

In addition, certain regions of gp120 (particularly a threonine-rich epitope called peptide T) have been reported to compete with neurotropic factors, such as neuroleukin (phosphohexose isomerase) and vasoactive intestinal polypeptide (VIP) (276, 1460, 2080), required for normal CNS function. This potential cause of pathology in the brain, however, has not received much attention recently.

Furthermore, as noted before (see Chapter 6), the envelope gp41 and Tat proteins have been found to be toxic to cells in culture (1645, 1791, 1792, 2320) (Table 9.15). Expression of gp41 is associated with elevated levels of nitric oxide synthase (18). Tat was neurotoxic when inoculated intracerebrally into mice (2320) (Table 9.15). This viral protein, like gp120, can cause an increase in expression of adhesion molecules on endothelial cells (see above), depolarization of cells, and degeneration of cell membranes. The mechanisms remain to be elucidated, but Tat is neuroexcitatory (via the NMDA receptor) and neurotropic (1645) and shows some homology to a neurotoxin (see below) (851). In addition, Tat was found to cause aggregation and fascicle formation in cultures of primary rat cortical brain cells (1343) (Table 9.15). Cell death did not occur, and the region of Tat involved was different from its transactivation domain.

Finally, sequence similarity between the HIV Nef protein and perhaps a portion of gp41 to scorpion toxin has been noted (852, 2861). Nef protein can affect normal cellular transmembrane conduction (2861) and appears to be selectively expressed in astrocytes in vitro (111, 271, 2690) and in vivo (2184, 2329, 2692). Nef could compromise the electrical potential and function of these cells. Thus, this viral product, along with gp120, gp41, and Tat, might play a role in the neurologic conditions observed with HIV infection. It is important to note, however, that some studies have not shown any cell toxicity with recombinant HIV-1 proteins, including gp120, p24, Nef, protease, and reverse transcriptase (890, 891, 2868).

E.   Autoimmunity

Autoimmune responses induced as a result of molecular mimicry (1978) could play a role in CNS disease (see Chapter 10), because HIV proteins resemble normal cellular proteins. Autoantibodies to peripheral nerves have been found in this infection

---

Table 9.15 Neurotoxic activity of Tat

1. Kills cultured rodent glioma and neuroblastoma cells (1645, 2320)
2. Acts on cell membrane and induces a large depolarization and a decrease in membrane resistance (1645)
3. Affects cell permeability (e.g., endothelial cells) (1092)
4. Increases expression of adhesion molecules (1403)
5. Shows homology to a neurotoxin (851)
6. Neurotoxic after intercerebroventricular injection of mice (2320)
7. Causes aggregation and fascicle formation in cultured rodent cortical brain cells (1343)

(590, 1301) and appear to be responsible for peripheral neuropathy (1301). Antibody levels to myelin basic protein in the CSF have also correlated with the severity of dementia (1602). The reported cross-reactivity of anti-gp41 antibodies with certain proteins in astrocytes (but not GFAP) could compromise the function of these brain cells (2546a, 2929). Moreover, the reaction of a V3 loop monoclonal antibody with human brain proteins (2716) suggests that molecular mimicry could be part of a pathogenic pathway. Furthermore, brain-reactive antibodies have been detected in the sera of infected patients (1384), particularly those with neurologic disease. The presence of these antibodies in immune complexes within the CSF has been noted as well (180). In addition, antiviral or anticellular CTL that are harmful to the brain could be generated in the CNS (1189).

F.   Copathogens

Several investigators have reported the presence in the CNS of other infectious agents, such as herpesviruses (e.g., CMV) and papovaviruses (e.g., JC virus), that could exacerbate the neuropathologic condition (1914, 1915, 2879). It is noteworthy that cells coinfected with HIV and CMV have been found (1915). Nevertheless, whereas herpesviruses and papovaviruses have been shown to activate the HIV LTR in a conventional chloramphenicol acetyltransferase (CAT) assay (580, 865, 884, 1078, 1089, 1440, 1851, 1997, 2182) (see Chapter 5), it is not known whether their infection in the brain has biological significance in terms of HIV replication and pathology. In some cell culture studies, for example, CMV increased HIV replication (2520); in others, the opposite effect was noted (1364). Many findings suggest that opportunistic infection, when present, can be the primary cause of the neurologic disease. Other observations, however, such as the improvement in a patient's dementia after zidovudine (AZT) therapy (125, 609, 2123, 2124), suggest that HIV directly or indirectly plays a major role as well.

G.   Conclusions

Because certain neurologic findings are primarily found to be associated with HIV infection (e.g., multinucleated cells vacuolar myelopathy) (2086), the concept that neuropathogenesis depends on infection of the brain by a neurotropic HIV strain is now widely accepted. This virus would evolve from a circulating virus that replicates sufficiently in endothelial cells and particularly in astrocytes to cause damage to the blood-brain barrier (Figure 9.11). Alternatively, it could pass through intercellular fenestrations to reach astrocytes lining the blood-brain barrier or infect these cells after transcytosis (246). Support for this hypothesis comes from the fact that the non-macrophage-tropic strains from the blood infect glioma (astrocyte) cell lines (427, 1367) and brain capillary endothelial cells (1852). Finally, activated infected CD4$^+$ lymphocytes and macrophages can traffic through the CNS and introduce virus to the brain by this means.

It would appear that astrocytes are a key factor in CNS disorders. They produce cytokines that help maintain the blood-brain barrier or could be harmful to the

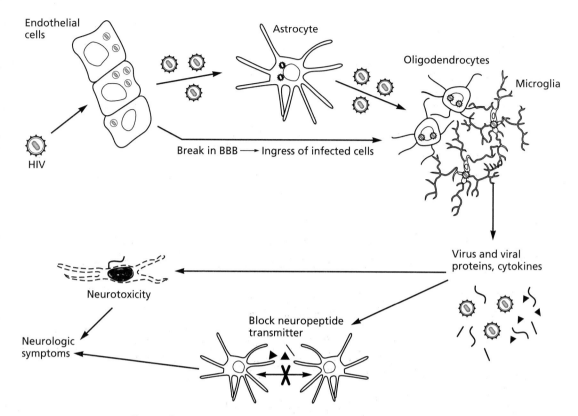

Figure 9.11   HIV neuropathogenesis. It is proposed that the virus infects capillary endothelial cells of the brain and passes via the basolateral surface of these cells to astrocytes lining the blood-brain barrier (BBB). Infection of both these cell types leads to a breakdown in the blood-brain barrier and ingress of infected T cells and macrophages. The ultimate result is an infection of other brain cells (e.g., oligodendrocytes and microglia) by HIV. Production of HIV and its viral proteins ensues, as does the release of various cytokines (e.g., TNF-α and low-molecular-weight substances). These products could lead to an interruption of cell-to-cell transmission through a blockage of neurotropic factors. Direct infection of cells, as well as high levels of viral proteins (e.g., envelope glycoproteins, Tat, and Nef) and cytokines, could lead to direct neurotoxicity through detrimental effects on the cell membrane.

brain (e.g., IL-1β and TNF-α), and they inactivate neurotoxins (Figure 9.10). Astrocytes, as well as microglia, play an important role in antigen presentation and can have phagocytic activity (2494). HIV infection of astrocytes could produce many of the sequelae leading to neuropathogenesis (Table 9.16). Therefore, the role of these cells in CNS disease merits increased attention (for a review, see reference 172).

The compromise in the function of the blood-brain barrier brought about by HIV infection leads to disease within the CNS through the ingress of virus and infected cells as well as toxic products (Figure 9.11). Subsequently, through mutations, the neurotropic strain that replicates well in macrophages, perhaps microglia and other brain cells (see Chapter 4), emerges and produces viral proteins (e.g.,

Table 9.16   Role of astrocytes in the CNS

1. Maintenance of the blood-brain barrier
2. Antigen presentation
3. Cytokine production (PGE^a, IL-1)
4. Decrease the effects of neurotoxins

^{a} PGE, prostaglandin E.

gp120, gp41, Tat, and Nef) that can be toxic to cells. Moreover, these viral products could compete with neurotropic factors to inhibit cell-to-cell communication. This macrophage-tropic virus might also pass most easily to other brain cells such as oligodendrocytes, producers of myelin needed for nerve transmission, and even to neurons. The many features of a macrophage-tropic virus that associate it with neurovirulence are listed in Table 9.17. In this regard, the loss of neurons observed in the frontal cortex in HIV disease (725, 1282) could result from the viral infection itself (1957) or its sequelae.

Specific infection of macrophages or other cells in the brain (e.g., astrocytes) could also favor enhanced production of toxic cellular factors (Tables 9.12 and 9.13; Figure 9.9) that damage other brain cells and myelin (Color Plate 10, following p. 188). Eventually, any approach to limiting HIV replication and spread should decrease neurologic symptoms. Such a response has been reported with some patients receiving AZT treatment; symptoms of AIDS-related dementia have been markedly reduced, at least for some period of time (125, 2123, 2124). This encouraging observation has been attributed to an anti-HIV and/or anti-cytokine effect of AZT. The fact that the dementia is reversible with AZT argues for at least an initial noncytolytic effect of HIV (and its proteins) or the presumed induced cytokines.

Autoantibodies also appear to be involved in some neurologic disorders, primarily peripheral neuropathy, as shown by immunohistochemical staining and successful treatment by plasmapheresis (1302). The role of other viruses, if not primary, could also be contributory in many cases. Finally, abnormal vitamin B_{12} metabolism in HIV infection has led some investigators to suggest that this deficiency can be responsible for some abnormal neurologic findings (1313).

Table 9.17   Evidence that macrophage tropism is associated with neurovirulence

1. Virus isolated from the CSF and brain in neurologic disease is macrophage tropic.
2. Virus isolated from the brain in animals dying of AIDS in the absence of neurologic disease is not macrophage tropic.
3. Intracerebral inoculation of macrophage-tropic SIV gives rise to severe encephalitis.
4. Neuroadaptation of SIV_{mac239} in macaques leads to encephalitis, and that virus is a macrophage-tropic virus.
5. Lymphotropic, non-macrophage-tropic SIV can cause persistent infection of the brain without disease.
6. HIV-infected macrophages produce high levels of neurotoxins.

III. Gastrointestinal System

Along with the CNS disorders observed during some acute HIV infections, bowel symptoms have been reported soon after infection, but they then subside (2679). The subsequent chronic malabsorption, malnutrition, and diarrhea occurring several years later have generally been attributed to the opportunistic infections in the bowel as a result of immune deficiency (667, 1355); however, HIV might be directly involved (see below). In Africa, this gastrointestinal problem has been termed "slim disease" (2452) because of the substantial loss of weight resulting from the infection. Generally, the gastrointestinal tract shows only subtle histologic changes during HIV infection, unless an opportunistic infection such as CMV infection, cryptosporidiosis, *Mycobacterium avium* complex, or microsporidium infection is present (1355). Thus, the permeability changes reflected by diarrhea and malabsorption may not be readily apparent in a bowel biopsy specimen.

Malnutrition is considered to be present in a patient with a weight loss of more than 10% of normal body weight and greater protein wasting than is observed in other cases of starvation (443, 1355). This malnourishment in HIV infection can result from anorexia or nutrient malabsorption secondary to intestinal damage and inflammation (667, 1355). Deficiencies in micronutrients, particularly vitamins A and B_{12}, have been associated with disease progression (155). Moreover, metabolic abnormalities, such as hypertriglyceridemia, have been observed in HIV-infected individuals (957), but their role in the wasting syndrome is not known. The latter condition is most probably related to the high cytokine production in HIV infection (958).

Studies investigating the cause of gastrointestinal disturbances have demonstrated the presence of HIV itself in the bowel mucosa of patients with intestinal disorders, as well as in asymptomatic individuals (1047, 1356, 1696, 1916) (Color Plate 7, following p. 188). In several cases, it is the only pathogen found in the bowel. Thus, the virus can "home out" in this organ as well as in the brain. Its presence in enterochromaffin cells in the bowel mucosa (1516, 1916) is noteworthy. These hormone-producing cells are distributed throughout the intestinal tract and are responsible for normal motility and bowel function (2110). The lamina propria has also shown evidence of HIV infection, most probably in infected macrophages (782, 1356, 1916), since very few $CD4^+$ lymphocytes are present in the gastrointestinal tract at the time of bowel symptoms (309, 1550, 1551, 2581).

HIV pathogenesis in the bowel has not yet been explained, and, as with HIV infection of the CNS, certain mechanisms have been considered (Table 9.18). As in the brain, when opportunistic infections are present, it is difficult to determine whether they caused the initial disease or are contributing to an HIV infection. In

Table 9.18 Factors potentially involved in HIV pathogenesis in the bowel

1. HIV infection of bowel cells
2. Induction of toxic cytokines (e.g., IL-1β and IL-6)
3. Toxicity of viral proteins (e.g., gp120 and Tat)
4. CTL activity

symptomatic individuals in whom no other bowel pathogen can be found, direct infection of the bowel mucosa by HIV (e.g., enterochromaffin cells) should be considered (1516). In further support of this conclusion, bowel-derived HIV strains with some properties that can distinguish them from viruses recovered from the blood of the same individual have been described (see Chapter 7, Table 7.7); these viruses are often macrophage tropic (141). Moreover, SIV isolates from the bowel and the brain of the same monkey have shown genetic features that suggest independent evolution of the virus variants in these tissues of the animal (1329).

As with CNS disease, however, other investigators argue that an indirect effect of HIV infection is involved. They believe that infection of macrophages and T cells in the intestines of HIV-infected patients induces production of cytokines that have destructive toxic effects on the bowel mucosa. In the primate model, for example, SIV infection of intestinal lymphoid tissue (macrophages and T lymphocytes) was associated with abnormalities in absorption, even before the onset of clinical disease (1048). The results may reflect the known effect of cytokines (presumably produced by the infected cells) on the morphology and function of gastrointestinal cells (1626). As noted above, macrophage-tropic HIV strains are readily isolated from bowel tissue (141) and could influence the cytokines produced. Differences in cytokine secretion by intestinal mononuclear cells from AIDS patients as compared to uninfected subjects have been noted (2581). However, in these cases, IL-1β and IL-6 production was increased but levels of TNF-α (generally a toxic cytokine) were decreased. In these studies, the number of CD4$^+$ cells in the lamina propria of the AIDS patients was reduced, but the possible role of cytokines released by other cells in the intestinal mucosa was not considered. Furthermore, the reduced level of APC (e.g., activated DC) in the bowels of HIV-infected individuals could contribute to a loss of immune response and the occurrence of opportunistic infections in these tissues (1551).

As noted above, histochemical studies of the gastrointestinal tract show chronic inflammation (1355, 1916) that is not unlike that in bowel disorders caused by a variety of infections and toxic agents. Nevertheless, the extensive diarrhea and malabsorption observed in AIDS does suggest a direct effect of the virus on intestinal cell membrane integrity, perhaps in the handling of sodium ions and water (see Chapter 6). The watery diarrhea often observed could be the effect of a toxin, perhaps a product of infected cells or a viral protein. As in the CNS disease, the potential role of the envelope glycoproteins, or of Tat or Nef, on cell viability and physiologic function should be considered (Section II.D). Finally, an increased number of CTL have been found in the small intestines of HIV-infected patients (2528). Although no relationship between the cell number and presence of diarrhea has been found, some tissue injury may result from the presence of these cells (see Chapter 11).

A strain of SIV, PBJ, has been characterized that induces severe diarrhea in infected rhesus macaque monkeys within 10 to 21 days (808). An increase in lymphoid tissue is found in the bowel, a pathology not commonly seen with HIV. Whether cytokine production by immune cells or direct toxic effects of the virus or viral proteins on bowel epithelium are responsible for the disorder is not yet known. IL-6 production was found to be associated with the inflammatory process (215). Studies of this unusual animal model might uncover the cause of gastrointestinal disorders associated with HIV infection in humans.

IV.   Other Organ Systems

HIV has been detected in the hearts of patients with cardiomyopathy (1562), the kidneys of individuals with tubular glomerulopathy (492), the lungs of patients with pneumonia (608), and the joint fluid of arthritis patients (2899); it has also been recovered from the adrenal glands of infected individuals (2811a). In the adrenal glands, cytokines expressed by infected hematopoietic cells could be involved in decreased adrenal function (947). Fetal adrenal cells in culture have been found to be susceptible to HIV (133), but most evidence suggests that, in vivo, CMV and not HIV causes the cell destruction noted in this tissue (940, 2152). Nevertheless, a role of HIV in other endocrine disorders by a variety of mechanisms merits further study (947).

It is not yet clear how HIV could play a role in the disorders of the heart, kidneys, lungs, and joints. However, the known effects of gp120 on membrane permeability (see Section II.D, also Chapter 6) could explain some of the electrophysiologic abnormalities that accompany heart disease. In the kidneys, direct infection of the endothelium or mesangial cells might produce the tubular destruction observed in this HIV-associated condition (492, 938, 1293, 2186). It is noteworthy that immune complex glomerulonephritis occurs rarely in HIV infection but has been described with IgA-containing complexes (for a review, see reference 1293). A variety of potential virologic and immunologic mechanisms for HIV-associated nephrology have been presented (2187) and require more study.

In the lung, changes in permeability or other toxic effects of viral proteins should be considered, especially in the childhood pneumonias. A role of anti-HIV CTL in this tissue could be involved (106, 2102). Visna/maedi virus causes pneumonitis in sheep (Table 1.1) (1980). Moreover, lung fibroblasts can be infected by HIV (2103), and HIV isolates from the lung and blood of the same individual can be distinguished (1169). This finding suggests a possible pathogenic role of certain HIV strains in this tissue. Finally, the presence of HIV antigens in joint fluid and synovial membranes (716, 2899) merits further consideration of the potential role of HIV in associated arthropathies. The caprine lentivirus counterpart, CAEV, causes rheumatoid arthritis-like disease in goats (537, 1726).

Chapter 9   **SALIENT FEATURES**

1. HIV infection is associated with suppression of hematopoiesis, as reflected by reduced growth of bone marrow cells in culture. The infection of bone marrow endothelial cells and stroma could be involved.

2. HIV infection is reflected by changes in the subset number and phenotype of lymphocytes. Activated cells are increased, $CD4^+$ cells are reduced, and a loss of naive lymphocytes occurs over time.

3. B-cell abnormalities include polyclonal activation and a lack of response to new antigens.

4. Abnormalities in the function of macrophages, NK cells, and DC are reflected in cytokine production, reduced phagocytosis, cytotoxicity, and decreased antigen-presentation ability. Loss of expression of the B7 costimulatory molecule on DC and macrophages can be involved.

5. A decrease in $CD4^+$ lymphocyte function is demonstrated by the reduced proliferative responses to recall antigens, alloantigens, and mitogens. Potential reasons for the loss in $CD4^+$ cell number and function include both direct and indirect mechanisms, such as the effect of viral proteins, disturbance in signal transduction, loss of noninfected cells (e.g., bystander effects), cytotoxic cells, immune suppressor factors, and antilymphocyte antibodies.

6. Cytokines released as a result of HIV infection can determine the maturation of $CD4^+$ cells and their function. They can influence the extent of HIV replication and the strength of the antiretroviral immune response.

7. HIV most probably infects lymphoid tissues first or very early in infection and gradually causes a disruption in the architecture and function of this organ system. Virus particles are visualized on FDC, and eventually germinal centers are destroyed, leading to the decrease in immune activity. Destruction in the normal function of lymphoid tissue presages progression to disease.

8. HIV infection in the CNS is determined by a variety of factors, including how the virus enters cells through the blood-brain barrier, which cells it infects, development of neuropathic strains, toxic cellular and viral products, autoimmune phenomena, and other cofactors, such as concurrent viral infections. Infection of astrocytes may cause CNS disorders by disturbing their function in antigen presentation and as inactivators of neurotoxins.

9. Infection of the gastrointestinal system may result from direct HIV infection of bowel cells or from a disturbance in cytokine production, leading to poor absorption and lack of control in handling of salts and water.

10. HIV may have effects on several organ systems, such as the heart, kidneys, lungs, joints, and adrenal glands. HIV has been isolated from several of these tissues. Immune responses to the virus could play a role in the disorders observed.

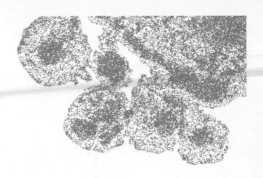

Humoral Immune Responses to HIV Infection

10

T HUS FAR, WE HAVE DISCUSSED THE BASIC BIOLOGIC FEATURES OF HIV and its heterogeneity. How certain characteristics could play a part in the pathogenic pathway has also been considered. We review in the next two chapters the immune responses of the host that could influence HIV-induced disease (for further reviews, see references 135 and 1943). The effect of HIV on the immune system was considered in Chapter 9, and the heterogeneity in virus sensitivity to antibodies was reviewed in Chapter 7. These features have relevance to the following two chapters.

I.   Detection of Anti-HIV Antibodies

Shortly after the discovery of HIV, different tests were developed to detect antibodies to the virus. As noted in Chapter 4, these antibodies are made soon after acute infection. The isotype distribution of these HIV-specific antibodies can reflect their function. Antibody-dependent cellular cytotoxicity (ADCC), complement-dependent cytotoxicity, and neutralizing and blocking abilities reflect specific antibody classes (e.g., IgG1). These molecules circulate in the blood or are secreted at mucosal surfaces. They can be detected in genital as well as other body fluids.

Antibodies to a variety of viral proteins can differ in their isotype. For some antiviral responses (e.g., Gag), several subclasses may be present. In others, such as anti-envelope-specific antibodies, one major type is present (135). Cytokines present at the time of exposure of B cells to a specific viral protein can influence the type of antibodies produced (135). In general, IgG antibody levels in serum are lower in AIDS patients than in asymptomatic infected individuals (102). IgG1 is the dominant subclass in all clinical stages and can be found at similar titers (1573). Levels of other antibody classes (e.g., IgM, IgA, IgG2, IgG4, and IgD) can vary depending on the clinical stage (for a review, see reference 135). IgM and IgA levels can be higher in AIDS patients. However, some studies suggest that the antibody isotype pattern does not correlate with clinical state (1717).

One of the first techniques described for the detection of anti-HIV antibodies was an indirect immunofluorescence assay in which acetone-methanol-fixed virus-infected T cells are incubated with an individual's serum and fluoresceinated anti-human antibodies are subsequently added to detect specific antibody binding (146, 1230, 1510). Other early approaches included an enzyme-linked immunoabsorbent assay (ELISA) and immunoblot methods (for review, see (135, 142, 2409).

The standard procedure for rapid detection of anti-HIV antibodies is an ELISA technique. The results are confirmed by supplemental testing, either by immunoblotting (359) or by an indirect immunofluorescence assay. The ELISAs have now gone through several generations and in most cases can detect antiviral antibodies within a few days to a few weeks after acute infection. Some concern for sensitivity when a clade O virus is involved in the infection has been raised, since only about 80% of individuals with this virus will be detected by present ELISA procedures (2381). Improvements are expected to make the ELISAs sensitive to all clades.

Other approaches to detect infection in individuals without requiring blood samples include the examination of urine and saliva for anti-HIV antibodies. Recent

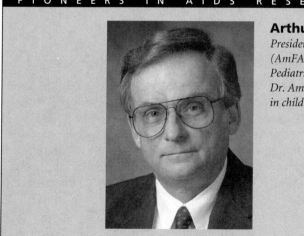

results have been encouraging, and both approaches are approved for use by the U.S. Food and Drug Administration. The saliva testing gives up to 99% sensitivity in a large number of cases evaluated (832), and the urine testing has a similar accuracy (193, 1585a). Other methods for screening large numbers of individuals without requiring venipuncture have included a needlestick assay, in which blood is added to small cotton blots that are analyzed for antibodies by an enzyme reaction (161). This procedure is also sensitive and is currently being used for home testing (1761). Home testing, while controversial, is considered important for informing reluctant individuals of their infection status (2606). However, measurement of antibodies in plasma or serum by the most recent ELISAs is still the most sensitive routine method for the detection of HIV infection.

II. Neutralizing Antibodies

A. General Observations

A conventional response of the host against viral infection is the production of antibodies that attach to the virus and inactivate (neutralize) it. The HIV envelope is the major target for such humoral antibody responses. As discussed previously (see Chapter 7), the viral proteins believed to be primarily involved in antibody neutralization have been localized to the envelope gp120 and the external portion of gp41 (295, 400, 564, 990, 1584, 1699, 2161; for review, see references 323a, 2255, and 2996) (Table 10.1).

The presence of anti-HIV neutralizing antibodies in infected individuals has been reported by several investigators. Whereas some sera show high levels of antiviral activity against common laboratory strains, sera from infected individuals have not consistently demonstrated strong neutralizing activity against their homologous strain (421, 1102, 2846). In our laboratory, when the antibodies are present, titers of only 1:10 to 1:100 are usually found (1102). The observations could reflect "escape" from humoral immune response (31, 80, 1732, 2214, 2247) (see

Table 10.1   Regions of HIV sensitive to antibody neutralization[a]

1. Viral envelope gp120
   V3 loop (PND)
   CD4 binding domain
   V1 region
   V2 region
2. Viral envelope gp41
3. Viral p17 (?)
4. Carbohydrate moieties
5. Cellular adhesion molecules?

[a] All regions can have linear or conformational epitopes, but the CD4 binding domain is generally conformational and the epitopes in gp41 (and p17) are usually linear.

Chapter 7), a greater affinity of the virus for its cellular receptor than for antiviral antibodies, or the method used to assay for neutralization (2997). Moreover, with progression to disease, neutralizing antibodies can be replaced by enhancing antibodies (1102) (Section III).

Why certain laboratory strains, passed for months or years in vitro, are very sensitive to neutralization by a variety of heterologous sera is not clear. With some HIV-1 strains (e.g., SF2 and MN), a common envelope epitope (i.e., in the V3 loop) can be involved, but with others (e.g., LAI) an antigenic similarity among many isolates is not evident. Moreover, we have some long-term-passaged laboratory strains that are resistant to neutralization and others that are more sensitive to antibody-mediated enhancement (Section III) (1104, 1321). Different antibody binding affinities seem to be involved (1321, 2759). Thus, as noted previously (see Chapter 7), other factors besides prolonged growth in culture can determine the antibody sensitivities of various HIV strains.

Usually, sera from HIV-1-infected individuals can neutralize HIV-1 but not HIV-2 strains. In contrast, sera from HIV-2-infected individuals have been reported to cross-react with and neutralize some HIV-1 strains (2847); they also cross-neutralize SIV strains (2244). This latter finding emphasizes further the reported similarities in envelope structure of these two human lentiviruses. In addition, immunization of animal species (e.g., rodents, guinea pigs, rabbits, goats, monkeys, and baboons) with HIV envelope proteins has induced antibodies that neutralize the immunizing strain and are type specific. With several booster inoculations, the antibodies produced are no longer type specific but can react with other diverse HIV-1 strains, suggesting a broadening of the humoral immune response (988, 1191). What governs this cross-reactivity is not clear but could reflect antibodies to conformational epitopes on the viral envelope, especially those related to the CD4 binding site (Section II.B) (2584). Finally, the mechanism for neutralization has not yet been well defined. Some studies suggest that it does not involve agglutination of virus or dissociation of the envelope protein (2571), as has been described for this immunologic reaction with other virions (640). Possibly there is a disturbance in the flexibility of the envelope that is required for virus entry into the cell (1718). Several studies have indicated that neutralization of HIV can involve virus attachment, fusion, or a step following virus:cell fusion (1727a).

B.   Neutralization Epitopes on HIV

By comparing a variety of strains, conserved (C) and divergent or variable (V) regions of the envelope gp120 of HIV-1 have been identified (1479, 2577, 2883, 2887). Five C and five V domains have been recognized. Moreover, by using monoclonal antibodies, the structure of gp120 can be defined in terms of naturally exposed or covered epitopes (1836). The latter appear to be primarily conserved determinants (1836) (Color Plate 1, following p. 188). Recognition of these regions has helped to identify domains in the envelope gp120 that are sensitive to neutralizing antibodies. In general, these epitopes are associated with gp120 oligomers and not monomeric forms of the viral envelope (2365).

Most studies of neutralization sites on HIV indicate that at least five regions of the viral envelope could be involved in HIV neutralization: four portions of gp120

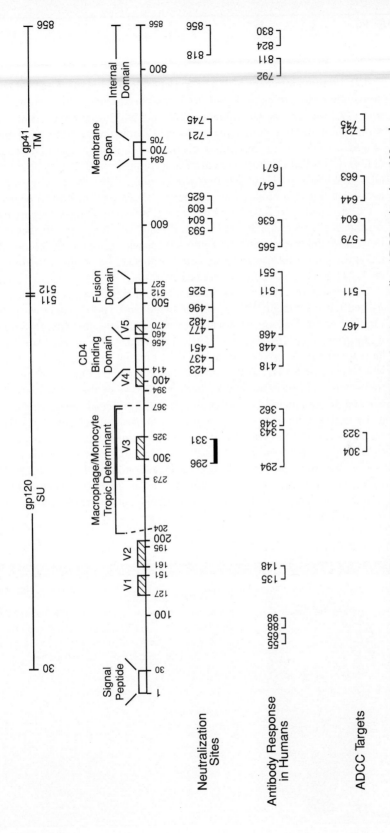

Figure 10.1 The envelope region of HIV-1 with some neutralization domains as well as ADCC regions in gp120 and gp41 demonstrated. For the most up-to-date summary of these parameters of the immune response, consult the Internet at http://hiv-web.lanl.gov/immuno/. Figure courtesy of J. Bradac.

233

and an immunodominant region of gp41 (Table 10.1) (400). A second conserved domain in gp41 (amino acids 647 to 671) has been suggested but needs confirmation (295; for reviews, see references 272 and 1938) (Figures 3.2, 3.4, and 10.1). Moreover, a specific region in the conserved C4 domain of gp120 (1902) may be involved. The C4 region contains a major CD4 binding domain (see Chapter 3) (1434) (Color Plate 1). Further neutralizing epitopes on gp120 may be best revealed after HIV binds to CD4 (1234, 1641, 2571, 2668). Other observations suggest that additional linear or conformational envelope epitopes sensitive to neutralization will be detected. Antibodies to the p17 core protein have also been reported to show neutralizing activity (2358, 2458). This finding, which requires further confirmation (2236), may represent cross-neutralization with anti-gp41 antibodies (318). Finally, the pattern of glycosylation could influence the results of antibody assays (167, 741, 855) (see Chapter 7) (see below).

A very important immunodominant neutralizing domain of gp120, the principal neutralizing domain (PND), is found in the central portion or crown of the third variable region (V3 loop, amino acids ~308 to 322), located approximately in the midportion of gp120 (295, 296, 1191, 1192, 1433, 1699) (Color Plate 1). The V3 loop appears to be involved in a post-CD4 binding step (i.e., with a coreceptor), which is needed for HIV entry into cells (see Chapter 3). One mechanism for neutralization could be inhibition of envelope cleavage by the antibodies (2859) (see Chapter 3). Although V3 is a variable region, the principal neutralizing domains of many strains differ only slightly in amino acid structure (Figure 7.11). Thus, immunization with this region of gp120 will, with time, induce antibodies that neutralize a large number of HIV-1 strains that share this envelope domain (188, 912, 1191). This cross-reactivity can reflect a linear epitope as well as a conformational structure common to many viral strains. The latter can be recognized by a wide variety of conformation-dependent neutralizing antibodies (910; for a review, see reference 2583).

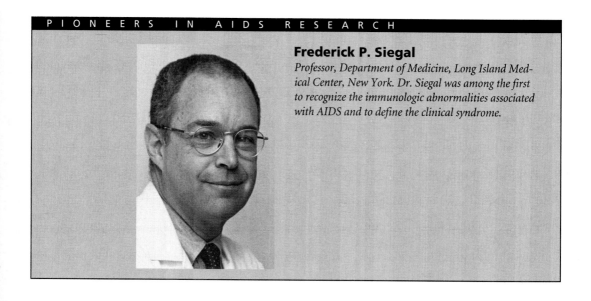

PIONEERS IN AIDS RESEARCH

Frederick P. Siegal

Professor, Department of Medicine, Long Island Medical Center, New York. Dr. Siegal was among the first to recognize the immunologic abnormalities associated with AIDS and to define the clinical syndrome.

The V3 loop-directed neutralization does not appear to involve the CD4 binding domain (1560, 2518), but changes in this domain and other envelope regions might alter the antibody interaction with the V3 loop and vice versa (2096). In some cases, neutralization is enhanced (2096); in others, it is reduced (see below). In this regard, a synergy in neutralization has been demonstrated by using antibodies against the CD4 binding region and the V3 domain (2676).

The V3 loop can have both neutralizing and nonneutralizing epitopes, since sera with high-titer antibody to V3 peptides do not always neutralize the homologous HIV-1 strain (2825). Moreover, as noted in Chapter 7, work with "escape" mutants has indicated that regions within the V3 loop (2908) or outside it (1732, 2214, 2828, 2883) can reduce antibody neutralization (for a review, see reference 2583). Some of these mutants have the same V3 loop sequence but contain changes distal to this envelope region (1309, 2883). The other sites can apparently alter the conformation of the V3 loop, permitting "escape" of the virus from neutralization. Thus, as noted above, the V3 region can present both linear and conformational determinants for antibody recognition.

A second major neutralizing region on gp120 is the CD4 binding domain, a large, complex conformational region of the envelope (1730) (see Chapter 3). Polyclonal antibodies that cross-neutralize a large number of strains (both primary and laboratory adapted), including those with different V3 regions, are directed against this domain (1235, 1434, 2095, 2584, 2615). The determinant is generally conformation dependent, and antibodies are frequently found in sera of infected individuals (1080, 1830, 2584).

Neutralizing monoclonal antibodies that recognize discontinuous epitopes on gp120 that are involved with CD4 receptor interaction have been derived from HIV-infected individuals (2666). The antibodies are thought to block the ability of the HIV strains to attach to the major cellular receptor. Because several regions of the HIV envelope are involved, neutralization by monoclonal antibodies alone may not show a broad antiviral activity (910). Perhaps for this reason, neutralizing monoclonal antibodies to the V3 loop are often more active than those to the CD4 binding site (2667, 2922). Other studies have indicated that point mutations in gp41 as well as the V3 loop can affect this neutralization (and that of other anti-gp120 antibodies), most probably as a result of conformational changes in gp120 (112, 1309, 1730).

The third and fourth major neutralizing sites on gp120 can be found in the V1 and V2 regions (811, 990, 1734, 2491) (Color Plate 1). As with the V3 loop, both linear and conformational determinants appear to be involved (1734, 2491). These regions are recognized by antibodies directed at both glycosylated and nonglycosylated epitopes (1078). Whether the V4 and V5 regions contain domains that induce neutralizing antibodies, as was suggested by work with deletion mutants (990), remains to be determined.

The neutralizing antibodies directed against gp41 have received less attention. Nevertheless, immunization of laboratory animals with the amino-terminal portion of the envelope (a common fusion domain) has elicited antibodies to the homologous and heterologous strains (400, 564). Monoclonal antibodies to gp41 have also shown anti-HIV activity; they interact with the ectodomain (amino-terminal region) of this viral protein (1885) and can have broad reactivity (2157). The immunodominant portion of gp41 has been recognized particularly after HIV inter-action with CD4; removal or displacement of gp120 is assumed to have occurred (2364) (see Chapter 3). Anti-idiotype neutralizing antibodies have been made as well by using portions of gp41 (2980).

A region suggestive of a V3 loop in HIV-2 strains has also been identified (220, 238, 604) but needs further evaluation. Moreover, studies with the HIV-2 envelope protein have defined epitopes in the C1, V1/V2, and V3 envelope regions that react with neutralizing antibodies. As with HIV-1, some of them are conformation de-pendent, whereas others react to linear regions of the envelope (1736).

Recent reports indicate broad neutralizing activity against carbohydrate re-gions of the viral envelope (167, 741, 1002). Whether these antibodies reflect con-formational epitopes or true anti-carbohydrate reactions is not clear. Glycosylated forms of the HIV-1 envelope can be better recognized by immune sera than by nonglycosylated proteins (577, 988, 2583, 2584). Likewise, carbohydrate side chains (e.g., N-linked glycans) may interfere with the interaction of virus with neutralizing antibodies (43, 113). Since intracellular modification of HIV envelope glycosylation has been observed (see Chapter 8), whether "escape" variants using this mechanism would be easily formed needs to be explored. Finally, antibodies to the adhesion molecule LFA-1, detected on the surface of virions, may enhance the neutralization of HIV-1 by antiviral antibodies (906). Antibodies to other cell surface molecules (e.g., ICAM) found on the virion (see Chapter 3, Section VI) might also participate in virus neutralization (2241).

C.   Clinical Relevance

The clinical relevance of these neutralizing antibodies remains unclear. In many in-fected subjects, neutralizing antibodies against earlier virus isolates and not against the isolate present at the time of plasma collection have been found (1102, 1825, 2704, 2789). The results suggest selective pressure or delayed recognition of HIV-1 by the immune system (1637, 2917). A similar observation has been made with neu-tralizing antibodies to equine infectious anemia virus (EIAV) (1823, 2341). An ef-fective antiviral antibody response would have value when elicited by a vaccine, but the potential effect of neutralizing antibodies in controlling viral spread after infec-tion is not clear. Genetic sequence differences in one envelope region have been used to classify HIV-1 into clades (see Chapter 7, Section VI). The relevance of this subgrouping to potential cross-neutralization and future vaccine development is an important question. Generally, the HIV-1 genotype does not necessarily correspond to the neutralization phenotype. The extent of virus neutralization depends on the isolates and the antibodies present in the individual's serum (see Chapter 7).

Initially, levels of neutralizing activity appeared to correlate with the clinical state (2245, 2439, 2789, 2856), but patients, including those with AIDS, were found to have substantial titers of neutralizing antibodies, as measured with laboratory strains of HIV-1 (2245). In most cases, however, their antiviral response to the auto-logous strain, which would be clinically relevant, was not evaluated. Some studies with autologous strains have indicated a loss of neutralizing antibodies with pro-gression to disease (1102, 2704).

As noted above, some observations (1102) suggest that AIDS patients often elicit antibodies that enhance rather than neutralize infection by the virus found in the patient (Section III). Moreover, as discussed in this section and Chapter 7, the virus undergoes changes during immunologic responses to "escape" neutralization (80, 1102, 1732, 1907, 2245). Thus, the induction of neutralizing antibodies would appear to be beneficial early in the course of HIV infection and to have less influence in later stages.

Passive therapy with human immunoglobulins with neutralizing activity has prevented HIV infection of chimpanzees after a low-dose (10 chimpanzee infectious doses to infect 50% of the animals [CID_{50}]), but not after a high-dose (100 CID_{50}) challenge (2146, 2147). These IgGs have protected SCID-hu mice from infection by the strain used to elicit the immune response (114). Moreover, anti-V3 specific antibodies have protected chimpanzees from infection (75 CID) when given 1 day before virus inoculation or within a few minutes after exposure to the virus (701). However, this protection has not been seen after longer periods of delay before treatment (2145a) (see Chapter 14, Section I). In some SIV studies, passive immunization had no effect and may have enhanced the infection (see below) (846). In other studies, anti-SIV antibodies delayed progression of disease (989).

Some concern has been raised about whether antibodies made against one viral strain will suppress the ability of B cells to make antibodies to a different viral strain. This concept of "original sin" was first described by Francis (786) and has been recognized with a variety of viruses, including the toga-, paramyxo-, and enteroviruses, as well as influenza virus (1905). The humoral immune response to a variety of antigens may be limited in HIV-1 infection, as revealed by some evidence in animal models (1335, 1905). The mechanism appears to be a paralysis by B-cell clonal dominance resulting from the reaction of B cells to the initial infecting virion (1336). The hypothesis deserves further study, particularly in relation to vaccine development.

III.   Enhancing Antibodies

A.   Complement- and Fc-Mediated Responses

We have previously discussed the presence in HIV-infected individuals of antibodies that can enhance viral infection via either the complement or Fc receptors (see Chapter 3, Figure 3.8) (1104, 2256; for a review, see reference 2255). Enhancing antibodies are often evident after dilution of a serum past the level showing neutralization. This observation may reflect a greater population of antibody species with less binding affinity for the viral target (Section III.C) (1321). That possibility, if proved, would suggest that as antibody levels decrease in an infected individual over time, the enhancing antibody might be preferentially conserved. The potential role of these antibodies in enhancing subsequent infection needs consideration. The results with various sera also suggest that at any given dilution, the overall effect on the virus in cell culture would reflect the net effect of neutralizing and enhancing antibodies. With some sera, however, only a neutralizing antibody or an enhancing antibody for a specific virus strain has been noted (1103, 1104, 1321).

In complement-mediated antibody-dependent enhancement (ADE), the complement receptors CR1, CR2, and CR3 appear to be involved (2257, 2670). In Fc-mediated ADE, two receptors have been identified. FcRI was shown to be the antibody binding site in the U937 monocyte cell line (2632). In primary macrophages, the FcRIII receptor appears to be involved (1103, 2708). This receptor, identified by antibodies to CD16, is found on natural killer (NK) cells and a variety of other human cells that conceivably could also be infected by antibody:HIV complexes.

IgA-mediated enhancement of virus infection has also been demonstrated with sera from HIV-infected patients (1186). Some studies suggest that these patients produce more IgA than IgG antibodies with enhancing activity (1371). This response may be important at the mucosal level of infection.

As reviewed in Chapter 3, the role of CD4 in ADE is controversial. Some studies (2076, 2213, 2257, 2702, 2971) have suggested that enhancement via the complement receptor depends on CD4, since monoclonal antibodies to CD4 can block viral enhancement. Others (2632) drew the same conclusion with Fc-mediated enhancement. In contrast, in studies with peripheral blood macrophages, ADE via the Fc receptor took place in the presence of blocking antibodies to CD4 (Leu 3a) as well as after pretreatment of the virus with large quantities of soluble CD4 (1103). Likewise, studies of ADE in cultured human syncytiatrophoblast cells showed that complement-mediated enhancement of infection required CD4 but the Fc-dependent process did not (2695). Thus, different mechanisms on the same cells can be involved in these two ADE processes observed with HIV infection in vitro. In further support of a non-CD4 mechanism is the experiment with HIV:antibody complexes demonstrating that HIV can replicate in CMV-infected fibroblasts lacking CD4 but expressing the Fc receptor (1733).

If CD4 is involved in ADE, most investigators conclude that the enhancement occurs because the virus:antibody complexes are brought closer to the CD4 molecule after attachment to Fc or complement receptors. Alternatively, if CD4 is not involved, perhaps HIV is brought to the cell surface via Fc receptor binding. Then the virus interacts with a coreceptor or fuses directly with the cell membrane (see Chapter 3).

B.   Virus Epitope Determinants of Antibody-Dependent Enhancement

In contrast to the identification of several viral domains involved in neutralization (Section II), only limited regions on the virion thus far have been linked to ADE. Antisera made in animals to peptides have suggested the process can be mediated by several regions on the envelope gp120 and gp41 (1202, 2708). However, the relevance of these induced antibodies to naturally produced antibodies requires further evaluation. In the complement-mediated ADE process, two domains (amino acids ~579 to 613 and ~644 to 663) at the amino-terminal end of gp41 appear to be the reactive sites (2253, 2254) .

In the studies examining the viral envelope region responsible for Fc-mediated ADE, polyclonal antibodies against regions in gp120 and monoclonal antibodies directed against the V3 region of some HIV-1 strains have been helpful (2996). Polyclonal anti-gp120 and anti-V3 loop antibodies have shown both neutralizing and enhancing effects, depending on the HIV-1 strain and on the concentration of the antibodies used (553, 1203, 1321). Moreover, some monoclonal antibodies to gp120 were found to neutralize HIV, whereas other antibodies enhanced it (1321, 2631). These studies helped to narrow the possible regions on gp120 (particularly within the V3 loop) that mediate Fc-directed ADE (1321, 2631). Moreover, a human monoclonal antibody that also reacts with the amino-terminal region of gp41 has been found to enhance HIV-1 infection in the absence of complement (680).

C.

Relation of Envelope Sequences to the Anti-HIV Effect of Antibodies

A noteworthy observation was the presence in some human and animal sera of antibodies that neutralize one HIV-1 strain and enhance another (1104, 1321). Moreover, two human monoclonal antibodies and one murine monoclonal antibody that react with the V3 domain of HIV-1$_{MN}$ were found to neutralize the SF2 and MN strains of HIV-1 but to enhance the SF128A strain (1321) (Figure 10.2). They had no effect on the SF162 strain, which was resistant. These monoclonal antibodies were shown to bind to the gp120 cloned from all of these viral strains, but the affinity of the binding was reduced with the viral strains that were resistant or enhanced in infectivity (1321). Since, among the three affected strains (SF2, SF162, SF128A), only one amino acid differed in the epitope on the V3 loop recognized by the monoclonal antibodies, very few amino acid changes in the viral envelope seemed to affect sensitivity to enhancement or neutralization. This possibility was supported by molecular studies. The SF128A strain, which was enhanced, has an asparagine (N) at position 311 of the V3 loop; SF2, which was neutralized, has a tyrosine (Y), and SF162, the resistant strain, has a threonine (T) at this position (Figure 10.2). By site-directed mutagenesis, the tyrosine in SF2 was changed to a threonine, and the resulting virus was found to be resistant to neutralization by the monoclonal antibodies. A change in that position in SF2 from tyrosine to asparagine also resulted in an antibody-resistant strain. Thus, sensitivity to enhancement could not

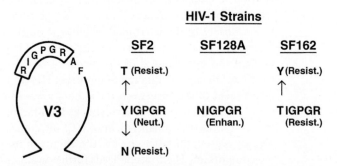

Figure 10.2 The V3 loop in virus:antibody neutralization versus enhancement. By using a monoclonal antibody to a small epitope in the HIV-1 V3 loop, differences in response of various virus strains can be appreciated. Some are neutralized (Neut.), others are enhanced (Enhan.), and still others are resistant (Resist.). As demonstrated, only one amino acid change appears to affect the serologic response, but the results are strain specific. If the amino acid is modified by site-directed mutagenesis (arrows), the mutant virus appears to become resistant. Data from reference 1321.

Figure 10.3   HIV-1$_{SF162}$ with the amino acid substitutions (present on HIV-1$_{SF2}$) that make this strain neutralizable by an anti-HIV-1$_{SF2}$ monoclonal antibody (see Figure 10.2).

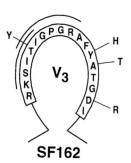

SF162

be induced. Finally, a change of the threonine in SF162 to tyrosine did not alter the resistance of this strain (Figure 10.2). Nevertheless, when three other amino acids in the carboxyl-terminal portion of the V3 loop of SF162 were changed to those of SF2, a neutralizable strain was obtained (Figure 10.3) (1319a). These latter changes were outside the epitope recognized by the monoclonal antibodies.

These and other observations have suggested that, in general, production of a strain sensitive to neutralization or enhancement will involve several regions on the virus envelope and not just one amino acid. In further support of this conclusion, findings with interviral recombinants of the SF2 and SF128A strains indicate that envelope regions in addition to the V3 loop determine the consequence of the virus:antibody interaction. Exchange of an envelope region encompassing the CD4 binding and fusion domains of SF128A with that of SF2 rendered the SF2 virus resistant to neutralization by a V3 monoclonal antibody. Furthermore, only the exchange of a larger region that included the V3, CD4 binding, and fusion domains of SF128A resulted in enhanced infection with the SF2 recombinant virus (1319a). Once again, the data reviewed above underline the importance of envelope conformation in this biologic property.

Additional studies with recombinant strains should help to clarify further the envelope epitopes responsible for the serologic properties observed. The findings with monoclonal antibodies, however, suggest that the extent of attachment to a virion surface could determine the biologic outcome. One hypothesis under consideration is that high-affinity binding of the antibody leads to virus neutralization, perhaps through removal or displacement of the gp120 (1834) (Figure 10.4). In contrast, low-affinity binding might bring HIV to the cell surface and subsequent detachment of the virus from the antibody would permit infection of the cell. In some ways, this hypothesis involving gp120 binding mirrors the one proposed for inactivation versus enhancement of HIV infection with sCD4 (1834) (see Chapter 3). However, in the latter process, the affinity of the gp120:CD4 attachment seems most important. The concept needs further evaluation.

D.   Clinical Relevance

The clinical importance of ADE is not known, but its association with HIV disease (see Chapter 7, Figure 7.12) (813, 1102) suggests a role in pathogenesis. Circulating infectious virus:antibody complexes have been described in HIV infection (1328,

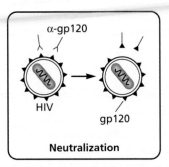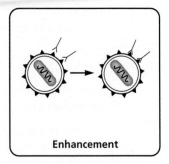

Figure 10.4   Mechanisms for neutralization versus enhancement. The concept is proposed that neutralization involves a strong binding of antibody to the viral envelope with the subsequent removal of gp120, resulting in virus inactivation. Enhancement would involve binding to the virus without removal of the envelope glycoprotein. Conformational changes would subsequently occur that enhance infection by the virus, presumably via virus:cell fusion.

1849). It is surprising that these virus:antibody complexes are infectious rather than being destroyed in the macrophage lysosomes. The reason could be the relative affinity of antibodies for the HIV envelope protein and how the complexes are dissociated within the cell.

The potential clinical relevance of ADE in vivo has been evaluated in animal model systems. In EIAV infection, ADE was recognized in vaccine studies. Horses immunized with a baculovirus-expressed recombinant envelope glycoprotein of one strain were protected from infection by that strain, but disease developed more rapidly when a heterologous strain was used as the challenge strain (1165, 2822) (see Chapter 15). Enhancement was also found in cats immunized with certain envelope glycoprotein subunits (2498). The presence or absence of enhancing antibodies also correlated with clinical disease in primates infected with SIV (1820) and in one study reduced the beneficial effects of an SIV gp160 vaccine (1797). High-titer enhancing antibodies also correlated with failure of passive immunization to protect from SIV infection (846). Complement-mediated ADE was also noted in acute primary infection of macaques and was detected before the appearance of neutralizing antibodies (1819). As the extent of ADE activity decreased, neutralizing antibodies appeared, reflecting the comment noted above that a balance between these two responses determines the overall immunologic effect. Further serologic studies with HIV-infected individuals and lentivirus-infected animals are needed to address the question of the clinical relevance of ADE.

Results showing no biologic significance of ADE (2454) or no correlation with disease progression (1817) have been presented. Nevertheless, an increase in symptoms of disease linked to ADE has been observed with dengue virus, coronaviruses, and other viruses (147, 520, 993, 1320, 1925, 2059, 2065, 2139). The process has been reported with retroviruses (1463), including, most convincingly, the caprine (CAEV) (1726) and equine (EIAV) lentiviruses (1165). Finally, antibodies that enhance infection of certain HIV-1 strains in vitro have been detected in some recipients of a vaccine consisting of a recombinant gp160 from a different HIV-1 strain (e.g., IIIB)

(1319a, 1815). Thus, the risk of this type of immune response should be considered in treatment approaches and vaccine development (see Chapters 14 and 15).

E. Conclusions

Certain important conclusions can be drawn from these early findings on antibody responses to HIV infection.

1. Neutralizable HIV strains can mutate to be resistant to or enhanced by the same antibody species.
2. Immunization of individuals with a particular viral strain might induce neutralizing antibodies to the immunizing virus but enhancing antibodies to a different viral strain (1203, 1321).
3. Defining envelope regions that will induce only neutralizing-antibody responses and not enhancing-antibody responses could be very difficult. A highly conserved envelope domain, without which HIV infection could not take place, must be identified.

Thus far, regions in gp41, as well as gp120, have been associated with both types of humoral immune reactions. It is particularly noteworthy that some studies suggest that only a small change at a critical region, perhaps in one amino acid, might determine the sensitivity of a virus to antibody neutralization or enhancement. Nevertheless, the overall conformation of the viral envelope appears to be the most important determinant.

IV. Antibody-Dependent Cellular Cytotoxicity and Antibody-Dependent Cytotoxicity

Antibodies (primarily IgG1 isotypes) to both the gp120 and gp41 envelope proteins induce ADCC (723, 1359, 1572, 1573, 1944, 1976, 2272). In this process, the antibody-antigen-coated cells are recognized by effector NK cells or by monocytes/macrophages (1200) bearing Fc receptors (see Chapter 11). They are killed by a cytolytic mechanism, either perforin mediated or via apoptosis (for reviews, see references 184 and 2925). Certain epitopes on HIV envelope proteins must induce this response (for review, see references 272 and 1938) (Figure 10.1), since not all anti-Env antibodies produce this activity. The ADCC immunoglobulins can be distinguished from neutralizing antibodies (259, 2791), but not in all cases (2791). This observation most probably reflects the presence or absence of a neutralization epitope on the viral envelope expressed on the cell surface. Cross-reactivity of antibodies mediating ADCC with HIV-1 and HIV-2 strains has been demonstrated (1944).

The ADCC process is active in destroying herpesvirus-infected cells early after virus transmission (2490). Whether ADCC is clinically relevant in HIV infection is not known; conflicting data on its association with an asymptomatic state have been presented (723, 1573, 2370). A recent report has shown a significant association of ADCC with a healthy state and loss of this response with progression of disease (154). Since anti-envelope antibodies are present at substantial titers throughout the course of the infection (723), the extent of effector cell function would appear to be the most important parameter influencing the ability of the ADCC process to control HIV infection (277, 2625, 2730). One detrimental effect of this process during HIV infection could be the release, by cell destruction, of large quantities of infectious particles, with subsequent spread in the host. At that time, neutralizing antibodies should play an important antiviral role.

In principle, ADCC would seem most valuable soon after infection to kill incoming or postentry virus-infected cells. Induction of the ADCC response by vaccines would then be an important objective, and this response might be helpful in preventing mother-child transmission. Thus, ADCC could be another reason to consider passive immunization with anti-HIV envelope antibodies for recently exposed individuals or infected mothers before delivery.

By another process, anti-HIV antibodies in chimpanzees directly kill infected cells via a complement-mediated mechanism (1906). Antibody and complement attach to virus-infected cells and can bring about cell death without effector cells. This antibody-dependent cytotoxicity has not been generally observed in humans, although studies with certain cell lines lacking CD55 and CD59 expression have demonstrated this activity (2399). The general absence of this process in humans has been cited as one possible reason that infected chimpanzees have not developed HIV-induced disease.

V. Complement-Fixing Antiviral Antibodies

Some studies have indicated that certain neutralizing and nonneutralizing antibodies can lyse HIV via complement fixation (2543, 2544). With the neutralizing antibodies, the antiviral titer can sometimes be increased 10-fold by the addition of high levels of complement to the assay (2542). This response could counter the ADE observed, since only low levels of complement initiate this response.

VI. Complement

Activation of complement during HIV infection can also lead to destruction of the virus by two antibody-independent mechanisms (Table 10.2). By the first process, the complement components can bind to the virion or infected cells and become activated by the alternative pathway (2533). During HIV infection, this process is increased because molecules that inhibit complement activation (e.g., decay accelerating factor and CD59) are made in lower concentrations in infected individuals than in seronegative ones (1459, 2844). By the second mechanism, activation of complement by the classical pathway can occur directly from an interaction with gp120 (2617). Recent evidence suggests that this viral lysis occurs in vivo from antibody binding to complement proteins on virions. This process could be a reason for the rapid virus clearance from plasma (2612). In addition, any mechanism by which gp120 expression on infected cells is increased will enhance complement-mediated lysis (for a review, see reference 135).

The levels of complement components in serum appear to be stable through-

Table 10.2 Potential role of complement in HIV infection

Direct
    Lysis of virions in association with antibodies (2543, 2544)
    Binding to virions and activation of the alternative complement pathway (2533)
    Binding to gp120 and activation of the classical complement pathway (2617)
Indirect
    Lysis of $CD4^+$ cells carrying envelope proteins (815, 1678, 2617)
    Participation in antibody-dependent enhancement of HIV replication (2257)
    Induction of direct lysis of cells expressing complement receptors through interaction
      with NK cells (2938)

out the course of HIV infection (for a review, see reference 815). Activation of complement is reflected by the presence of complement by-products (e.g, C4d, Ba, and C3d) that are elevated in HIV-infected individuals as well as the by-products from both the alternative and classical pathways regardless of the stages of infection. Complement components therefore do not appear to play a major role in the development of disease.

Complement can also affect the HIV virion by other mechanisms besides direct interaction (Table 10.2). First, if the viral envelope proteins (particularly gp41) are bound to the surface of uninfected $CD4^+$ cells, complement can fix to the cells and lyse them (815, 1678, 2617). Second, as noted above, complement can play a role in ADE. Third, complement activated by the alternative pathway can induce direct lysis of cells (infected and uninfected) expressing complement receptors through their interaction with NK cells (2938). This latter process appears to result from the decreased levels of complement inhibitors in the blood of infected people (1459, 2844).

VII.   Autoimmunity

Since HIV disturbs the balance of the immune system, it is not surprising that autoimmune disorders (e.g., Reiter's syndrome, systemic lupus erythematosus, Sjögren's syndrome, vasculitis, and polymyositis) accompany this viral infection (334, 2745; for reviews, see references 1848, 2383, and 2991). Vasculitis has been linked in HIV infection to immune complexes (334), but immune complex glomerulonephritis is not commonly found. An autoreactive cellular immune response could be involved in HIV-associated autoimmunity (566) but has not been found in AIDS (60). The report of anticellular cytotoxic T lymphocytes (CTL) in the central nervous system needs further study (1189), as does the anti-Env CTL activity described in uninfected individuals (1091).

In some early studies of AIDS patients, antibodies, often associated with clinical disorders, against platelets, T cells, and peripheral nerves were detected (see also Chapter 9) (for a review, see reference 1848). More recently, autoantibodies to a large number of normal cellular proteins have been found in HIV-infected individuals (Table 10.3) (16, 79, 236, 392, 868, 934, 1301, 1307, 1602, 1638, 1874, 2340,

Table 10.3 Autoantibodies detected in HIV infection[a]

Antibodies to:	Associated clinical condition
Lymphocytes	Loss of CD4$^+$, CD8$^+$, and B lymphocytes
Platelets	Thrombocytopenia
Neutrophils	Neutropenia
Erythrocytes	Anemia
Nerves (myelin)	Peripheral neuropathy
Nuclear protein (antinuclear antibody)	Autoimmune symptoms
Sperm, seminal plasma	Aspermia
Lupus anticoagulant (phospholipid; cardiolipid)	Neurologic disease (?), thrombosis (?)
Myelin basic protein	Dementia; demyelination
Collagen	Arthritis (?)
CD4	CD4$^+$ cell loss
HLA	Lymphocyte depletion
Hydrocortisone	Addison's-like disease
Thymic hormone	Immune disorder
Cellular components (Golgi complex; centriole; vimentin)	Immune disorder
Thyroglobulin	Thyroid disease

[a] See Section VII for references.

2672, 2836). Their role in disease has been considered but has been documented in only a few cases (see below). The reason for these autoimmune sequelae is not clear, but they could reflect the presence of cellular membrane proteins on HIV particles (89, 1028, 1115, 1747, 2411). The potential influence of these cellular products on vaccine development is discussed in Chapter 15. The mechanisms of autoantibody production involving processes besides T-cell dysregulation are discussed below (Table 10.4).

A.   B-Cell Proliferation

A lack of T-cell regulation during HIV infection can lead to a proliferation of B cells with resultant polyclonal activation and antibody production (see Chapter 9). These kinds of reactions have been reported in other viral infections (e.g., Epstein-Barr virus) in which hypergammaglobulinemia and autoimmune disorders are described (1057). Polyclonal B-cell activity has been observed in HIV-infected individuals (1175, 2017, 2487) and is associated with high levels of antibody production, particularly in children (59). These hyper-B-cell responses can result from the presence of viral proteins (see Chapter 9) or from increased production of cytokines (interleukin-6 [IL-6] and IL-7) by HIV-infected or reactive macrophages or B cells (261, 275, 2326; for reviews, see references 1697 and 2284). B-cell growth could also result from tumor necrosis factor alpha (TNF-α) production by HIV-infected CD4$^+$ cells (2411), particularly if this cytokine, like TNF-β, is expressed on the cell

Table 10.4 Potential mechanisms for induction of autoimmunity by retroviruses

1. T-cell dysregulation
2. B-cell activation
3. Molecular mimicry
4. Carrier-hapten
5. Anti-idiotype antibodies

surface (1261); Tat also induces TNF-α and IL-6 in T lymphocytes (315, 2194). Finally, some of the altered B-cell functions could be secondary to enhanced production of type 2 cytokines (2475) (see Chapter 11). Among the immunoglobulins released by activated B cells are autoantibodies.

B.   Molecular Mimicry

When an organism shares nucleotide sequence, amino acid homology, or conformational form with a normal cellular component, molecular mimicry can result (1978). In this regard, similarities between HIV proteins and normal cellular proteins could elicit antiviral antibodies or cellular immune responses that cross-react

Table 10.5 Regions of HIV that resemble normal cellular proteins[a]

Normal cellular protein	HIV region	Relation
HLA (MHC)	gp120	Sequence
	gp41	Serology
	nef, p17	Sequence
IL-2	gp41	Sequence
	LTR	Sequence
IL-2R	*nef*	Sequence
Thymosin	p17	Serology
Interferon	LTR	Sequence
Vasoactive intestinal polypeptide	gp120 (peptide T)	Sequence; serology
Neuroleukin (phosphohexose)	gp120	Sequence; serology
Immunoglobulin	gp120	Sequence
Neurotoxin	*nef, tat*, gp41	Sequence
Protein kinase	*nef*	Sequence
Epithelial cells	p17	Serology
Astrocytes	p17, gp41	Serology
Platelet glycoprotein	gp120	Serology
Platelets	p24	Serology
Brain	Env (V3 loop)	Serology
Fas	gp120	Sequence

[a] See Section VII.B for references and discussion.

Figure 10.5 HIV molecular mimicry and autoimmunity. If the viral envelope protein has a similarity to an MHC domain (e.g., class I or II), antibodies (Abs) to this portion of the viral envelope could induce an anti-MHC reaction at the cell surface even with uninfected cells.

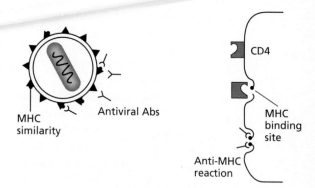

with normal cellular proteins (219, 1978) (Table 10.5). Evidence in favor of this possibility includes the presence of IL-1, IL-2 receptor, major histocompatibility complex (MHC) classes I and II, and interferon-like sequences in the HIV genes as well as epitopes on certain portions of the viral envelope (566, 851, 901, 1494, 1910, 2206) (Figure 10.5). Sequence homology between gp120 of HIV-1 and Fas, a protein involved in apoptosis (2624), may also have clinical relevance if anti-Fas antibodies are found in infected individuals.

Similarities of some regions of the viral Gag, Tat, and Nef proteins to normal proteins have also been described (849, 851, 852, 2045, 2347, 2402). Molecular mimicry may also explain the loss of platelets in HIV infection. Cross-reactive antibodies recognizing HIV gp120 envelope protein and platelet glycoprotein have been observed in individuals with thrombocytopenia purpura (200). Moreover, a murine anti-Gag (p24) monoclonal antibody has reacted with human platelets (1097).

Most notable are the studies by Golding and coworkers (227, 901), who have shown that some antibodies to the carboxyl-terminal domain in HIV gp41 cross-react with regions found on the human leukocyte antigen (HLA) class II molecule, particularly the beta chain. Antibodies to HLA class II proteins are found in HIV-infected individuals. They bind to "native" class II HLA antigens molecules and interfere with normal activation of $CD4^+$ T cells; they also have the potential to induce lysis of MHC class II-expressing cells by ADCC (Figure 10.5) (227). The presence of these anti-HLA antibodies in asymptomatic individuals correlates with a subsequent loss of $CD4^+$ cells (227).

Observations by others (1300) indicated that immunization of animals with murine peripheral blood mononuclear cells (PBMC) can lead to the production of antibodies that bind to the surface of normal human lymphocytes and neutralize HIV. Similarly, the discovery of anti-HIV antibodies (including those mediating ADCC and virus neutralization) in the sera of autoimmune MRL/*lpr* mice and in a subset of autoimmune human patients (657) presents additional support for molecular mimicry involving cellular proteins and the viral envelope (1583). Such antibodies (most likely to have shared HLA-like regions on the cell surface), as noted above, could contribute to the loss of uninfected $CD4^+$ cells observed during HIV infection (566, 2991). Recently, an AIDS-like disease, consisting of lymphoproliferation, a decrease in $CD4^+$ lymphocytes, impaired immune responses, and tumor development (Kaposi's sarcoma and B-cell lymphomas), was induced in crosses of mice differing in HLA type after immunization with paternal lymphocytes. The resemblance of this syndrome to AIDS placed further focus on autoimmune reactions to MHC antigens and CD4$^+$ cells as possible mechanisms for development of human AIDS (2654).

Finally, antibodies to the amino-terminal region of gp41 have been found to react with normal rodent brain astrocytes, perhaps by the same mechanism (2929). Similarly, antibodies to the immunodominant region of HIV-1 gp41 have been demonstrated to bind to a 100-kDa protein on the surface of human astrocytes (2546a). In addition, a monoclonal antibody to an epitope in the V3 region cross-reacts with a human brain protein (2716). These observations do suggest that molecular mimicry could represent a possible source of some pathogenic autoimmune responses.

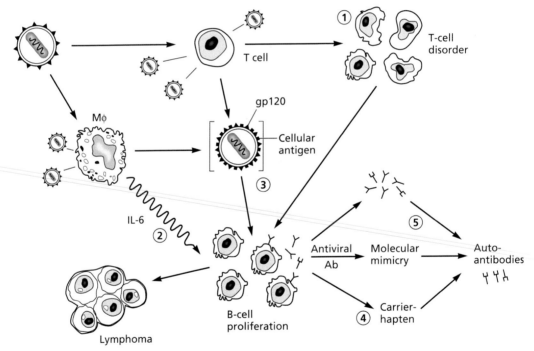

Figure 10.6 Possible mechanisms for autoimmune responses in HIV infection. HIV infection of T cells could lead to T-cell disorders (step 1) with subsequent loss of T-cell control of B-cell proliferation. Similarly, infection of macrophages by HIV could lead to enhanced production of IL-6 with resultant B-cell proliferation (step 2). B-cell proliferation could eventually lead to lymphomas through chromosome changes and establishment of a transformed state. The presence of viral antigens on the surface of T cells or B cells (step 3) might induce immune responses against nearby normal cellular antigens (step 3) in a carrier-hapten fashion (1554) (step 4), leading to autoantibodies or autoimmune cellular reactions. Antiviral responses by B cells could also lead to autoantibodies through molecular mimicry (step 5). By this phenomenon, viral proteins may resemble normal cellular proteins sufficiently to cause an autoimmune response against these cellular components.

C. Carrier-Hapten Mechanism

As shown in other viral systems, HIV could, after infecting the cell, uncover cellular proteins that are not normally recognized as "foreign" by the immune system (1554). By linkage with an HIV protein (e.g., envelope) acting as a hapten, these cellular proteins could become immunogenic and elicit an immune response in the host. This phenomenon reflects a carrier-hapten mechanism (1554). The subsequent production of autoantibodies leads to the sequelae recognized. This possibility has been examined with antiplatelet and anti-T-cell antibodies. Although HIV infection is associated with production of antibodies that react with lymphocytes (see above) (654, 1325, 1874), these antibodies do not react with a viral protein (1505a). Moreover, while infection of megakaryocytes has been reported (3001), an association of the anti-platelet antibodies to a viral protein or virus:cell protein complex has not been shown (1505a). Instead, other immune processes may be involved in thrombocytopenia (1246). Finally, via a carrier-hapten mechanism, some autoantibodies might be induced by HLA molecules incorporated onto the surface of virions during budding (89, 1115, 1747, 2411). Such proteins can be the source of some nonspecific false-positive results encountered during ELISA screening for anti-HIV antibodies (2372). In summary, however, the carrier-hapten mechanism does not appear to be involved in HIV-associated autoimmunity.

D. Anti-Idiotype Antibodies

One concept that has received some popular support as a mechanism for autoimmunity involves the network of antibodies produced after introduction of an antigen into the host. Besides making antibodies to the incoming antigen, antibodies to the anti-antigen antibodies may be induced. These anti-idiotype antibodies should be mirror images of the epitope against which the initial antibody was produced (663). Thus, antibodies to the HIV envelope gp120 might induce autoantibodies against the CD4 epitope to which the gp120 attaches. While the possibility for these antibodies to form and be detrimental to the host has been proposed, evidence for such a phenomenon has not been shown. The anti-CD4 antibodies produced (2672) are not against the epitopes involved in the binding site to HIV-1 gp120. Nevertheless, anti-idiotype antibodies mirroring a region on the envelope gp120 have been implicated in autoimmune thrombocytopenia (1246). This observation places new attention on this immunologic phenomenon in HIV pathogenesis but is still in need of further confirmation.

E. Conclusions: Potential Importance of Autoimmune Responses

While the role of autoimmunity in HIV-induced disease is still somewhat theoretical, the presence of this type of immune response in HIV infection should be considered a potential cofactor in the pathogenesis observed. The possible mechanisms involved are reviewed in Figure 10.6. Autoimmune responses have been linked to the loss of neutrophils and platelets and to peripheral neuropathy (1301, 1302). One explanation for the reduction in CD4$^+$ cells in HIV infection has also been the induction of anti-T-cell antibodies or antibodies to CD4 (654, 1874, 2672, 2836). The use of plasmapheresis in HIV-infected patients has supported the role of autoantibodies in the loss of neutrophils and platelets and in peripheral neuropathy but not in the loss of T cells (1302). In treated individuals, neutrophils and platelets return and the neuropathy is ameliorated; no change in $CD4^+$ cell count is observed (1300a). The potential contribution of autoreactive cells in HIV infection merits further study.

On another note, a potential danger in vaccination with HIV proteins could be the eliciting via molecular mimicry of immune responses that deplete $CD4^+$ cells, compromise the immune system further, or induce autoimmune pathology in other tissues. Measuring this response, therefore, should be part of the evaluation of any approach at preventing HIV infection (Chapter 15).

Chapter 10   SALIENT FEATURES

1. Antibodies to HIV can be detected as early as a few days after primary infection but generally within 1 to 3 months. In rare cases, several months are needed. Antibodies can be measured by ELISA, immunofluorescence, and immunoblot procedures.

2. The IgG1 subclass is dominant in all clinical stages. Other antibody classes can vary depending on the clinical stage.

3. Antibodies can be detected in urine and saliva. A home kit is now available for detecting anti-HIV antibodies in plasma.

4. Inducing neutralizing antibodies to the autologous virus strain provides the most clinically relevant response. Generally, these antibodies are at low levels and appear at a time when the initial autologous virus has mutated.

5. Antibodies that bind to the virus and enhance virus replication have been demonstrated, particularly in individuals who progress to disease. The difference between neutralization, enhancement, and resistance to both processes appears to be related to the affinity of binding of the antibody to the virion.

6. Neutralizing antibodies could have relevance for vaccines to prevent entry of infectious virions. After infection, antibodies might be helpful in killing cells by ADCC. Generally, levels of antibodies in the host have not correlated with a particular clinical state.

7. HIV can mutate to become resistant to neutralization and enhancement and can undergo changes to become sensitive to enhancement.

8. ADCC can have clinical relevance by destroying virus-infected cells, but the process appears to depend mostly on the function of host effector cells (e.g., macrophages and NK cells).

9. Complement can play a role in the antiviral response by enhancing antibody-mediated lysis of virions or by destroying virus and virus-infected cells through binding and activation by the classical or alternative pathways. Complement can also interact with complement receptors on NK cells to cause direct lysis of both infected and uninfected cells.

10. HIV is associated with a variety of autoimmune disorders, particularly those involving blood vessels, muscles, and joints.

11. Autoimmunity can occur as a result of B-cell proliferation, molecular mimicry, or carrier-hapten mechanisms. Autoantibodies can be made to several normal cellular proteins and can produce clinical symptoms such as reduction in platelets and neutrophils and a peripheral neuropathy. Anti-idiotype antibody production might also play a role in autoimmune disease syndromes.

12. Plasmapheresis of HIV-infected patients has produced reduction of symptoms in people who have decreased levels of neutrophils and platelets or have neuropathy associated with autoantibody production.

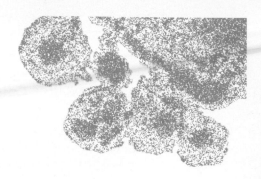

Cell-Mediated Immune Responses in HIV Infection

11

Natural Killer Cells

Cytotoxic T Lymphocytes

CD8⁺ Cell Noncytotoxic Anti-HIV Activity

Cell-Mediated Antiviral Immune Responses in Uninfected, HIV-Exposed High-Risk Individuals

Antiviral Responses at Mucosal Surfaces

Rᴇᴠɪᴇᴡᴇᴅ ɪɴ ᴛʜɪꜱ ᴄʜᴀᴘᴛᴇʀ ᴀʀᴇ ᴄᴇʟʟᴜʟᴀʀ ɪᴍᴍᴜɴᴇ ᴀᴄᴛɪᴠɪᴛɪᴇꜱ ᴛʜᴀᴛ appear to be directed against HIV through recognition of viral proteins associated with the virus or virus-infected cells. Since HIV infection disturbs the immune system, some of the findings cited in Chapter 9 also have direct relevance to this discussion. In most viral infections, the cell-mediated immune response plays a vital role in arresting or eliminating the infectious agent. The activities include cytotoxic responses of NK cells as well as CD8⁺ and CD4⁺ cells. These observations have been made in human diseases caused by agents such as herpesvirus, paramyxovirus, and influenza virus (332, 644). An effective response of the cellular immune system depends on efficient functioning of antigen-presenting cells (APC). The roles of macrophages and dendritic cells as APC are considered in Chapter 9.

Other mechanisms for virus control, particularly locally (e.g., oral, anal, and genital cavities), might involve nonspecific killing by polymorphonuclear leukocytes (PMN) using the myeloperoxidase system (1312). The potential contribution of antibody-dependent cellular toxicity (ADCC) activity by PMN has also been reported (2625).

I.   Natural Killer Cells

A major component of the overall cellular immune response to viruses is the natural killer (NK) cell, which recognizes and kills the virus-infected cells in a non-major histocompatibility complex (MHC)-dependent manner. The extent of decreased MHC class I expression on virus-infected cells determines the susceptibility of these cells to NK cell killing (for a review, see reference 303). Recently, a decoy mechanism was described by which cytomegalovirus (CMV) (and probably other herpesviruses), which can down-modulate MHC class I expression on the cell surface (see Chapter 13), can code for a molecule that resembles an MHC (733, 2220). By having this deceptive viral protein expressed on the cell surface, the virus-infected cell (also not expressing the true MHC molecule) could escape both cytotoxic T-lymphocyte (CTL) and NK cell killing. To what extent this process relates to other viruses and has clinical relevance merits attention.

In HIV infection, the NK cell has been found to have decreased function, particularly when infected individuals progress to disease (333, 776). This effect may result from HIV infection of NK cells (412) (see Chaper 9, Table 9.1). The observations appear to reflect a reduction in NK cell cytotoxic factor production (247) and a defective distribution of tubulin (2516). These findings correlate with a decrease in the number of $CD16^+$ $CD56^+$ NK cells concomitant with an increase in the number of NK cells in which the expression of these markers is substantially decreased (1121). These latter cells show less cycotoxic activity. Recent studies suggest that NK cells may be lost during ADCC, either directly or via apoptosis (1201).

Decreased NK cell activity can also affect $CD8^+$ cell responses, since NK cells produce gamma interferon (IFN-γ), which increases $CD8^+$ cell activity. The reduced NK cell function in HIV infection noted in vitro has been countered by the addition of interleukin-12 (IL-12) to the assay mixture (412). Production of this cytokine may be reduced because of HIV infection of dendritic cells and macrophages (see Chapter 9). Alternatively, the decreased production of IL-12 may result from a direct effect of IFN-α and IFN-β, whose levels are found to be increased in HIV infection (2795). These cytokines, while enhancing the NK response, can down-regulate IL-12 expression (2858; for a review, see reference 214) (Figure 11.1). This effect could enhance antibody production and decrease cell-mediated immune responses. Since $CD8^+$ cell antiviral activity appears to be important in controlling HIV replication (Sections II.C and III), the potential benefits of IL-12 for therapy are under consideration (see Chapter 14).

NK cells probably eliminate HIV-infected cells through ADCC as well. By this process, HIV-infected cells are killed by NK cells through the recognition of antibodies bound to the viral envelope proteins on the infected cell surface. Most ADCC studies, measuring levels of antibodies to the HIV envelope proteins, have not shown a correlation with the clinical state; anti-gp120 antibody levels do not differ substantially in most symptomatic or healthy HIV-infected individuals (see Chapter 10). If, however, the number of active effector cells in the infected individual is considered, a reduction in ADCC can be demonstrated with disease progression (277, 2625, 2730). Finally, as noted previously, NK cells carrying complement receptors may kill infected as well as uninfected cells through an interaction with complement on the cell surface (2938).

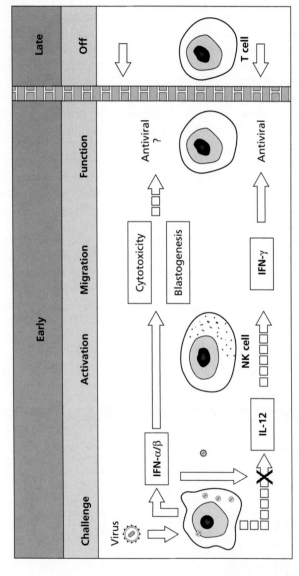

Figure 11.1 Regulation of NK cell activation and function during viral infections. Soon after many acute viral infections, IFN-α/β is induced by infected cells to activate NK cell-mediated cytotoxicity and blastogenesis (open arrows pointing to the right in the top pathway). Some, but not all, viral infections also spontaneously elicit detectable IL-12 production (broken arrows pointing to the right in the bottom pathway). If IL-12 is present, NK cell production of IFN-γ is induced. The IFN-γ response contributes to antiviral defense primarily by activating cell-mediated immune responses. IFN-α/β acts to block or inhibit IL-12 expression and can cause a lack of detectable IL-12 during certain viral infections. This process, by reducing IFN-γ production, could affect the extent of cell-mediated response induced by IFN-γ. Once T-cell responses are activated, they then can act to turn off the NK cell response. (From reference 214 with permission.)

II.   Cytotoxic T Lymphocytes

A.   General Observations on T Lymphocytes

CD8$^+$ and CD4$^+$ T lymphocytes showing cytotoxic (CTL) activity usually respond to the presentation of epitopes in association with MHC class I or class II molecules, respectively. Recognition with class I molecules appears to be more precise, not only because of limitations to the length of the peptides (8 to 10 residues), but also because the ends of the peptide (amino-terminal and carboxyl-terminal) must fit into defined pockets at opposite sides of the grooves in the MHC class I locus (for reviews, see references 380 and 2180) (Color Plate 12, following p. 188). The peptides in the MHC class II grooves can be longer (12 to 24 residues) and thus more heterogeneous. Therefore, the diversity of antigenic determinants presented to CD4$^+$ cells by MHC class II molecules can be greater than that presented to CD8$^+$ cells by class I molecules (380).

An antigen is recognized by means of the T-cell receptor (TCR), which is a heterodimeric cell surface molecule that interacts with the foreign antigen presented as short peptides with MHC class I or class II molecules on the surface of cells (Color Plate 12). The TCR is composed of either α, β, γ, or δ chains, although the vast majority of circulating T lymphocytes express $\alpha\beta$. Human leukocyte antigen (HLA) background and environmental factors can influence the diversity of the mature T-cell repertoire (for a review, see reference 2864). Alterations in the T-cell repertoire (as reflected by different TCR subunits) could come about by superantigen effects of HIV (see Chapter 6, Section V, and Color Plate 9, following p. 188), expression of other viral antigens that induce selective cell expansion or cell death, molecular mimicry by regions of gp120 that resemble HLA (2763), or HLA molecules incorporated into the viral envelope (89). The overall result is an imbalance in the diversity of the CD8$^+$ cell or CD4$^+$ cell responses, which could have clinical relevance (2864). As will be noted in Section IIIC, costimulation of T lymphocytes

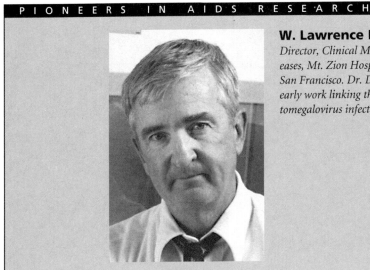

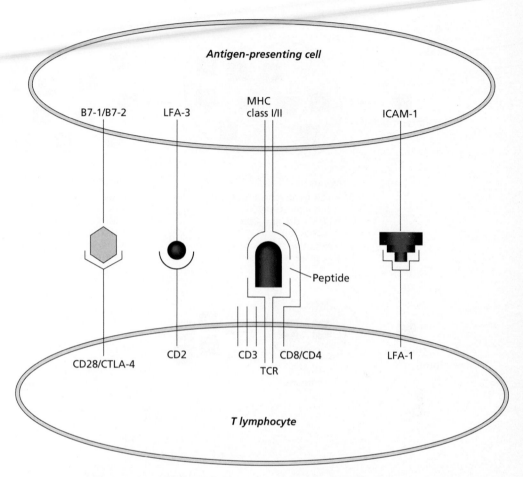

Figure 11.2   T-lymphocyte surface markers and their corresponding ligands on the APC. Cell-to-cell contact between a CD8$^+$ (MHC class I-restricted) or a CD4$^+$ (MHC class II-restricted) T lymphocyte and an APC involves the binding of several surface molecules to their specific ligands on the APC surface. (Figure courtesy of S. Stranford.)

through the CD28:B7 interaction enhances their response. Other T-lymphocyte cell surface markers can play a role in enabling the efficient communication between a T lymphocyte and an APC (Figure 11.2). Some of these cell surface molecules are found on virus particles (e.g., LFA and ICAM) and may serve as an alternative method for virus attachment to cells (see Chapter 3).

Some investigators maintain that when the T-cell repertoire is limited, immunologic response can be compromised (Figure 11.3), particularly when new antigens are encountered (see Chapter 9) (698, 2268). The diversity of this T-cell repertoire response during primary infection may predict the clinical outcome (see Chapter 13) (2033). In particular, in studies of HIV-infected people, CD4$^+$ and CD8$^+$ cell expansions can be clonal or oligoclonal. Because these expansions are not necessarily concomitant, spaces or "gaps" in the T-cell repertoire can exist and become exaggerated with disease progression (2268). The alterations result in either

a

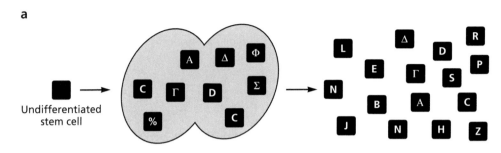

Thymus
- TCR gene rearrangement and expression
- CD8, CD4, and CD3 expression
- Negative selection
- Positive selection

Cells of the T-cell pool
- Recognize self MHC antigen
- Do not recognize self MHC alone
- Have a predefined specificity
- Are "naive" until they encounter antigen

b

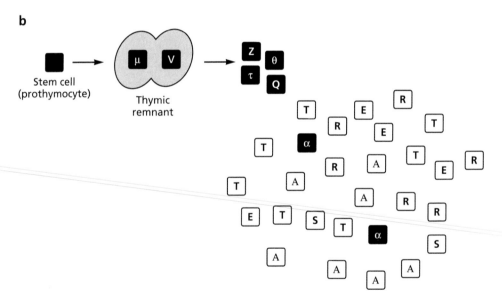

c

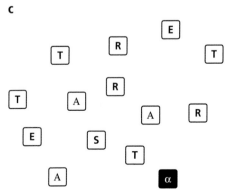

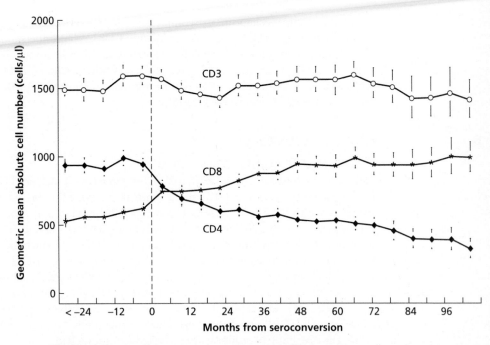

Figure 11.4   T-cell homeostasis. Geometric means of absolute numbers of circulating T-cell subsets ($CD3^+$, $CD4^+$, and $CD8^+$ lymphocytes) as a function of seroconversion in a large cohort of individuals monitored over time (MAC study). Numbers of observations beginning at <24 months before seroconversion are provided. In this figure, observations on subjects who developed AIDS have been excluded. Note the level of $CD3^+$ cells (total T lymphocytes) resulting from the alteration in production in $CD4^+$ and $CD8^+$ cells. (From reference 1666, with permission.)

protective or deleterious responses if the cells have CTL activity (2268). Absence or reduction in certain T-cell specifications may decrease the resistance to infection and malignancy (2268, 2864) (Figure 11.3).

Other studies have suggested that there may be a physiological regulation of T lymphocytes in the host (22). A loss of $CD4^+$ lymphocytes appears to be compensated for by an increase in the number of $CD8^+$ lymphocytes (Figure 11.4). This $CD8^+$ cell lymphocytosis could interfere with regeneration of $CD4^+$ cells (1666). If

Figure 11.3   Generation of the T-cell repertoire. (a) Generation of the T-cell pool through differentiation. Undifferentiated lymphoid stem cells (prothymocytes), as they pass through the thymus, express CD4 and CD8 molecules. Their TCR genes are rearranged and expressed, and the resulting thymocytes undergo negative and positive selection. T-cell clones released into circulation have a diverse T-cell receptor pattern (illustrated by letters and symbols), indicating their potential for polyclonal responses. (b) Regeneration of the T-cell pool following therapeutic intervention. With destruction of T cells by HIV, a limited T-cell repertoire may exist which, when allowed to regenerate through a variety of therapeutic interventions, may not recover the entire repertoire initially present in the host. (c) "End-stage" T-cell pool. The end-stage T-cell repertoire may be limited so that it cannot react quickly to a particular antigen. In a sense, as shown here, the T-cell repertoire could not respond in a way that would require the spelling of ZEBRA. Nevertheless, by other processes, it might be able to respond (although more slowly) by recognizing the antigen as "a horse with white and black stripes." (Ideas derived from figures and discussions provided by H. Cliff Lane).

such homeostatic mechanisms exist, approaches in HIV-infected individuals to increase the number of CD4$^+$ cells by modulating CD8$^+$ cell numbers might be possible. Some studies suggest that a failure to maintain this homeostasis is associated with progression to disease (1666). Nevertheless, further evaluation of human systems needs to be undertaken (952a) before approaches for modifying this potential mechanism would be considered feasible.

B.   CD4$^+$ T Lymphocytes

1. CD4$^+$ HELPER CELL CLASSIFICATION

Similar to the murine system (1861, 1862), human CD4$^+$ T-helper (TH) cells can be separated into TH1 and TH2 subsets (480, 481, 2270, 2271, 2475; for a review, see reference 1597). These cell subsets have been distinguished by a variety of features discussed in this book (Table 11.1) (see also Chapters 4 and 9). TH1 cells secrete IL-2, IFN-γ, and tumor necrosis factor alpha (TNF-α), which are important for strong cell-mediated immunity; TH2 cells produce IL-4, IL-5, IL-6, IL-10, and IL-13, which increase antibody production. The cytokines produced by the TH1 and TH2 subsets also cross-regulate one another (2270, 2271). For example, IFN-γ, a product of TH1 cells, can inhibit the generation of TH2 cells (824), whereas IL-10, a product of TH2 cells, can inhibit cytokine production by TH1 cells (603) (Figure 11.5). The effect of IFN-γ appears to be linked to a suppression of IL-1 production (1989). The inhibitory effect of IL-10 appears to reflect a block of IL-12 synthesis by macrophages (551) (see below). In one report, macrophages of HIV-infected symptomatic patients were found to have increased production of IL-1 and decreased production of IL-12 (446). These findings, suggesting an inhibitory effect of IL-1 on type 1 cytokine production, could explain a shift from a type 1 to type 2 immunologic pattern with advancement to disease.

Most recently, the differential expression of the IL-12 β receptor on CD4$^+$ cells has provided a possible means of distinguishing TH1 (present) and TH2 (absent) cells (1682)(Table 11.1). Apparently, IL-4 inhibits the expression of this receptor

Table 11.1   Characterization of CD4$^+$ cell subsets

Characteristics	CD4$^+$ cell subsets	
	TH1	TH2
Cytokines	IL-2, IFN-γ	IL-4, IL-5, IL-10, IL-13
Cytokines that enhance their development	IL-12	IL-4
IL-12β receptor expression	+	−
CCR-3 expression	−	+
Sensitivity to apoptosis	+ +	−
Cytokine effect on apoptosis	Protect	Accelerate
CD95L expression[a]	Normal	Decreased
Relative sensitivity to HIV infection	+	+ +
CTL activity	+	−
Function	Increase cell-mediated immunity	Increase antibody production

[a] CD95L is involved in Fas-mediated apoptosis.

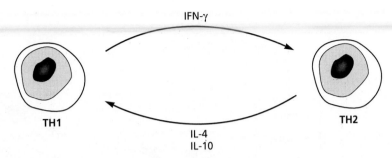

Figure 11.5 Cross-regulation of the TH1 and TH2 subsets of CD4$^+$ cells. The production of certain cytokines by TH1 and TH2 cells can suppress the production of cytokines by the corresponding cell subset (2270). (From reference 1491 with permission.)

and can thereby induce the development of TH2 cells (1682). IFN-α and IFN-γ can maintain the presence of this IL-12 receptor and restore the ability of the cells to respond to IL-12, which is part of the TH1 pathway (2267, 2623, 2858). Importantly, IL-12 induces IFN-γ production by NK cells (214), and thus the interplay among these different cytokines can be appreciated (Figure 11.1). The information on cytokine production may be helpful in evaluating the prognosis of HIV infection and in defining the factors influencing a switch from TH1 to TH2 cytokine patterns. In this regard, some studies suggest that TH1 cells are less susceptible to productive infection by HIV-1 (particularly SI strains) than are TH2 cells (1644, 2797). These differences, if confirmed, might be related to selective expression of chemokine receptors on human TH cells (234, 2343a) (Chapter 3). This possibility, however, would not easily explain the emergence of SI strains and the shift from TH1 to TH2 cytokine production that appears to be associated with progression to disease (Chapter 7).

Because similar cytokines can be produced by other cells in the body, the terminology of type 1 and type 2 responses has also been used when the specific cells producing the cytokines are not identified (2270, 2271). It is important to note that the separation of TH CD4$^+$ cells into TH1 and TH2 cells and the interactions of type 1 and type 2 cytokines (481, 1597, 2433) provide a helpful concept but that the system is more complex. For example, unlike in the murine system, IL-10 can be made by both TH1 and TH2 cell clones (380, 612, 2270, 2271), although the dominant cell type releasing IL-10 is TH2 (612). Moreover, both type 1 and type 2 cytokines can increase immunoglobulin production, although specific differences can be appreciated (e.g., IgE production by type 2 cytokines) (481, 2270). Furthermore, while TH1-like cytokines (e.g., IFN-γ and IL-2) may increase cellular immune anti-HIV responses, the same cellular factors can augment HIV-1 production (see Chapter 9, Table 9.5) (1635, 1697, 2113). In contrast, the TH2-like cytokines (e.g., IL-4 and IL-10) suppress HIV expression (1635, 1697, 2113) but reduce CD8$^+$ cell response (138, 380, 2270, 2271). The suppressing effect of IL-10 could be linked to its inhibition of the production of TNF-α, an up-regulator of HIV replication. Because of these dual roles of cytokines (decreasing or increasing CD8$^+$ cell response and decreasing or increasing HIV production), their clinical use may present problems in terms of the dominant effect observed in the infected person (see Chapter 14).

With regard to CD4$^+$ cells, the TH subsets appear to represent terminally differentiated cells derived from a precursor (or TH0-type) cell capable of expressing many different cytokines (2837). Differentiation of TH0 into TH1 and TH2 cells can occur in response to antigens (2602) or the type of cytokine present at the time

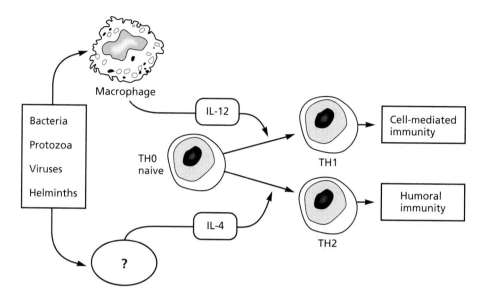

Figure 11.6 Cytokine-driven TH cell differentiation. Bacteria, protozoa, probably viruses, and helminths can induce the production of IL-12 by macrophages or other cells. The IL-12 then induces the differentiation of naive or TH0 cells into a TH1 subset, which encourages cell-mediated immunity. Other pathogens, particularly helminths, stimulate IL-4 production by cells not yet defined, but most likely T cells. IL-4 induces TH0 cells toward TH2 cell differentiation. The TH2 cells mediate help for antibody production. What determines the predominant TH1 or TH2 response in the host is not known. Modified from reference 2433 with permission.

of differentiation. The induction process cannot change an already committed TH1 or TH2 cell (2639). IL-12, for example, induces TH1 cell development from TH0 cells while down-regulating TH 2 cell cytokine expression (e.g., IL-4) (1654, 2433, 2436; for a review of IL-12, see reference 2706) (Figure 11.6). IL-12 inhibition of TH2 development may occur indirectly through the stimulation of IFN-γ synthesis (214, 2706) (Figure 11.1). IL-1, produced by macrophages, can selectively stimulate TH1 cells (2891); IL-4 and, perhaps more so, IL-13 stimulate the development of TH2 cells (1349, 2998), which in turn produce IL-4, which can down-regulate TH1-type cytokine expression (481).

2. CD4⁺ HELPER CELL RESPONSES

CD4$^+$ cell functions that may influence anti-HIV responses have been found to be reduced early in HIV infection before the occurrence of a substantial decrease in CD4$^+$ cell number (483, 961, 1420, 1781, 2275, 2469). They can be prognostic of the clinical course (483, 961, 1420, 1781, 2275, 2469) (see also Chapter 9). Clerici and Shearer (483, 2469) have categorized the activities that decrease over time by measuring cell proliferation and IL-2 production after exposure to recall antigens (e.g., tetanus and influenza A), irradiated HLA disparate leukocytes (allo response), and phytohemagglutinin (mitogen response) stimulation (Figure 9.2). Approximately one-third of asymptomatic individuals have responses to all three stimuli; those who have no response to the stimuli progress more rapidly to disease. The decrease in proliferative responses to alloantigens can be found in both CD45RA$^+$ and CD45RO$^+$ subsets of CD4$^+$ T cells.

Based on studies of HIV-infected individuals over time, a hypothesis has been presented that cytokines produced by TH1 and TH2 cells can play an immune regulatory role in HIV infection and affect progression to disease, as has been observed in studies of other infectious agents (481, 858, 1643, 2469, 2475). The findings suggest that TH1 responses are found primarily in healthy asymptomatic HIV-infected individuals, whereas a predominance of the TH2 subset response occurs during the symptomatic stage of disease (Figure 11.7) (473, 481, 2469).

This concept was derived from observations that peripheral blood mononuclear cells (PBMC) from asymptomatic individuals early in disease produce type 1 cytokines (e.g., IL-2) while those progressing to disease produce type 2 cytokines (e.g., IL-4 and IL-10) (473, 481). A reduction in IL-2 production has also been observed with purified CD3$^+$ and CD4$^+$ cell populations from symptomatic patients in comparison to healthy infected subjects, concomitant with an increase in the number of IL-4-secreting cells (137a, 924). The results confirm, by intracellular staining (924, 1317a) and other techniques, the shift from type 1 to type 2 cytokine production with advancement to disease. The data suggest that the TH1-type response is protective against disease in an individual (473, 481).

Studies with uninfected high-risk individuals have supported this conclusion (472, 475, 2183) (Section IV) (see Chapter 13), since a TH1-type response is observed. Moreover, the data suggest that progression to disease in adults and children is associated with a type 2 response (1149, 1188, 2270, 2271), which may be responsible for suppressing the type 1 response. Not only can increased production of type 2 cytokines, such as IL-4 and IL-10, reduce the production of type 1 cytokines nec-

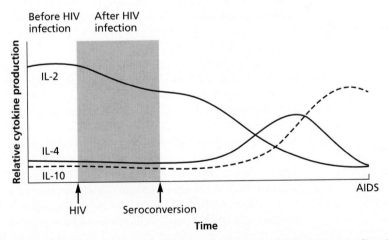

Figure 11.7   CD4$^+$ cell cytokine production before and after HIV infection. Studies of cultured PBMC suggest that, prior to HIV infection, the dominant TH cell subtype is TH1, with production of such cytokines as IL-2 and IFN-γ. During the early stages of HIV infection, the TH1 subset predominates, but with advancement to disease, it is replaced by the TH2 subset, reflected in the production of the cytokines IL-4 and IL-10. (Data from reference 480. Adapted from reference 1491 with permission.)

essary for maintaining cellular immune cell function, but also they could directly decrease the antiviral responses of CD8$^+$ effector cells (Section III.B).

These observations on responses of TH cell subsets during HIV infection suggest how other infectious agents or allergy (e.g., TH2 cytokines) could affect immune responses to HIV (see Chapter 13). For example, infection of individuals by *Schistosoma mansoni* has been shown to elicit a TH2-like response to tetanus toxoid antigens, whereas uninfected subjects showed a TH1- or TH0-like response (2321). Likewise, some parasitic diseases, because of a TH2-like dominant state, may be associated with a poor prognosis for HIV infection (171).

Potentially, the findings for type 1 and type 2 cytokine expression can offer new approaches for immune modulation in this disease (see Chapter 14). For example, IL-12 has been shown to restore the proliferative responses of PBMC from HIV-infected individuals (476). Moreover, antibodies to IL-4 and IL-10 added in vitro restored production of IL-2 by PBMC from infected patients (473, 484). These results suggest that inducing a type 1 response directly or indirectly can help elicit cellular immune responses to HIV (see Chapter 14).

A correlation of cytokine and chemokine production by CD4$^+$ cells to the clinical state has also been suggested in primate studies. With infection by the *nef*-deleted attenuated SIV, there was a preferential type 1 pattern of cytokine production. With infection by the pathogenic SIV, higher levels of chemokines were made in association with type 2 cytokine production (2999). This observation counters that of other studies (2416) that suggested that a type 1 immune response is associated with β-chemokine production in humans. In addition, individual β-chemokines have been reported to influence cytokine production by CD4$^+$ cells (Section III.G). For example, macrophage inflammatory protein 1α (MIP-1α) enhances IFN-γ production, whereas macrophage chemotactic protein 1 (MCP-1) enhances IL-4 production. Thus, besides playing a role in lymphocyte trafficking, these cellular factors could participate in the induction of type 1 or type 2 responses (1247). The findings are preliminary and need further evaluation, certainly in terms of clinical relevance (Section III.G).

3. CYTOTOXIC CELL ACTIVITY

As noted in Chapter 9, some CD4$^+$ cells can have CTL activity directed either at infected or uninfected CD4$^+$ cells or at cells expressing HIV peptides in association with the MHC class II molecule (613, 999, 1388, 1796, 1988, 2093). This response is usually found with TH1-type CD4$^+$ cells (613) and is virus strain specific (999), mediated by perforin (1796) or Fas:Fas ligand (Fas L)-induced apoptosis (2093). Recent evidence suggests that CD8$^+$ cells play a role in the development of CD4$^+$ cell cytotoxic activity (2891a). Therefore, while these types of CD4$^+$ cells, by their CTL activity, may help in cell-mediated responses against HIV, they also could have a detrimental effect on uninfected cells. Some investigators also warn that the rapid lysis observed between CD4$^+$ cells and infected target cells (1796) could appear to be a result of CTL activity but may be related to cell-to-cell contact and syncytium formation (1044).

C.   Cytotoxic CD8$^+$ Cells

1. GENERAL OBSERVATIONS

The other cell type, besides NK, that commonly reacts against virus-infected cells is the cytotoxic subset of CD8$^+$ T lymphocytes. Some evidence suggests that the extent of response of CD8$^+$ cells to HIV infection, mirrored by the TCR repertoire pattern, can influence the clinical course (932, 2033, 2034) (see Chapters 9 and 13). By functional and flow cytometry analysis, cytotoxic cells have been shown to have a CD8$^+$ CD11b$^-$ phenotype while suppressor cells (which can down-modulate immune responses) have a CD8$^+$ CD11b$^+$ phenotype. Recently, depending on expression of the CD28 molecule, a distinction has been made between CD8$^+$ cells that have anti-HIV CTL activity (CD8$^+$ CD28$^-$ cells) and those that have a non-cytotoxic antiviral response (CD8$^+$ CD28$^+$ cells) (136, 255, 757, 1416) (Table 11.2). Some results suggest that the CD8$^+$ cells lacking CD28 are at an end stage in the replicative cycle. They have reduced telomere lengths (685) and are relatively unresponsive to mitogen and to anti-CD28 antibodies, since they lack the CD28 molecule (255). A possible influence of this process on HIV pathogenesis (e.g., enhanced aging) has been considered (685) (see Chapter 13).

The TH classification of CD4$^+$ cells by cytokine production (Table 11.1), discussed above, has suggested a similar classification for CD8$^+$ cells. In this case, T1 and T2 type cells (or Tc1 and Tc2) could define distinct subsets (1862, 2270, 2271). Some studies suggest that type 2 CD8$^+$ cells have decreased CTL activity (1642), perhaps reflecting their reduced production of IL-2, which is needed for CD8$^+$ cell function (138).

2. ANTI-HIV CYTOTOXIC RESPONSES

Classically, the CD8$^+$ cell cytotoxic response is HLA restricted and antigen specific and requires cell-to-cell contact (Table 11.2). It appears to be very important in the control of certain viral infections (332, 644). In culture, this cellular cytotoxicity is demonstrated by a high input of CD8$^+$ cells, typically a CD8$^+$ cell/target cell (E/T) ratio of 25:1 to 100:1, and is measured in a 4-h ^{51}Cr release assay. However, CD8$^+$ CTL clones can show this activity at much lower E/T ratios (e.g., 1:1). Moreover, as expected, the cytotoxicity is observed only with viral protein-expressing cells that have the same MHC class I phenotype as the CD8$^+$ cells. A unique observation of CTL-mediated lysis of HIV-infected cells is that stimulation of the CTL with viral antigen before evaluation of their ability to lyse their target is often not necessary. However, the response is generally weaker than that of HIV-stimulated CTL (1358).

Studies of this antiviral response have shown that CD8$^+$ lymphocytes can kill cells expressing (via a variety of vector systems) peptides from several different HIV

Table 11.2 Anti-HIV responses by CD8$^+$ T cells

Characteristic	Cytotoxic response	Noncytotoxic response
MHC-restricted	Yes	No
Mechanism	Perforin/granzymes or *fas*-mediated apoptosis	Soluble antiviral protein
Antigen specificity	Fine	?Broad
Clinical relevance[a]	Develops early after infection but lost with progression to disease	
Vaccine-inducible	Yes	?

[a] With cytotoxic response, clinical relevance is most evident when levels of precursor CTLs are measured.

proteins, including reverse transcriptase, envelope, core, and some accessory proteins (e.g., Vif and Nef) (1091, 1388, 2102, 2238, 2809; for a review, see references 1938 and 2295). Estimates of the frequency of peptide-specific CTL clones range from 0.2 to 1% of T cells (1866). In some cases, the CTL clones persist in vivo for at least 5 years (1866); in others, they are replaced (see below).

Some investigators have attempted to determine by mathematical modeling the extent of CTL activity and viral production in HIV infection (1319). Considering the turnover rate of infected cells subjected to CTL activity as well as viral cytopathicity, the half-life of a $CD4^+$ cell target appears to be about 17 h. The major cytotoxic effect is on productively infected cells; the influence on latently infected cells remains to be determined. CTL response can affect viral loads in the blood by killing virus-infected cells. The overall effects on the half-life of all infected cells, however, may not be great, since so many cells contain virus in a latent state (see Chapter 5). An escape from CTL activity would subsequently permit renewal of viral production and high levels of circulating virus particles (see below).

The cytotoxic $CD8^+$ cells also have a high expression of CD38 and HLA-DR, indicating their activated state (1087, 1416). The mechanisms for cytotoxicity appear to involve both a lytic molecule, perforin, and the induction of apoptosis via Fas:Fas L interaction (for a review, see reference 184). Similar CTL responses have been identified in SIV infection and can be important in controlling virus replication during acute infection (see Chapter 4) (2934; for a review, see reference 1938). Studies with cell clones have shown that $CD8^+$ CTL can be more cross-reactive with divergent HIV-1 strains than are $CD4^+$ CTL (Section II.B) (see Chapter 9) (999). The findings most probably reflect the different epitope presentation mechanisms (MHC class I versus class II) for these two lymphocyte subsets.

3. CLINICAL RELEVANCE

When evaluating the clinical relevance of $CD8^+$ cell cytotoxic activity, a distinction should be made betweeen CTL function measured without stimulation (effector CTL [CTLe]) or after stimulation (precursor CTL [CTLp]). The $CD8^+$ cell cytotoxic activity associated with precursor cells can be found at relatively high levels during the asymptomatic period but then appears to decline in individuals with progression to disease (361, 1091, 1317, 2232; for reviews, see references 914 and 2295). However, in some studies, no change in CTLp levels was observed (871, 931, 2235). In most studies the CTLe but not the CTLp activity has been found in all stages of HIV infection and does not substantially decline with the development of AIDS (202, 361, 933, 1091, 1210, 2032, 2232, 2235, 2238). In studies of children, the opposite has been noted: CTLe has been found to decrease in symptomatic children, but the CTLp responses were consistently detected at all stages of the disease (326).

Whether the CTLe or CTLp frequency has clinical relevance is therefore not certain, but as noted above, high levels of CTLe to HIV peptides have not prevented the development of disease (2235). Moreover, the number of virus-infected cells in the blood of some subjects studied has been found to increase despite a high level of anti-Gag-specific CTL (1317). Finally, the induction of CTL responses has not protected monkeys from SIV-induced disease (2934).

In general, CTL can be found that react with several epitopes on Gag, in particular, three conserved regions of the protein (326). In contrast, CTL against the HIV envelope protein have been identified for only a few epitopes (2809a). These observations may be important in the control of HIV-1 infection (see below). It is noteworthy that the decrease in HIV-specific CTL activity may occur in AIDS patients without a reduction in $CD8^+$ cell cytolytic functions directed at other pathogens (e.g., anti-Epstein-Barr virus activities) (361, 871, 2032). Similarly, T-cell proliferative responses to HIV proteins can be reduced in HIV-infected patients at the same time that these responses to CMV and herpes simplex virus (HSV) proteins are maintained (2803). Recently, in a well-documented study of an infected laboratory workers, group-specific and type-specific anti-Gag CTLp responses to the homologous virus proteins were noted initially. This response appeared to broaden over time (2515a). Since the individual remains asymptomatic, a protective role of this $CD8^+$ cell activity is implied.

In some cases, the CTL response to some viral peptides (e.g., Gag) may decrease with progression to disease while this activity against other HIV proteins (e.g., Env) does not (1973, 2237, 2803). These results suggest a selective loss of the anti-HIV CTL (2032) that can have clinical relevance. Recently, CTL to a variety of epitopes from the Nef protein were identified and the dynamics of the response indicated that the immune system was quite flexible and could adapt to react to multiple HIV variants. Such a phenomenon could play a role in maintaining a long-term asymptomatic state (978). In these studies, however, the expression of some viral epitopes persisted, despite the presence of CTL. Most surprising is the presence of anti-HIV Env CTL in normal uninfected subjects (1091). This observation suggests a cross-reactivity of certain viral proteins with cellular proteins (see Chapter 10, Section VII).

For the above reasons, it is difficult to assess conclusively the clinical relevance of CTL in HIV infection. Although this type of antiviral activity has prevented virus spread in some animal model systems (332, 644), the role of CTL in HIV infection is not clear. Despite some correlation of CTL activity with a healthy clinical state (361) (for reviews, see references 914 and 1938), as noted above, progression of disease with increasing numbers of HIV-infected cells and small numbers of $CD4^+$ cells occurs in the presence of $CD8^+$ cells as effector cells (978).

4. HIV RESISTANCE TO CTL ACTIVITY

Some observations have suggested mechanisms by which HIV-infected cells could escape CTL activity (Table 11.3). Conceivably, suppression of viral antigen expression by the $CD8^+$ cell antiviral factor (Section III) leads to the lack of recognition by CTL (1515). Alternatively, the ability of CTL to lyse cells may be compromised by HIV.

Table 11.3 Possible mechanisms of cellular resistance to anti-HIV CTL activity

1. Cellular factor that blocks CTL response (1210)
2. Mutation in viral peptide (254, 927, 2091, 2143)
3. Mutant peptide that can inactivate the CTL (i.e., TCR antagonism) (1318, 1748)
4. High levels of circulating free peptides
5. $CD8^+$ cell suppression of HIV antigen expression (1515)
6. Down-modulation of MHC expression (1273, 2390)

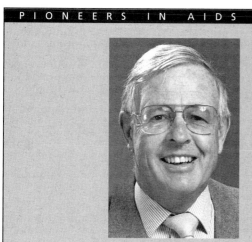

Murray B. Gardner
Professor Emeritus, University of California, Davis. Dr. Gardner played an important role in determining the participation of SIV in immune deficiency and in defining differences among HIV and SIV strains.

A cellular factor that blocks the CTL response has been identified in symptomatic individuals (1210). This inhibitor, produced by $CD8^+$ cells, binds lectin; is heat, trypsin, and acid resistant; and is about 20 to 30 kDa in size (2325). It could be directly involved in a pathogenic pathway that results from a depression in the control of HIV by cytotoxic $CD8^+$ cells.

Some reports, but not others (419, 1767), suggest that HIV strains can escape the CTL response by mutational events (254, 927, 2091, 2143) (see Chapter 7). This phenomenon could occur early in primary infection (254, 2143), reflecting selective pressure by the immune system. It could be involved in progression to disease (927). However, escape from CTL activity at a limited level seems an unusual reason for a pathogenic course, since CTL to multiple viral antigens are usually present. The resiliency of the CTL response and its ability to recognize variants appear to be determined by HLA profiles (2893). This finding could explain the protection from infection in some exposed, uninfected individuals (781).

One recently described mechanism for escape from CTL activity is the masking of an epitope recognized by the CTL through alterations in its peptide structure. Certain class I epitopes in the form of small peptides can inhibit normal lysis of target cells presenting the original epitope (i.e., cells infected with the original virus). This T-cell repertoire antagonism has been described in several systems (1184), as well as in HIV infection (for reviews, see references 1319 and 1748). The exact mechanism is not known but is somewhat reminiscent of the paralysis to B-cell clonal proliferation (see Chapter 10). In the latter case, however, it is the original virus and not the subsequent virus that prevents a sufficient response to a different strain. These TCR antagonists may induce anergy in CTL clones (196). Thus, HIV could escape this immune reaction either by replacement of the normal epitope within the HLA class I molecule with a mutant peptide or by the action of the mutant peptide as an antagonist inactivating the CTL. In support of the latter mechanism, incubation of CTL with mutant virus-infected cells reduces CTL killing of cells expressing the wild-type virus (196). Moreover, as would be expected, a large variety of circulating free peptides could tie up the CTL present and prevent them from interacting with the target cell.

Another mechanism by which HIV could escape CTL activity is through down-modulation of the MHC antigen. Several viruses, including herpesviruses, coronaviruses, paramyxoviruses, and adenoviruses, have been known to decrease both class I and class II antigen expression on cells (for a review, see reference 2234). HIV infection is associated with reduced HIV MHC expression on CD4$^+$ cells (1112, 1273, 2390); both the Tat (1112) and Nef (2428) proteins could be involved. Nevertheless, some studies suggest that this mechanism is probably not important in affecting CTL activity in HIV infection (2931). Moreover, reduced MHC expression can increase cell susceptibility to lysis by NK cells (Section I) (303). Finally, HIV particles bound to follicular dendritic cells may escape CTL lysis because the viral antigens are not associated with MHC class I molecules.

D. Diffuse Infiltrative Lymphocytosis Syndrome

In reference to these CD8$^+$ cell responses to HIV infection, the description of a diffuse infiltrative lymphocytosis syndrome may reflect some anti-HIV activity of these cells (1166, 1257). This syndrome is characterized by an infiltration of salivary glands, lungs, gastrointestinal tract, and kidneys by CD8$^+$ cells. An increase in the number of circulating CD8$^+$ lymphocytes is noted, and B-cell lymphomas can develop. These patients have a delay in CD4$^+$ T-cell loss. The cellular immune response appears to be stimulated by HIV antigens and is found in individuals who have survived a long time with infection. A similar symptom complex has been described in children experiencing long-term survival, particularly those infected around the time of delivery (594). How this syndrome relates to CD8$^+$ cell function is not clear.

E. Potential Detrimental Effects of CTL Activity

This CTL activity in response to HIV infection may appear to provide a beneficial effect in some studies, but in others these cells seem to be part of the pathogenic pathway (Table 11.4) (see Chapter 13). In some infected individuals, CTL have been

Table 11.4 Possible evidence for detrimental effects of CTL activity in HIV infection[a]

1. Lysis of autologous or heterologous activated uninfected CD4$^+$ lymphocytes (205)
2. Lysis of APC (1326, 1765)
3. Continued presence in AIDS patients (932, 2235)
4. CTL infiltration of lymph nodes (436, 2281)
5. Found in the cerebrospinal fluid of symptomatic patients (1189)
6. Associated with Sjögren's syndrome
7. Involved in lung lymphocytic alveolitis (106)
8. Absence of CTL responses in disease-free primates, naturally infected with simian lentiviruses (1504)
9. CTLs are harmful in other viral infections (e.g., lymphocytic choriomeningitis, Theiler's virus) (252, 2261)

[a] See also references 1515, 1780, and 2993.

found that can lyse autologous or heterologous activated uninfected CD4$^+$ lymphocytes (205). Thus, this non-MHC-restricted cytotoxic activity may have a role in the loss of CD4$^+$ cells in the HIV-infected individuals. The findings are reminiscent of other CTL activities in autoimmune diseases (1581, 2949) and those described in previous work with HIV-infected subjects (2963). A detrimental role of CD8$^+$ cells has been demonstrated with lymphocytic choriomeningitis virus and Theiler's virus infections in mice (252, 2261). Destruction of virus-infected dentdritic cells was involved (Chapter 13, Section II.E). Moreover, the absence of CTL responses in healthy chimpanzees chronically infected with SIV$_{cpz}$ and other disease-free primates naturally infected with simian lentiviruses has suggested some relationship between this activity and HIV pathogenesis (1504, 1515) (see Chapter 13). Finally, a detrimental role of CD8$^+$ cell CTL in HIV-related Sjögren's syndrome (i.e., autoimmune response) and lung lymphocytic alveolitis has been considered (106).

III. CD8$^+$ Cell Noncytotoxic Anti-HIV Activity

A. General Observations

In addition to having anti-HIV cytotoxic activity associated with CD8$^+$ cells, a subset of these T cells can suppress HIV replication in CD4$^+$ cells (Tables 11.2 and 11.5) without killing the cells. Initially, this cellular antiviral activity was recognized by studying individuals who were asymptomatic and did not yield HIV from their cultured PBMC. When their CD8$^+$ cells were removed from the blood sample by panning with monoclonal antibodies to CD8, high levels of virus were released from the CD4$^+$ cells remaining in the culture (2812). The replacement of CD8$^+$ cells in this culture at levels that were far below those used to demonstrate CTL activity ($<$1:1) led to complete suppression of virus replication. Subsequent removal of the CD8$^+$ cells again revealed virus-releasing cells. While the effect appeared to be most evi-

Table 11.5 Characteristics of the CD8$^+$ cell noncytotoxic anti-HIV response[a]

1. Property of CD8$^+$ T cells, not CD4$^+$ cells, NK cells, or macrophages
2. Exhibited predominantly by the CD8$^+$ HLA-DR$^+$ CD28$^+$ human cell subset
3. Blocks HIV replication in naturally or acutely infected CD4$^+$ cells
4. Can block HIV replication at low CD8$^+$/CD4$^+$ cell ratios ($<$0.05:1)
5. Correlates directly with clinical status and high CD4$^+$ cell counts
6. Active against strains of HIV-1, HIV-2, and SIV
7. Dose dependent
8. Not HLA restricted
9. Nonlytic mechanism
10. Blocks HIV replication at viral transcription
11. Observed with CD8$^+$ cells from infected nonhuman primates
12. Mediated (at least in part) by a soluble factor (Table 11.9)
13. Optimal activity with cell:cell contact
14. No effect on activation or proliferation of CD4$^+$ cells

[a] Measured by in vitro assays. For review, see references 1515 and 1629.

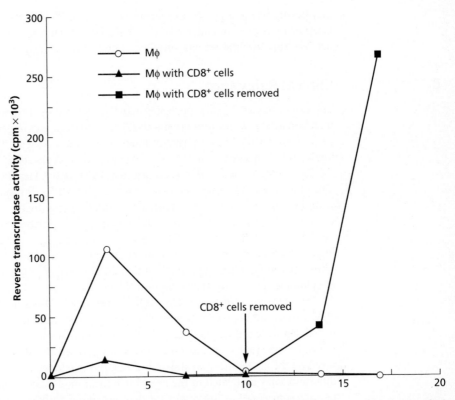

Figure 11.8 CD8$^+$ cell suppression of HIV replication in macrophages. Purified macrophages (Mφ) were inoculated with the macrophage-tropic strain HIV-1$_{SF162}$. After 1 h the macrophages were washed and CD8$^+$ cells were added to some of the cultures. After 10 days, the CD8$^+$ cells were removed from some cultures. Virus replication was measured by monitoring the reverse transcriptase activity in the culture fluid. The figure shows that when CD8$^+$ cells are cultured with infected macrophages, virus replication does not take place, but when CD8$^+$ cells are removed, virus replication occurs. (Adapted from reference 136a with permission.)

dent when effector and target cells were MHC compatible (2812), non-MHC-restricted suppression was readily demonstrated.

These and other observations indicate that the CD8$^+$ cells can suppress virus production without affecting the proliferation or expression of activation markers on CD4$^+$ cells and without killing the virus-infected cells (1515, 1629, 2814, 2900). This noncytotoxic, non-MHC-dependent antiviral response can be measured with naturally infected CD4$^+$ cells obtained from infected individuals (endogenous assay) as well as with normal CD4$^+$ cells obtained from seronegative individuals and acutely infected in culture with HIV (acute infection assay) (2810; for a review, see reference 1515). Suppression of virus replication in both CD4$^+$ lymphocytes and macrophages has been demonstrated (136a, 1515, 1847) (Figure 11.8). Moreover, these CD8$^+$ cells show similar responses against many different isolates of HIV-1 (including the cytopathic strains), HIV-2, and SIV (Table 11.5) (1636, 2814). CD8$^+$ cell clones with this activity have been described (1120, 2694), and some cell clones may have both CTL and noncytotoxic activities (325). The latter function may be important in preventing harmful effects of CTL (1515) (see Section II.E and Chapter 13). Cells from infected children show a similar response and a relationship between this antiviral activity and their clinical state (1505a, 1511a, 2100, 2116).

B.   Clinical Relevance

The extent of CD8$^+$ cell-suppressing activity, revealed by the endogenous or acute infection assays, varies among subjects (2813) and decreases in patients with disease (905, 1416, 1636). In many asymptomatic individuals, a CD8$^+$/CD4$^+$ cell ratio as low as 1:20 is needed to suppress endogenous virus replication; in AIDS patients, this ratio often is increased to 4:1 or greater (1515, 1629). Healthy infected individuals monitored over time also show a loss of this CD8$^+$ cell response concomitant with the onset of symptoms (1416). This reduction in antiviral response correlates with the observed decrease in the CD8$^+$ CD28$^+$ cell population associated with disease progression (286, 1416, 2276). Moreover, purified CD8$^+$ CD28$^+$ cells show the highest level of this anti-HIV response (136, 1416) and production of IL-2 (286). Thus, the cellular phenotype of this antiviral CD8$^+$ cell population differs from that of cytotoxic cells (1515, 1629) (Section II.B).

In one study utilizing an acute infection system, CD8$^+$ cell noncytotoxic anti-HIV activity did not correlate with clinical state (139), but the use of cocultured infected dendritic cells and uninfected CD4$^+$ cells in that system may have influenced the results. In that study, gamma irradiation blocked the suppressing activity assayed by the acute infection system but not by the endogenous system (139). This difference may be related to the need for activation of CD8$^+$ cells in culture. This requirement is not as important for demonstrating antiviral responses in the endogenous system (139, 1416).

CD8$^+$ cells from several uninfected subjects have also demonstrated this response (139, 287, 1629, 2814). However, their reactivity occurs only with naturally infected CD4$^+$ cells, not with acutely infected cells, and generally only at a CD8$^+$/CD4$^+$ cell ratio of 0.5 or higher (1629, 2814). Although two studies have suggested that CD8$^+$ cells from uninfected people can reduce HIV-1 replication in the

Table 11.6   The potential clinical value of CD8$^+$ cell noncytotoxic antiviral activity in HIV infection

1. Could ensure long-term survival
2. Not affected by viral heterogeneity (HIV-1 and HIV-2); cytopathic and noncytopathic strains are sensitive
3. Can prevent several log units of virus replication in vitro (and possibly 3 to 5 log units in vivo)
4. Can prevent emergence of drug-resistant strains and immune "escape" mutants by blocking virus replication
5. Can prevent dual infection by HIV
6. Does not affect activation and proliferation of CD4$^+$ cells
7. Prevents effects of CTL activities that could be destructive to the host (i.e., death of uninfected as well as infected cells)

Table 11.7 Possible mechanisms for the loss of
CD8$^+$ cell noncytotoxic anti-HIV activity

1. Loss of CD8$^+$ CD28$^+$ cells (e.g., by apoptosis)
   (922, 1764, 2148)
2. Reduction in type 1 cytokines (138)
3. Reduction in CD28 costimulation (136)

acute infection assay (121, 2285), definite proof that CTL activity was not involved
was not provided.

The potential clinical value of the CD8$^+$ cell noncytotoxic antiviral response includes several features besides its association with long-term survival (Table 11.6).
The response appears to affect both cytopathic and noncytopathic (SI and NSI)
strains and can reduce virus replication by several log units. By its suppressing activity, it can prevent the emergence of drug-resistant strains, and it does not appear
to affect the activation or proliferation of CD4$^+$ cells. Thus, it may in fact permit
normal function to return to CD4$^+$ cells. Perhaps importantly, the suppression of
viral antigen expression on cells by this antiviral response could prevent the detrimental effects of CTL activities that might be present in HIV-infected individuals
(Section IIE) (Table 11.4) (1515).

C.   Loss of the CD8$^+$ Cell Noncytotoxic Anti-HIV Response

Why CD8$^+$ cell noncytotoxic antiviral activity is lost over time is not known, but the
phenomenon may reflect the reduction in a particular activated cell subset (e.g.,
CD8$^+$ CD28$^+$ cells) (1416) or loss of its function (Table 11.7). Perhaps the difference in survival of CD8$^+$ cells in culture (2148) and the known presence of apoptosis of CD8$^+$ cells in HIV infection (922, 1525, 1574, 1764) could explain this phenomenon. Since apoptosis appears to be related to the cytokines produced (see
Chapter 6, Section IV), a shift from type 1 to type 2 cytokines may be partly responsible for this loss in CD8$^+$ cell function (479).

1. ROLE OF CYTOKINES

The possible effect of cytokines on CD8$^+$ cell antiviral activity has been studied in
approaches to determine the reason for a reduced anti-HIV response by CD8$^+$ cells.
As reviewed in Section II.B, it is known that TH1-type CD4$^+$ cells increase cell-mediated immunity whereas TH2-type CD4$^+$ cells are associated with weak cellular
and strong antibody responses. Since cytokines from each cell type can cross-regulate each other, whether particular cytokines might influence the CD8$^+$ cell anti-
HIV activity was evaluated. In these studies, CD8$^+$ cells were stimulated in the presence of various cytokines. The effect of these cytokine-treated CD8$^+$ cells on
HIV-infected CD4$^+$ target cells was then assessed. The studies demonstrated that
the type 1 cytokines (e.g., IL-2) increased the CD8$^+$ cell antiviral activity whereas
the type 2 cytokines (e.g., IL-4 and IL-10) suppressed the CD8$^+$ cell antiviral activity (Figure 11.9) (138, 1297). IL-12 showed no effect. The results reflected the importance of IL-2 for this response. IL-4 and IL-10 down-modulate IL-2 production

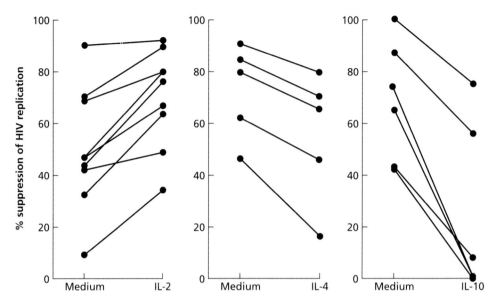

Figure 11.9 Effect of cytokines on the CD8$^+$ cell noncytotoxic anti-HIV response. CD8$^+$ cells were stimulated in the presence of type 1 or type 2 cytokines for 3 days. After being washed, they were tested for their ability to suppress HIV replication in acutely infected CD4$^+$ lymphocytes. (From reference 138 with permission.)

(138, 2324). IL-4 can also decrease the expression of the CD28 molecule (1574), which is involved in this response (136) (see below). IL-10 can decrease B7 expression on APC (2882) and thereby reduce the costimulatory process involved in activating CD8$^+$ cell function (see below). These observations indicate how cytokines can influence this antiviral response. Similar observations have been made with CTL activity: type 1 and not type 2 responses have correlated in vivo with strong CTL activity (2826). The potential role of these cellular factors in pathogenesis and long-term survival is discussed in Chapter 13.

2. CD28 COSTIMULATION

In further studies examining the reduction in CD8$^+$ cell noncytotoxic anti-HIV activity over time, the importance of costimulation via the CD28 molecule in maintaining CD8$^+$ cell function was evaluated. The lymphocyte response is optimal when stimulation occurs both through the TCR interaction with antigen within the MHC molecule and through the interaction of the CD28 molecule with the B7 molecule on APC (e.g., macrophages and dendritic cells) (for reviews, see references 1559 and 2211). This effect appears to be mediated by increased IL-2 production and expression of the IL-2 receptor (Figure 11.10) (387, 1946). It involves the transcription of the IL-2 gene through the activation of an enhancer element within the IL-2 promoter (790a). The process appears to involve the NF-κB pathway (1009).

When CD8$^+$ cells from HIV-infected individuals were stimulated in the presence of macrophages, their noncytotoxic antiviral response was markedly increased (136). When an agonist for B7 (e.g., CTLA-4 immunoglobin) was added to the cul-

Figure 11.10 Costimulation of CD8$^+$ T cells. The lymphocyte response is optimal following the interaction of the TCR with an MHC class I molecule associated with antigen, together with the interaction of the CD28 molecule on the T cells with the B7 molecule on APC (e.g., macrophages and dendritic cells). The response appears to be mediated by increased IL-2 production and expression of the IL-2 receptor (IL-2R) (387, 1946).

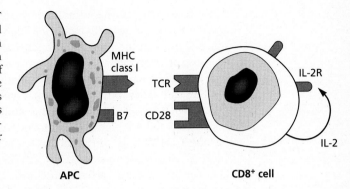

ture, activity was abrogated. When antibodies to IL-2 were added, a similar inhibition of the enhanced antiviral response was noted. The CD28 costimulation also increased IL-2 receptor expression on the cell surface. These latter results supported those of earlier studies indicating the importance of IL-2 for this CD8$^+$ cell antiviral suppressing activity (138) (Figure 11.9). Subsequent studies demonstrated that the use of anti-CD28 antibodies increased CD8$^+$ cell noncytotoxic responses in both asymptomatic and AIDS patients (Figure 11.11). Once again, this costimulation was mediated by IL-2 (136). The findings underline potential approaches for immune therapy in HIV infection (see Chapter 14).

In studies with infected CD4$^+$ cells, CD28 costimulation increased endogenous production of HIV (2526), but this observation was strain specific (SI and not NSI

Figure 11.11 When CD8$^+$ cells are stimulated in the presence of antibodies to the TCR complex (anti-CD3 antibody [Ab]) together with the costimulatory molecule CD28, their ability to suppress HIV replication in infected CD4$^+$ cells is increased in asymptomatic individuals and particularly in AIDS patients (progressors). (From reference 136 with permission.)

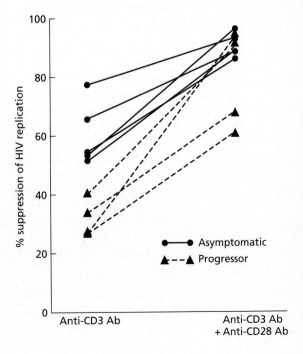

type) (1486). The reason for this finding could be that the observation of CD3:CD28 costimulation of CD4$^+$ cells blocks infection of cells with NSI but not SI strains, presumably through the production of chemokines (2231a) and down-regulation of CCR-5 expression (369). Whether a comparable activation event in vivo would produce a relatively resistant cellular state merits further study. However, the interaction of CD28 antibodies with CD4$^+$ cells has presented conflicting results on the relative infection of these cells by HIV. In some studies, infection by NSI as well as SI viruses is enhanced and not blocked (137a). For example, in a recent study, stimulation of memory CD4$^+$ T cells with antibodies to CD3 and CD28 blocked replication in naive CD4$^+$ T cells, but not memory CD4$^+$ T cells (2263). The issue needs further evaluation. Finally, low CD4$^+$ cell responses to CD28 costimulation also appear predictive of advancement to disease (2276). The finding could reflect the decrease in CD28$^+$ cells noted in infected individuals over time (see also Chapter 3).

D.   Superinfection

Another finding related to CD8$^+$ cells that potentially affects the clinical outcome is the resistance of PBMC from asymptomatic individuals to superinfection by other strains of HIV-1. Despite the known presence of many uninfected CD4$^+$ cells in their cultured PBMC, no acute infection by NSI or SI viruses can take place unless the CD8$^+$ cells are first removed (137, 1239). HIV enters and integrates but is not produced by the infected cells (137). CD8$^+$ cells prevent the superinfected PBMC from releasing virus. With PBMC from symptomatic patients, superinfection can be demonstrated. The replication of both the endogenous and exogenous viruses by these PBMC reflects the absence of a strong CD8$^+$ cell antiviral response (137).

E.   Animal Studies

This CD8$^+$ cell noncytotoxic antiviral activity has been demonstrated as well in the SIV system with rhesus macaques (1238, 2136) and sooty mangabeys (2136) and in HIV-infected chimpanzees (374, 1143) and naturally infected chimpanzees (1279). It has also been observed in HIV-2-infected baboons (225). CD8$^+$ cell suppression of feline immunodeficiency virus replication has been described as well (1199). These animal models may provide approaches for further evaluation of this antiviral response. It is noteworthy that a similar type of noncytotoxic suppression of virus expression has been described for hepatitis B virus antigens in transgenic mice. The CTL function through secretion of TNF-α and IFN-γ (964). Finally, most recently, the possibility that allo-stimulated lymphocytes have a similar noncytotoxic suppressing activity of HIV replication has been reported (302). A soluble mediator was found to inhibit HIV replication (2467a). Its relevance to the antiviral factor produced by CD8$^+$ cells from infected individuals is under study.

F.   Mechanism of CD8$^+$ Cell Antiviral Activity: the CD8$^+$ Cell Antiviral Factor

How CD8$^+$ cells suppress HIV infection has been investigated. Suppression appears to take place before RNA transcription (1632). Naturally infected CD4$^+$ cells, when mixed with CD8$^+$ cells, have a marked reduction in viral protein and RNA synthesis. However, at the time of suppression, the number of infected CD4$^+$ cells re-

Figure 11.12 Quantity of CAF produced by CD8$^+$ cells. Dilutions of CAF-containing fluid from cultured CD8$^+$ cells from an asymptomatic individual indicate that a 1:4 dilution will still show a 50% reduction in HIV replication as measured by reverse transcriptase (RT) activity in the culture fluid. Fluids from CD8$^+$ cells of normal individuals or those with AIDS do not show evidence of CAF production.

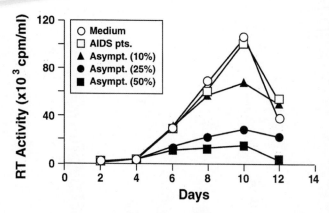

maining in the culture is almost equal to that in control cultures. Thus, no loss of infected cells takes place, whereas virus expression is reduced. Recently, the block in HIV infection has been shown not to affect early steps in reverse transcription or integration (1636a). CD4$^+$ cells transfected with a long terminal repeat:chloramphenicol acetyltransferase (LTR:CAT) construct have also shown suppression of CAT production by this CD8$^+$ cell response (415, 516, 1463a). These findings support an effect of the CD8$^+$ cells on virus transcription.

A soluble factor produced by the CD8$^+$ cells is involved at least in part in this CD8$^+$ cell anti-HIV response (287, 2811). Cell-to-cell contact, however, is the most efficient method for suppressing HIV production. Whether it reflects a different antiviral mechanism is under study. The presence of this CD8$^+$ cell antiviral factor (now called CAF) can be shown by adding supernatants from CD8$^+$ cell cultures directly onto infected CD4$^+$ cells (1629, 2812). Virus replication is substantially reduced without any effect on cell viability or proliferation. Nevertheless, the amount of CAF produced by CD8$^+$ cells is small; only up to a 25% dilution will still show 50% reduction of HIV replication (Figure 11.12). The level of CAF produced correlates with the clinical state (1629, 2811). The highest production is by CD8$^+$ cells cultured from healthy individuals with high CD4$^+$ cell counts.

CAF blocks viral transcription, as has been described for the coculture system with CD8$^+$ cells (1632) (Figure 11.13). In some studies, the factor has reduced CAT expression mediated by the LTR from HTLV and Rous sarcoma virus (516). Similar findings in the SIV system with rhesus macaque CD8$^+$ cells (2135) also suggest that the antiviral activity involves an effect by CD8$^+$ cells on LTR transcription. In other studies, CD8$^+$ cell culture fluids added to 1G5 cells, a Jurkat T-cell line carrying the HIV LTR linked to the luciferase reporter gene, suppressed luciferase production induced by HIV-1 (1630) and a simian virus 40 (SV40) *tat* construct (1515). The affected site in the LTR could be NFAT-1 and/or NF-κB, depending on whether the LTR is activated by Tat or by mitogen, respectively (516, 517).

By function and antigenic features, CAF lacks identity to other cytokines, including the IFNs, TNF, and the chemokines (288, 1631, 1634, 1635) (see below and Tables 9.5 and 11.8 for the cytokines evaluated). The known characteristics of CAF are listed in Table 11.9. It is a small protein that is heat stable and pH resistant. The identification and complete characterization of this novel lymphokine and the elucidation of its function are under study.

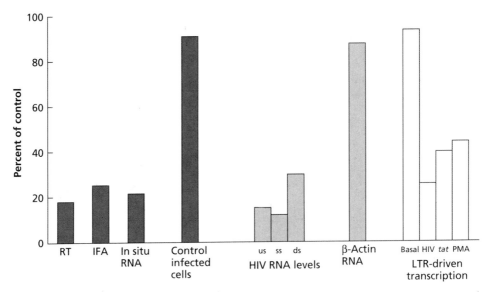

Figure 11.13   Effect of CD8$^+$ cells or CAF on parameters of HIV replication. The CD8$^+$ cell noncytotoxic antiviral response blocks viral replication, as indicated by decreased reverse transcriptase (RT) activity, viral protein expression measured by immunofluorescent antibody (IFA) techniques, and in situ RNA production. This activity has no effect on the number of infected cells in the culture. The antiviral effect is observed as well by reduction in unspliced (us), single-spliced (ss), and double-spliced (ds) HIV RNA levels compared to a normal expression of β-actin RNA. Finally, the suppressing effect of CD8$^+$ cells or CAF does not affect the basal-level expression of HIV LTR-driven transcription but blocks induction of this transcription by HIV, an SV40 *tat* construct, or phorbol myristate acetate (PMA) using cells in which the HIV LTR has been linked to a reporter gene (1632).

G. Antiviral Activity of Chemokines

In attempts to define the nature of the antiviral factor, investigators have examined cytokines produced by CD8$^+$ cells. One in vitro study identified three β-chemokines, RANTES, MIP-1α, and MIP-1β, as important anti-HIV factors produced by CD8$^+$ cells that do not kill the infected cells (487). Chemokines are a family of structurally related proteins that induce migration of specific subsets of leukocytes to sites in the body and are involved in the generation of cellular inflammation (15, 1985) (see Chapter 3, Table 3.2). These chemoattractant cytokines are also made by a large number of cell types that are sensitive to HIV infection, including CD4$^+$ lymphocytes, NK cells, and macrophages (15, 1985).

Cell culture studies with the β-chemokines have indicated that they can act individually in blocking HIV replication, but the presence of all three at amounts ranging from 500 pg to 500 ng is most effective (487, 1633a). The block appears to take place at the cell surface by competitive inhibition of the viral envelope protein for the β-chemokine receptor, CCR-5 (see Chapter 3). These cellular proteins do not block viral LTR transcription (1473, 1633a), which is suppressed by CAF (1632). Differences in virus sensitivity to these cytokines can be observed.

Table 11.8 Cytokines lacking identity to CAF

IL-1 to IL-13, IL-15, IL-16

TNF-α, TNF-β

IFN-α, IFN-β, IFN-γ

TGF-β

GM-CSF

G-CSF

RANTES

MIP-1α, MIP-1β

MCP-1, MCP-2, MCP-3

GRO-α, GRO-β

LIF

IP-10

Lymphotactin

Macrophage-tropic NSI viruses are sensitive, and T-cell-line-tropic viruses are not (487, 1187, 1631). The variance can be explained by the fact that only the NSI viruses use CCR-5 for virus entry (see Chapter 3). In addition, the NSI strains can differ in their relative sensitivity to the β-chemokines (i.e., 500 pg to 500 ng) (1633a). The reason for this finding is not known.

The clinical relevance of the β-chemokines in preventing disease progression has been questioned (1187, 1630), because NSI as well as SI viruses can be found in individuals progressing to AIDS. Moreover, no significant difference has been found in levels of chemokine production by activated CD8$^+$ cells from HIV-infected individuals regardless of their clinical state (231, 470, 1630, 2301). Likewise, whereas higher levels of chemokines were produced by CD4$^+$ cells from infected individuals than by those from uninfected individuals, no relation to the clinical condition was found (470, 1630). In addition, endogenous production of HIV or acute infection by HIV does not substantially change the kinetics of chemokine production by the CD4$^+$ cells. In general, high levels of chemokines are produced shortly after stimulation and then low levels are made until day 10 to 13 of culture, when moderate amounts can be detected (up to 4 ng/ml) (1630). Based on the evidence

Table 11.9 Characteristics of the CD8$^+$ CAF

1. Produced only by activated CD8$^+$ T cells
2. Active against HIV-1, HIV-2 and SIV
3. Resistant to trypsin; sensitive to *Staphylococcus* V8 protease
4. Lacks identity with other known cytokines
5. Blocks HIV replication in naturally and acutely infected CD4$^+$ cells
6. Blocks HIV replication by inhibiting LTR-driven transcription
7. Does not affect CD4$^+$ cell activation or proliferation
8. Stable at high temperature
9. Stable at low pH

that 5 ng or more of chemokines is generally needed for an antiviral effect, the lack of an influence of β-chemokine production on endogenous virus replication in CD4$^+$ cells is not unexpected (1630, 2301). Furthermore, chemokine production appears to be increased following acute infection of CD4$^+$ cells with NSI strains and decreased after infection with SI strains (1630). This result does not support a clinical antiviral role of the β-chemokines that act only on NSI viruses (Table 11.10). Finally, levels of β-chemokines in serum do not distinguish patients with AIDS from asymptomatic individuals (1735, 2962).

The production of CAF by CD8$^+$ cells appears to be most important in controlling HIV infection. High levels of the β-chemokines do not affect acute infection of CD4$^+$ cells by SI strains, but both SI and NSI strains are sensitive to CAF. Moreover, infection of dendritic cells with NSI or SI strains is not inhibited by the β-chemokines (2301). Furthermore, when CD8$^+$ cells are cultured with CD4$^+$ cells infected by either SI or NSI subtypes, neutralizing antibodies to the β-chemokines do not block the suppression of HIV replication (136, 416, 1298, 2022, 2301). In addition, neutralizing antibodies to the β-chemokines do not affect the antiviral activity of CAF-containing fluids in CD4$^+$ lymphocytes (1473, 1631) and macrophages (136a). All these findings indicate that CAF is not a chemokine and that CAF is the major cellular factor inhibiting HIV replication. Nevertheless, when antibodies to the chemokines were added to cultured, stimulated, naturally infected CD4$^+$ lymphocytes, there was a shorter period before virus replication began in these cells (1298, 1630, 2301). Since other cytokines, such as TNF-α and IFN-β, might increase virus production in CD4$^+$ lymphocytes, a balance in the production of these various cellular factors could determine the extent of HIV replication in infected individuals (1298). Nevertheless, the findings do not support a role of β-chemokines in vivo in influencing HIV infection (1630) (Table 11.10).

In the search to identify CAF, another group cited IL-16 as a potential anti-HIV factor (127). The identification of IL-16, another chemokine-like protein, was made because of its known interaction with CD4 (545). Thus, a block of HIV at the cell surface might be expected. However, other studies with purified recombinant IL-16 and antibodies to IL-16 have demonstrated that human CD8$^+$ cells do not make a sufficient amount of this chemokine to block HIV replication. Furthermore, neutralizing antibodies to IL-16 do not affect the antiviral effects of CAF (1634). Finally, levels of IL-16 production by CD8$^+$ cells do not differ among HIV-infected individuals in different clinical states (231).

In summary, based on several observations in the laboratory, CAF is neither IL-16 nor a β-chemokine, and these latter substances, released by CD4$^+$ and CD8$^+$

Table 11.10 Evidence for a lack of clinical relevance of β-chemokines in HIV infection

1. Production of β-chemokines does not correlate with the clinical state.
2. Sensitivity of HIV strains to β-chemokines is strictly related to the biological phenotype (NSI) and not the clinical state; AIDS patients have NSI viruses which are β-chemokine sensitive.
3. Production of β-chemokines by naturally infected CD4$^+$ cells is not affected by HIV production.
4. Production of β-chemokines is increased following acute infection with NSI strains and decreased or not affected following infection with SI strains.

cells (505), do not appear to play a major role in vivo in controlling HIV replication (Table 11.10).

IV.   Cell-Mediated Antiviral Immune Responses in Uninfected, HIV-Exposed High-Risk Individuals

A variety of studies have been published suggesting that some individuals were exposed to infectious virus or viral antigens but have not had an established infection (see also Chapters 9 and 13). The high-risk exposed people include sexual partners of infected individuals, intravenous drug users, children born of infected mothers, and health care workers with needlestick injuries (176, 437, 472, 473, 475, 482, 1262, 2098, 2183; for reviews, see references 2297 and 2470). In a few subjects, the absence of the viral coreceptor (e.g., CCR-5) has been noted (607, 2346), but the possible presence of anti-HIV immune responses in these individuals has not yet been reported. HIV antigen-specific production of IL-2 by PBMC can be demonstrated in some high-risk uninfected subjects (176, 482, 1262). In one study, the pattern of the TCR repertoire appeared to reflect a response to HIV but without infection (201). In other studies, CTL responses to HIV epitopes have been observed in exposed, uninfected adults (201, 1426, 2296) and in children born to HIV-1-infected mothers (437, 592, 2296). Finally, antibodies to HLA proteins shared by the HIV envelope have also been noted in high-risk uninfected people (176).

We have noted CD8$^+$ cell noncytotoxic anti-HIV activity in 27 of 54 high-risk adults (sexual partners of infected individuals) (2601a) (Figure 11.14) and in 19 of 31 HIV-negative infants born to HIV-positive mothers (1491, 1511a). Most dramatic was the finding of CD8$^+$ cell antiviral responses in an uninfected monozy-

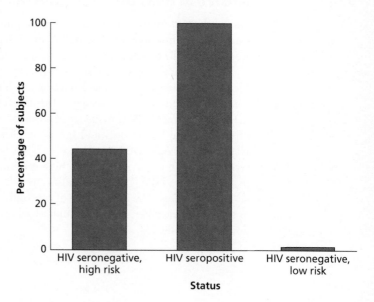

Figure 11.14 CD8$^+$ cell noncytotoxic antiviral response in high-risk uninfected individuals. In a study of more than 50 high-risk adults (sexual partners of infected individuals), up to 50% showed evidence of CD8$^+$ cell HIV-suppressing activity that could not be detected in normal low-risk individuals (2601a). This activity, as noted in the text, is found in all asymptomatic infected individuals. (Figure courtesy of S. Stranford.)

gotic twin whose sister was infected by HIV (1491). Evidently, both twins were exposed to viral antigens and mounted cellular immune responses, but only one twin had established infection. Whether the other twin warded off the infection or was exposed to an amount of infectious virus too small to establish infection is not known.

These observations on the subjects studied have been considered potential evidence that a predominant type 1 immune response occurred after exposure to HIV, and that infectious virus was eliminated by cellular immune activity before the infection was widespread and before antiviral antibodies were produced. Alternatively, perhaps insufficient viral antigens were presented to the host so that an antibody response was not elicited.

This possibility has been evaluated in preliminary experiments with two rhesus monkeys originally inoculated with low doses of SIV. Antibodies to the virus were not produced, but the proliferative responses of cultured T cells to SIV antigens were noted. These animals were then challenged with low doses of infectious SIV. In contrast to control animals, which were infected only once, these preexposed monkeys were protected (471). This preliminary evidence suggests that the two animals had a response that prevented SIV infection. Similarly, multiple exposures to viral antigens or to low-dose infectious virus might boost the cellular immune response and thus prevent an established infection. For this reason, antibodies are not produced. If this concept proves correct, vaccines containing low antigen doses could be useful (see Chapter 15) (2343).

Recently, IgA antibodies to HIV have been detected in urine and vaginal secretions of some high-risk uninfected individuals. IgA antibodies in some sera neutralized primary isolates (1703a). These findings of solely an IgA response are surprising and require confirmation. If confirmed, whether HIV is present undetected in tissues in these people will require further study.

V. Antiviral Responses at Mucosal Surfaces

One of the first indications that antiviral responses could be present in the vaginal canal came from studies of CTL in SIV infection (1580). SIV-specific precursor CTL from chronically infected monkeys and from acutely infected animals were found at higher frequency at this site. Likewise, virus-specific CTL have been recovered from the small intestines of SIV-infected macaques. Similar studies of HIV have not been completed, but recent results suggest that infected women might have CTL activity in the genital tract (1883). Evidence of humoral responses has also been found in the cervical/vaginal region. IgG and IgA antibodies to the envelope protein for both HIV-1 and HIV-2 have been found (86). IgA was more prominent in cervical secretions than in the blood and had high specific activity, suggesting local synthesis of antibodies to HIV (162). Antibodies have also been found in nasal (86) and rectal (1805) washes. The importance of mucosal immunity against HIV, particularly in relation to vaccines, has been emphasized (1762) and merits further consideration (see Chapter 15).

1. The cell-mediated immune response is generally the first immunologic reaction to a viral infection. In HIV infection, cytotoxic NK cells can kill virus-infected cells in a non-MHC-directed manner. Nonspecific killing can also occur via PMN directly or through ADCC.

2. CD4$^+$ cells respond to HIV infection through production of cytokines. These cells can be separated into type 1 and type 2 subgroups, depending on the pattern of cytokine release: e.g., IL-2 and IFN-γ for type 1 response, and IL-4 and IL-10 for type 2 response. Generally, type 1 responses are associated with strong cell-mediated immunity.

3. CD4$^+$ cytotoxic cells can also kill virus-infected or uninfected cells through perforin secretion or the induction of apoptosis.

4. Cytotoxic CD8$^+$ cells have been identified that react to a variety of viral peptides representing structural or regulatory gene products but primarily to the Gag and Env proteins. This response can be mirrored in the diversity of the T-cell population as measured by the TCR repertoire. Clonal or oligoclonal responses may indicate the inability of the host to respond to new foreign antigens.

5. The clinical relevance of CD8$^+$ CTL is still not certain. A stable level of effector CTL can be found even as individuals progress to disease, but a loss of CTL precursors (CTLp) appears to occur and may have clinical relevance. Some data suggest that CTL may play a detrimental role in HIV infection.

6. HIV may escape CTL killing by changes within the epitope recognized by CTL, by inducing anergy in the CD8$^+$ cells, by masking the epitope through alterations in peptide structure, or through down-regulation of MHC expression.

7. CD8$^+$ cells can control virus replication through a noncytotoxic mechanism involving a block in virus transcription. Suppression of virus replication is mediated in part by a CD8$^+$ cell antiviral factor (CAF). CAF lacks identity to all known cytokines, including the chemokines.

8. The CD8$^+$ cell noncytotoxic antiviral response correlates with the clinical state. It is strong in asymptomatic individuals and is lost with progression to disease. It is active against all types of HIV-1, HIV-2, and SIV isolates. This activity depends on IL-2 production.

9. Costimulation through CD28 can increase the CD8$^+$ cell noncytotoxic response and CAF production. This costimulation of CD4$^+$ cells has shown differential effects on HIV replication.

10. Chemokines show anti-HIV activity by blocking virus replication at entry. β-Chemokines suppress only certain types of HIV strains (i.e., NSI viruses). There is no correlation of β-chemokine production with clinical state.

11. Some cell-mediated anti-HIV responses can be detected in high-risk uninfected individuals, suggesting exposure to the virus without established infection.

12. Antiviral antibodies and CTL can be detected in secretions from mucosal surfaces.

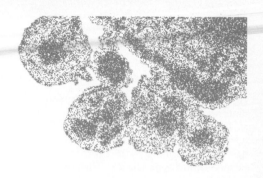

HIV Infection and Development of Cancer

12

I. Introduction

The development of malignancies is not unexpectedly associated with the immune system disorders caused by HIV infection. However, the finding that certain types of cancer (Kaposi's sarcoma [KS], B-cell lymphoma, and probably anal carcinomas) show an increased prevalence in HIV-infected individuals has led to an emphasis in elucidating their etiology (for reviews, see references 1617 and 2172). The first two cancers involve cells of the immune system: endothelial cells and B cells. Endothelial cells have characteristics of immune cells since they express Fc and C3 receptors and can also act as accessory cells in lymphocyte activation (92, 126).

In attempts to find a common link among these malignancies, the possibility of infectious agents has been raised. Cytomegalovirus (CMV), human papillomavirus (HPV), and hepatitis B virus have all been associated with KS (for a review, see reference 2291). None has been proved to be the direct cause. Recently, a new human herpesvirus, HHV-8, appears to be linked to this malignancy (see below). Epstein-Barr virus (EBV) has been found in up to 60% of B-cell lymphomas and in all lymphomas primary to the central nervous system (CNS) (1639, 2488, 2489). Nevertheless, although EBV appears to induce B-cell proliferation, it may not play a direct role in transformation (see below). Furthermore, HHV-8 has been

285

Figure 12.1   Tumor development appears to be a multistep phenomenon. A variety of agents can initiate the process, which is then promoted often by cellular products such as cytokines or hormones. Finally, a transforming event occurs which generally involves chromosome changes. This last event can be induced directly by virus.

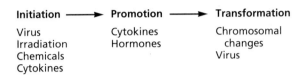

Initiation	⟶	Promotion	⟶	Transformation
Virus		Cytokines		Chromosomal
Irradiation		Hormones		changes
Chemicals				Virus
Cytokines				

found to be associated with lymphomas of the body cavity (see below) (388, 1344). Finally, HPV has been linked to carcinomas in the anus and the cervix. The development of malignancy in HIV infection could involve three distinct steps (initiation, promotion, and transformation) (Figure 12.1). A variety of factors could initiate the malignant process by causing disturbances in the immune or other organ systems. In the case of virus infection, the subsequent induction of cytokine (or hormone) production by the immune system could promote an increased proliferation of the target cell (i.e., endothelium, B cell, or epithelial cell). Finally, a clastogenic event leads to autonomous cell growth or transformation (1498) (Figures 12.1 and 12.2). Subsequently, the host immune system could influence the expression of these neoplasms. In some cases, a virus itself could be the transforming agent, but most evidence thus far suggests that viruses play a promoter role.

A leading hypothesis to explain the cancers associated with HIV infection is that immune suppression prevents the proper immune surveillance and inhibition of virus replication or growth of transformed cells. Another possibility linking immune disorders to cancer is that the malignancies take place secondary to the abnormal secretion of high levels of certain cytokines. These cellular factors would be

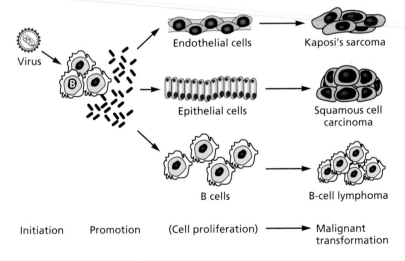

Figure 12.2   Potential role of viruses in induction of malignant disease. Virus can infect host cells, and in the case presented, immune cell cytokine production is induced that promotes the proliferation of certain target cells (e.g., endothelial, epithelial, or B cells). With increased replication of cells, other factors can cause chromosome changes leading to autonomous growth and malignant transformation. (Adapted from reference 1498, with permission.)

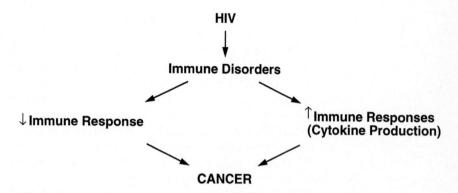

Figure 12.3 HIV infection and cancer development. HIV infection can lead to immune disorders that result in either an increase or a decrease in immune responses. Both processes could be involved in cancer development.

produced by hyperresponding cells resulting from the disrupted balance in the immune system. They could induce cell proliferation and perhaps virus activation (1498, 1522). Some lymphokines, for example, have angiogenesis-promoting activity and could be linked to KS development (103, 706, 1935).

The cancers in HIV infection could thus result from either depression or enhancement of the immune system. In any case, a disorder in the immune system is tantamount to the development of certain malignancies found in this infection, as it is for opportunistic infections and other clinical conditions in the host (Figure 12.3). One common observation is that cancers developing in the presence of HIV infection are much more aggressive than those found in noninfected patients (1617). Thus, immunologic response appears to be important in controlling the progression of cancer.

As individuals are living longer with HIV infection, other malignancies may eventually appear with increased prevalence. In this regard, the incidence of AIDS-associated neoplasms, more so than that of opportunistic infection, appears to increase with age (2771). An increase in other cancers has been suggested, such as Hodgkin's disease, multiple myelomas, and seminomas (1617) and leiomyomas and leiomyosarcomas in HIV-infected children (391). In the neoplasms involving the latter tissues, EBV may be involved (1705). The suggested increase in multiple myelomas may reflect an activation of HHV-8 and the induction of cell proliferation (2218) (see below). In this chapter, I will review studies of the four cancers frequently associated with HIV infection and comment briefly on other tumors that could become more prominent in the HIV-infected host.

II.   Kaposi's Sarcoma

A.   Introduction

KS, first reported by the Hungarian physician Moritz Kaposi in 1872 (1240), is a well-demarcated, angioproliferative, often multifocal malignancy that is usually observed in men over the age of 50, particularly those from Eastern Europe and the Mediterranean region (634, 917, 1378, 2992) (Color Plate 13, following p. 188). As the endemic type, it is found frequently in sub-Saharan Africa, at times in an aggressive form, and in men more often than in women, at relatively young ages (1378, 2291, 2992). Unless it is the aggressive form, KS rarely kills the affected person; it remains confined to the skin of the extremities, usually the feet (1378, 2992). For this reason, several groups have considered KS a benign tumor, at least in its initial stages (533, 1522). As noted above, its emergence, usually in cutaneous areas of the body, has been considered a reflection of overall disease expression (i.e., multifocal) and not metastasis (917, 1378, 2992). However, the latter conclusion has recently been reexamined (Section II.B).

With its increased prevalence in young HIV-infected men, KS received new attention (800, 917, 1675). Moreover, in virus-infected patients, KS presents as a more aggressive disease, with both mucocutaneous and visceral involvement (2992).

B. Pathology

The histopathology of KS is complex. The tumor can be divided into four histologic subtypes: nodular, florid, infiltrative, and lymphadenopathic (2327). These subtypes reflect the relative malignancy of the lesion, which appears to have an angiomatous origin. The skin tumors, especially in the early stage, consist of a mixture of cells. The KS lesions often have spaces lined by capillary endothelium with the cells appearing activated or atypical, not unlike vessels in an inflammatory milieu (Color Plate 14, following p. 188). More advanced tumors consist of spindle-shaped cells. The histologic range of endothelial cells, spindle cells, and inflammatory cells within the lesions may account for the controversy surrounding the actual cell of origin (2290, 2291).

Several other cell types besides endothelial cells are prominent in the KS lesions, including macrophages, dendritic cells, mast cells, and fibroblasts. Lymph nodes with KS lesions often contain a considerable number of plasma cells (1987). Conceivably, these cells are under cytokine control (e.g., interleukin-6 [IL-6]), as are perhaps the KS cells (1522, 1784) (Sections II.C and II.F).

As noted above, the origin of the cells characterizing the KS lesion is not conclusive. Many researchers link the endothelium to KS (159, 320, 1897, 2291, 2309). In some studies, the tumors are considered to be derived from the vascular endothelium (320, 1566, 2291) and in others the lymphatic endothelium (159) (for reviews, see references 2290 and 2291). Others have suggested that smooth muscle cells (37) and the dermal dendrocytes (1926) are the cells of origin. In this latter case, the properties of the cells could be those shared by macrophages.

The studies on defining the origin of KS have used antibodies to antigens expressed on specific cell types, including Factor VIII, Factor XIIIa, HLA-DR, and CD68, as well as binding to *Ulex europeus* and uptake of low-density lipoproteins. The results indicate that KS represents a proliferation of a heterogeneous population of cells, predominantly of the endothelial type but also with other spindle/dendritic cells (Factor XIIIa and CD68$^+$), macrophages, and mast cells. Whether these other cells contain an agent that stimulates the proliferation of the endothelial spindle cells and thus the development of KS is an important consideration. In sum-

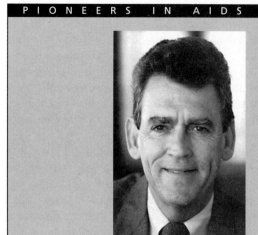

Marcus A. Conant
Clinical Professor, Department of Dermatology, University of California, San Francisco. Dr. Conant was among the first to recognize the presence of Kaposi's sarcoma associated with AIDS and has played an important role in defining antiviral therapies.

mary, most data support the hypothesis that this neoplasm originates from endothelium and that it is most probably of vascular origin (2291).

Recent genetic analyses of multiple lesions from the same patients have suggested that KS results from the dissemination of monoclonal spindle cells (2171). In this regard, spindle cells can be cultured from the blood of HIV-infected KS patients (301) and have been found positive for HHV-8 (224a, 2517) (Section II.E). The findings on clonality counter previous views that this tumor is multifocal and that different lesions on a patient do not reflect metastases (917, 1378, 2992). This issue will certainly be addressed in future studies.

C. Role of the Immune System

The occurrence of both classic KS and HIV-associated KS appears to reflect in part an immune suppression in the host (2802). The presence of high levels of antibodies to known viruses such as EBV and CMV in HIV-infected KS patients supports the presence of defects in cellular immune regulation. Moreover, in classic Mediterranean KS, this tumor occurs in men with increasing age and has been found to be associated with immune abnormalities (1693). The high prevalence of this cancer in immunosuppressed individuals being treated for kidney transplants (1029, 2070) also supports the importance of immune control in this malignancy (1522, 1693). In addition, if the immunosuppressive therapy is withdrawn, the KS lesions disappear (1029). A direct relationship of KS with immunologic dysfunction, however, is controversial (2290); some patients with endemic KS show no detectable immune disorder (1278).

The explanations for the potential role of the immune system in KS can be quite diverse. For instance, in transplant recipients, the restoration of immune balance could result in rejection of the tumor by an active immune system. Alternatively, the stimulus (e.g., cytokine production) for endothelial cell growth or "KS cell" replication in the patients could be eliminated once immune equilibrium is reached.

This latter possibility is based on the hypothesis that a deficiency in one arm of the immune system may lead to enhancement of the response by another part of the immune system (1522). KS could then be like a hormone-dependent tumor induced through immune enhancement (1522). Upon stimulation by certain angiogenesis-promoting cytokines (103, 1935), the normal endothelial cells (the suspected cells of origin for KS) would replicate continuously (Figure 12.2). In support of an immune system-based pathology is the observation that KS cells can die by apoptosis, suggesting an effect of cytokines on the tumor. The potential cytolytic effect of a productive virus infection should also be considered (Section II.E).

KS cells, although perhaps initially benign (533, 1522), might, if persistently stimulated, undergo karyotypic changes with mutations that establish a stable transformed state. Thus, KS lesions would appear in many parts of the body and, depending on the chromosome changes, could be relatively benign or frankly malignant. In support of this idea, KS lesions at different stages of transformation have been observed in the same HIV-infected individual (1508a, 2992). Moreover, the classic Mediterranean form is usually relatively benign (2992). In a sense, the induction of this malignancy by such a process of cytokine production could resemble the role of EBV in some B-cell lymphomas (711). The virus induces cell proliferation, and in some cases, these replicating activated B cells may evolve into lymphomas (Section III).

In summary, the finding of KS in HIV-infected patients (800, 1029, 1693, 2070) is consistent with the emergence of this cancer in individuals with immune disorders. Moreover, the involvement of other tissues besides the skin reflects the extensive immunocompromised state in AIDS (1378, 2992). However, whether the lesion results directly from an infectious agent, spontaneous growth in an immunocompromised host, or excessive stimulation by cytokines of certain cells in the immune system (e.g., lymphatic or vascular endothelium) is not well defined.

D.   Epidemiology

The geographical distribution of KS varies in different parts of the world and even within Africa (2988). It is most prevalent in men in the countries of Eastern Europe and around the Mediterranean basin and sporadically occurs in parts of North America and elsewhere. While present at higher frequency in homosexual men with HIV infection (see below), the overall prevalence in other populations can be equally distributed between men and women (955). In regions where KS is not endemic, KS develops in organ transplant recipients at a 400 to 500-fold greater rate than in the general population (207, 2069, 2082).

KS occurs in about 20% of HIV-infected men (2082) and in approximately 2% of infected transfusion recipients, hemophiliacs, and women in the United States. It has declined in prevalence in the cohort of infected homosexual and bisexual men observed in San Francisco from 1981 to 1989 (1253, 1540) and in other groups studied (174), presumably owing to a change in sexual practices. Transfer of an infectious agent is inferred. Nevertheless, this reduction in cases has not been observed in all cohorts (2082). Transfusion recipients with AIDS are three times more likely to have KS than are those individuals receiving blood via clotting factor concentrates (Table 12.1) (2082). Transfusion has also been associated with KS develop-

Table 12.1 Relationship of HIV transmission group and gender to the percentage of adult AIDS patients in the United States with KS[a]

HIV transmission group	Sex	No. of patients with KS/total no.	% with KS
Homosexual or bisexual	M	24,160/122,170	19.8
Homosexual or bisexual and injecting drug user	M	2,244/13,094	17.1
Born in Caribbean or Africa	M	110/1,849	6.0
	F	27/41	3.6
Heterosexual partner of person born in Caribbean or Africa	M	6/97	6.2
	F	4/78	5.1
Injecting drug user	M	909/33,276	2.7
	F	192/10,608	1.8
Blood transfusion	M	98/2,689	3.6
	F	35/1,647	2.1
Hemophilia	M	19/1,717	1.1

[a] Reprinted from reference 2082 with permission.

ment in women, but the risk is much lower than that associated with sexual contact (Table 12.2). Since hemophiliacs do not have a high prevalence of this disease (Table 12.1) (2170), a KS-inducing agent (if present in the blood) must be cell associated or inactivated by the clotting factor processes (2082). In this case, a herpesvirus would be a plausible etiologic agent (Section II.E).

Cases of KS in children are rare, except in the setting of endemic KS in Africa. It is noteworthy that one infant with this cancer was described in Kaposi's initial report (1240). In general, KS in an HIV-infected child is associated with the mother's being in a risk group (2082). In one unusual case, a 6-day-old boy developed AIDS-related KS, although his mother died without evidence of this cancer (972, 2082). Thus, as with other malignancies, the tumor could be clinically silent or expressed only under certain conditions.

HIV-infected individuals who present with KS as their first manifestation of AIDS generally live longer and have a less compromised immune system at onset than those with opportunistic infections (1378). This finding could reflect the path-

Table 12.2 Relation of partner's HIV transmission group to percentage of infected women with KS in the United States[a]

HIV transmission group		No. of women with KS/total no.	% with KS
Woman	Sexual partner		
Heterosexual	Bisexual man	22/852	2.6
	Injecting drug user	40/4,113	1.0
	Transfusion recipient	1/154	0.7
	Hemophiliac	0/98	0
Injecting drug use	Bisexual man	8/173	4.6
	Injecting drug user	27/1,815	1.5

[a] Reprinted from reference 2082 with permission.

ogenesis of this malignancy, which appears when the immune system is not completely suppressed (Section II.C); KS could reflect a response to immune enhancement. As noted above, the disease is characterized by the multifocal appearance of lesions and then spontaneous regressions (2201). This "waxing and waning" of KS lesions supports an influence of the immune system in controlling the emergence and subsequent growth of this tumor (157, 2201) or its causative agent (Sections II.C and II.E).

E.   Etiology

One of the first suggested causes of KS was the use of amyl butyl nitrate inhalants (800, 1034). This drug appears to disturb immune system cells, particularly T cells, perhaps through the production of cytokines that could induce the Kaposi's lesions in the multifocal pattern observed. However, a role of these drugs in this cancer has not been substantiated. An increased frequency of certain HLA-DR5 antigens was found in patients with KS in the New York area (800, 2117). This link to an immune response has not been observed in other cohorts (2291).

Because KS is common in HIV-infected homosexual men (174, 1675), is found on sexual organs (1436), and is prevalent in women with bisexual partners (174, 1436), the possibility that this tumor is a sexually acquired disease has been considered (174, 2290, 2291). Supporting this idea is that adoption of "safe sex" guidelines has correlated with a decrease in incidence of this cancer in HIV-infected individuals (174). Children and heterosexual individuals (including men over the age of 50 years) can develop KS, but the high association of this malignancy with sexual activity (particularly anal receptive intercourse) has suggested the idea that an infectious agent is the cause. These observations imply that the agent might be found in greater quantity in seminal fluid than in blood, although recipients of blood transfusion may also develop KS (Table 12.1) (174, 2083). Oral-fecal contact ("rimming") was initially considered a major risk factor (174, 2082), but this was not confirmed by other studies (1222).

The evaluation of KS biopsy specimens and KS cell lines (Section II.F) revealed no infectious agent for KS (1493, 2290, 2291, 2499) until recently. Whereas CMV was originally linked to this tumor (887) and was found in subsequent studies (1163), evidence for CMV has been lacking in most KS biopsy specimens and tumor-derived cell lines (1493, 2291). In one instance, hepatitis B virus DNA was detected in a tumor (2495), but this finding has not been confirmed. Moreover, a possible role of HPV in KS was proposed (1130, 2431) but not substantiated (206) by other studies. Nevertheless, a recent report suggests that the BK papillomavirus is latent in KS skin lesions and many KS-derived cell lines (1809). A possible role of this agent needs further study. Some investigators have reported the detection of retrovirus-like particles in KS lesions by electron microscopy (977, 2189, 2389) or as HIV-like sequences (1647). These findings need further evaluation but have not been noted in other electron microscopic studies of this tumor (1505a, 2291).

In 1994, Chang et al. (398) identified unique DNA sequences in KS tumors that were closely related to regions of the genome of EBV and herpesvirus saimiri, members of the gammaherpesvirus subfamily (Figure 12.4). The herpesviruses detected in KS lesions in earlier studies (887, 1163) could have been this agent, now called

Figure 12.4 Phylogenetic tree showing the relation of various herpesviruses based on a comparison of aligned amino acid sequences for single genes and combined gene sets. The tree, derived by bootstrap analyses, is shown in unrooted form with branch lengths proportional to the divergence between the nodes binding each branch. HSV, herpes simplex virus; EHV, equine herpesvirus; PRV, pseudorabies virus; VZV, varicella-zoster virus; HCMV, human cytomegalovirus; HVS, herpesvirus saimiri. (Adapted from reference 1500 with permission.)

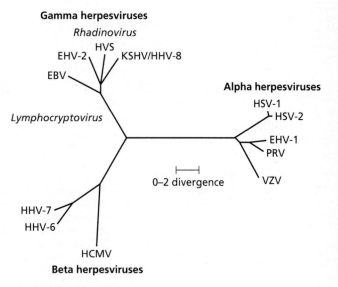

HHV-8 or KS-associated herpesvirus (KSHV). However, immunohistochemistry and in situ hybridization suggested the presence of CMV in these KS lesions. Further studies demonstrated the presence of these herpesvirus-like sequences in nearly all forms of KS in both HIV-infected and uninfected people in various parts of the world (for reviews, see references 1498 and 1500). They were also noted in B-cell lymphomas found in the body cavity (388, 1344), in lymphoid tissue from Castlemen's disease (2540), and most recently in dendritic cells from multiple myeloma patients (2218) (see below). An indirect role of the virus in the induction of multiple myelomas has been linked to production of the viral homolog for IL-6. The association of these herpesvirus-like sequences with an intact virion was demonstrated by phorbol ester treatment of cultured B lymphoma cells containing this virus (2215). Electron micrographs showed production of herpesvirus virions. The virus was found in peripheral blood mononuclear cells (PBMC) of KS patients (56, 2870), particularly in CD19$^+$ B cells (56). The virus has also been detected in peripheral blood cells resembling spindle cells (224a, 2517). The infectivity of HHV-8 was demonstrated by taking fluid from either activated peripheral blood B cells, B-cell lymphomas, or KS biopsy specimens in culture and showing replication in CD19$^+$ B cells (222) or in adenovirus-transformed human kidney cells (777).

A role of HHV-8 in KS has been implicated by the almost universal finding of the virus in KS lesions and within the endothelial cells, spindle cells, and monocytes present in these tumors (229a, 258, 1533, 1987). Viral DNA sequences have also been detected in the sensory ganglia of KS patients (524), suggesting a reason for the frequently symmetrical cutaneous distribution of KS lesions in patients. However, the HHV-8 sequences have not been detected in tumor-producing cell lines derived from Kaposi's tumors (56, 1606) Thus, whether this virus is a direct cause or a promoter of the malignancy remains to be elucidated.

While a transforming role for the virus has not been demonstrated, its genome does contain sequences that could be responsible for cell transformation. These

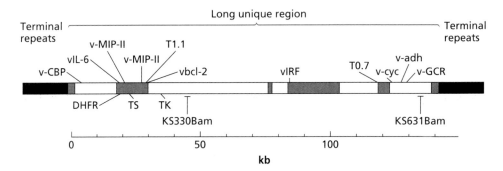

Figure 12.5   Schematic representation of the HHV-8/KSHV genome showing the 140-kb unique coding region containing all identified genes (2310). The long unique region is flanked by high-GC-containing 801-bp terminal repeat sequences (about 35 kb) at either end, which probably ligate together to circularize the genome during the cellular portion of the viral replicative cycle. The long unique region is divided into portions that have genes conserved among other herpesviruses (shaded bar) and regions unique to HHV-8 containing regulatory, cytokine, and DNA metabolism genes homologous to cellular genes (white bar). v-CBP, complement-binding protein homolog; vIL-6, IL-6 viral homolog; DHFR, dihydrofolate reductase homolog; TS, thymidylate synthase homolog; TK, thymidine kinase homolog; v-MIP, macrophage inflammatory protein homolog; vbcl-2, *bcl-2* homolog; vIRF, IFN regulatory factor homolog; v-cyc, D-type cyclin homolog; v-adh, adhesin-like molecule; v-GCR, G-coupled protein receptor resembling IL-8Ra. Also shown are T1.1 and T0.7 (2979a), two highly expressed mRNA transcripts, and KS330Bam and KS631Bam sequences, originally found by representational difference analysis of an AIDS KS lesion (398). (Adapted from a figure by R. A. Bohenzky, P. S. Moore, and Y. Chang; from reference 1500 with permission.)

viral regions include the sequence encoding cyclin D (399) (a cell cycle inducer) and a *bcl*-2-like sequence that could ensure dominance of a transformed cell by blocking apoptosis (1840, 2310). The virus also encodes certain cytokines and chemokine receptors that could help in resisting host responses (1840; for a review, see reference 1500) (Figure 12.5).

Serologic studies have indicated a close association of HHV-8 antibodies with the presence of KS. A variety of assays, including indirect immunofluorescence (1259, 1478), immunoblot (841, 1790), and recombinant protein approaches (578, 2511), have been utilized. Most of these studies show the presence of antibodies in about 1 to 2% of the normal population, but in these cases, they were measuring primarily the latent or nuclear protein expressed in transformed cells. In studies by Lennette et al. (1478), a seroprevalence of about 25% was noted in healthy adults in the United States when antibodies to the cytoplasmic (or viral replicative) antigens were measured. A similar frequency of antibodies to HHV-8 in healthy blood donors was noted in a recent serum evaluation by an ELISA to a minor viral capsid protein (578). This prevalence seems closer to the occurrence of HHV-8 in the normal population (rather than 1 to 2%), since the virus has been found in the blood and lymph nodes of healthy individuals without KS or HIV infection and in a normal blood donor (222). HHV-8 has also been detected in seminal fluids from normal men (1808, 2778) and in saliva and nasal secretions of KS patients (223, 242, 2870). These latter fluids would provide a means of transmission aside from the sexual route. The finding of HHV-8 in oral tissues supports its presence in saliva (628).

Importantly, the prevalence of antibodies to HHV-8 appears to increase at the time of puberty (1478), suggesting transmission primarily through the sexual route. This distribution pattern is similar to that of herpes simplex virus type 2 (for a review, see reference 1500). The sexual transmission of HHV-8 has been suggested by finding the virus in seminal fluid (970, 1111, 1552, 1808, 2778) and the prostate gland from KS patients and those without KS (1111, 1552, 1808, 2778). However, others have not confirmed these findings (56), particularly in relation to healthy subjects (523, 1111, 1456, 2646) (for a review, see reference 224). Since PCR procedures have generally been used to detect the virus, discrepancies in the results can be explained by artifacts introduced by this very sensitive technique. Certainly, the serologic studies suggest transmission by the sexual route. Moreover, non-PCR-based evidence of HHV-8 in the prostates of both HIV-infected and uninfected individuals has recently been reported (2578).

Further work is needed to determine to what extent HHV-8 is found in KS patients, HIV-infected individuals, and normal populations. The reactivity of sera to the latent antigen suggests that it represents a tumor-associated protein. Seroconversion to this antigen predicts the development of KS (841). Moreover, the prevalence of anti-latent antibodies appears to correlate with the overall incidence of KS in different populations (840, 1478).

In perhaps related studies, subcutaneous fibromatosis has been found in pig-tailed macaques (*Macaca nemestrina*) with an AIDS-like condition (2719). These tumors were initially linked to infection with a type D simian retrovirus (SRV-2), which gives rise to an immunodeficiency syndrome (2605, 2719). Recently, two new herpesviruses related to HHV-8 have been detected in these macaque tumors (2279). The relation of these herpesviruses and SRV-2 to the development of the KS-like tumors needs further study. Similarly, fibromas emerging from the muscular layer of blood vessels have been described in baboons developing AIDS from HIV-2 infection (144). In some studies, these tumors have also shown evidence of a herpesvirus with some relation to HHV-8 (1577a, 2279). These studies merit further attention since they could lead to animal models for studying KS.

F.   KS-Derived Cell Lines

In attempts to characterize the tumor and find the cause, cell lines were derived from KS tumors (521, 707, 1493, 1903, 2292, 2338, 2499). Cells obtained from tumors of HIV-infected patients stain with markers for endothelial cells, but their malignant nature is not pronounced. Most are reported to induce "angiogenic"-type lesions of murine origin in nude mice, and they have therefore been considered to have tumor-inducing properties. The KS-derived cells presumably produce growth factors that induce enhanced proliferation of murine endothelial cells in the inoculated animals. In our experiments with KS-derived cells, we also saw these types of lesions in nude mice, but they had the characteristics of granulomas often seen with inoculation of tumor cells, and they regressed, as in the other reports, within 4 to 5 days (1493).

In studies on the growth of KS-derived cells in culture, mRNAs for fibroblast growth factor (FGF) and IL-1 were detected (707, 1129). Moreover, KS cell lines derived by several laboratories have been induced to replicate by cell-secreted factors or cytokines such as IL-1, IL-6, β-FGF, and epidermal growth factor (EGF) and with fluid from HTLV-transformed cells (1903). In some studies, cytokines present in fluid from activated T cells induced normal vascular cells to acquire features of KS cells in culture (756). The HIV regulatory protein Tat induces KS cell growth and has angiogenic properties (36, 521, 705, 1784, 1903). This latter observation was cited as support for earlier work by Vogel et al. (2780) showing that the HIV *tat* gene introduced in transgenic mice induced skin lesions resembling KS. This finding, confirmed in part by other studies (519), needs further evaluation (1128). Recently, Tat was shown to induce HHV-8 replication (1019). A role for oncostatin M in the induction of KS has also been suggested by cell culture studies (1783, 1900). Nevertheless, the extent of replication of these cultured KS cells by cytokines is not dramatic (usually twofold), and conclusive evidence that these human cells are truly malignant and not normal replicating endothelial cells is lacking. As noted above, none of these lines, when examined, contained HHV-8.

In one instance, a KS cell line (SLK) induced angiogenic tumors in nude mice (1063, 2499). The SLK line was derived from an oral mucosa biopsy specimen from a KS lesion in a young man who was immune suppressed for a kidney transplant. The line readily grows in culture and has a variety of markers characteristic of capillary vascular endothelium (1063). No virus or HHV-8 sequences have been found to be associated with this tumor (56, 1063), although initially virus-like particles (including herpesviruses) were observed by electron microscopy in the early passages of the cultured cells (2499).

Another KS-derived cell line from an HIV-infected individual (Y1) induces metastasizing KS lesions in nude mice. This cell line differs biologically from SLK but is similar in lacking HHV-8 (1606). Aside from these two cell lines, other KS-derived lines require cytokines for any replicative capability and thus may reflect one of the processes needed to induce sustained growth of transformed cells (for reviews, see references 1498 and 2291). None of these cell lines contain HHV-8 (56, 766). The virus could have been the promoter of cell replication and subsequent transformation (Figure 12.1). In this case, similar to a "hit-and-run" process (836), the virus may have provoked the transformation event and then disappeared.

G.   Conclusions

Epidemiologic data suggest that an infectious agent is associated with KS. HHV-8 appears to be a proximal agent involved in the tumor, but it may act to promote the malignant process rather than to transform the cells directly (1498) (Figure 12.2). Such a process has been suggested for its role in multiple myelomas (2218). After stimulation of cell proliferation, transformation may occur by other, non-virus-related subsequent events, particularly those leading to chromosome changes, with the emergence of an independently growing cell. Similarly, for KS development, HHV-8 could, through infection of B lymphocytes, induce cytokines that enhance proliferation and subsequent transformation of endothelial cells (56) (Figure 12.1). Studies of the macaque herpesvirus might help elucidate the pathogenic pathway.

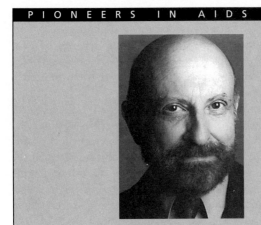

Alvin Friedman-Kien
*Professor, Departments of Dermatology and Microbiology,
New York University Medical Center. Dr. Friedman-
Kien was among the first to report the high prevalence of
Kaposi's sarcoma in homosexual men that led to the
recognition of AIDS.*

III. B-Cell Lymphomas

A. Introduction

HIV infection is associated with several B-cell abnormalities, including increased B-cell proliferation, polyclonal hypergammaglobulinemia, and enhanced production of certain B-cell cytokines (see Chapter 9, Table 9.1). These events can be linked to the reactive lymphadenopathy often seen early in HIV infection (6, 963). The most likely cytokines responsible for B-cell proliferation are IL-6 and IL-10, produced by many cells, particularly monocytes but also B cells, fibroblasts, endothelial cells, and cells in the brain (see Chapter 9). B-cell proliferation can be demonstrated with HIV particles (2017) and with the HIV envelope gp41 (439). It may be induced in some B cells via binding of the gp120 to a V_H3 immunoglobulin (175).

In one theory, this proliferative state of B cells has been considered a prelude to chromosomal changes that can establish a malignant process (Figures 12.1 and 12.2) (see below). This B-cell growth has been considered the cause of the large number of B-cell lymphomas in immunosuppressed transplant recipients (1295, 1315). Thus, B-cell lymphomas like KS are not an entirely unexpected finding in HIV infection. Immunosuppression, as in KS, can play a role in the development of lymphomas through a reduction in appropriate cell-mediated immunity. Likewise, increased production of cytokines (e.g., IL-6 and IL-10) could be involved (1677), as discussed for KS (Figure 12.2). The result is usually widespread disease involving sites outside the lymphoid organs (2989; for a review, see reference 1060).

B. Epidemiology and Pathology

Although B-cell lymphomas were reported in homosexual men at a time when AIDS was first being recognized (2989, 2990), it was not until 1985 that the Centers for Disease Control revised its guidelines to include lymphoma in the case definition of AIDS (385). B-cell lymphomas are 60 to 100 times more common in AIDS patients than in the general population (173). Between 8 and 20% of the 36,000 new cases in 1990 were estimated to be in HIV-infected individuals (820). In one report, 30% of AIDS patients before 1990 had been diagnosed with lymphoma (173). Furthermore, between 5 and 20% of individuals with AIDS could have B-cell lymphoma as their initial or subsequent diagnosis (996, 1060, 2064). Involvement of extranodal sites in the AIDS-associated lymphomas is common, with tumors found in the intestine, CNS, bone marrow, and liver (1060).

The HIV-related B-cell lymphomas are twice as common in whites as in blacks and occur in more men than women (173). They are more frequent in HIV-infected recipients of clotting factors than in those infected with HIV by heterosexual contact (173). These observations contrast with findings on KS and suggest that the lymphoma agent (if one exists) is not spread by a sexual route. When found in the peritoneal or other body cavities, these B-cell lymphomas have been given the name "body-cavity-based" or "primary effusion" lymphomas (1344) and are associated with HHV-8 infection (Section II.E).

HIV-associated lymphomas present with systemic or primary CNS involvement. Some studies suggest that there are three characteristic types of B-cell lymphomas associated with HIV infection: polyclonal, monoclonal, and monoclonal with EBV infection (216, 1725, 1745, 2066) (Figure 12.6). In one series, polyclonal lymphomas were found about as often as monoclonal lymphomas (1063), but the prevalence of polyclonal tumors remains controversial. Lymphomas of the monoclonal type are usually more common. Polyclonal proliferation of B cells most probably occurs before the development of the monoclonal lymphoma types. The polyclonal type is more similar in molecular diversity to the lymphomas observed in individuals who have been immunosuppressed for organ transplantation (1725). However, unlike the transplant-associated lymphomas, many HIV-associated lymphomas do not contain EBV.

The diffuse aggressive B-cell lymphomas, commonly seen in HIV disease, have been classified histologically as large cell (1393) and Burkitt's lymphoma-like (173, 1745, 2066; for a review, see reference 1060). The use of two subgroupings repre-

Figure 12.6 Emergence of B-cell lymphomas in HIV-infected individuals. Polyclonal proliferation of B cells can give rise to monoclonal lymphomas. The latter type may show evidence of c-*myc* translocation and/or EBV infection. The Burkitt type of lymphoma appears to develop from one malignant cell. EBV and c-*myc* may be detected in polyclonal lymphomas but at a reduced frequency. Figure courtesy of B. Herndier.

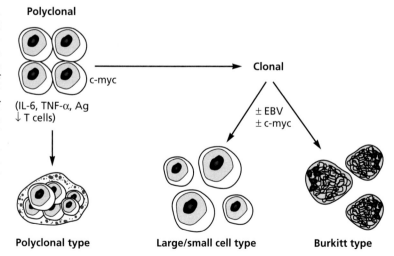

Table 12.3   Classification of lymphomas[a]

HIV infection	Conventional
Lymphoma	Non-Hodgkin's lymphoma
	Non-Hodgkin's disease (?)
Hodgkin's disease	Hodgkin's lymphoma
Large-cell lymphoma	Large-cell lymphoma
	Cleaved cell
	Noncleaved cell
	Sclerosing variant
	Large cell, immunoblastic
	Plasmacytoid
	Clear cell
	Polymorphous
	Epithelial cell component
Burkitt's lymphoma	Small noncleaved cell
	Burkitt's
	Non-Burkitt's
	Diffuse undifferentiated
	M3 (designation for Burkitt's leukemia)

[a] Reprinted from reference 1060 with permission.

sents a simplification of the several subclasses previously used for non-Hodgkin's lymphoma in non-HIV-infected patients (1060, 2989) (Table 12.3). Small noncleaved lymphomas associated with HIV infection are at least 1,000 times more common in AIDS patients than in the general U.S. population (173). About 20 to 30% of the lymphomas in HIV-infected patients are of this type, some of which are the Burkitt subtype. This finding contrasts with the incidence of this type of B-cell lymphoma in 1% of immune-suppressed transplant recipients (173).

Primary lymphoma of the brain, usually the immunoblastic or large-cell type (not Burkitt's), occurs to the same extent in all ages. It is found in up to 25% of patients with HIV-associated lymphoma (1060) and was reported in an AIDS patient younger than 1 year old (173). EBV is found in all the AIDS-associated primary lymphomas in the brain (538, 1639, 1745, 2488, 2527). HHV-8 has not been detected (818). Presenting symptoms for these tumors include seizures, headache, neurologic vocal abnormalities, cranial nerve palsies, and altered mental state. Although not common, patients have been described as undergoing personality changes (for a review, see reference 1484). Clinically, the patients with primary brain lymphomas do very poorly, and many are diagnosed only at autopsy (1484, 2529). Generally, the $CD4^+$ cell count in brain lymphoma patients is <50/μl (1060).

One characteristic shared by some HIV-associated lymphomas and lymphomas of patients immunosuppressed for organ transplant (1006) is the absence of c-*myc* rearrangements (1725, 2066, 2478, 2608). This feature, particularly for lymphomas in the brain, distinguishes these tumors from some peripheral lymphomas. Small noncleaved lymphomas in AIDS patients (some of the Burkitt type) often show this genetic abnormality (for reviews, see references 819 and 1060).

Moreover, EBV, often associated with endemic Burkitt's lymphoma (1057), is not required for lymphoma induction in HIV infection; only 40% of the tumors

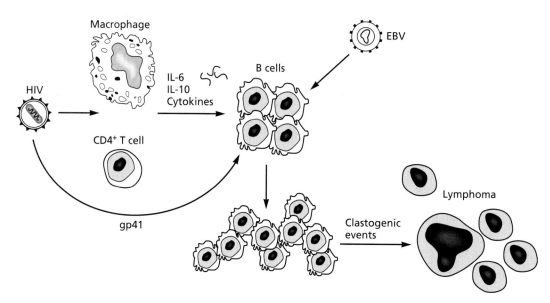

Figure 12.7   Potential mechanisms for transformation of B cells into lymphoma. HIV infection of macrophages or CD4$^+$ T cells can result in the production of cytokines that induce the proliferation of B cells. The HIV gp41 envelope protein and EBV can also be involved. The polyclonal activation and chromosomal changes (e.g., c-*myc* translocation) cause the emergence of an autonomously growing malignant cell.

outside the brain harbor the virus. In recent reports, the occurrence of EBV-associated diffuse large-cell lymphomas was linked to a loss of anti-EBV cytotoxic T lymphocytes and a rise in the EBV load (1276). EBV, once released from immune control, most probably plays a role in inducing the cell proliferation that can lead in some instances to transformation (see below) (Figure 12.7). With increased cell division, karyotypic changes can take place with selection of cells that grow autonomously (Figure 12.1). These events, perhaps directly linked to EBV, may occur preferentially in the brain. In other tumors, cytokine production could be the stimulus for proliferation (see below). One immunophenotypic feature of most AIDS lymphomas that could explain the absence of EBV is the lack of the viral complement receptor CD21 on the cell surface (2488).

Patients on long-term anti-HIV therapy appear to develop B-cell lymphomas in association with prolonged survival (2106). The duration from infection to lymphoma can be about 7 to 8 years, similar to that for opportunistic infections (173). It appears, however, that patients living longer with HIV infection may have a greater risk of developing this malignancy (2106, 2771).

C.   Pathogenesis

An increase in B-cell number associated with HIV is mirrored early in infection by the increased size of germinal follicles in the lymph nodes of infected individuals who present clinically with lymphadenopathy (see Chapter 9). This activation of B lymphocytes, observed in other viral infections, can result from HIV itself, a reduction in regulatory T-cell responses, or a response to cytokines such as IL-4 or IL-6.

The cause of the B-cell lymphomas is not known. As with KS, the cancers could reflect infection by a new agent, spontaneous growth of cells reflecting a lack of T-cell regulation, or response to cytokines released as a result of HIV infection. The last two possibilities most probably overlap, since controls on cytokine production are linked to a normal balance in other arms of the immune system (1498, 1522). Some investigators believe that these lymphomas occur as a result of germinal center destruction by a process of follicular lysis (1060). A lack of follicular dendritic cell (FDC) function as antigen-presenting cells renders B cells less sensitive to normal apoptotic processes (see Chapter 6), particularly those linked to cytokines. Thus, B cells survive longer and replicate (1060). Perhaps the predominant production of IL-10 by type 2 cells or B cells or expression of IL-10-like activity by EBV (1118) plays a role in this process (see Chapters 9 and 11). IL-10 prevents the spontaneous death of cultured germinal B cells, most probably by the induction of the bcl-2 protein (1523). A similar inhibitory effect on apoptosis by the EBV protein, latent membrane protein 1 (LMP-1), has also been described (1054).

Some data indicate multiple genetic changes in these lymphomas associated with HIV infection. Depending on the cell type, abnormalities in c-*myc, ras*, and p53 expression have been noted (128). The relationship of these changes to the initiation of the cancer is not known. Conceivably, the genetic alterations could have developed as a result of cell proliferation.

While the role of EBV in lymphoma development is unclear, as mentioned above, the induction by certain viral proteins (e.g., LMP-1 and BHRF1) of IL-10-like activity and expression of bcl-2 could be involved in inducing the tumor (1054, 1118). The expression of EBV is increased in HIV infection, and the presence of multiple variants in the same host has been reported (Table 12.4) (52, 216). The incidence of EBV in lymphomas outside the brain is low, although it can range from 20% to nearly 70% (average, 40%), depending on the cohort of subjects studied (2478). Most EBV-infected tumors are the large cell type (Table 12.3).

In some cases, EBV has been considered a proximal cause of the B-cell transformation, particularly in lymphomas in the CNS (216). This conclusion suggests a separate mechanism for development of this tumor in this compartment, perhaps reflecting some of the processes described above. The almost universal finding of EBV in lymphomas occurring in transplant patients has suggested immune suppression as a major component of pathogenesis (216). Thus, polyclonal B-cell proliferation from EBV activation, decreased apoptosis in association with EBV infection, and/or a lack of cellular immune control could be involved in development of brain lymphomas. Whether karyotypic changes (e.g., translocations) occur before or after polyclonal activation requires further study.

Most of the tumors in AIDS patients are monoclonal, suggesting the outgrowth of one transformation event (1060). In some cases, lymphomas appear to result from the clonal expansion of EBV-transformed B cells (2478). Nevertheless, the possibility that EBV has infected and spread in an already malignant B cell cannot be ruled out.

Table 12.4 EBV and HIV infection[a]

1. Increased levels of EBV in the saliva (10- to100-fold)
2. Increased levels of virus-infected cells in the blood (10-fold)
3. Increased EBV replication in the oropharynx
4. Can be reinfected with multiple EBV strains
5. Multiple EBV genome variants can be found in the same lymphoproliferative lesion
6. High antibody titers to the replicative proteins
7. Increased prevalence of brain lymphoma

[a] Data from references 52, 216, and 1789a.

Finally, HHV-8 has been detected in association with EBV in body cavity-based lymphomas (also called primary-effusion lymphomas [PEL]) (388, 1344) but also in the absence of EBV in these tumors (2215, 2328). As noted in Section II.E, since HHV-8 carries sequences associated with transformation and encodes an IL-6 homolog, its role in inducing these B-cell lymphomas (and perhaps multiple myelomas) (2218) merits further attention. It is curious that this virus is found predominantly in B-cell lymphomas of the body cavity and not elsewhere. In this regard, it is site specific, as EBV is somewhat for brain tumors. Why these B cells carrying particular viruses should proliferate in these locations in the body has yet to be elucidated.

For polyclonal lymphomas, similar events in transformation could be involved, but a role of cytokines seems important. Chronic stimulation by HIV, EBV, HHV-8, or other antigens could cause the proliferative responses observed (1725) in HIV-infected patients. Cytokines, including IL-1, IL-2, IL-4, IL-6, IL-7, IL-10, IFN-γ, and TNF-α, have all shown the ability to enhance B-cell proliferation (1196, 1197, 2326). In general, IL-6 and IL-10 seem mostly responsible for this proliferation, particularly since they can also be made by B lymphocytes (1691, 2937). Furthermore, reports have shown the induction of high levels of IL-6 production by monocytes in HIV-infected patients (1484, 1901, 2106). These cellular factors can maintain the proliferative phase of the lymphoma or B cells through continual growth in an autocrine fashion. Under these conditions, chromosomal changes might not be present and anti-cytokine approaches might offer effective therapy.

This possibility merits further study. In some ways, the polyclonal tumor resembles the murine model of AIDS (MAIDS), in which the proliferating CD4$^+$ cells are persistently stimulated by either viral antigens or superantigens, with cytokines playing a central role (1850).

D.   Conclusions

In general, the pathogenesis of B-cell lymphomas in HIV infection is considered a result of polyclonal B-cell activation secondary to HIV antigens (e.g., gp41), EBV, HHV-8, or T-cell dysregulation associated with cytokine production (Figure 12.7). In some cases, a virus (e.g., EBV or HHV-8) may be the direct transforming agent.

The induction of B-lymphocyte proliferation by cytokines or other processes can lead to clastogenic events, sometimes including c-*myc* translocation, which is linked to immortalization and outgrowth of clonal transformed B cells (Figures 12.2 and 12.7) (1315, 1646). The concomitant upregulation of c-*myc* and EBV transcripts has been cited by some to indicate a role for HIV in cell transformation (1442), but this finding needs further evaluation. The mutations in oncogenes or tumor suppressor genes associated with DNA rearrangements, as noted in Section IV for anal carcinomas, could also be involved in the development of the monoclonal B-cell lymphomas (817). Finally, normal regulation of B-cell replication may be disturbed by the loss of FDC function in lymphoid tissues (1060).

IV.   Anal Carcinoma

A.   Introduction

The incidence of anal carcinoma has been estimated to be 7 in 10^6 men and 9 in 10^6 women in the general population (2020, 2959). The increased prevalence in women is probably related to receptive anal intercourse as well as exposure to HPV in the nearby vaginal and cervical region (for reviews, see references 2020 and 3002). Nevertheless, there has been a rise in the incidence of anal cancers in both men and women, most probably secondary to the above factors and particularly in association with HIV infection (2020, 2021). In the latter instance, suppression of the immune system may be responsible for the initiation and promotion of the malignant process (see below). Even before the recognition of HIV infection, this cancer was more common among homosexual men; its prevalence was greater than that of cervical cancer in women (567, 2020).

The prevalence of anal cell dysplasia and HPV infection can be quite high in HIV-infected homosexual men. In one study, 55% of 285 seropositive men versus 23% of 240 seronegative men showed HPV DNA in anal cytology studies (1306). The detection of HPV was associated with dysplastic cellular regions. In this report, anal dysplasia was increased more than threefold among HIV-seropositive men with low $CD4^+$ cell counts compared to a seronegative group. Moreover, those with $CD4^+$ cell counts of $<500/\mu l$ had a sixfold increased risk of dysplasia compared to HIV-infected men with $CD4^+$ cell counts of $>500/\mu l$ (2020). This direct association suggests that HPV proliferation, dysplasia, and development of carcinoma are linked to the extent of immune compromise. Similarly, the prevalence of biologic abnormalities and HPV infection of the anus in women indicates a high prevalence in HIV-infected women (26%) versus uninfected women (7%) (1070).

Recent studies suggest that approaches similar to those used in cervical cancer screening (e.g., Pap smear) should be adapted to screening for dysplasia in the anal canal. Cytology would seem important, particularly in individuals at risk, such as HIV-infected men and women (2020). Based on findings thus far, stages in HPV infection can be defined and interpreted for risk of developing carcinoma (Table 12.5).

Table 12.5   Stages in human papillomavirus infection

Phase 1: HIV-negative/early HIV infection
  Low-level HPV infection
  Low prevalence of disease
  Low-grade disease
Phase 2: Late asymptomatic HIV infection
  Active HPV replication
  Increasing prevalence of low-grade disease
Phase 3: Symptomatic HIV infection
  HPV replication
  Increasing prevalence of low-grade disease
  Increasing prevalence of high-grade disease

B.   Pathogenesis

Anal cancer, like cervical cancer, often arises in areas of squamous metaplasia near the glandular epithelium. A progressive course can be observed histologically from mild dysplasia to severe dysplasia (i.e., carcinoma in situ) (2020) (Figure 12.8). Most cervical and anal cancers develop from intraepithelial neoplasia called CIN or AIN, respectively (Color Plate 15, following p. 188). These latter lesions appear to be increased in HIV infection (1868a, 2172). On cytologic examination, enlarged nuclei and irregular shapes and coarse chromatin are noted (Figure 12.9). HPV has been found associated with both cervical and anal cancers, and these malignancies are quite similar histologically (2959, 3002).

The development of cancer in the anal canal (as well as the cervix) is greatly increased in the presence of HPV, particularly the high-risk strains HPV 16 and 18 (3002). A common finding is mutations in the cellular p53 tumor suppressor gene or binding and inactivation of this protein by HPV proteins (e.g., E6 and E7) (2387, 2862). This process is more efficient with the high-risk strains of HPV. The HPV early-gene product (E7) also inactivates the retinoblastoma (RB) gene product (677, 2386), another tumor suppressor protein that regulates the extent of cell replication. These findings on the effects of E6 and E7 on p53 are mirrored in HPV-negative cervical cancer, in which mutations in p53 have been noted (542, 2924). These tumors are usually found in older individuals.

The role of the immune response in HPV expression is reflected in the known appearance in immunosuppressed individuals of warts associated with cancer or organ transplants (2068). Many homosexual men have florid condylomata accumulata. The onset of the anal cancer may therefore reflect inadequate cellular immune reactions to HPV or to transformed cell antigens. Alternatively, cytokines produced by HIV replication or immune imbalance (Section I) could influence cell growth and susceptibility to HPV gene transformation.

C.   Conclusions

The findings suggest that HPV infection promotes the expression of anal or cervical carcinoma through the suppression of cellular proteins (e.g., p53 and RB) that control cell division. With increased cell replication, chromosome aberrations and

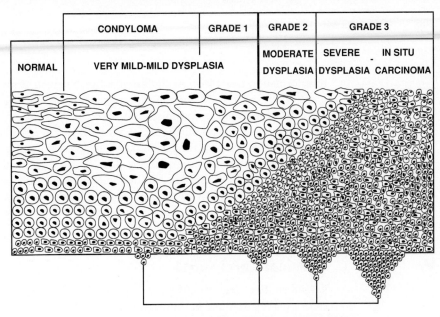

		CONDYLOMA	GRADE 1	GRADE 2	GRADE 3

NORMAL	VERY MILD-MILD DYSPLASIA	MODERATE DYSPLASIA	SEVERE DYSPLASIA - IN SITU CARCINOMA

MICROINVASIVE CARCINOMA

Figure 12.8 Schematic presentation of different grades of AIN. AIN grade 1 is characterized by 20 and 25% replacement of the epithelium with immature cells with a high nucleus/cytoplasm ratio. AIN grade 2 has approximately 50% replacement with immature cells, and grade 3 has complete or nearly complete replacement of the normal epithelium with immature cells. Microinvasion, shown at the bottom of the figure, takes place when cells traverse the basement membrane. Microinvasion usually occurs with AIN grades 2 to 3, as indicated. Reprinted from reference 2020 with permission.

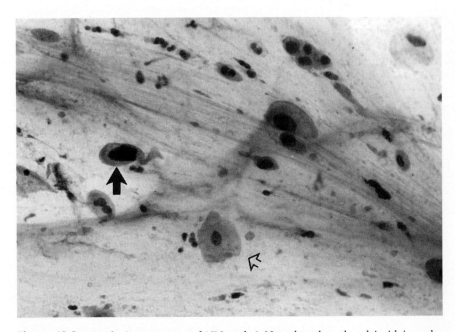

Figure 12.9 Cytologic appearance of AIN grade 2. Note the enlarged nuclei with irregular shape (dark arrow) and cross-chromatin. A normal cell with a low nucleus/cytoplasm ratio is seen nearby (open arrow). Magnification, ×455. Reprinted from reference 2020 with permission.

305

transformation take place. As discussed above, a similar explanation for development of KS and B-cell lymphomas has been considered (Figures 12.1, 12.2, and 12.7). In an immunocompromised host, HPV replication as well as the growth of malignant cells could be enhanced (for a review, see reference 3002) (Figure 12.10). It is for this reason that these HPV-associated carcinomas reach much more advanced stages in the immunosuppressed hosts (1649). Nevertheless, anal carcinomas, like cervical carcinomas, can develop, although rarely without evidence of HPV infection (2020). In these cases, the role of cytokines should be further examined.

V. Cervical Carcinoma

Several studies (1648, 1649) have emphasized that an advanced state of cervical carcinoma can be found in women who are HIV positive. The aggressive tumors are present in those subjects with a poor immune status, as measured by $CD4^+$ cell counts. Variability in response also seems to be directly related to whether women are infected by HIV.

Although not yet statistically significant, cervical neoplasia in HIV infection appears to be increasing in prevalence and severity. HIV-infected women have twice the risk of abnormal cytologic results on cervical smears as uninfected women and have a high prevalence of persistent HPV infections (1795). However, whether there is an increased incidence of invasive cervical cancer in HIV-infected women compared to uninfected women is controversial and may depend upon socioeconomic factors. In certain populations, identification of cervical cancer is the AIDS-defining illness of HIV infection (1648), and its presence, in its invasive form, is now part of the diagnosis of AIDS (376). The pathway leading to transformation resembles that of anal-rectal carcinoma; likewise, the role of HPV in this tumor is not yet fully defined. While the interaction of HPV with tumor suppressor genes seems apparent, why these tumors are more prominent in the immunocompromised individual is not known. Conceivably, as discussed with B-cell lymphomas, cytokines could be produced that increase the proliferation of epithelial cells and enhance HPV replication (Figure 12.11). As noted above, HPV is not needed, as virus-negative cervical carcinomas have been detected (542, 2924). These tumors emphasize the molecular aspects of the carcinogenic process, with the viral agents most probably acting as cofactors in the induction of the malignancy (Figures 12.7 and 12.11).

VI. Other Lymphomas

Herndier et al. (1062) have described T-cell lymphomas lacking HTLV in HIV-infected patients. Whether HIV is responsible for the transformation or whether it infected the cells associated with the tumor after transformation remains to be determined. In one case, HIV was found in the transformed $CD4^+$ cells; in three other tumors, the virus was detected in the macrophages associated with the lymphoma (2489). The common finding that the retrovirus was integrated adjacent to the c-*fps/fes* oncogene complex suggests an example in humans of retroviral insertional

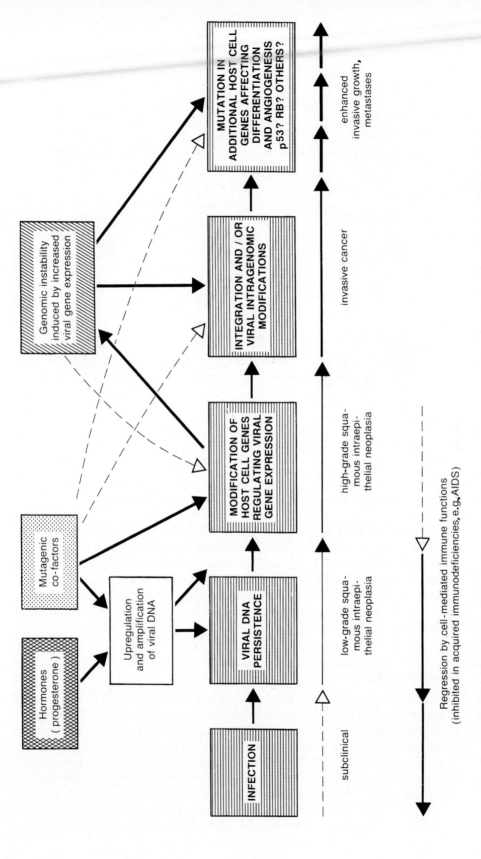

Figure 12.10 Proposed schema of pathogenesis of anal-genital cancer. Subclinical infection with HPV establishes viral persistence, and various factors interact to lead to a final transformation event. As with other malignancies, chromosome changes caused by genomic instability would be involved. Control or regression could be mediated by cellular immune responses that are absent in HIV infection. Reprinted from reference 3002 with permission.

307

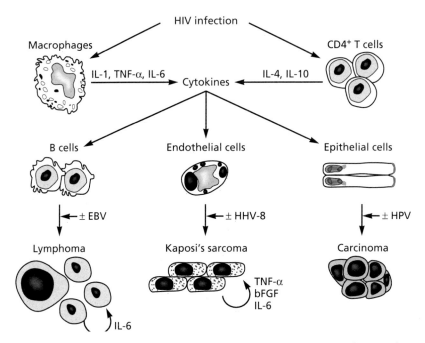

Figure 12.11 Induction of cancers in HIV infection. Virus infection of macrophages, CD4$^+$ cells, or other cells could lead to production of cytokines that enhance the proliferation of certain target cells, such as B cells, endothelial cells, and epithelial cells. The enhanced replication of these cells, either through apocrine cytokine production or through subsequent viral infection (EBV, HHV-8, HPV), could lead to the eventual development of the malignancies noted. In some cases, such as B-cell lymphomas and KS, ongoing cytokine production by the tumor cells maintains the malignant state. (See also Figure 12.7.)

mutagenesis (2489). Whether an increased prevalence of T-cell lymphomas will appear over time in HIV-infected individuals remains to be seen (for a review, see reference 1484). Since HTLV is associated with T-cell leukemia and lymphoma and since the agent is present in many HIV-infected individuals, the lack of a high prevalence of HTLV-induced leukemias is noteworthy. Moreover, the absence of liver cancers despite the high prevalence of hepatitis B virus infection in HIV-infected men (983) is surprising.

VII.   **Summary**

HIV infection can set off a chain of events that lead to development of KS, B-cell lymphomas, and probably anal carcinomas (and cervical cancers) in the infected individual. Other cancers may emerge at high frequency in the future. For instance, Hodgkin's disease, potentially involving EBV in several cases (1061); multiple myelomas, related to HHV-8 infection (2218); and seminomas are beginning to show an increased incidence in HIV infection (1617). The mechanisms involved could include immune suppression or immune enhancement associated with virus infection (Figure 12.3; Table 12.6). A major consideration, because of the potential approaches to therapy, is the role of cytokines in these diseases (Figures 12.1, 12.2,

Table 12.6 Disorders induced by HIV infection that could promote cancer development

1. Loss of antibodies to "oncogenic" virus (EBV and HPV)
2. Loss of antibodies to cancer cells
3. Loss of cytotoxic $CD8^+$ T cells (anticancer, antiviral)
4. Loss of NK cell function (anticancer, antiviral)
5. Release of growth-promoting cytokines (increase cell proliferation)
6. Release of cytokines that block apoptosis

12.7, and 12.11). B cells, endothelial cells, and epithelial cells could proliferate as a result of cytokine production and could give rise to lymphomas, KS, and anal carcinomas. The chromosomal changes that take place can result from this stimulated growth or directly from an infectious agent, and eventually the malignancy is established. In some cases (e.g., polyclonal B-cell lymphoma), the persistent growth into a cancer could be caused solely by cytokine production. In the presence of immunologic disorders, tumors, such as cervical carcinoma, could spread more readily. The mechanism, although suggestive of reduced immune response, is not yet defined.

Chapter 12	**SALIENT FEATURES**

1. Malignancies develop in HIV-infected individuals, either through a loss of anticancer immune activity or through hyperactive immune responses that increase proliferation of target cells.

2. The steps involved in transformation could involve increased proliferation of target cells, activation of an oncogenic agent and/or a clastogenic event, and subsequent cell transformation.

3. Kaposi's sarcoma (KS) is the most common malignancy observed in HIV infection and appears to involve endothelial cells, most probably of vascular origin.

4. HHV-8 appears to be a proximal agent involved in KS and perhaps in body cavity-based lymphomas. Its direct role in transformation has not yet been demonstrated.

5. Serologic studies suggest that HHV-8 is present in all KS patients and patients with body cavity-based lymphomas. The virus is found in saliva, nasal secretions, and semen. Antibodies to the virus can be found in up to 25% of the normal population.

6. Diffuse aggressive B-cell lymphomas occur at various sites during HIV infection. The peripheral B-cell lymphomas can have c-*myc* rearrangements. Some peripheral lymphomas and all those primary to the brain contain EBV. Lymphomas in the body cavity have either EBV and HHV-8 or HHV-8 alone. Some B-cell lymphomas contain neither HHV-8 nor EBV, indicating that transformation does not require infection by these viruses.

7. The incidence of anal carcinomas is increased in HIV infection in both men and women. These carcinomas are linked to HPV infections.

8. Anal dysplasia is increased more than threefold in HIV-positive men when they show decreased CD4$^+$ cell counts. This finding suggests a link of HPV activation to dysplasia and the eventual development of cancer.

9. Cervical cancer can be the AIDS-defining illness in some women. It is associated with persistent HPV infection.

10. HPV may promote the development of anal or cervical carcinoma by its suppression of certain cellular proteins (e.g., p53 and RB) that control cell division. With increased cell replication, chromosome aberrations and subsequent cell transformation take place.

11. HPV-associated carcinomas (anal and cervical) reach more advanced stages in immunosuppressed (HIV-infected) hosts.

12. Cervical carcinoma appears to be much more advanced in women who are HIV positive than in those who are not. These women have twice the risk of abnormal cervical smears and a high prevalence of persistent HPV infections.

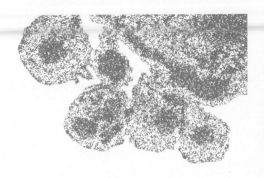

Overall Features of HIV Pathogenesis: Prognosis for Long-Term Survival

13

HIV PATHOGENESIS REFLECTS THE VARIOUS PROPERTIES OF HIV AND the host's immune response to the virus. The differential expression of these two major components of HIV infection determines the final outcome: long-term survival or development of AIDS with its associated opportunistic infections and cancers. How these features of HIV pathogenesis, covered in the previous chapters, influence survival from HIV infection becomes an important consideration.

I. Cofactors in HIV Infection and Disease Progression

A. General Observations

Whether factors other than HIV itself determine HIV infection and pathogenesis has been an important question under study (Table 13.1). From the initial discussion on HIV transmission, earlier in this volume, it is evident that multiple sexual contacts and sexually transmitted diseases, particularly those leading to genital ulcers, are cofactors in HIV infection of the host and can enhance transmission of the virus. In addition, the use of alcohol

Table 13.1 Potential cofactors in HIV infections and pathogenesis

1. Genetic background
2. Sexually transmitted diseases
3. Other viruses (e.g., herpesvirus, HTLV)
4. Other infections (e.g., tuberculosis, parasites)
5. Age
6. Antigenic stimulation (e.g., mycoplasma, immunization)
7. Immune suppression (e.g., cytokines, drugs, toxins)
8. Alcohol and drugs (can increase risk of HIV transmission; they may enhance virus replication in $CD4^+$ cells or decrease cellular immune response)
9. Lifestyle (e.g., smoking, depression, stress)

and drugs can increase the risk of HIV transmission by compromising mental status.

After infection has occurred, factors other than the AIDS virus itself appear to influence progression to disease. This conclusion is based on the variation in time from infection to the development of symptoms and AIDS among different individuals, even those receiving the same contaminated blood. Genetic differences in the host are an obviously important variable. Age has also been recognized as having an influence on progression to disease (Section III). In addition, the extent of activation of $CD4^+$ cells needed for efficient infection and spread of HIV has been considered. Thus, the potential roles of other viruses (e.g., herpesviruses and papovaviruses), foreign antigens, and cytokines that increase immune activation (and thereby the ability of HIV to replicate in cells of the host) have been proposed. Finally, additional immune suppression, resulting from other infectious agents, drugs, or toxins, could be a potential contributing event. Thus far, no specific factor, besides the genetic makeup of the individual, appears to be a consistent determinant of disease progression.

B.   Infection by Other Viruses

A possible cofactor in HIV pathogenesis is infection by another virus. Some investigators reported enhanced HIV replication following infection with certain herpesviruses (e.g., cytomegalovirus [CMV], herpes simplex virus [HSV], human herpesvirus 6 [HHV-6]) in cell culture studies (370, 899, 1610, 2520) (Table 13.2). Some strains of HHV-6 are reported to induce the CD4 molecule on the surface of $CD8^+$ cells and even natural killer (NK) cells (1609, 1611). Thus, this herpesvirus could permit HIV infection of these cells. However, other HHV-6 strains do not show this biologic property (1505a). Others have shown that HHV-6, Epstein-Barr virus (EBV), and CMV suppress HIV replication when cultured cells are coinfected with these viruses (365, 1190, 1364, 1513). The conflicting data could reflect the cell types or the virus strains used. In addition, HHV-7 uses CD4 as its cellular receptor (1612) and could interfere with HIV infection of T cells and macrophages (544). Previous EBV transformation of B cells (1051) increases the replication of HIV in

Table 13.2 Herpesviruses and cofactors in HIV infection

1. Suppression of immune responses (2293)
2. Cause of genital ulcers; enhancement of HIV transmission (340, 1105, 2107)
3. Destructive effects on brain and other tissues (2877a, 2879)
4. Induction of hairy leukoplakia (i.e., EBV) (943)
5. Link to HIV-associated malignancies: KS (i.e., HHV-8); B-cell lymphoma (i.e., EBV) (398, 1057)
6. Effects on HIV replication: enhancement or inhibition (365, 370, 1513, 1610)
7. Induction of complement and Fc receptors on infected cells—potential role in antibody-mediated enhancement of infection (1733, 1742)
8. Phenotypic mixing (2986)

these cells (see Chapter 5). Recently, infection of T cells in culture by EBV enhanced HIV-1 production, possibly via expression of EBNA-2 (2978).

As discussed in Chapter 3, herpesviruses can also induce the Fc receptor on the surface of cells and may therefore permit HIV infection via antigen:antibody complexes (1733). Since CMV infects astrocytes and can be found together with HIV in brain cells (1915), such a mechanism could be involved in HIV entry and spread in the brain. The recent report that CMV can induce a chemokine coreceptor in infected cells that could be used by HIV for entry (2105) may also have relevance but requires further study. Coinfection of lymphocytes by HIV and CMV appears to be very rare in vivo (197).

Clinically, several instances of concomitant infection of the host by different herpesviruses can be cited as evidence for their role as cofactors in HIV infection. One study suggested that CMV infection was associated with a more rapid progression toward AIDS in hemophiliacs (2833). Another report showed dual infection of keratinocytes with HIV and HSV-1 in nongenital herpes lesions (1055); in the absence of HSV-1, no HIV infection was detected. These findings suggested a possible means of increased transmission of HIV during herpesvirus infections (see Chapter 2).

Herpesviruses could also play a role in HIV pathogenesis through their association with Kaposi's sarcoma (KS), B-cell lymphomas, and hairy leukoplakia (see Chapter 12) (388, 398, 943, 1057) and through their causation of genital ulcers that could enhance HIV transmission (340, 2107) (Table 13.2). Acute HSV infection can cause an increase in HIV viremia (1805a). Finally, some cell culture studies and observations in vivo (see Chapter 5) (1055) suggest that HIV itself might be a cofactor in herpesvirus infections by enhancing or suppressing the replication of these viruses (356, 1089, 1513, 2520), possibly through cytokine production.

HIV replication can also be increased after coinfection of cells with HTLV (1008) or after their exposure to HTLV antigens in vitro (2955). In some cases, these effects on HIV were mediated by cytokine production (see Chapters 5 and 9) (765, 1697). In one of the first examples of viral interactions studied in vitro, CD8$^+$ cells established by HTLV-1 infection into a continuous line were found to be susceptible to HIV infection, even without expression of CD4 on their cell surface (619). The mechanism for this phenomenon is still not known.

In this regard, some investigators have reported an increase in the development of AIDS in HTLV-1-infected subjects (149, 2014). In contrast, other observations suggest that HTLV-2 infection in $CD8^+$ cells (992) might delay the course of disease (2776). These issues require further study.

Further evidence supporting viruses as potential cofactors in AIDS comes from molecular studies. When herpesviruses, adenovirus, hepatitis B virus (HBV), or papovaviruses or specific genes from these viruses were introduced into cells transfected with a construct of the HIV long terminal repeat (LTR) linked to the chloramphenicol acetyltransferase (CAT) gene, the production of the CAT protein increased (see Chapter 5). The early-gene products of these DNA viruses appear to be primarily responsible for this effect on the HIV LTR in a variety of promoter regions that can be different from those responsive to Tat, SP1, and NF-κB (38, 580, 875, 1268, 1896, 1997; for a review, see reference 1440). The Bel-1 protein of the human spumavirus was also shown to activate HIV gene expression via a new target sequence in the LTR U3 region (1266).

Despite these in vitro findings suggesting that other viruses could be cofactors in HIV pathogenesis, clinical studies of individuals have not yet indicated a contributory role for specific viruses. The viruses could produce the opportunistic infections or tumors observed in some patients, but an association with enhanced progression to HIV-related disease has not been well documented. How dual infection by HIV-1 and HIV-2 (722, 869, 2062, 2195) will affect the clinical outcome is not known, but previous infection with HIV-2 has been reported in one study to prevent HIV-1 superinfection (see Chapter 7) (2701). All these issues need to be evaluated by observing several clinical groups over longer periods.

Hepatitis C virus (HCV) is commonly found in HIV infection, since both viruses share the same routes of transmission, but HCV does not have an effect on HIV disease progression (3004). However, HCV infection can be more severe in people coinfected with HIV and treated with antiretroviral drugs (2765a). Likewise, HBV does not affect the course of HIV infection, but HIV can influence the natural history of chronic HBV infection (883). In the presence of HIV, the extent of inflammatory liver disease due to HBV is reduced (883). The latter finding might reflect a less aggressive anti-HBV response of the cellular immune system.

C.   Other Infectious Agents and Foreign Proteins

1. MYCOPLASMAS

Certain reports have suggested that agents other than viruses could play a role in the pathology observed in HIV infection. A mycoplasma was found associated with KS tissue (*Mycoplasma incognitas*, a variant of *M. fermentans*) (1575) that induced immune deficiency and death in primates (1576). Antigens of this agent have been detected in HIV-infected individuals with renal disease (153), and its DNA sequences were found in the blood of 6 of 55 HIV-seropositive individuals (1035). T cells from HIV-infected individuals have been shown to respond actively to mycoplasma antigens (1475), and their potential role as superantigens has been proposed (see Chapter 6). Most evidence suggests, however, that mycoplasmas do not play a major role in HIV pathogenesis.

2. OTHER POTENTIAL COFACTORS

Some immunologic studies on HIV-infected individuals with tuberculosis have suggested that the increased immune activation observed with this infection may enhance progression to AIDS (2816). In this regard, immune activation from long-term exposure to a variety of antigens or infectious agents may enhance the activation state in individuals and may therefore increase their susceptibility to HIV infection and spread. Such consideration has been given to HIV-negative Africans who have shown high levels of immune activation markers in their sera (2240). Moreover, when female sex workers were compared with mothers enrolled in HIV vertical transmission studies, the sex workers had a faster clinical course, perhaps reflecting exposure to sexually transmitted diseases (330).

Several studies suggest that postinfection immunization procedures will enhance HIV release through antigenic stimulation (807). An increase in HIV levels in plasma has been noted after pneumococcal vaccine challenge (281). Moreover, both influenza and tetanus immunizations have led to a transient increase in viremia in most studies (1964, 2575, 2576) but not in all (892). The latter finding may be due to measuring viremia at 7 days, since the highest increase in viral replication usually occurs in the first few days after immunization. While the above reports have raised the issue of whether or not infected individuals should be vaccinated, the short duration of the rise in viral load and the importance of protection against several of the infectious agents argue for continuation of immunization in seropositive individuals.

In terms of affecting immunologic reactions, evidence from other infectious diseases suggests that TH2-type responses can result from infections with helminth or other parasites and allergens (10, 2271, 2433) (see Chapter 11). In this regard, allergy has been associated with enhanced CD4$^+$ cell loss in some infected individuals (635), perhaps secondary to interleukin-4 (IL-4) release by mast cells (273). Since TH2-type cytokines can suppress the production of TH1 cytokines (see Chapter 11), cell-mediated anti-HIV immune responses might be diminished by concurrent infections or allergies (10). While this possibility is still a hypothesis, studies need to be continued to determine whether allergic reactions or coinfection by certain agents such as parasites could influence HIV disease by selective production of cytokines (171). Finally, in other reports, the purity of Factor VIII concentrates was found to correlate directly with the total number of CD4$^+$ cells. This finding suggested that antigenic stimulation of the immune system in hemophiliacs by impurities in the concentrates could increase HIV pathogenesis (2451). High-purity Factor VIII concentrates, however, have not been found to delay the development of AIDS (895).

D.   Lifestyle Factors

Certain studies have examined the effect of lifestyle factors on virus expression in peripheral blood. Alcohol intake was found to increase the sensitivity of the subjects' peripheral blood mononuclear cells (PBMC) to HIV infection and growth (118). Alcohol also appeared to have a toxic effect on CD8$^+$ lymphocyte function (115). In other reports, cocaine enhanced HIV replication in cultured PBMC (121, 2085), most probably via transforming growth factor β (TGF-β) or tumor necrosis factor alpha (TNF-α) production (2085). Moreover, morphine sulfate increased SIV replication in T cells (448) and decreased cellular and humoral antiviral immune responses in rhesus monkeys infected with SIV (449). These findings contrast with those of studies of HIV-1 infection in vivo that suggest no role of alcohol and other psychoactive drugs in enhancing progression to disease (1250). Smoking has been found to reduce the accessory cell function of alveolar macrophages in HIV-infected individuals. Cigarette smoking also increases the susceptibility of those cells to HIV-1 infection (3). These effects could influence HIV-related disease (1933, 2729).

The association of clinical depression with a decrease in CD4$^+$ cell counts and progression to disease has been reported by some groups (316) but not by others (1614, 2173). Acute exercise has induced a transient rise in the number of lymphocytes but not other cells in HIV-positive men (2737). Further studies on this issue need to be conducted. Since emotional states, such as stress, can affect hormone and immunologic functions (498, 572, 1285), this possibility should be evaluated further. In this regard, corticosteroids do not affect HIV growth in vitro (1447), suggesting that short-term treatment with these hormones will not be harmful.

E.   Animal Studies

Our laboratory has directly investigated the cofactor hypothesis in chimpanzees by examining whether another agent, after coinfection of a host, would compromise the immune response and enhance the HIV pathology. For these studies, we inoculated HIV-1-infected chimpanzees with a chimpanzee CMV and monitored the animals for signs of disease. Whereas no evidence of pathology ensued, the chimpanzees began to release HIV-1 in their blood, a characteristic not observed in these animals for over a year previously (374). Whether immune enhancement or suppression brought about this change in viral control is not known, but increased levels of antibodies to HIV were noted at the time of virus recovery.

Other studies in animals on the potential role of cofactors in HIV pathogenesis involved the inoculation of anti-Leu 2a (anti-CD8) antibodies into HIV-infected chimpanzees to determine if a reduction in CD8$^+$ cell count would bring about renewed HIV replication in vivo (374). This approach was based on the observations of CD8$^+$ cell suppression of HIV production (see Chapter 11). Animals treated for 7 to 14 days with anti-Leu 2a monoclonal antibody showed a decrease in their CD8$^+$ cell number, and their PBMC released HIV within 2 months (374). No HIV had been recovered from these chimpanzees for 15 to 40 months previously. Neither of the two animals treated showed any symptoms of HIV infection, but they recovered their CD8$^+$ cell number within weeks after the administration of anti-CD8$^+$ antibody. Both these evaluations of potential cofactors indicated that other agents and effects on CD8$^+$ cells (e.g., by type 2 cytokines) could permit HIV replication from a relatively suppressed state (Section II).

F.   Conclusions

HIV is the proximal cause of AIDS, but other infectious agents or environmental factors could influence the progression to disease (Table 13.1). How these cofactors could work in the infected individual is not clear. They might induce cytokines or intracellular factors (see Chapter 5) that promote HIV replication or compromise

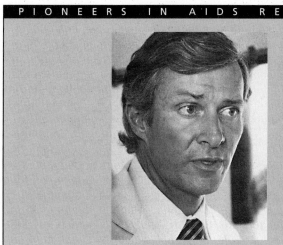

John L. Ziegler

Professor, Department of Medicine, University of California, San Francisco. Dr. Ziegler was among the first to define the cancers (B-cell lymphomas and Kaposi's sarcoma) associated with HIV infection.

immune responses. They might modify the production of cytokines (type 1 and type 2) that can affect immune function (see Chapter 11). They could stimulate the immune system abnormally, leading to increased HIV spread or autoimmune responses. Alternatively, cofactors might reduce the cellular antiviral activity and permit the escape of HIV from host immunologic control. For this series of events to occur, a continual compromise of the individual's normal immune function would presumably be needed. Generally, it appears that other factors, including opportunistic infections, can affect the overall health of the infected individual but that only the inherited genetic make-up of the host is important in determining the direct pathogenic effects of HIV itself. Genetic factors can influence cell susceptibility to HIV infection (Chapters 3 and 4) and host immune antiviral response (Chapter 11). However, if left unchallenged, HIV appears to be primarily responsible for the disease progression observed, either by direct infection of cells or by an indirect effect on the immune system of the host.

II.   Features of HIV Pathogenesis

A.   Early Period

Given the viral and immunologic factors in HIV infection, the following hypothesis can be proposed about the events involved in HIV pathogenesis (Figure 13.1). The virus initially enters an individual primarily by infecting activated $CD4^+$ T cells, resident macrophages, dendritic cells, or mucosal cells lining the bowel or uterine cavity. Few activated $CD4^+$ lymphocytes are circulating in the blood, and peripheral blood monocytes are not very susceptible to infection (see Chapters 3 and 5). Therefore, aside from cells in the mucosa, the first cells infected via the blood are most probably tissue macrophages (particularly in lymph nodes or spleen) that are in a differentiated state ready to replicate the virus (see also Chapter 2). These cells pass virus to T cells after their activation. In the initial days following acute infection,

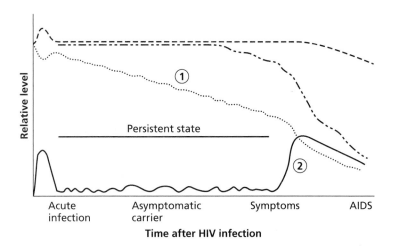

Figure 13.1   Schematic diagram of events occurring after HIV infection. Prior to sero-conversion, high levels of virus (———) can be detected in the blood. Subsequently, this viremia is reduced to low levels with episodic release of varying amounts of virus over time (phase 1). Concurrent with the onset of clinical symptoms, a second high level of viremia occurs and remains raised throughout the terminal period (i.e., development of AIDS) (phase 2). The CD4$^+$ cell number (••••) decreases during acute (primary) infection and then returns to a level somewhat below normal. A slow decrease in CD4$^+$ cell count, estimated to be approximately 60 cells/μl per year (1422), occurs over time (the persistent period) (phase 1). Subsequently, in some individuals developing symptoms, a marked decrease in CD4$^+$ cell counts can be observed concomitant with reemergence of high levels of viremia (phase 2). The number of CD8$^+$ cells (– – –) rises during primary infection, as is commonly seen in viral infections. Their number then returns to just above normal and stays elevated until the final stages of disease. In contrast, the CD8$^+$ cell anti-HIV responses (– ••• –) begin to decrease prior to or around the time of symptoms (late in phase 1) and then to decrease steadily as progression to disease occurs (phase 2). (Modified from reference 1497 with permission.)

high-level virus replication takes place in the activated lymphocytes in the lymph nodes and is reflected in a few days by p24 antigenemia and high viremia titers. Up to 5,000 infectious particles/ml, or 10^7 viral RNA molecules per ml of plasma, can be detected (see Chapter 2); the extent of virus production could reflect the intrinsic susceptibility of the individual's PBMC to the entering virus (see Chapter 3). Evidence for this scenario has been provided by SIV animal studies. Shortly after intravaginal inoculation, virus is detected first in mucosal cells (primarily dendritic cells), then in the draining lymph node within 2 days, and in the peripheral blood after 5 days (2554). CD8$^+$ cell numbers rise, as observed in other viral infections (235). It is during this period, before an antiviral response develops, that large numbers of cells become infected in lymphoid tissues and other cells in the host.

Generally, within weeks after acute infection, viremia is reduced substantially (see Chapter 4), most probably as a result of immune reaction in response to HIV. In the lymph node as well as in the blood, only a small percentage of infected cells (<1%) actively produce virus. After 10 to 14 days, up to 200 billion CD4$^+$ cells could be infected (696). Cellular immune responses appear to be the first effective antiviral activity produced, since CD8$^+$ cell anti-HIV responses have been noted early and in some cases even before seroconversion (253, 472, 1357, 1637) (see Chapters 9 and 11). Moreover, virus levels in plasma appear to be reduced before neutralizing antibodies can be detected in recently infected individuals (1357, 1637). During the acute period, before strong immune responses occur, replication of a predominant HIV strain can be detected as a relatively homogeneous virus population. With the decrease in viremia during the persistent period, the virus population becomes heterogeneous, probably reflecting the ongoing emergence of variants in the face of anti-HIV immune responses (1716) (see Chapter 4).

B.   Persistent Period

At 3 to 4 months after the primary virus infection, $CD4^+$ cell numbers usually rise to near-normal levels. They then generally decrease steadily at a rate estimated by some at 25 to 60 cells/μl per year (1422) (Figure 13.1). Why this cell loss occurs over time is one of the unsolved mysteries of this infection (see Chapter 9). We surmise from the SCID-hu animal studies that apoptosis could be a major cause of this $CD4^+$ cell death induced by noncytopathic (non-syncytium-inducing [NSI]) macrophage-tropic strains (see Chapter 6). Alternatively, if syncytium-inducing (SI) strains are present, some direct cytopathology by the virus could be involved. Over the ensuing months to years (the persistent period), the $CD8^+$ cell number remains slightly elevated. During the asymptomatic period, virus replication in the body continues but generally at a low level, particularly in lymph nodes. As discussed in Chapter 4, only 1 in 300 to 400 infected cells in the lymph node may be releasing infectious virus (see Color Plate 6, following p. 188) (696). Peripheral blood contains, in 1 ml, about 1 to 100 infectious particles and 1 to 100,000 infected cells. We believe that the suppression of HIV replication during the persistent period is mediated by antiviral $CD8^+$ cells (1515).

C.   Symptomatic Period

By the time the individual develops symptoms, $CD4^+$ cell counts have usually dropped below 300 cells/μl and the HIV in the blood and lymph nodes has again risen to high levels compared to the levels detected in blood during the asymptomatic state. At the same time, a reduction in antiviral $CD8^+$ cell responses can be demonstrated (1416, 1636) (see Chapter 11). The latter is probably also reflected in the increased expression of HIV mRNA in $CD4^+$ cells that is detected up to 2 years before the development of disease (2335). In some cases, the $CD4^+$ cell numbers drop precipitously (e.g., up to 200 cells/μl) in just a few months, most probably mirroring a return to high-level virus production (726, 1497, 2388) (Figure 13.1). This event presages the development of disease. Similar events occur in the lymph node, where virus replication increases concomitant with destruction of the lymphoid tissue, including follicular dendritic cells (FDC) (for reviews, see references 738 and 2037), and disruption of the normal architecture (see Chapter 9, Section I.F, and Color Plates 10 and 11, following p. 188). The cause of these changes in the lymph nodes is not defined and may represent the effect of the virus or an overactive cellular immune response (see below). The overall change in clinical course appears to be directly related to the cellular immune response, particularly $CD8^+$ cell antiviral activity (1491).

During the symptomatic period, and certainly when the individual develops AIDS, the HIV population in the blood once again becomes relatively homogeneous. As observed in primary infection, when antiviral immune responses are absent or low, a predominant strain emerges. This latter virus (often with the SI phenotype) has properties associated with virulence in the host that include an expanded cellular host range, rapid kinetics of replication, and CD4$^+$ cell cytopathicity (Table 7.8). It also appears to resist neutralization and becomes sensitive to enhancing antibodies (see Chapter 10). This virus, emerging later in the host, is related to the early virus at the genomic level (>97%) (429), but certain molecular changes in the regulatory regions (e.g., *tat*) and envelope regions are associated with these altered in vitro biologic properties (see Chapter 8). In addition, in some cases, the HIV strains appear to evolve within the host into neurotropic variants or viruses causing pathology in other organ systems (Chapters 7 and 9).

D.   Two Phases of HIV Pathogenesis Reflected by CD4$^+$ Cell Loss

Based on observations of changes in viral variants, the pathogenic pathway could be divided into two major phases (Figure 13.1). In the first phase, CD4$^+$ cell number and immune function decrease in association with the slow but persistent replication of relatively noncytopathic, usually macrophage-tropic strains. These viruses reduce the CD4$^+$ cell number either by direct cytotoxicity or, more probably, by an indirect means such as apoptosis (see Chapter 6). This gradual loss of CD4$^+$ cells is observed in infected individuals from all risk groups, including blood and clotting-factor recipients, intravenous drug users, and heterosexual contacts (158, 649, 726, 2445).

When the CD4$^+$ cell number is decreased to a level too low to support strong cell-mediated immunity, CD8$^+$ cell antiviral activity becomes compromised. HIV replication then returns to its high levels, which is the second phase of pathogenesis (Figure 13.1). In this phase, a more virulent cytopathic strain emerges that is associated with the ultimate demise of the host. In the terminal stages, CD8$^+$ cells, as well as CD4$^+$ cells, decrease in number, perhaps in part because of the loss of IL-2 production by CD4$^+$ cells. Apoptosis of both cell types can also be involved (see Chapter 9). Included in this pathogenic pathway is the disruption in the normal immune balance reflected in lymph node structure and associated with development of severe opportunistic infections and malignancies (Chapter 9). Moreover, as noted above, the possibility that cytokine production and hyperresponsiveness in the immune system (e.g., autoimmunity) also contribute to the final outcome needs to be considered.

How the "virulent" viruses evolve or emerge in the host is not yet known. One possibility is that a virulent strain, present early in infection, is suppressed or eliminated by an active antiviral immune system but a less cytopathic strain remains. After the reduction in immune response, either by the loss of antiviral activity or the presence of escape mutants, a strain that has the characteristics of increased virulence re-emerges or redevelops through genetic changes (Table 7.8). An alternative possibility is that the initial virus is relatively nonpathogenic in the infected individual, but with increased replicative cycles, resulting from reduced immune anti-

HIV activity, it mutates over time to a virulent strain. Evolution of NSI to SI strains has been commonly observed, but in some cases an incoming SI strain is replaced by an NSI strain (530). AIDS can develop from either virus biotype but is most commonly associated with SI strains (see Chapter 7).

Emergence of the more virulent strains appears to depend on an already compromised immune system. These strains are not usually found in individuals with CD4$^+$ cell counts of >500/μl. Studies in our laboratory have shown that CD8$^+$ cell antiviral responses are active against all strains of HIV and that this activity decreases with progression to disease. A drop in this antiviral response has been observed just before a major reduction in CD4$^+$ cell number (1491) and a return of high viremia levels (Figure 13.2). Thus, it would seem that the cytopathic strains emerge when sufficient antiviral cellular responses are no longer present. Nevertheless, it is still not clear if these virulent strains are actively responsible for the development of AIDS or if they reflect events that have permitted increased HIV replication and their eventual emergence in the host. In the latter case, the virulent strains are a result of immune loss and not the cause; they would not be needed to progress to AIDS. In this regard, as noted previously, AIDS can develop in adults and children in the absence of a detectable cytopathic strain (919, 1216, 2229) (see Chapter 7).

This concept of two phases in the pathogenesis of HIV infection fits many of the observations on the virus reported by several groups. Nevertheless, the relevance of the in vitro findings to the true pathogenic role of the virus requires further study with animal model systems.

E.   Events Responsible for Immune Deficiency

The processes leading to a reduction in anti-HIV immune responses, mirrored by the loss of CD4$^+$ cells and CD8$^+$ cell responses, are also not yet well defined (Table 13.3). Most probably, multiple factors are involved and no one factor predominates as the major cause of decreased control of HIV infection. The potential effects of direct infection of CD4$^+$ cells by HIV, an immunologic imbalance, and CD8$^+$ cell cytolytic responses should be considered (see Chapter 9). Since larger numbers of CD4$^+$ lymphocytes have now been found to be infected, a direct effect of HIV could be responsible for the CD4$^+$ cell loss, even though very few infected cells show suf-

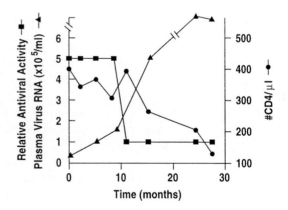

Figure 13.2   CD8$^+$ cell anti-HIV activity in an HIV-infected individual monitored over time. In this subject, the loss of CD8$^+$ cell response, reflected by the relative ability to suppress virus replication (*y* axis, left), decreases prior to a loss of CD4$^+$ cell number (*y* axis, right). Virus production (▲) resumes at time of reduced CD8$^+$ cell antiviral response. (Modified from reference 1491 with permission.)

Table 13.3 Possible factors responsible for immune deficiency

1. Direct infection by HIV
2. Immunologic imbalance: cytotoxic disorders lead to apoptosis, decreased antiviral immune responses
3. ADCC: killing of CD4$^+$ cells carrying gp120
4. CTL activity against normal CD4$^+$ cells

ficient virus replication to lead to cell death (see Chapter 4). Without dying, the virus-infected cell could still be compromised in its function, including the production of cytokines necessary for normal immune activity (see Chapter 9).

The balance in type 1 and type 2 cytokine production can influence CD4$^+$ cell counts and the dominant viral phenotype. The type 1 cytokine pattern has been associated with higher CD4$^+$ cell counts and an NSI strain. A high ratio of IL-2 to IL-10 identifies individuals with a good prognosis (469). Thus, strengthening of a type 1 response (i.e., cell-mediated immunity) could help in controlling HIV infection (see Chapter 11).

Normal immune reactions that have gone aberrant, such as apoptosis, antibody-dependent cellular cytotoxicity (ADCC), and cytotoxic T-lymphocyte (CTL) responses, as well as autoreactive cells and autoantibodies, can all play a role in an immunopathogenic pathway. In this regard, as noted in Chapter 11 (Table 11.4), hyperactive CTL activity in HIV-infected individuals could contribute to the immune abnormalities that ultimately lead to AIDS (1515, 1780, 2993). For example, CTL responses could destroy antigen-presenting cells (APC) and prevent the normal cellular immunity needed to maintain an asymptomatic state (1326, 1515, 1765). Infiltration of lymph nodes by CTL may reflect destruction of this tissue in vivo (436, 2282). Furthermore, in one report, antiviral CTL activity was found only in infected people who showed clinical symptoms during primary infection (1411). In fact, one individual who did not have CTL activity maintained high CD4$^+$ cell numbers and an asymptomatic clinical course (748). In this connection, in one disturbing report, an HIV-seropositive individual received autologous CTL directed against the HIV-1 Nef protein. The individual's clinical state worsened, with a decline in the number of CD4$^+$ cells, and the viruses isolated were resistant to these CTL (1330). The administration of CTL, not necessarily the emergence of the resistant virus, could have been responsible for the change in clinical state.

Moreover, no CTL activity has been found in long-term healthy viremic monkeys naturally infected with SIV. The monkeys have, however, shown the CD8$^+$ cell noncytotoxic antiviral response (2136, 2774; reviewed in reference 1504).

Finally, some CTL may react against cells that produce neutralizing antibodies, as has been reported with lymphocytic choriomeningitis (LCM) virus in mice. Infection of B cells by a noncytopathic LCM virus led to destruction of the cells and a persistent infection by these types of viral strains (2101). A similar mechanism might be responsible for the emergence of the NSI viral phenotype and merits evaluation. In one HIV-infected subject, neutralizing antibodies to an SI virus led to the switch to an NSI virus after seroconversion (1437).

The importance of humoral immune reactions in preventing disease progression is unclear. When autologous strains are tested, neutralizing antibodies can be found throughout the course of the infection, albeit generally only at low levels (see

Figure 13.3 Balanced immunogenicity. In this model, sufficient noninfected or non-virus-releasing CD4$^+$ cells are present to make IL-2, which maintains the production of CAF by CD8$^+$ cells. CAF in turn suppresses HIV production and prevents the loss of the CD4$^+$ cells and their function.

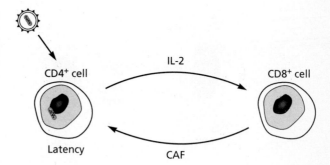

Chapter 10). The role of these antibodies would appear to be most important during the early phase of HIV infection, when destruction of virus-infected cells (via ADCC) could be effective in preventing HIV spread in the host.

With these possible processes in mind, the overall conclusion is that suppression of HIV replication in the host is the most important factor in preventing the progression to disease. Both inhibition of noncytopathic strains (which could cause a slow loss of CD4$^+$ cells by an indirect mechanism) and suppression of more virulent strains, in which direct cell killing is associated with rapid progression to disease, depend on a strong antiviral cell-mediated immune response. A compromise in this activity appears to be a major determinant for progression to disease. Importantly, maintenance of this antiviral activity depends upon cytokines produced by the very cells that HIV infects, the CD4$^+$ lymphocytes (see Chapter 11) (Figure 13.3).

These features of HIV infection indicate that an immunologic balance reflected by sufficient functioning of both CD4$^+$ and CD8$^+$ cells is needed to control HIV pathogenesis (Figure 13.3). The loss of IL-2 or CD8$^+$ cell antiviral factor (CAF) production could lead to the release of virus from its "latent" state, with the known pathogenic sequelae (Figure 13.4) (see Chapter 11). Maintenance of an asymptomatic state appears to depend on an adequate production by CD4$^+$ cells of type 1 cytokines, such as IL-2, that are needed for CD8$^+$ lymphocyte antiviral activity (138). The CD8$^+$ cells ensure suppression of HIV replication, whether of the nonvirulent or virulent strains, and thus ensure normal CD4$^+$ cell function and a long

Figure 13.4 Immune pathogenesis. CD4$^+$ cells produce cytokines such as IL-2 that maintain the production of CAF by CD8$^+$ cells. CAF inhibits CD4$^+$ cell release of HIV. If an inhibitory event prevents IL-2 production by CD4$^+$ cells (pathway 1) or blocks CAF production by CD8$^+$ cells (pathway 2), HIV production takes place.

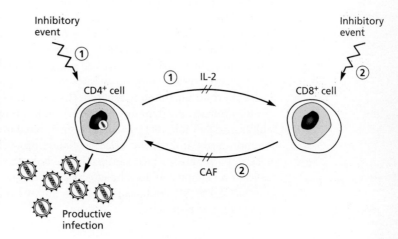

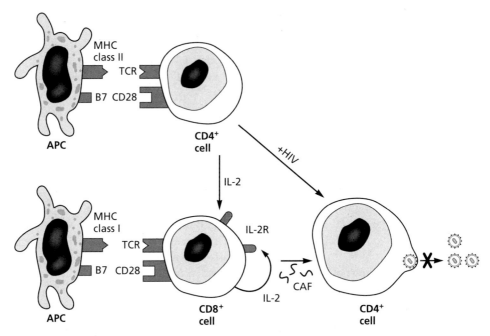

Figure 13.5   APC (e.g., dendritic cells), through their expression of MHC molecules and B7 proteins, help in the stimulation of CD4$^+$ and CD8$^+$ cell responses. The ultimate result is an increase in IL-2 production and IL-2 receptor expression. In terms of HIV infection, this costimulation can lead to an increase in the CD8$^+$ cell antiviral response and thereby control of virus replication (136).

asymptomatic course. A breakdown in this antiviral activity of CD8$^+$ cells as a result of a change in type 2 cytokine responses (e.g., IL-10 production) could permit the emergence of HIV from a relatively latent state and progression to disease (Section IV). What causes a decrease in IL-2 production (or CAF release) is not known and is under study. Since APC, such as dendritic cells, play an important role in elucidating and maintaining both CD4$^+$ and CD8$^+$ cell responses (Figure 13.5), abnormalities in this cell type merit attention (see Chapter 9). In this regard, evidence in our laboratory has indicated that CD28:B7 costimulation of CD8$^+$ cells is needed for an efficient CD8$^+$ cell antiviral response (136). If B7 expression is decreased on APC (669) or if dendritic cells are removed more quickly from blood and tissues than they can be renewed, as has been suggested (1326), a compromise in immune function could result. Thus, approaches to restoring APC function may be very important in restoring immune function (Chapter 14).

   In summary, the steps involved in HIV infection and progression to disease are multifactorial (Table 13.4). Each has been covered in some detail in this book. The common factor influencing delay in disease progression is the inherited genetic makeup of the host, which can determine both the susceptibility of cells to HIV replication (Chapter 3) and the effectiveness of the antiviral cellular immune response (Chapter 9). Youth can also be an important influence, probably reflecting strong immune responses.

Table 13.4 Steps involved in HIV infection and pathogenesis

1. Virus attachment to cellular receptor(s), fusion, and nucleocapsid entry into cells (Figure 3.5)
2. Virus replication in cells (influence of intracellular factors)
3. Acute virus infection with spread primarily to lymphoid tissues (and peripheral blood cells)
4. Virus replication controlled by cellular immunity (CD8$^+$ cell response) (Figure 13.2)
5. Dominant TH1 responses enhancing cell-mediated immunity (Figure 11.9)
6. Most virus-infected cells placed in a latent state
7. Gradual loss of CD4$^+$ cell function and number (role of noncytopathic, macrophage-tropic HIV strains?) (Figure 13.1)
8. Switch from type 1 to type 2 cytokine responses (direct role of HIV?) (Figure 11.7)
9. Loss of CD8$^+$ cell antiviral responses (Figure 13.2)
10. Release of infectious virus and increased numbers of virus-infected cells (lymphoid tissue and peripheral blood)
11. Enhanced virus replication
12. Emergence of cytopathic strains (Figure 7.14)
13. Further loss of CD4$^+$ cells and function (Figure 13.2)
14. Onset of symptoms and progression to AIDS

III.   Prognosis

Several studies have attempted to define those factors that might be useful in predicting the clinical course (Table 13.5). The most common finding associated with disease progression has been a low CD4$^+$ cell count (1751, 1752; for a review, see reference 2588). Recently, viral RNA levels were found to be a better predictor for clinical progression than was the CD4$^+$ cell number (825, 1751, 1752). However, both markers considered together are the most helpful for prognosis (1752). Furthermore, high-level expression of viral transcripts in PBMC has been used as a predictor of progression to disease (124, 2335). Importantly, high levels of circulating free virus (assessed as viral RNA) or virus-infected cells following seroconversion have correlated with a more rapid clinical course (see Chapter 4) (Figure 13.6) (1058, 1461, 1751, 1752, 2767).

Infants with a rapid rise in plasma viremia soon after infection, without the expected decline in HIV levels within 4 to 6 weeks, have shown a poor prognosis (596). In this regard, as might be expected, severe immune defects in the first year of life in children with HIV infection predict rapid progression to disease (440). Furthermore, as noted previously, viral heterogeneity correlates with a slower progression to AIDS (607). These parameters appear to reflect the strength of the immune response shortly after primary infection (1058).

Among other parameters associated with a poor prognosis are such features of immune activation as high levels of β_2-microglobulin, soluble IL-2 or TNF receptors, and soluble CD8 in the blood; high levels of neopterin in the urine; and increased numbers of CD8$^+$ CD38$^+$ cells (210, 960, 1541, 1803, 1945, 1996, 2203). Other prognostic factors associated with disease progression include elevated levels of p24 antigen or infectious virus in the blood; low antibody titers to p24 or p17 Gag

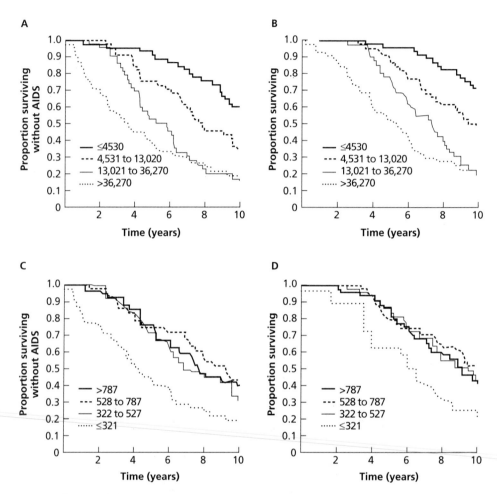

Figure 13.6 Relations between baseline markers and prognosis following acute HIV infection. Kaplan-Meier curves for AIDS-free survival (A) and overall survival (B), stratified by baseline HIV-1 RNA quartiles (molecules per milliliter), and for AIDS-free survival (C) and overall survival (D), stratified by baseline CD4$^+$ T-cell quartiles (cells per microliter). (Adapted from reference 1752, with permission.)

proteins (404, 777a, 1094, 1201a, 1423a, 1424, 2438, 2832a); cytopathic strains of HIV (429, 1346, 2659); decreased dehydro-3-epiandrosterone levels in serum (1179); and decreased delayed-type hypersensitivity reactions (2970) (Table 13.5). The introduction of acid dissociation has increased the sensitivity of p24 antigen assays for these evaluations (244). Nevertheless, viral RNA is a better predictor of the clinical course than is the antigen assay (1873). Its measurement is more sensitive, and p24 is not necessarily associated with intact virions (262). Cytokines produced during immune activation and low antibody titers to HIV have also correlated with the highest chance of developing AIDS (1461, 2473, 2767). The role of an activated immune system in predicting disease progression is supported by finding the largest antigen-specific CD4$^+$ T-cell proliferative responses to HIV, CMV, and HSV antigens in people who subsequently progress to disease (2415).

Table 13.5   Parameters suggesting progression in HIV infection[a]

 1. Low CD4$^+$ cell number (604a, 728a, 2088a)
 2. High β_2-microglobulin level in serum (1541)
 3. High soluble IL-2 receptor level (1945)
 4. High soluble CD8 level in serum (1996)
 5. High soluble TNF receptor level in serum (894a)
 6. Low antibody titers to p24 or p17 Gag proteins (777a, 1201a, 1423a, 1424, 2438, 2832a)
 7. Plasma p24 antigenemia (619, 1424, 2233, 2438)
 8. High viremia level (512, 1081)
 9. Cytopathic HIV strain (429, 1346, 2659)
10. Decreased dehydroepiandrosterone level in serum (1179)
11. Reduced CRI (complement receptor) expression on erythrocytes (494)
12. High neopterin level in urine (2203)
13. Reduced delayed-type hypersensitivity reactions (2970)
14. Reduced CD8$^+$ cell antiviral response (1636)
15. Reduced number of activated CD8$^+$ cells (1416)
16. Specific MHC phenotype (1167, 1251a, 1659, 2579a, 2864) (Table 13.6)

[a] See Section III for discussion and other references.

As reviewed above, the nature of the infecting virus can have a prognostic value. The SI strains are more closely associated with a rapid progression to disease than are the NSI viruses (see Chapter 7) (429, 1931, 2274, 2658). However, a switch from the NSI to the SI phenotype is not necessarily seen with progression to disease (530, 555, 919, 1094, 1216, 2318). NSI strains are present in up to half of AIDS patients in some studies (919, 2318) (see Chapter 7). Importantly, in some individuals studied over time, a switch from an NSI to an SI virus has not led to increased viral RNA levels in serum (1216, 1254). The findings emphasize the fact that viral load or phenotype alone is not the sole parameter for progression to disease and may not carry the worst prognosis. The overall state of the immune system is the major determinant. In terms of the virus, deletions in the *nef* gene and in the region of overlap of *nef* with the U3 portion of the LTR can be associated with slow progression to disease (605, 1303). Some of these infected individuals have been healthy for up to 14 years.

With regard to virus phenotype, inoculation of SI strains (and not NSI strains) into thymus-implanted SCID-hu mice leads to lymphoid destruction (1232). In contrast, in PBMC-implanted SCID-hu mice, NSI strains induce the fastest CD4$^+$ cell loss, most probably from apoptosis (1859). Thus, in some clinical situations, the SI strain may be responsible for direct lytic activity in thymus and lymph nodes, leading to cell depletion. In others, the NSI strain can lead to the immune disorder, perhaps by an indirect means (Section II). The *nef*-deleted viruses in this system show a delay in CD4$^+$ cell loss, but it still takes place (965).

Attention has also been given to the possible relation of certain major histocompatibility complex (MHC) class I or class II phenotypes (e.g., HLA-B5 and HLA-A1B8,DR3) to disease progression (1167, 1168, 1251, 1251a, 1316, 1659, 2579a, 2864) (Table 13.6). The outcome of HIV infection may depend on the MHC, human leukocyte antigen (HLA) types, and the relative expression of the variable gene repertoire of the T-cell receptor. Thus, these two regions have been examined for possible roles in disease progression. In addition, TAPs (transporters associated

Table 13.6 HLA association with HIV disease progression

Fast progressors
  A1, A9, A11, A23, A28 + TAP2.3, A29 + TAP2.1; B8 + DR3, B35 + Cw4, DR2, DR5
Slow progressors/long-term survivors
  A9, A25 + TAP2.3, A26, A32, B5, B14, B18, B27, B51, B57, BW4, DR,5, DR6, DR7,
    DRB1*0702 + DQA1*0201, DR13
High-risk exposed HIV-seronegative individuals
  A2, A28, DR13

^a Adapted from reference 2864 with permission.

with antigen processing) have been recognized as perhaps playing a role in the clinical course (1251) (Table 13.6). This protection could result from the most effective presentation of antigen in the context of MHC molecules. Thus, a strong CTL or cell-mediated immune response is generated. An alternative reason may be protection following frequent sexual exposures to HLA proteins that are present on the surface of virions or on cells that carry the infectious virus (Chapter 3, Section VII). However, no conclusive evidence of a link with a particular HLA type is available.

Older age (>25 years), particularly in hemophiliacs, has been associated with faster progression (158, 364, 573, 726, 2764). Moreover, in hemophiliac children, oral candidiasis was the strongest predictor (727). High CD8$^+$ cell counts and high immunoglobulin A (IgA) levels in hemophiliacs in the first years after seroconversion also predict future progression to disease (2089). Another important prognostic factor is CD4$^+$ cell proliferative responses to a variety of stimuli. As noted earlier in this book (see Chapter 9), a loss of response to recall antigens and alloantigens and to mitogens presages development of disease (481, 483, 2415).

Based on our studies, the level of CD8$^+$ cell antiviral noncytotoxic activity would also be a good marker of risk for disease progression (1636), but cannot be quickly measured in a laboratory. In this regard, the finding of increased HIV mRNA levels in CD4$^+$ cells up to 2 years before the development of symptoms (2335) could reflect a decrease in the CD8$^+$ cell antiviral response (see Chapter 11). When a monoclonal antibody against CAF is developed, measuring the number of CAF-producing cells in the blood by flow cytometry may be helpful. Some studies suggest that flow cytometric analyses of CD8$^+$ cell subsets (e.g., CD38$^+$) might be useful in defining phenotypic markers associated with progression to disease (886, 1416, 1482). In addition, observations by some researchers suggest that a rise in levels of myelin basic protein or antibodies to this central nervous system protein might predict the development of dementia (1602). The presence of activated CD69$^+$ macrophages in the peripheral blood may also predict neurologic disease (2153) (see Chapter 9).

In summary, several of the findings cited above are controversial, and the parameters for predicting progression to AIDS need further evaluation. The use of CD4$^+$ cell counts as a surrogate marker for prognosis can be misleading if the individual is coinfected with HTLV; high CD4$^+$ cell counts can be observed in advanced disease (2384). Viral RNA levels are the best predictor for clinical progression (825, 1751, 1752). A decline in HIV-1 RNA levels during the early period of infection correlates with a better clinical course and is independent of the viral phenotype and CD4$^+$ cell count (1216, 1752) (Figure 13.6). Increased levels of HIV-1 DNA in the PBMC,

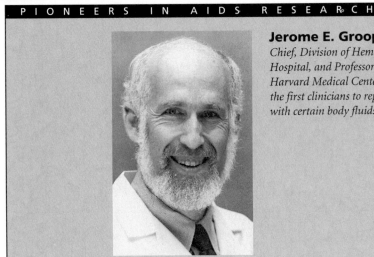

Jerome E. Groopman
Chief, Division of Hematology/Oncology, Deaconess Hospital, and Professor, Department of Medicine, Harvard Medical Center. Dr. Groopman was among the first clinicians to report on the association of HIV with certain body fluids and clinical syndromes.

as well as high numbers of HIV-1-producing CD4$^+$ cells, correlate with disease progression (969). In general, most investigators today rely on viral RNA levels combined with CD4$^+$ cell numbers as prognostic markers (1752). Particular attention has been given to viral RNA levels at the time of seroconversion, when a sharp decrease can portend a long asymptomatic course (Figure 13.6). Importantly, CD4$^+$ cell numbers, and in some cases viral RNA levels, may not be predictive of immune competence (or prognosis) after antiviral therapy has been instituted (see Chapter 14).

IV. Differences in Clinical Outcome

As reviewed by Haynes et al. (1037), one group of infected individuals consists of typical progressors, whose immune functions appear to be intact early in infection but whose immunologic control weakens within 8 to 10 years, with progression to disease. Another clinical group consists of rapid progressors, who show a very quick decline in CD4$^+$ T-cell numbers, usually within 2 to 5 years after primary infection (2474). They are characterized by low levels of antibody to HIV proteins and poor HIV-1 neutralizing activity (354, 2040). They may also have enhancing antibodies (1102). Importantly, CTL activity may be present in the rapid progressors (2235), who may have larger numbers of activated CD8$^+$ CD38$^+$ HLA-DR$^+$ cells (886) (see Chapter 9). This feature underlines the stimulated immune state associated with a poor prognosis (see above). The most characteristic feature of rapid progression is a high viral load that does not decrease substantially after primary HIV infection (1216, 1751, 1752). In these individuals, homogeneity in HIV isolates is found. In contrast, for typical progressors, a change from viral homogeneity to heterogeneity and back to homogeneity at the time of disease is usually observed. Viral homogeneity most probably reflects a poor host antiviral immune response.

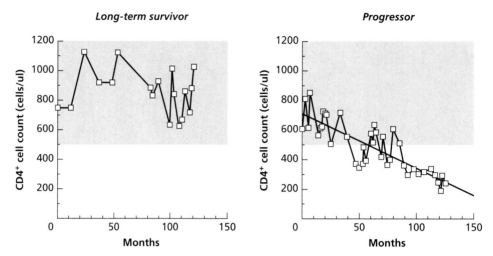

Figure 13.7 CD4$^+$ cell counts in long-term survivors and progressors. Over a 10-year period, CD4$^+$ cell counts remained within the normal range (shaded area) for long-term survivors but persistently decreased in progressors. (Figure courtesy of E. Barker.)

A third category of infected individuals consists of the long-term survivors, also called long-term nonprogressors, who have remained healthy with normal CD4$^+$ cell numbers for at least 10 years (Figure 13.7). Some groups have predicted that up to 13% of homosexual/bisexual men infected at a young age will remain asymptomatic for more than 20 years (1877). The usual percentage of these long-term survivors is 8 to 10% of the total number of infected people (308, 2311) (Figure 13.8) (Section V). These asymptomatic people can also be found among infected hemophiliacs (2772), intravenous drug users, heterosexual contacts (1502), and newborn children (see below for references).

The long-term survivors maintain a very low viral load, both in plasma and in PBMC (354, 1491, 1502, 2772), and usually have a less cytopathic (NSI) strain, but

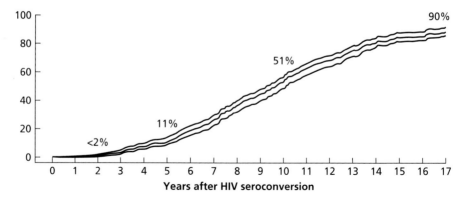

Figure 13.8 Progression to AIDS with time. In the San Francisco city cohort, individuals known to be infected have been monitored since 1978. The results through 1995 show that it takes about 10 years for 50% of the individuals to develop AIDS; 69% of the infected subjects develop the disease within 14 years (307a, 308, 1539). (Figure courtesy of S. Buchbinder.)

Table 13.7 Characteristics of long-term survivors

1. There is a low virus load (measured by plasma viremia; infected PBMC).
2. The HIV strain present is of a relatively nonvirulent type.
3. Antibodies to the HIV strain present in the individual do not enhance infection.
4. Type 1 cytokine production by PBMC is demonstrated.
5. Cellular CD8$^+$ cell antiviral response is strong.

occasionally SI strains are present (Table 13.7). In some cases, the kinetics of viral replication is lower in these subjects (354). They can have neutralizing antibodies to the autologous strain but no enhancing antibodies (1102, 1491). Antibodies to the viral envelope V3 region do not correlate with this slow progression to disease (1094). Moreover, CD4$^+$ cell proliferative responses to HIV and antiviral CTL in long-term survivors have been noted in other studies (481, 1016, 2040, 2275). The long-term survivors show a strong CD8$^+$ cell noncytotoxic antiviral response (1491, 1502) and can have a high frequency of precursor CTL (1017, 2040). Furthermore, the structure of the lymph node is more intact in long-term survivors, there is a low level of virus replication in PBMC and the lymph nodes, and the function of the lymphoid cells is maintained at a high level (226, 2040). Finally, the diversity of HIV strains in long-term survivors is heterogeneous, in contrast to the homogeneity noted in the rapid progressors. Again, these observations on viral heterogeneity most probably reflect an active anti-HIV immune response in which different "escape" variants can emerge until they are recognized by the immune system (Section V).

In children, a similar distinction in clinical course can be appreciated (for a review, see reference 2880). About 10 to 25% of infected newborn children develop AIDS within the first 2 years of life, whereas the rest can have a slower progression to disease, with some remaining healthy for several years (104, 229, 2698). Moreover, central nervous system disorders in children appear to follow a course very similar to that in adults (2880). Similar to adults, very high viral loads in the months soon after infection correlate in newborn children with an increased risk for rapid progression of disease (2478).

Some studies suggest that a poor clinical course in the mother correlates with faster development of AIDS in the baby (2696). The data could reflect transmission of either virulent strains or increased amounts of virus to the child (see Chapter 2). As noted in Chapter 2, the same kind of association has been made for recipients of blood transfusions (2075). In newborn children, progression to disease is generally more rapid than in adults. Low birth weight, an early decrease in CD4$^+$ cell counts, high viral loads, and clinical symptoms (lymphoadenopathy, splenomegaly, and hepatomegaly) are predictors of this progression (831, 1702). These symptoms suggest intrauterine infection (see Chapter 2). Progression is also more rapid in infants infected in the perinatal period than in neonates infected from a blood transfusion (306, 791).

Finally, another group of infected individuals has an unusual clinical presentation. They remain free of illness and AIDS symptoms for more than 3 years after their CD4$^+$ cell counts have dropped below 200 cells/μl. They have been called low CD4$^+$ cell long-term survivors. These infected people have a slower decline in

CD4$^+$ cell count and T-cell reactivity than conventional progressors (1259a). The reason for this lack of progression in the absence of treatment has not been explained but could be related to other immune system cells (e.g., NK cells) that are active in defense against the virus (1106) or against the opportunistic infections (2501) (see Chapter 11).

V.   Factors Involved in Long-Term Survival

The discussion in this chapter underlines an important question considered in this book on HIV pathogenesis: what is the cause of the wide variations in progression to disease observed among infected individuals? For example, the San Francisco study of HIV infection in a cohort of 622 subjects with well-defined dates of HIV seroconversion (308, 1539, 2311) revealed that 87% of the individuals had developed AIDS (384) 17 years after HIV seroconversion (307a, 308) (Figure 13.8). In evaluating the entire cohort with long-term HIV infection at the end of 1995 ($n = 594$, 10 to 18 years after HIV seroconversion), 15% of the cohort remained healthy and 4% of the cohort had normal CD4$^+$ cell counts (307a, 308). These healthy individuals have laboratory markers and clinical histories indicating a slow progression of disease (2474). Although relatively few subjects are in this category (8 to 10%), the reasons for their long-term survival could provide insights into possible therapeutic interventions for others. A lack of exposure to sexually transmitted diseases or recreational drugs did not explain the long-term asymptomatic course (308).

As reviewed above, long-term survivors often show no infectious virus and very low levels, if any, of viral RNA in plasma (354). Only after depletion of CD8$^+$ cells can virus be recovered from the PBMC and lymph node cells of some subjects (226, 354). Importantly, long-term survivors have shown no evidence of resistance of their CD4$^+$ cells to HIV infection, but they have a strong CD8$^+$ cell noncytotoxic antiviral response (354, 1491) (Figure 13.9).

Our findings on long-term survivors indicate five major characteristics discussed in this book (Table 13.7). First, they have a low viral load, as reflected by the relatively small number of infected CD4$^+$ cells and free infectious virus in the peripheral blood and lymphoid tissues. Second, the viruses recovered from PBMC are

Figure 13.9 Suppression of HIV replication by CD8$^+$ cells. CD8$^+$ cells at different input ratios were added to acutely infected CD4$^+$ cells. The relative extent of suppression was determined. The smallest number of CD8$^+$ cells needed to suppress virus replication by more than 90% was determined. The strength of the CD8$^+$ cell response in long-term survivors was significantly greater than that in progressors ($P = 0.001$). (Figure courtesy of E. Barker.)

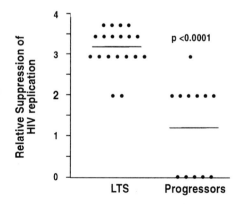

"nonvirulent" HIV strains that grow to low titer, are not cytopathic, and do not replicate in established T-cell lines. They are often macrophage tropic and, as studied in the SCID-hu animal system, appear to lead to $CD4^+$ cell death slowly through an indirect mechanism, most probably apoptosis (1855, 1859). Third, as discussed above, neutralizing, and not enhancing, antibodies to the virus are found in the blood of long-term survivors (1102). Fourth, their PBMC show a type 1 response in cytokine production (IL-2, IFN-γ) (see Chapter 11). Finally, whereas $CD8^+$ cell responses (both cytotoxic and noncytotoxic) are decreased in individuals progressing to disease, the $CD8^+$ cell noncytotoxic activity in both PBMC and lymphoid tissue remains strong in long-term survivors (138, 226, 914, 1491, 1636) (Figure 13.9). In terms of virus suppression, 1 $CD8^+$ cell can inhibit virus replication in as many as 20 $CD4^+$ cells from asymptomatic individuals. In contrast, some AIDS patients can require up to 100 times more $CD8^+$ cells to control HIV replication (1515).

As cited above, some studies indicate that long-term survivors are infected by slowly replicating defective viral mutants, in particular those lacking Nef expression (605, 1303) (see above). However, this finding does not account for nonprogression in most of these subjects (1127). Viruses from long-term survivors also show no abnormal *vif*, *vpr*, or *vpu* sequences (529, 2975).

In addition, some long-term survivors may have a reduced expression of the CCR-5 receptor on $CD4^+$ cells (see Chapter 3) as a result of one deleted allele for this coreceptor (607, 1568, 2346). This heterozygosity could influence the viral spread and pathogenicity of NSI strains, but the finding needs additional epidemiologic evaluation (2). In the most recent evaluation of polymorphisms in chemokine receptor genes, some studies (2522a) but not others (1773a) suggest a mutation in CCR-2b on one allele is associated with a slower progression to AIDS in infected individuals. Moreover, further work is needed to determine whether there is also a reduced expression of the CXCR-4 receptor in some of these individuals. In this regard, long-term survivors do not show substantial differences from progressors in the production of β-chemokines after stimulation of their PBMC or $CD4^+$ cells in vitro (1630, 2772) (see Chapter 11, Section III).

In terms of the humoral immune response, certain studies have shown that neutralizing antibodies to heterologous viral strains correlate with a healthy clinical state (354, 1590). Some investigators have found that neither neutralizing antibodies nor complement-mediated antibody-dependent enhancement is associated with long-term survival or disease progression (1818). We have commonly detected neutralizing antibodies to the autologous and heterologous strains in long-term survivors. This humoral immune response is not consistently detected in progressors, who, as noted previously, can have enhancing antibodies (1102). Nevertheless, in general, the humoral immune response does not appear to be a major determinant of long-term survival.

These observations on long-term survivors strongly suggest that low viral load, the noncytopathic nature of the virus, and the absence of viruses sensitive to enhancing antibodies all reflect the anti-HIV effect of $CD8^+$ cells, which reduce the ability of HIV strains to replicate and thus mutate in the host. The importance of the $CD8^+$ cell anti-HIV response is reflected in the reduced viral load in asymptomatic individuals and long-term survivors even when SI strains are present in the blood and lymph nodes (226). As noted above, this $CD8^+$ cell activity depends on strong type 1 cytokine production (Figure 11.9). It would appear that most in-

Table 13.8 Factors influencing long-term survival

1. Infection with an attenuated HIV strain (*nef*-mutated) showing a reduced replicative ability[a]
2. Strong cell-mediated anti-HIV immune response, particularly CD8$^+$ cell noncytotoxic antiviral activity; depends on type 1 cytokine production
3. Genetic background (immune response)
4. Neutralizing antibody[a]
5. Young age
6. Lack of one CCR-5 allele[a]

[a] In some studies.

fected individuals initially have this CD8$^+$ cell antiviral response. It can be demonstrated sometimes very shortly after infection, before antibody production, and is detected before neutralizing antibodies are seen (see Chapters 4 and 11) (1637). A loss of CD8$^+$ cell anti-HIV activity appears to presage the development of disease. This cellular immune response is probably reduced before substantial virus production takes place, since decreased CD8$^+$ cell noncytotoxic antiviral activity can be demonstrated before a major reduction in CD4$^+$ cell counts occurs and viral RNA production rises (1491) (Figure 13.2).

The reason for the decrease in CD8$^+$ cell antiviral response that permits increased virus replication and progression to disease remains to be elucidated (Section II) (Table 13.8). As with other viruses, one major influence can be the genetic makeup of the individual; protection can come from strong immune responses and reduced inherent sensitivity of the host cells to virus replication. For example, people infected with the same or different HIV-1 strains showed a similar rate of change in CD4$^+$ lymphocyte number and viral RNA levels. These findings support the conclusion that host factors, rather than the virus, are most important in determining HIV-1 disease progression (1983a). A recent report of HIV infection in monozygotic triplets also illustrates the importance of the genetic background on host response to the virus. All three children, receiving the same virus through transfusion of a common unit at birth, showed very similar immunologic profiles during several years of infection and developed the same opportunistic infections (2367). In addition, younger age groups can have slower progression perhaps secondary to a more vigorous immune response. An important factor is the extent of cytokine production needed to maintain a strong CD8$^+$ cell response (Figure 13.3). As discussed in Chapter 11, the relative levels of type 1 and type 2 responses appear to be directly involved (138), and what influences the switch from type 1 to type 2 responses is an important question (481) (Section IV).

Progression to disease does not correlate with a reduction in total numbers of CD8$^+$ T cells (1515, 1629). The level of this lymphocyte subset often remains ele-

Table 13.9 Possible reasons for lack of HIV infection in high-risk individuals

1. Exposure to killed virus or viral antigens
2. Low viral load of partner (seminal fluid, vaginal fluid, blood)
3. Inherited resistance of host cells to HIV (e.g., mucosa, lymphocytes, decreased coreceptor expression)
4. Strong immunologic response against HIV that eliminates infection shortly after it occurs

vated until the late stages of disease (1422, 1497). The emergence of a virulent strain that cannot be controlled by CD8$^+$ cells also does not seem to be the cause. In cell culture, CD8$^+$ cells demonstrate high antiviral activity against HIV-1 and HIV-2 strains, whether cytopathic or not (137, 1515). Thus, it appears that an intrinsic reduction in CD8$^+$ cell activity is involved. Why this antiviral response is lost over time is an important unanswered question. The loss could reflect a shift from type 1 to type 2 cytokine production (Section VII), which may be related to dysfunction of dendritic cells and other APC (1515) (Section IV).

VI.   High-Risk Exposed Seronegative Individuals

As reviewed in Chapter 11, some individuals with a history of exposure to HIV on several occasions are not infected by the virus (1491, 2297, 2470). The possible reasons for this resistance to infection need to be defined (Table 13.9). The seronegative individuals have the following two characteristics. (i) Some lack CCR-5 expression (homozygous for the deletion mutation) (see Chapter 3) (1568, 2346). (ii) Several (50% of those we studied) have CD8$^+$ cell noncytotoxic activity against HIV (1491, 2601a) (see Chapter 11, Section VI; Figure 11.14). This latter feature does suggest that the subjects were exposed to live virus but have controlled the infection. Some investigators have reported CTL responses against HIV in this group (2296; for reviews, see references 1426, 2297, and 2470), while others have reported T-cell proliferation with exposure to viral antigens (475, 2297) (see also Chapter

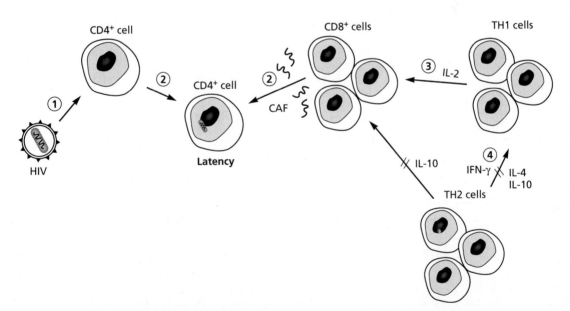

Figure 13.10   Viral and immunologic events in the persistent stage of HIV infection (long-term survivors). HIV infection of CD4$^+$ cells (step 1) is placed into a relatively latent state by the action of CD8$^+$ cells and their antiviral factor (CAF) ($\sim\sim$) (step 2). This CD8$^+$ cell anti-HIV response is increased with the production of cytokines (i.e., IL-2) secreted by TH1-type CD4$^+$ cells (step 3). The TH1-type cytokines also suppress the potential inhibitory effects of TH2-type cytokines on this control of HIV infection by CD8$^+$ cells (step 4). (Modified from reference 1491 with permission.)

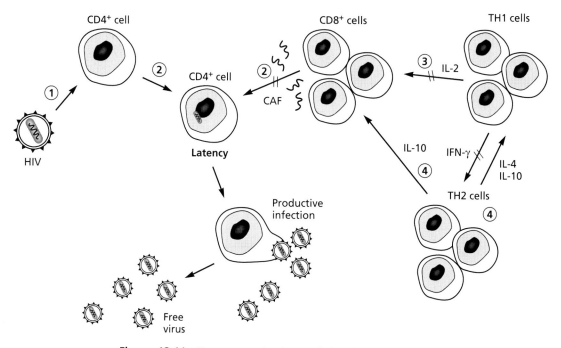

Figure 13.11   Events occurring in HIV-infected individuals progressing to disease (progressors). The events described in the legend to Figure 13.10 are changed by a predominant expression of the TH2-type versus the TH1-type cytokine response. Cytokines such as IL-4 and IL-10 (step 4) can suppress cytokine production by TH1-type cells and thereby affect the CD8$^+$ cell antiviral activity. Moreover, these cellular factors can directly suppress CD8$^+$ cell antiviral responses (Figure 11.9). The result of the loss of CD8$^+$ cell antiviral activity is release of HIV from latency and production of virus in lymph nodes and peripheral blood. These events lead to development of disease. (Modified from reference 1491 with permission.)

11). Some evidence that previous exposure to low levels of viral antigen induces this immunologic resistance comes from studies of monkeys receiving small doses of infectious SIV. These animals, which did not seroconvert or have detectable virus, were protected from a low-dose viral challenge that infected the naive control animals (471).

VII.   Conclusions: Viral and Immunologic Features of HIV Pathogenesis

In summary, long-term survival (or nonprogression) of HIV infection appears to depend on dominant type 1 responses of CD4$^+$ cells (138, 481). Cytokines, such as IL-2, support cell-mediated immunity and enhance CD8$^+$ cell antiviral responses and the production of CAF (see Chapter 11) (Figures 13.3, 13.9, and 13.10). Likewise, the production of TH1-type cytokines (e.g., IL-2 and IFN-γ) in long-term survivors helps maintain CD8$^+$ cell anti-HIV activity (Figure 11.9) and other immune functions (see Chapters 10 and 11). In contrast, in progressors, TH2-type cytokines (e.g., IL-4 and IL-10) suppress CD8$^+$ cell antiviral responses (see Chapters 9 and 11) (Figure 11.9). Thus, individuals progressing to disease could reflect a shift from a

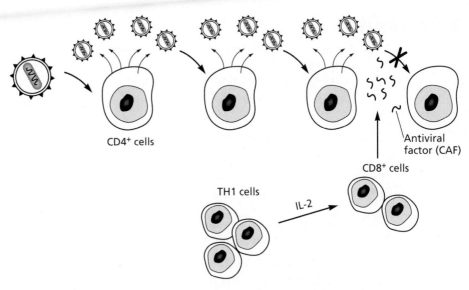

Figure 13.12   Cellular immune responses in long-term survival: approaches to controlling HIV pathogenesis. Methods directed at increasing CD8$^+$ cell anti-HIV activity such as IL-2 therapy (e.g., increasing production of the CD8$^+$ cell antiviral cytokine [CAF]) or enhancement of TH1-type cell responses would suppress HIV infection and maintain a long asymptomatic state. Administration of CAF, once purified, might also be beneficial. (Modified from reference 1491 with permission.)

TH1- to a TH2-type cell response. The type 2 cytokines subsequently produced not only turn off the type 1 cytokines needed for strong cell-mediated immune responses but also can directly affect the antiviral responses by CD8$^+$ cells (Figure 13.11). The reason for this shift in dominant cytokine production is not known but may reflect damage to dendritic cells (1515).

When sufficient numbers of CD4$^+$ cells are lost by direct or indirect mechanisms (see Chapter 9), the levels of cytokines such as IL-2 that are needed to maintain the functions of CD8$^+$ cells will be reduced (Figures 13.3 and 13.4). The resultant loss of CD8$^+$ cell antiviral activity and CAF production then leads to the emergence of HIV from many "latently" infected cells in both lymph nodes and peripheral blood (Figure 13.4). The noncytopathic strains will induce further CD4$^+$ cell loss by indirect mechanisms. With increased HIV production, the mutations associated with formation or emergence of the "virulent" strains can eventually take place.

If this concept of HIV pathogenesis is correct, a major question is: What approaches can be made to maintain the TH1-type responses and thus prevent replication of HIV (Figure 13.12)? The possibilities under consideration are the use of type 1 cytokines directly, of IL-12, or of neutralizing antibodies to certain type 2 cytokines such as IL-4 and IL-10 (see Chapters 9, 11, and 14) (476, 484). Moreover, the importance of CD8$^+$ cells in controlling the infection has been explored through the administration to infected individuals of autologous CD8$^+$ cells previously grown in large quantities ex vivo (see Chapter 14) (1088, 1323). It is hoped that approaches to increase CD8$^+$ cell antiviral responses in the host or the use of CAF directly will bring long-term survival to all HIV-infected individuals.

1. Cofactors that might play a role in HIV pathogenesis include the genetic makeup of the host, infection by other viruses or infectious agents, sexually transmitted diseases, immune-stimulating processes such as allergens, and other factors that influence cytokine production.

2. Lifestyle factors, particularly alcohol, smoking, drugs, and stress, are possible cofactors in HIV pathogenesis, particularly in their effect on mental capacity.

3. HIV pathogenesis involves three major clinical stages of infection: an early period in which high virus production takes place, a persistent period when virus is maintained at a lower threshold primarily by the immune system, and a symptomatic period when viral production has reemerged and presages the development of disease. At these various clinical stages, the virus shows homogeneity, heterogeneity, and then a return to homogeneity, respectively.

4. Two phases of HIV pathogenesis can be reflected by a slow turnover of $CD4^+$ cell numbers during the persistent period and a rapid loss of these cells in the symptomatic period. The nature of the replicating virus (NSI or SI) can influence this process.

5. The factors involved in the decrease in immune function include loss of $CD4^+$ cells by direct killing or by indirect effects such as apoptosis; relative changes in type 1 or type 2 cytokine production that can influence cell-mediated immunity; aberrant immune responses, such as autoreactive T cells; autoantibodies; and an inadequate production of IL-2. A possible detrimental role of CTL should be considered.

6. In the absence of therapy, a delay in progression to disease correlates with low viral RNA levels and high numbers of $CD4^+$ cells in the blood. Several other parameters reflecting immune activation, virus phenotype, and reduced immune function may be predictive of the risk for progression to disease.

7. Three clinical outcomes of HIV infection can be distinguished: a typical progression over 8 to 10 years, a rapid progression within 2 to 5 years, and a long-term survival or nonprogression in which an individual remains healthy for more than 10 years. One other group, patients with an AIDS diagnosis (<200 $CD4^+$ cells/μl), may not develop terminal disease for several years.

8. Factors involved in long-term survival can include infection with a virus with reduced cytopathic effects and low replicative ability; an absence of enhancing antibodies; a strong $CD8^+$ cell antiviral noncytopathic response; and a dominant TH1-type cytokine pattern. Loss of $CD8^+$ cell noncytotoxic antiviral activity presages progression to disease.

9. Long-term survival appears to depend on sufficient production of IL-2, which maintains the $CD8^+$ cell anti-HIV response and other immune functions that protect the host from disease. A basic determinant would appear to be normally functioning APC (e.g., dendritic cells).

10. High-risk exposed seronegative individuals represent a clinical group that has probably been protected from infection by a strong cellular immune response.

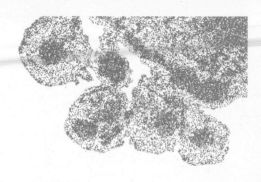

Antiviral Therapies

14

Wᴴɪʟᴇ ᴛʜɪѕ ʙᴏᴏᴋ ᴄᴀɴɴᴏᴛ ᴄᴏᴠᴇʀ ɪɴ ᴅᴇᴛᴀɪʟ ᴛʜᴇ ᴍᴀɴʏ ᴛʜᴇʀᴀᴘᴇᴜᴛɪᴄ approaches being evaluated to control HIV infection, some review of work in this field is appropriate and important. Several steps in the viral infection cycle discussed in the early chapters (Figure 5.1) have been targeted for antiviral action (for reviews, see references 1208 and 2222). Many drugs have been evaluated over the past decade (Figure 14.1; Table 14.1). A brief historical account is provided in this chapter and is followed by an update on present therapies. Recently, antiviral drugs, when used in combination, have shown real promise in controlling HIV infection. The effect of these therapies on neurologic disorders is covered in Chapter 9.

I. Anti-HIV Therapies

A. Reverse Transcriptase Inhibitors: Monotherapy

Recognizing the causative agent of AIDS as a retrovirus led to an immediate emphasis on arresting the replicative cycle of the virus. It is not surprising, therefore, that the first successful drug found

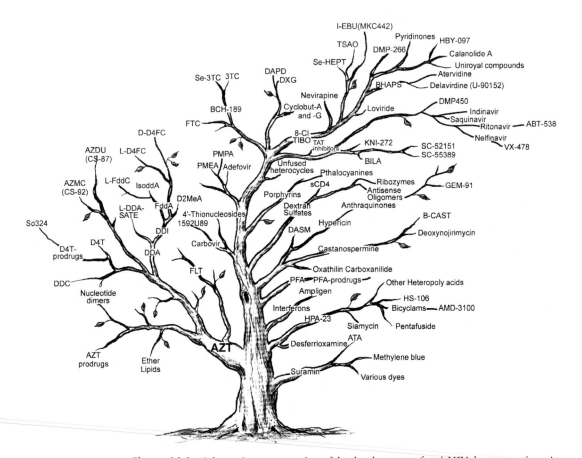

Figure 14.1 Schematic representation of the development of anti-HIV drugs over time. At the left side are the nucleoside analogs. At the right side are the nonnucleoside drugs. The tree presents several different approaches directed at the replicative cycle of HIV. (Revised from original figure in reference 2390a and provided by R. Schinazi).

was an inhibitor of the required reverse transcription. A compound that had been previously synthesized for potential use against cancer, 3′-azido-3-deoxythymidine (AZT) (zidovudine or Retrovir), inhibited viral reverse transcriptase (RT) and HIV replication in vitro (1798). Its mechanism of action, evaluated in the laboratory, appears to involve both a termination of viral DNA production and a competition for nucleosides used by the viral polymerase. Nevertheless, the exact mechanism(s) for AZT activity in vivo is not known.

AZT was immediately evaluated clinically and was soon reported effective in preventing the onset of symptoms (656, 2933). At first, large doses of the drug were administered (1,500 mg/day) and were associated with frequent side effects, especially toxicity to the bone marrow (758). Subsequently, the amount of AZT prescribed was reduced to 500 to 600 mg/day. This level resulted in fewer harmful side effects (500). In many patients, this drug decreased symptoms of the disease and in some cases delayed progression. Nevertheless, it did not prevent the emergence of syncytium-inducing (SI) strains (1455), which are more commonly encountered in

Table 14.1 Potential approaches to therapies for HIV infection

Anti-HIV virions	Postintegration
sCD4	Anti-Tat (Ro 24-7429)
Neutralizing antibodies (polyclonal, monoclonal)[a]	Antiprotease
	Antisense nucleotides
Virus entry	Hypericin
CD4 analogs	Ribozymes
Galactosyl ceramide analogs	CAF
Neutralizing antibodies[a]	Cytokines (immune modulation)
Saliva glycoprotein	**Virus budding**
Sulfated polysaccharides	Glycosylation inhibitors
Peptide T	(castanospermine)
Early steps prior to integration	Interferons
Anti-RT, e.g., nucleoside analogs (e.g., AZT, ddI, ddC, d4T), nonnucleoside inhibitors (e.g., TIBO, nevirapine, foscarnet)	**Anti-infected cells**
	Trichosanthin (compound Q)
	Antiviral antibodies—antibody-dependent cellular cytotoxicity
Antinucleotides (e.g., MPA, hydroxyurea)	rCD4 toxin
Anti-integrase	Anti-gp120 toxin
Interferons	UV-A plus psoralen
Hypericin	CD8$^+$ cells
Anti-RNA (e.g., hammerhead RNA)	

[a] By either passive immunotherapy or active immunization.

patients with disease (see Chapter 7). Whether AZT therapy used alone prolonged survival was controversial (see below). Moreover, for many asymptomatic individuals, even those on low doses, a reduction in quality of life negated the benefit of any delay in disease progression (1477). Based on the early reports, therapy was recommended for asymptomatic individuals with a CD4$^+$ cell count of <500 cells/μl (2786), but that recommendation was later challenged (2441). Some studies suggested that AZT treatment offered less benefit to asymptomatic subjects than to symptomatic patients (1164). The effect of the drug was short-term and appeared to be greatest late in the clinical course (2138).

In a noteworthy clinical trial lasting 3 years and involving several cohorts in Europe (the Concorde study), AZT was not found to prolong survival or delay disease progression (2441). The study also showed that CD4$^+$ cell counts were not predictive of drug efficacy. Similarly, AZT treatment of asymptomatic adults with ≥500 CD4$^+$ cells/μl did not prolong either AIDS-free or overall survival (2785). The conclusion from these reports was that the decision to initiate AZT therapy should be made according to when the clinical benefit would be greatest, which seemed to be when symptoms developed (2352). Today, however, since other antiviral drugs have shown clinical value in combination with AZT, the early use of drugs is being reconsidered (see below).

Over the past 3 to 5 years, other nucleoside analogs that compete with the viral RT have been introduced into treatment (Table 14.2). Like AZT, many need to be activated by intracellular phosphorylation. 2′,3′-Dideoxyinosine (didanosine [ddI]) and 2′,3′-dideoxycytidine (zalcitabine [ddC]) appear to be effective and less toxic to bone marrow than AZT (328, 2222, 2472, 2932). Nevertheless, their administration has been associated with pancreatitis and peripheral neuropathy. Another

Table 14.2 Anti-HIV drugs[a]

Drug names[b]	Studied most in combination with:	How given	Side effects
RT inhibitors			
Retrovir (zidovudine, AZT)	ddI, ddC, 3TC, saquinavir, ritonavir, indinavir, nevirapine	Two or three times daily	Anemia, granulocytopenia
Videx (didanosine, ddI)	AZT, d4T, indinavir, nevirapine	Twice daily, 1 h before or 2 h after eating	Pancreatitis, peripheral neuropathy
Hivid (zalcitabine, ddC)	AZT, saquinavir	Three times daily 1 h before or 2 h after eating	Peripheral neuropathy, pancreatitis
Zerit (stavudine, d4T)	ddI, 3TC, nelfinavir	Twice daily	Peripheral neuropathy
Epivir (lamivudine, 3TC)	AZT, d4T, AZT plus 3TC; is well studied with all protease inhibitors	Twice daily	Adults: mild headache, nausea, fatigue; children who have had pancreatitis should use AZT plus 3TC only if they cannot take other anti-HIV drugs
Viramune (nevirapine)	AZT, AZT plus ddI	Once daily for first 2 weeks, then twice daily, with or without food	Rash, usually transient
Rescriptor (delavirdine)	AZT, ddI, AZT plus ddI	Three times daily	Rash, usually transient
Protease inhibitors			
Invirase (saquinavir)	AZT, ddC, AZT plus ddC, ritonavir	Three times daily	Mostly mild; nausea, diarrhea
Norvir (ritonavir)	AZT plus 3TC, AZT plus ddC, saquinavir	Twice daily, with meals if possible	Nausea, numbness around mouth, diarrhea common, especially in first weeks of therapy; advised to start with 300 mg twice daily, then build up to the full dose, 600 mg twice daily, within 2 weeks
Crixivan (indinavir)	AZT, AZT plus 3TC, AZT plus ddI	Three times daily, 1 h before or 2 h after eating, or with a light low-fat meal	Painful kidney stones (high water intake lowers the chance of this side effect)
Viracept (nelfinavir)	d4T, AZT plus 3TC	Three times daily with food	Diarrhea, usually transient

[a] Adapted from reference 1672a, with permission.

[b] The first drug name in each group, spelled with a capital letter, is the brand name, i.e., the official name approved by the FDA. The second name, spelled without a capital letter, is the generic name, i.e., the one used during later studies of a drug. The nucleosides are usually referred to by abbreviation of the chemical names of the drugs (i.e., AZT, ddI, ddC, d4T, 3TC). For therapy, AZT, d4T, and nevirapine can pass the blood-brain barrier; ddI, ddC, and 3TC are most active in quiescent infected cells.

anti-RT drug, 2',3'-didehydro-3'-deoxythymidine (stavudine [d4T]) (300), has shown less toxicity than the other drugs, with some indication of stabilization of $CD4^+$ cells. In patients previously receiving AZT, d4T showed a moderate effect in delaying disease progression, compared to the progression in those who continued taking AZT (2558). The nucleoside analog (−)-2'-deoxy-3'-thiothiadine (lamivudine [3TC]) was found to have activity against HIV-1 strains resistant to AZT. However, monotherapy with 3TC soon gives rise to resistant strains. Nevertheless, the common mutation in the HIV-1 polymerase gene at the 184 Met codon that confers resistance to the drug maintains or restores the sensitivity of the virus to AZT (714). Thus, 3TC and AZT are often used in combination (Section I.C).

Nonnucleoside RT inhibitors (NNRTIs) such as nevirapine and the thiobenzimidazolone (TIBO) agents have also been described (Table 14.2). They affect the hydrophobic pocket within the polymerase domain of the p66 RT subunit. The TIBO compounds selectively inactivate the RT of HIV-1 and not HIV-2 (2222), probably because of their specific predilection for the end chain of the HIV-1 polymerase (2482). These drugs, even given in lower doses than AZT, can be toxic and have not been effective in clinical trials because of the rapid development of drug resistance (2226, 2316). However, the use of the NNRTI nevirapine in combination with nucleoside analogs has shown dramatic antiviral effects (1893). Recently, a thiocarboxyanilide NNRTI (UC781) has been described that can render cells refractory to HIV infection and that inactivates the polymerase enzyme within the virion (249). This drug and related second-generation NNRTI therapies (2302) are under further study.

B.   Protease Inhibitors

The protease inhibitors block the action of another HIV enzyme, which is also encoded by the *pol* gene. Protease autocatalyzes its own precursor protein and then

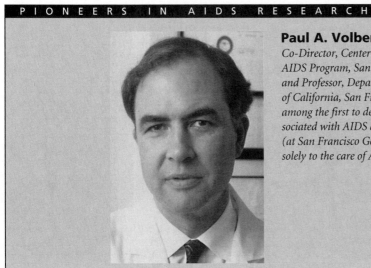

PIONEERS IN AIDS RESEARCH

Paul A. Volberding

Co-Director, Center for AIDS Research and the AIDS Program, San Francisco General Hospital, and Professor, Department of Medicine, University of California, San Francisco. Dr. Volberding was among the first to define the clinical syndromes associated with AIDS and established the first ward (at San Francisco General Hospital) dedicated solely to the care of AIDS patients.

cleaves other polypeptides to bring viral proteins into functional units. In general, this activity occurs within the virion during or after budding from the cell surface (Figures 5.1 and 14.2). Similar to the advancement made with crystallization of RT (1337), the crystal structure of the protease enzyme (1909, 2901) helped in the development of these antiviral drugs. Computer modeling was able to identify compounds that could fit into the active site at the base of a cleft present in the dimeric form of the functional HIV-1 protease (712, 2249).

Thus far, the U.S. Food and Drug Administration has approved four protease inhibitors for treatment of HIV infection: sequinavir mesylate (Invirase), ritonavir (Norvir), indinavir sulfate (Crixivan), and nelfinavir mesylate (Viracept) (Table 14.2). These drugs have provided a major boost in the management of HIV infection and have influenced the concepts of treatment along the lines of those used in anticancer therapies (for reviews, see references 611 and 2897). In essence, adding the protease inhibitors to drugs with different antiviral effects (e.g., retroviral RT inhibitors, either nucleoside or nonnucleoside) has led to promising results on the persistent control of HIV replication in the body and restoration of an asymptomatic clinical course (Section I.C).

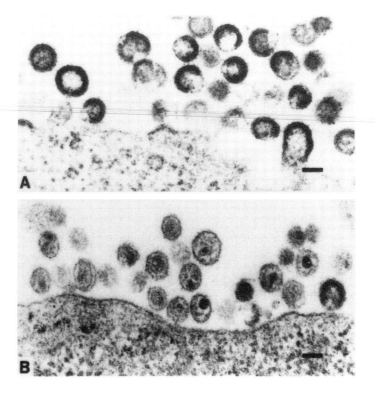

Figure 14.2   (A) Donut-shaped HIV-1 particles from a T-cell line infected with a protease-deficient virus (1228). The morphology of the particles resembles that of viruses released from protease inhibitor-treated cells. (B) For comparison, the wild-type virus released from the T-cell line is presented. Bar, 100 nm. (Figure provided by K. Ikuta.)

Each of the drugs, however, can cause substantial adverse effects and can interact with other medications. Thus, several factors need to be considered when prescribing protease inhibitors, including their interaction with various analgesics, antibiotics, anticoagulants, and other antiretroviral drugs (611). If the protease inhibitors are not used according to the recommended timing (e.g., Crixivan every 8 h), viral resistance that often shows cross-reactivity with other protease inhibitors could quickly emerge (Section I.E). Adherence to the protocol is important, leading to some discussion about not giving these drugs to those who might not be compliant (e.g., intravenous drug users). Such individuals could be a source of resistant strains in the environment. Importantly, however, some studies suggest that nelfinavir has limited cross-resistance with other protease inhibitors (2047).

A notable concern is the oral bioavailability of certain protease inhibitors (especially sequinavir) and their capacity to cross the blood-brain barrier to enter other reservoirs for the virus in the body. For example, none of these drugs thus far has shown efficient passage into the cerebrospinal fluid (because of the high degree of protein binding), and the development of drug-resistant strains in these sanctuaries must be considered. It is also noteworthy that protease-defective HIV particles produced in the laboratory can induce apoptosis of human peripheral blood mononuclear cells (PBMC) (1228). The effect of these protease-deficient virus particles on the viability of $CD4^+$ cells in vivo merits further consideration.

C.   Combination Therapy

Because the antiviral effects of the RT inhibitor monotherapies were limited, the use of two or three drug therapies was begun, and the results are now being reported (Table 14.2). Initially, AZT, ddI, ddC, and combinations of these drugs were attempted in two-drug therapy trials (997, 1219, 2357). In general, adding another nucleoside analog increased the efficacy of the treatment, but often resistance resulted and persistent control of virus replication was not achieved. One of the most effective approaches has been dual treatment of HIV-infected individuals with AZT and 3TC. The doses are well tolerated, and the dual treatment shows better improvement in $CD4^+$ cell counts and viral levels than treatment with either of the drugs alone (714). Most importantly, the lack of emergence of a resistant strain in this combination can be explained by the 3TC-induced mutation in codon 184 of the viral RT. This mutation appears to prevent the emergence of resistance to AZT (associated with a codon 215 mutation) (1432) by increasing the fidelity of the polymerase enzyme (2807).

The most dramatic effect on viral RNA levels has come with triple-drug therapy, in which two anti-RT drugs are combined with a protease inhibitor (611). Recent statistics suggest that a decline in death rate from AIDS in individuals with <100 $CD4^+$ cells/µl can be credited to the use of such antiretroviral drugs in combination (1095). As noted above, protease inhibitors given alone quickly give rise to resistant strains, some of which become cross-resistant to other protease inhibitors. However, in combination with other anti-HIV drugs, they add an antiviral effect that can lead to undetectable levels of virus in the plasma for many months. In short-term therapy, there appears to be no substantial toxicity. Common clinical findings are fatigue, diarrhea, and nausea (501). An important consideration is the interaction that can occur when multiple drugs are used concomitantly. For example, ritonavir is a strong inhibitor of cytochrome P-450, which is involved in the metabolism of protease inhibitors by the liver. If it is used along with sequinavir, toxic levels of sequinavir can result (1760). Alternatively, since sequinavir has poor oral bioavailability, ritonavir can increase its therapeutic potential.

| D. | ## Other Antiviral Approaches |

Integrase, a third viral enzyme, is essential for productive virus infection (2898) (see Chapter 4). This enzyme has been purified and its crystal structure identified at 2.5 Å (676). Like protease, it has a dimeric form. In macrophages but not CD4$^+$ lymphocytes, limited replication of an HIV integrase-defective mutant has been achieved (358). Macrophage-specific factors must help in the transcription of unintegrated viral DNA. However, in general, without the function of integrase, HIV is not infectious. Thus, future drugs targeted to integrase should also help control HIV replication.

Another direction in antiviral therapy has been the utilization of nucleotide analogs, a new class of RT inhibitors that contain a phosphate group and thus are less dependent on cellular kinase activity for activation. As an example, 9-(2-phosphonomethoxypropyl)adenine (PMPA) has shown promising results in preventing disease development (2755). Moreover, if given soon after virus transmission, the drug can block the establishment of infection (2718). While resistance to this compound can occur, its use after early exposure to the virus is receiving increased attention. A similar drug, adefovir dipivoxil (PMEA), has shown anti-HIV activity in phase II trials (610).

Attention has also been given to blocking some of the intracellular enzymatic properties that are needed for maturation of the virus. For example, analogs of myristic acid, which is necessary for the myristoylation of the Gag and Nef proteins, have reduced HIV replication (304). The addition of two hydroxy fatty acids to the regimen of antiviral drugs might also provide a different antiviral approach (1014). However, the potential effect of these treatments on normal cellular function involving these enzymes makes their use unlikely.

Most recently, the compound 2-hydroxy-3′-dideoxymethyl cystidine (BEA-005) has shown very effective antiviral activity in culture (2619) and in monkeys inoculated with SIV or HIV-2 (260). Animals receiving either virus by the intravenous or rectal route were protected from infection if the drug was administered before or up to 3 h after exposure. Complete protection from transmission appeared to result, since the animals could be infected subsequently with virus. Thus, presumably their immune systems had not previously encountered the virus. This new drug, like PMPA (above), offers promise for use after needlestick injury and for therapy for individuals who have recently been exposed to the virus by other means.

Other directions for antiviral therapy have included attacks on the viral cellular receptor by using recombinant CD4 (rCD4); blocking of virus attachment with sulfated polysaccharides (107, 1710); the use of interferons (1079, 1770, 1775); therapies directed at regulatory proteins or regions (e.g., Tat and the long terminal repeat [LTR]) (1119, 1530, 1969); viral envelope proteins (602, 1912, 2875); Gag and nucleocapsid proteins (2222, 2727); and approaches that destroy the virus-infected cells (217, 1441) (Table 14.1). In the last case, anti-gp120 antibodies, anti-CD4 antibodies, or soluble CD4 (sCD4) linked to ricin or other toxins (e.g., pseudomonas, pokeweed antiviral protein) have been tried in culture alone and in combination with AZT (94, 1664, 2179, 2964). More recently, efforts to develop small molecules to block virus attachment to the HIV coreceptors (CCR-5, CXCR-4) have been evaluated (2509). They offer promise because they do not appear to induce chemotaxic signaling (2509). Nevertheless, since HIV can use a variety of different coreceptors (Chapter 3), decoys for a particular coreceptor may select for viruses that will find other means of cell entry. The risk of HIV evolving to home out in other cells or tissues must be considered.

Ribozymes, antisense molecules, and attempts at gene therapy with intracellular *trans*-dominant inhibitors have been proposed after promising results were observed in vitro (740, 2067, 2287; for a review, see reference 282) (Table 14.1). Many of these theoretical approaches, nevertheless, need a means of drug delivery. The recognition of the three-dimensional structures of the HIV MA protein (1692) and the ectodomain portion of gp41 (393, 2849) may permit the development of therapies against these molecules. In addition, drugs against glycosylation have been considered (959, 2192). For example, castanospermine disrupts the glycosylation of the viral envelope and makes the virus noninfectious. Some investigators have considered using immunosuppressive drugs such as cyclosporine because of the possible detrimental effects of hyperactive immune responses in HIV pathogenesis (2430) (see Chapter 11). Furthermore, analogs of this drug lacking immune system-suppressing activity may be useful because they block cyclophilin A association with the Gag (p24) protein (211, 270, 787, 2663) (see Chapter 4). They are believed to prevent the opening of the viral capsid after virus entry and its transport to the nucleus. Thus, infection cannot take place. In addition, drugs that block the zinc finger motif of the NC protein have been considered (2223, 2727).

Compounds that prevent the incorporation of nucleotides into DNA and act on autoreactive immune cells have also been evaluated. Mycophenolic acid (MPA), at nontoxic concentrations that can be reached in the blood, inhibited HIV-1 and HIV-2 replication in cultured $CD4^+$ lymphocytes and macrophages (1151). Hydroxyurea also reduces the formation of deoxynucleoside triphosphate substrates (842, 1769). The addition of hydroxyurea to RT inhibitors has shown synergistic effects in inhibiting HIV replication in culture (1653) and a moderate effect in vivo (1814). *N*-Acetyl-L-cysteine, the antioxidant compound, has been proposed as a safe therapy in HIV infection (1561, 2264). It reportedly inhibits intracellular factors and cytokines that enhance HIV replication. Glutathione has been shown to block HIV replication by decreasing virus budding and release (2018). All these ideas require further examination and evaluation. Finally, as with other incurable diseases, many unproved approaches to therapy for HIV infection have been tried (4) with inconclusive results (317).

E.   Drug Resistance

One notable problem with antiviral treatments has been the emergence of resistant virus strains (839, 926, 1431, 2227). The most common genetic alteration linked to AZT resistance is a 2-bp modification leading to a change from threonine to tyrosine or phenylalanine at position 215 (1370). At least five genetic alterations associated with AZT resistance have been identified (1263, 1431, 2227). Reversion to an AZT-sensitive strain after cessation of therapy appears to take several months (35). The resistant strain is not necessarily more virulent (1161). Resistance to ddC, ddI, and 3TC and to protease inhibitors has also been reported (504, 764, 2227, 2559, 2807).

Fortunately, viruses from patients on monotherapy have not shown concomitant resistance to related anti-RT drugs, so that changes in therapy can be instituted, at least for a while (2227, 2228, 2273). With time, however, even with alternating therapies, resistance to multiple RT inhibitors can occur (763, 926, 1171, 2455).

In terms of cellular viral load, subjects who had received AZT for long periods of time and had ddI added to their therapy showed a reduction in viral RNA in plasma but no change in viral load as measured by PBMC DNA. Importantly, if wild-type and resistant strains were found in the plasma before therapy, only the resistant virus strain was noted in the plasma after therapy whereas the PBMC DNA maintained both types of virus (1101). This finding emphasizes that antiretroviral drugs affect only de novo infection and that the majority of circulating virions represent the product of such infection. Cells containing virus before treatment begins can be long-lived and unaffected by the therapy (1492). Certain studies have demonstrated, however, that the viral load in lymph node tissue can decline with single-drug therapy (1397), suggesting a gradual loss of infected cells. Moreover, effective elimination of many HIV-infected cells from lymphoid tissues has been achieved recently with combination therapies (see below) (379, 2072).

Sometimes cells such as macrophages are refractory to the antiretroviral effects of AZT because of decreased formation of AZT triphosphate, decreased phosphorylation of thymidine triphosphate, and/or decreased levels of thymidine kinase activity (1744, 2230). Cell-to-cell transmission of HIV in cultures containing AZT has also been noted (968). The role of these factors in the emergence of resistant strains remains to be determined.

In the laboratory, strains with resistance to four different anti-RT drugs have been identified (1171, 1430). Importantly, in one infected patient treated sequentially with five nucleoside RT inhibitors and one NNRTI, drug-resistant mutations produced a strain resistant to all of the dideoxynucleoside analogs tested and many NNRTIs (2396). Thus, this therapy did not prevent the appearance of multidrug-resistant viruses that maintain a stable replication rate.

Viral resistance to protease inhibitors has been recognized frequently in both in vitro and in vivo studies (504, 2278). These resistant viruses can even be found in untreated individuals (1458). Mutations in the protease gene that confer resistance have been described for all the currently available protease inhibitor drugs (504, 611). The flexibility of structure and function in the protease enzyme may make resistance more easily attainable than with the other viral enzymes. Sustained concentrations of the protease inhibitors need to be maintained to avoid the emergence of this resistance (611), which occurs less frequently when the drugs are used in combination with other antiretroviral therapies. With some of the mutations, cross-resistance to five structurally different protease inhibitors was found (504). One protease inhibitor (nelfinavir, Viracept) may not share its resistance pattern with other antiprotease drugs (2047). Thus, when resistance to Viracept occurs, the other protease inhibitors may still be effective. However, if resistance to the other protease inhibitors develops first, there is usually also resistance to Viracept.

In one study, two distinct viruses, resistant to either a protease inhibitor or AZT, were used to coinfect T-lymphoblastoid cells in culture. A recombinant virus was recovered that was resistant to both AZT and the protease inhibitor (1869). These observations indicate that genetic recombination could be contributing to the high level of multidrug resistance observed during treatment. All these results suggest that combination therapy may not prevent the development of resistance and that previous therapy with one drug might limit the effect of other treatments. Moreover, resistant viruses may remain in certain tissues and be unrecognized in the blood. Later, they could emerge and spread in the individual receiving therapy. AZT-resistant strains have been detected in the lungs, but not the blood, of treated patients (854). Finally, the detection of AZT-resistant variants of HIV-1 in genital fluids and the association of drug-resistant viruses with sexual transmission (1160, 2806) emphasize the potential spread of resistant strains among populations.

F. Effects of Antiretroviral Therapy on Virus in Other Tissues

One of the major challenges of antiretroviral drugs besides plasma bioavailability is their distribution in other tissues, particularly the lymph nodes, brain, and testes. The brain and testes maintain compartments that can be somewhat separated from the blood (134). Whether present antiviral therapy will reduce viral load in genital fluids sufficiently to decrease spread of infection remains to be determined. Some studies have suggested a reduction in virus shedding during antiviral therapy (882a, 969a) (see Chapter 2).

Studies of AZT monotherapy showed that while decreases in the viral levels in plasma were noted, no effect on the viral load in PBMC and lymph node cells could be appreciated (496, 651, 1398). However, when ddI was added to the AZT regimen, a decrease in virus replication in lymph nodes was comparable to that seen in the plasma (497). In another report evaluating these two drugs, a reduction in the level of circulating free virus was noted in blood and lymph nodes but the number of infected cells remained unchanged in these tissue sites (2031).

Recent studies, however, have indicated that present combination therapies including protease inhibitors can markedly reduce the levels of virus and virus-infected cells in both blood and lymphoid tissue (379, 2029, 2072). With tonsil tissue as a mirror of the effect of combination therapy on lymph nodes, PCR procedures indicated that productively infected lymphocytes were initially rapidly reduced for a half-life of 1 day and the amount of HIV-1 RNA on follicular dendritic cells (FDC) decreased at a similar rate (379). After 6 months of combination therapy, both lymphoid mononuclear cell and FDC-associated virus levels were reduced by several log units. Moreover, the established half-life of FDC HIV RNA (1.7 days) indicated that fresh virus is constantly being attached to the FDC (379).

In brief, studies determining the loss of HIV-infected cells over time during combination antiviral therapy suggest that there are two phases. The data provide some estimates on the potential turnover rate of cells in the host (Table 14.3). One phase leads to a loss of productively infected cells within 2 days (379, 2072, 2073), and the other requires activation of latently infected cells. This second phase has been

Table 14.3 Estimated turnover rate of infected cells in HIV-infected individuals[a]

Cell	Half-life (days)[b]
Productively infected CD4$^+$ lymphocytes	1.1
Latently infected CD4$^+$ lymphocytes	8.5
CD4$^+$ lymphocytes with defective virus	145
Virus-infected macrophages/dendritic cells[c]	14.4

[a] Summarized from references 2072 and 2073.
[b] The plasma virus half-life has been estimated at 6 h.
[c] Or other long-lived cells.

estimated to have a half-life of up to 2 weeks (Table 14.3) (2072, 2073). CD4$^+$ lymphocytes with defective viruses have been estimated to turn over every 145 days, whereas infected macrophages/dendritic cells can take 2 weeks (2072, 2073) (Table 14.3). For asymptomatic HIV infection, the extent of replication can vary substantially. Whereas cell-free virus is found to undergo rapid turnover, latently infected CD4$^+$ T cells have a much lower rate of turnover and can therefore maintain viral persistence during therapy (2593a). Based on these characteristics of virus loss, at best 2 to 3 years is needed for elimination of HIV-1 from lymphoid tissues (2072). Removal of HIV from reservoirs in other tissues (e.g., the brain) could take considerably longer or be unattainable. The accuracy of these estimates requires further study.

In this regard, drug-resistant viruses could emerge in the lymph nodes or brain of treated patients before these viruses are detectable in the blood (1396, 1723, 2437). However, in some studies, viruses isolated from the cerebrospinal fluid and blood of patients receiving AZT therapy have shown similar resistant genetic profiles, suggesting communication between the drug and the viruses within these two compartments (629, 2876). This issue of efficient drug penetration into various tissue sites in the body remains a major concern in antiviral therapies.

Despite these advances in reducing the levels of free virus in the blood and lymph nodes, several HIV-infected cells can still remain in lymphoid tissue sites (379, 497a, 2029, 2072). After discontinuation of therapy, high-level HIV replication can return as rapidly as is observed in acute infection (2029). Thus, this reservoir of infected cells that are poorly susceptible to antiviral therapy is a challenge to present treatment approaches. Since the available anti-HIV drugs cannot readily eliminate the large reservoir of virus-infected cells, whether prolonged reduction in de novo HIV infection will gradually reduce these cells to a limited and controllable number remains to be seen.

If an analogy to cancer can be drawn, the number of virus-infected cells may be sufficiently reduced that many infected cells surviving the therapy will die by normal processes. However, like single cancer cells surviving chemotherapy, the remaining long-lived infected lymphocytes, macrophages, or other cells in the body can be the source from which resistant strains can emerge and spread. Eventually, viruses within the remaining infected cells can reset the biologic clock to the time (during primary infection) when virus replication took place unchallenged. However, now the virus is perhaps less well handled by the host, since the immune system has been compromised by previous antiviral therapy.

G.   Therapy for Acute Infection

Administration of AZT or other antiviral drugs during acute HIV infection is being assessed (2682) after some indication of a possible positive effect (1296, 1937). A reduction in clinical symptoms and a smaller decline in the CD4$^+$ cell number have been noted (for a review, see reference 1937). Recently, a combination of AZT, ddI, and 3TC given 5 to 28 days after the onset of acute symptoms decreased viral loads in the blood and lymph nodes of the treated individual (1399). Immediate AZT treatment protected SIV-infected newborn monkeys against a rapid clinical course (2756). However, antiviral drugs, including AZT, have been shown to decrease PBMC proliferative responses to mitogen (1041) and might blunt the immune response to HIV if used too late after acute infection (1505a, 2274, 2678). Further studies of therapy during primary infection are needed, particularly now that combination therapy offers the possibility of markedly reducing viral loads.

In connection with exposure to HIV, AZT use after needlestick injuries has reduced the infection rate eightfold (1801). In this case, the timing (within hours and not days) after infection could be the important parameter. AZT is currently the drug of choice for acute exposure because of its demonstration of a 79% reduction in seroconversion (1840a). AZT therapy should be initiated preferably within 1 to 2 hours after suspected exposure, but the time when it will no longer be useful has not been defined. A 4-week course of therapy should be administered, since this period has been shown to be most effective (1840b). 3TC should be added to increase antiviral activity in the case of suspected resistance, and a protease inhibitor could be used for exposure to the highest risk of transmission.

H.   Summary and Conclusions

There are seven nucleoside or nonnucleoside RT inhibitors presently available—AZT, ddI, ddC, 3TC, d4T, delavirdine, and nevirapine—and four protease inhibitors—sequinavir, ritonavir, indinavir, and nelfinavir (see below) (Table 14.2). Of these, indinavir appears to be the most widely used to date (611). Additional anti-HIV drugs are expected to be developed, and combinations will be examined in trials similar to those performed with anticancer therapies. Clinicians are advised not to add a protease inhibitor to a drug regimen that is not working, since resistance to the other drugs administered will permit low-level replication of viruses that will eventually become resistant to the protease inhibitor. In clarifying this issue of therapy, physicians caring for HIV-infected people in the United States and Great Britain have published guidelines for treatment (Table 14.4). The two reports are similar in recommending the monitoring of the viral load in plasma and the CD4$^+$ cell count, the use of therapy to prevent the onset of immune deficiency, the attempt to sustain undetectable virus levels in the blood, and the selection of new antiviral drugs when viremia returns in the subject (363, 857). Two-drug or preferably three-drug therapy is recommended for all infected individuals with CD4$^+$ cell counts of <500 cells/µl or with viral loads of 5,000 to 10,000 copies of RNA/ml. Monotherapy with any drug is no longer recommended (Table 14.4).

The enthusiasm for the great reduction in viral RNA levels by three-drug therapy (one of which is a protease inhibitor) has led to trials examining the use of these

Table 14.4 Considerations for initiating antiretroviral therapy—1997[a]

1. Therapy is recommended for all patients with HIV RNA levels above 5,000 to 10,000 copies/ml of plasma

2. Therapy should be considered for all HIV-infected patients with detectable HIV RNA in plasma

3. For patients at low risk of progression (low HIV RNA level in plasma and high CD4$^+$ cell count), particularly those who are not committed to complex antiretroviral regimens, therapy might be safely deferred. These patients should be reevaluated every 3–6 months.

[a] From reference 363 with permission.

drugs soon after primary infection or early in the symptomatic course. Physicians need to consider the adverse effects of these drugs, especially protease inhibitors, on other medications taken by patients, particularly antibiotics, anticoagulants, and other anti-HIV drugs. Conventionally, until very recently, AZT and 3TC were considered to form a good combination for initiation of therapy, since 3TC can reduce the resistance to AZT. Subsequently, therapies with other RT inhibitors and a protease inhibitor would be considered. Some clinicians are advocating the initiation of triple therapy for all infected people in hopes of reducing the emergence of resistant strains (1423). However, the long-term clinical benefit of two versus multiple drugs has not been determined.

Whether treatment should begin early in the infection needs further evaluation. The toxicity of the drugs versus the emergence of resistant strains should determine how soon an individual is treated. The initial findings with AZT led to its administration to many healthy individuals sooner than was needed (Section I). Some infected individuals and some clinicians are reluctant to begin early therapy for HIV infection because they fear that resistance will emerge and no further antiviral drugs will be available. However, many companies are announcing the development of new RT and protease inhibitors, as well as treatments eventually aimed at the other viral enzyme, integrase. In addition, other approaches for limiting viral replication (e.g., the use of Gag antagonists) might provide alternative directions for controlling the virus.

It will take time, as well, to determine if the reduction of HIV-1 RNA levels in plasma and lymph nodes and the increase in CD4$^+$ cell counts observed with present treatment regimens are associated with slower clinical progression and perhaps longer life in all treated people (1095, 1965). In 1996, the number of AIDS cases diagnosed in the United States had already decreased after a steady increase in over 16 years, and a decrease in deaths from AIDS has been recently noted (1095). In this regard, with the lack of adequate antiretroviral therapy in most parts of the world, a difference in survival from AIDS will become evident. Whereas initially the time from infection to disease appeared similar in individuals infected in the Western countries and in Africa (Chapter 13), this pattern will change with the lack of treatment in developing countries. Nevertheless, there are yet no data suggesting that early or more aggressive treatment improves the clinical outcome. If combination therapy is used, it may reduce the value of some of the drugs later. Importantly, the probability of drug resistance remains a constant challenge. Already some reports are indicating up to a 50% failure in the control of HIV replication in individuals on protease inhibitor and combination therapy (610b, 735a). New therapies for controlling the virus are needed, as well as treatments that do not show toxic effects on the body and do not require multiple doses each day. A less toxic RT inhibitor, 1592U89 (abacavir) (568a), and DMP-266 (Sustiva), an NNRTI, are in final clinical trials, and AZT in a 300-mg pill has become available. Moreover, a combination of AZT and 3TC in one pill has been developed. These innovations should help in treatment and compliance.

Adherence to therapy is important in warding off resistance; studies have shown that people taking medicine more than twice a day have difficulty maintaining the schedule (Figure 14.3) (939). The timing of medication can be very difficult to follow (Figure 14.4). A single daily planner from one such subject underlines this problem (Figure 14.5). Timed-release capsules, other creative drug delivery systems, or pills containing more than one drug would be helpful and are in development. Without compliance, resistance to therapies can quickly develop.

Importantly, despite an increase in CD4$^+$ cell numbers during antiviral therapies, the nature and function of these immune cells remain to be elucidated. Based on telomere lengths, the initial return of CD4$^+$ cells most probably results from redistribution of cells from sequestered sites in the body and not from renewal (685, 2911). The slow rise in the CD4$^+$ cell number could be explained by a block in generation of fresh CD4$^+$ cells through infection of stromal cells, events in the microenvironment, or infection of precursor CD4$^+$ cells (2911). The increased turnover of CD8$^+$ T cells in HIV infection (2911) argues against a block in precursor formation and in support of a peripheral expansion in the number of these cells (see Section IV). Some studies suggest that the replenished CD4$^+$ and CD8$^+$ cells lack the diversity in their repertoire to be effective in immunologic responses to new agents (510, 2029) (see Chapter 11, Figure 11.3). There is a limit to the number of naive lymphocytes produced, usually depending on the number existing before therapy (510). Some studies have also demonstrated a reduced function of the restored CD4$^+$ cells (510). Moreover, the number of CD4$^+$ cells in an individual following therapy cannot be considered to predict the same clinical outcome as the number present during the natural history of HIV infection. Cytomegalovirus (CMV) retinitis has developed in treated individuals whose CD4$^+$ cell counts had risen to almost

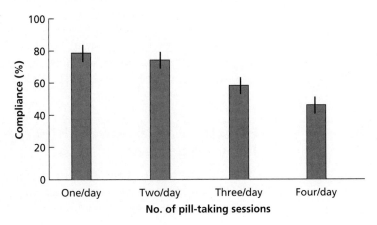

Figure 14.3 Studies on the ease of compliance in taking pills at regular times during the day. It is obvious that the need to take a smaller number of pills results in a much greater compliance. (Reproduced from reference 939 with permission.)

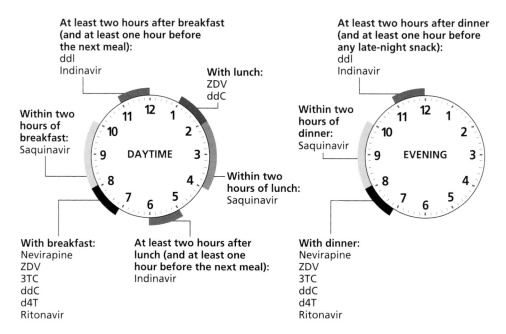

Figure 14.4   Daily dosing schedule for patients on combination therapy. A standard maintenance therapy is demonstrated for adults on two or three different antiretroviral drugs. (Modified from *AIDS Care* with permission.)

200/µl (1180). *Pneumocystis carinii* pneumonia has been observed in treated patients with $CD4^+$ cell numbers above 200/µl (1704). Thus, restoring the immune system to an effective antiviral state must be the optimal direction for therapies in HIV infection (1492) (Sections III and IV).

In this regard, one danger is the assumption in therapeutic approaches that mirroring the virologic parameter of low viral load in asymptomatic individuals is sufficient to ensure long-term survival. This concept lacks the understanding of the mechanism (i.e., the immune response) by which the untreated healthy individual controls virus replication. Unless the immune system is permitted to return to a normal state, the treated individual retains reservoirs of virus-infected cells that can destroy the immune system further in an indolent fashion and eventually induce a compromised immune state. For this reason, approaches to restore the immune response must be considered, with attention to control of the reservoir of virus-infected cells (1492, 1499) (Sections III and IV).

II.   Effects of Antiretroviral Therapy on the Immune System

Several studies have examined the effects of antiretroviral therapies on immunologic function (Table 14.5). Early studies with AZT-treated individuals suggested that these therapies reduced cell proliferation and would be toxic to the immune

TWO DAILY SCHEDULES		
Ritonavir/AZT/3TC	Time of day	Indinavir/AZT/3TC
	05:00	Fasting
	06:00	
	07:00	Indinavir 800mg/AZT 200mg/3TC 150mg
		Fasting
Bkfst/ritonavir 600mg/3TC 150mg/AZT 300mg	08:00	Breakfast – 500 cc fluids
	09:00	
	10:00	
	11:00	
Lunch	12:00	Lunch – 500 cc fluids
	13:00	Fasting
	14:00	
	15:00	indinavir 800mg/AZT 200mg
	16:00	Fasting
Supper	17:00	Supper – 500 cc fluids
	18:00	
	19:00	3TC 150mg
Ritonavir 600mg/3TC 150mg/AZT 300mg	20:00	
	21:00	Fasting
	22:00	
	23:00	Indinavir 800mg/AZT 200mg
	24:00	Fasting
	01:00-06:00	

Figure 14.5 A daily planner for times of therapy for an individual with HIV infection. The various times and conditions (with food or without food) are demonstrated. (Reproduced from reference 939 with permission.)

system. AZT and 3TC interfere with the proliferation of T cells (1041, 1565). In several situations, however, there has been improvement in cell-mediated immunity, as reflected by delayed-type hypersensitivity skin reaction, interleukin-2 (IL-2) production, T-cell proliferative responses, antibody production (2960), cytotoxic T-lymphocyte (CTL) activity (474, 559), and noncytolytic CD8$^+$ cell anti-HIV responses (1633). Other improvements include a reduction in immune activation. The results suggest that the antiviral drugs, either by decreasing virus levels or by acting directly on the immune system, provide a beneficial response. For example, AZT-resistant strains have been found in treated individuals who continue to have a reduced viral load (1588). Cellular immune response against HIV must be involved. Some studies also suggest that AZT can reduce tumor necrosis factor alpha (TNF-α) production (539). However, whether this finding reflects a direct or indirect effect of the antiviral activity has not been determined.

With protease inhibitors, an increase in the number of CD4$^+$ cells expressing the CD28 molecule has been noted as well as an enhanced proliferation of these cells to mitogens, recall antigens, and HIV core proteins (1265; for a review, see reference 1264). Nevertheless, short-term treatment with protease inhibitors does not seem to repair abnormalities in the T-cell repertoire (510; for a review, see reference 1264). As noted in Section I, the response of lymphocytes to antiretroviral therapies has

Table 14.5 Effects of antiviral therapy on the immune system

1. Reduced T-cell proliferation (1041, 1565)
2. Improved delayed-type hypersensitivity and IL-2 production, T-cell proliferative responses, and antibody production (474, 476, 1265, 2960)
3. Improved CTL activity (559)
4. Improved CD8$^+$ cell noncytotoxic antiviral activity (1633)
5. Reduced immune system activation
6. No immediate repair in T-cell repertoire (510)

been primarily an expansion of the existing pool of memory and naive cells and not the generation of new naive cells. The percentage of naive cells before therapy is the same as that after therapy (510). Thus, an expansion of the proliferating pool of cells already present in the infected individual takes place, and low CD4$^+$ cell counts usually correlate with the decreased regenerative capacity of these cells (2587). Nevertheless, most recent studies have suggested that prolonged use of highly active antiretroviral therapy (HAART) can give a late rise in the number of naive CD4$^+$ lymphocytes (105a). Moreover, a decrease in activation markers (HLA-DR and CD38 expression) on CD4$^+$ and CD8$^+$ T cells, and a return in response to recall antigens (e.g., CMV) but not to HIV antigens (105a), have been observed. Thus, some notable improvement in immune function has been observed and needs to be further evaluated. Therefore, a recovery of a full T-cell repertoire usually does not take place, although certain proliferative and cytotoxic responses may be restored. In summary, with limited increases in the CD4$^+$ cell count to 100 to 150 cells/μl, full improvement of immune function cannot be expected, at least in the short term. With immune therapeutic approaches, however, some benefit might be achieved (for reviews, see references 1264 and 2029) (Section III).

III. Immune System-Based Therapies

Direct attempts at restoring immune function affected by HIV infection are being considered (for reviews, see references 282, 698, and 2029) (Table 14.6). A return of the CD4$^+$ cell count may be obtained with antiviral therapy, but specific anti-HIV responses do not appear to improve substantially (2029). Moreover, the use of multidrug therapy for several years could be poorly tolerated and compromised by toxicity, noncompliance, and development of drug-resistant virus strains. Thus, immune system-based therapies need to receive further attention as an approach for controlling HIV.

With the recent appreciation that disease progression and HIV infection may be influenced by particular cytokines, some manipulations of these cellular products are being considered. The administration of IL-2 in 5-day cycles every 2 months or daily is under study, based on encouraging results in early clinical trials (575, 1176, 1361, 1363, 2653). After 1 year of therapy, CD4$^+$ cell numbers were maintained and no increase in the level of viral RNA in plasma was noted (1363). Some studies have suggested that IL-2 in combination with alpha interferon (IFN-α) may transiently increase CD4$^+$ T-cell numbers and reduce HIV replication in vivo

Table 14.6 Potential immune-based therapies for HIV infection

1. Anti-TNF-α drugs (pentoxifylline, thalidomide, antibodies) (406, 626, 2345)
2. IL-2 administration (575, 1176, 1363)
3. IL-12 therapy[a] (476, 1415)
4. Antibodies to IL-4 and IL-10[a] (484, 1415)
5. IL-10 therapy[a]
6. Thymopentin[a]
7. Thymus replacement[a] (1360, 1671)
8. CD8[+] cell administration[a]
9. Passive antibody administration

[a] Under consideration

(2408). The nature of these CD4[+] cells needs to be evaluated, since they may not have normal function (510, 698). Naive cells go to the lymph node, where they encounter new antigens and can react. With IL-2 therapy, it would be important to know the nature of the CD4[+] cells whose numbers are expanded. CD4[+] cells that enhance cell-mediated immunity (TH1 type) would be a preferred result.

The use of pentoxifylline against TNF-α is also being evaluated to reduce HIV replication and thus disease progression (626). Thalidomide (2345) and anti-TNF-α antibodies (406) have also shown some promise in blocking the production of TNF-α. These approaches might also improve symptoms related to high levels of TNF-α (1697), such as wasting syndrome (2221). Nevertheless, paradoxically, the successful treatment of oral ulcers with thalidomide was associated with increased TNF-α and HIV-1 levels (1178). Moreover, in a recent report, pentoxifylline has increased CMV replication in HIV-infected people (2561).

Other cytokine manipulations in the host are also being evaluated in cell culture studies. Cell-mediated immune responses of cultured PBMC, as measured by proliferation to recall and allogeneic antigens and to mitogens, have been restored by the addition of IL-12 to the cells (476, 1415). This cytokine, produced by macrophages, is known to induce the differentiation of TH0 cells into TH1 cells (see Chapter 11). IL-12 also could act to compensate for the inhibitory effects of IL-10 on IL-12 production by macrophages (380, 551, 2433). A similar restorative effect on PBMC cultures from HIV-infected subjects was observed with antibodies to IL-4 and IL-10 (484, 1415). Other findings have indicated that for some patients, cytokines can improve abnormalities in T-cell proliferation (230). The observations demonstrating in vitro that type 1 cytokines increase the CD8[+] cell antiviral response (Figure 11.9) may have been involved in the above results observed with IL-2 (138, 1297). With suppression of HIV replication, the proliferative response of the CD4[+] cells could have returned. Conceivably, IL-12 or the anti-type 2 cytokine antibodies induced a TH1-type response that increased the CD8[+] cell antiviral activity. Antibodies to type 2 cytokines can increase type 1 cytokine production (2504).

With the known effect of IL-12 on natural killer (NK) cell activity as well (see Chapter 11), the possible use of this cytokine and others in therapy for HIV infection is under consideration. Since IL-10 reduces HIV-1 replication in vitro, probably via its anti-TNF-α activity, some clinical trials may soon evaluate its potential use for HIV infection (738a). Obviously, however, a balance in the beneficial and detrimental effects of these immunologic factors needs to be considered; for example, IL-10 can inhibit CD8$^+$ cell responses (137, 1297). Other immunologic approaches include the use of thymopentin (1755) and IFN-α, although resistance to IFN-α has been noted (1390) (Table 14.6). IFN-γ might also have some antiviral potential, since it decreases the cell surface expression of the HIV-1 receptor galactosyl ceramide on bowel cells (2928) and increases cell-mediated immunity. However, thus far, clinical trials with these cytokines have been disappointing. Finally, the administration of antiviral drugs or cells along with cytokine therapy (460), as is done in some anticancer protocols (2041), should be considered. In the case of HIV infection, cytokine gene-transduced CD8$^+$ cells might be useful. In summary, a combined approach of antiviral drugs and immune-based therapy seems to be the most appropriate approach to regaining control of HIV (1499, 2029) (Section VI).

IV.   Immune Restoration

Thymopoiesis is important in regeneration of peripheral T cells and is dependent on both the age and immune status of the host (856). The thymus directs T-cell repertoire formation during ontogeny. Later, thymus-independent pathways are needed to replenish the turnover of mature T cells (CD45RO$^+$). Aging is characterized by replacement of naive T cells by memory cells and an accumulation of functional defects within the cells (1794). Expansion of already formed T cells may not always permit a full repertoire of cellular responses. In the absence of the thymus, it is estimated that peripheral T-cell numbers can expand 100,000-fold in vivo (2258) if the right cytokines are available, but new naive cells are not regenerated. The overall survival of individual cells (and their repertoires) depends on the extent of self-renewal versus apoptosis associated with activation (1794).

Studies evaluating the life span of lymphocytes in humans have projected various survival curves, with memory cells lasting for several years (797, 1628, 1779, 2557). These results have provided estimates of cell proliferation rates. Naive lymphocytes appear to divide once every 3.5 years and memory lymphocytes every 22 weeks (1628). It also appears that in the absence of persistent exposure to antigen, some memory lymphocytes can revert to a naive phenotype (1049, 1779) but only, on average, after 3.5 years in the memory cell class.

Results with individuals undergoing intensive chemotherapy also suggest that thymus-dependent regeneration of CD4$^+$ T lymphocytes can occur in children but that deficiencies are found in young adults lacking a normal functioning thymus. Recovery can be demonstrated by the number of CD45RA$^+$ CD62L$^+$ CD4$^+$ T lymphocytes (naive cells) and can take a long time (1628). Other studies have shown that T-cell recovery after immune suppression (e.g., for autologous bone marrow transplant) is due to proliferation of mature T cells and not naive ones (586). These estimates on the length of time that naive and memory cells live within a host and cycle between these stages of maturity need to be considered in modeling immune system restoration in HIV-infected individuals.

Recent data have made it possible to estimate the level of recycling T cells by measuring the prevalence of a mutation in the hypoxanthine-guanine phosphori-

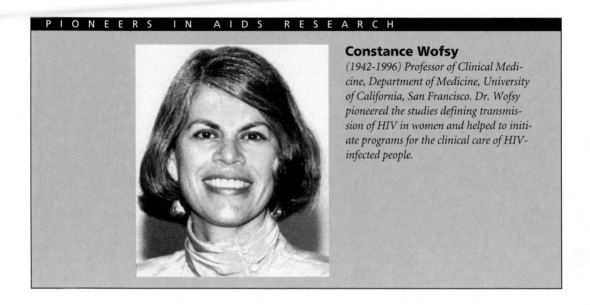

Constance Wofsy
(1942-1996) Professor of Clinical Medicine, Department of Medicine, University of California, San Francisco. Dr. Wofsy pioneered the studies defining transmission of HIV in women and helped to initiate programs for the clinical care of HIV-infected people.

bosyltransferase (HPRT) locus. The estimated rate assumes a recycling of about 5% per day or an accumulation of six mutations per million cells per year. Based on these computations, an elevated frequency of mutations was found in CD4$^+$ cells of most infected patients with <200 CD4$^+$ T cells/μl. These results support an elevated and continually increasing division rate in both T-cell subsets (2013). However, in the earlier stages of infection, the frequency of mutations can be lower than that observed in healthy control subjects. Thus, less recycling appears to be taking place. Overall, continuous postthymic T-cell expansion occurs in people with HIV infection. Whether this mechanism explains the rebound of the CD4$^+$ cell number after the use of antiviral drugs is uncertain, but this would most probably be involved after the first month, when redistribution appears to be a less feasible explanation.

Redistribution as part of the immediate return of CD4$^+$ cell numbers needs to be appreciated. As noted above (Section I.H), in some studies of anti-HIV therapy, the telomere length in T cells has suggested that the early return of memory or mature cells results primarily from migration of cells from tissue reservoirs (2911). Measuring the loss of telomere length in CD4$^+$ and CD8$^+$ cells from HIV-1-infected people has suggested in fact that an enhanced aging process takes place, particularly in CD8$^+$ CD28$^-$ cells (685, 1822). This cellular aging, mirrored by a reduction in telomere length, appears to be limited to CD8$^+$ cells, since CD4$^+$ cells maintain a telomere length expected for healthy populations (2911). Unless these cells have increased telomerase activity, which seems unlikely, the CD4$^+$ cells in infected individuals (even on therapy) appear to be turning over at a normal rate.

This finding on telomere length supports the conclusion that the initial increases in CD4$^+$ cell counts after antiviral therapy result from a redistribution of cells (1519, 2911) and not from de novo generation of fresh cells. Thus, in HIV infection, CD4$^+$ cells may not be rapidly destroyed but may be slowly released into the circulation. A disorder in CD4$^+$ cell migration from tissue sites could be involved.

Studies of the Vβ repertoire have also suggested that with treatment there is not a return to heterogeneous CD8$^+$ or CD4$^+$ cell responses with efficient immunologic activity (510) (Section II).

Whether immune function can be restored in people on antiviral therapy remains to be determined (698). An important question is how naive lymphocytes can be generated in the absence of a thymus. Most research studies indicate that the functioning thymus disappears by age 18 and that new T cells must come from other reservoirs in the body (586, 1628). The evidence suggests that T-cell populations can be maintained after thymic atrophy but that regeneration depends on some residual thymus-like function (1628). Recent findings suggest that sufficient residual thymus may be present to help restore T cells (1711a). Other studies indicate that certain cytokines, such as oncostatin M, a member of the IL-6 subfamily of cytokines expressed by hematopoietic tissues and cells, can stimulate the accumulation of immature T cells in the lymph node (465). The results have suggested an extrathymic T-cell developmental pathway. Disease progression in HIV-infected adults is linked to a loss of the independent regenerative capacity of the thymus (856). In children, marked thymic deficiency, secondary to destruction by HIV infection, is strongly associated with more rapid progression to disease (1360) (see Chapter 3).

Recent approaches are aimed at determining whether thymus-independent mechanisms can generate naive T cells in HIV-infected individuals. In this way, lost T-cell repertoires as well as the ability to respond to new antigens can be recovered. It is surmised that most naive cells in normal adults come from pools present in lymphoid tissues throughout the body. In HIV-infected individuals, this naive population becomes greatly reduced secondary to the cytopathicity of HIV and the activation of the immune system against the virus. Thus, if an extrathymic pathway cannot be utilized, approaches at thymus (explant) restoration (1360, 1671) or bone marrow stem cell therapy merit consideration (Table 14.6) (for a review, see reference 856).

Finally, based on the observation that CD8$^+$ cells can suppress HIV replication or function as CTLs, some groups have evaluated whether CD8$^+$ cells, grown in large quantities in culture, can be administered as therapy to restore immune function. Preliminary studies on ex vivo-cultured autologous CD8$^+$ cells showed no obvious toxicity in patients (1088, 1538a). A remission in Kaposi's sarcoma lesions was noted in two patients (1324). The administration of CD8$^+$ cells along with IL-2 and the use of CD8$^+$ cells genetically engineered to produce this cytokine (2041), as well as the administration of CD8$^+$ cell antiviral factor, should be studied. Conceivably, therapies directed at stimulating CD8$^+$ cell anti-HIV responses can be developed (e.g., CD28 engagement) (136) (see Chapter 11). This cellular approach to immune system modulation, in addition to cytokines, anticytokine antibodies, and anticytokine drugs, merits increased attention (Table 14.6).

V.   Postinfection Immunization

The suggestion that postinfection therapy could involve immunization with a viral protein (2342) has been evaluated. This approach should not be considered a vaccination, since this term is properly reserved for prevention strategies. Postinfection immunization is an attempt at immune system stimulation. In early studies, HIV-infected individuals received immunizations with envelope-depleted virus still containing the HIV-1 Gag proteins. One reason for this approach was to increase levels of p24 antibodies, which are reduced in symptomatic patients (see Chapter 13). After 5 years, no toxicity from the immunizations was noted (1485) and an increase in cell-mediated antiviral immune cell responses, a reduced rate of increase in the viral load, and a reduced rate of CD4$^+$ cell decline were noted (2700). Phase III clinical trials are now being conducted to determine the efficacy of this approach. Preliminary studies suggest that only certain infected people respond to this antiviral therapy. In other studies of infected people, immunization with recombinant p17/p24 Ty virus-like particles had no effect on the level of antibodies to the Gag protein (2762).

Following a similar concept, some investigators (2204) immunized infected individuals with recombinant gp160 (MicroGeneSys) produced in the baculovirus system. No obvious toxicity was noted, and T-cell proliferative responses were noted in vaccinees who had stabilized CD4$^+$ cell counts. Higher levels of antibodies to certain HIV envelope peptides were found in the subjects, and neutralizing antibodies measured in a few individuals were increased. In one study, HIV-1 envelope-specific CTL responses were also increased in immunized HIV-seropositive individuals (1387). However, the potential value of postinfection immunization was questioned after a randomized trial showed no clinical effect (713). Moreover, immune stimulation under some circumstances might be harmful by increasing the spread of virus in the host (807, 2576) (see Chapter 13).

VI.	**Passive Immunotherapy and Use of Antibody-Based Approaches**

Some investigators have considered the possibility that passive immunotherapy with plasma or purified immunoglobulins from HIV-seropositive individuals who are asymptomatic (1245, 2159) would be helpful (Table 14.6). The potential use of human anti-V3 loop monoclonal antibodies has received attention (701, 2996). It appears that several monoclonal antibodies with different epitopes would be needed, particularly if the noncontiguous viral CD4 binding site is the target (see Chapter 3).

The initial trials with anti-HIV plasma in AIDS patients showed some success, as measured by improvement in clinical status and stabilization of CD4$^+$ cell counts (1245, 2777). The effect could result from HIV neutralization, antibody-dependent cellular cytotoxicity, or nonspecific stimulation of the immune system of the recipient. Other studies have not demonstrated a clinical benefit in AIDS patients (1177). Large doses of monoclonal antibodies directed against HIV antigens appear to be needed to show a substantial increase in neutralizing activity in the host serum. Protection of cats from feline immunodeficiency virus infection by passive antibody administration has been reported (1096, 2150), as has protection of chimpanzees (2147) and SCID-hu mice (114). In rhesus macaques, possible transfer of antibodies against human cellular antigens protected the monkeys from infection by SIV$_{mac251}$ grown in human cells. No effect of anti-SIV neutralizing antibodies was noted (846). Recently, increased survival of SIV-infected macaques was achieved by passive treatment with antiviral antibodies (989).

A major concern is whether the immunoglobulins inoculated into a host will enhance rather than neutralize the HIV strain present in that infected individual. This result was suggested by the SIV studies cited above (846) (see Chapter 10). Experimentation with the isolated strain before clinical use might be warranted to avoid a potential danger in this therapy. If passive immunization is effective, immunoglobulins can be produced (perhaps by monoclonal antibody procedures) to use in individuals after needlestick injuries or in mothers around the time of delivery (see Chapter 2). Finally, as noted in Section I, antibodies linked to ricin or other toxins have been suggested for use in killing infected cells (1664, 2179). The viral envelope or cell surface molecules are targeted.

VII.   Summary

Substantial emphasis has been placed on finding therapeutic modalities for attacking the virus itself or virus-infected cells (Figure 14.1). Information on many different drugs showing anti-HIV activity in vitro appears regularly in the literature, but their clinical efficacy awaits further evaluation (Section I). Unfortunately, many drugs have shown organ system toxicity that cannot be evaluated in the laboratory. Most clinicians conclude that combination therapy, similar to the approaches taken to the treatment of malignancies, will be universally utilized to avoid toxicity and drug resistance. Therapies targeted against virus-infected cells must be given particular attention. Attempts at enhancing the immune response of the host against the virus and the virus-infected cells should be emphasized (Sections III and IV). In this regard, the influence of cytokines should be appreciated. Presently, in untreated individuals, the immune system, particularly the $CD8^+$ cell antiviral response, maintains control of HIV replication by suppressing virus production by the infected cells (Figure 14.6A). When the $CD8^+$ cell anti-HIV response (e.g., production of the $CD8^+$ cell antiviral factor [CAF]) decreases, virus is released (Figure 13.4), and loss of $CD4^+$ cells occurs. At this point, antiretroviral drugs have been very helpful in blocking de novo infection of fresh cells by the virus released from infected cells (Figure 14.6B). By this second approach, however, unless virus production is completely arrested, resistant strains can develop over time and reinstitute the infection within the host. Importantly, the present antiretroviral drugs do not directly attack the several billion virus-infected cells in the body, some of which are long-living macrophage and dendritic cells and latently infected $CD4^+$ cells that can eventually release virus particles in the host. Therefore, the optimal situation for control of HIV infection would be a combination of immune-based therapies and antiretroviral drugs (Figure 14.6C). Through immune system modulation, $CD8^+$ cells, for example, can be induced to produce CAF, which would block virus production by virus-infected cells. The antiretroviral drugs would prevent any fresh infection of cells by virus particles that are circulating in the host or have been released from some cells not yet controlled by the cellular immune system. The end result would be a persistent, long-term asymptomatic course (Figure 14.6C). In all antiviral therapies, the biologic and molecular features of HIV need to be considered (Table 14.7).

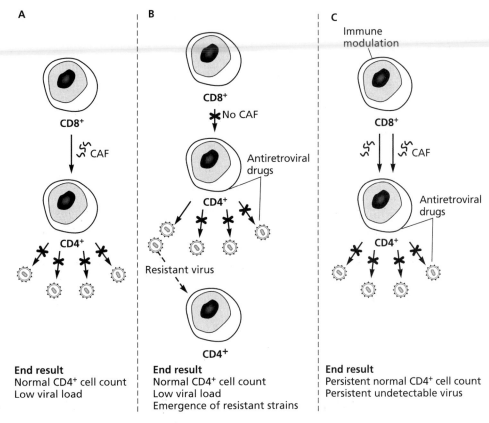

Figure 14.6 Therapeutic approaches for controlling HIV infection. (A) In untreated infected individuals who remain asymptomatic and have normal CD4$^+$ cell counts, control of HIV replication in infected CD4$^+$ cells appears to be mediated by CD8$^+$ cells, particularly those releasing the CD8$^+$ cell antiviral factor (CAF). (B) When this cell-mediated immune response decreases (secondary to a variety of factors suggested in the text), HIV is produced. Present combination therapy prevents this released virus from reinfecting fresh cells and can restore CD4$^+$ cell levels. The viral load is reduced. However, resistant strains can emerge if this arrest in virus replication is not complete. (C) The optimal control of HIV infection would come from a dual approach in which immune system modulators are used to enhance CD8$^+$ cell antiviral response and antiretroviral drugs are administered to prevent infection of fresh cells by the free virus remaining in the host.

Table 14.7 Biologic and molecular features of HIV that affect antiviral therapy

1. Infected cells are a major source of HIV transmission and pathogenesis.
2. Infected T cells, B cells, and macrophages can be circulating reservoirs for HIV. Tissue macrophages and stromal cells can be resident reservoirs that persistently release virus.
3. Integrated virus can be latent and remain unaffected by the immune response and antiviral therapy.
4. Virus can spread by cell-to-cell transfer.
5. Virus can infect brain cells: astrocytes and oligodendrocytes. Therapeutic agents must pass through blood-brain barrier.
6. Virus can "escape" neutralizing antibodies; in some cases, virus infection is sensitive to enhancement by antibodies.
7. Antigenic variations occur widely among HIV-1 and HIV-2 strains.
8. Sequence mutations can occur early in the regions coding for the HIV envelope and regulatory genes.

1. Anti-HIV therapies initially began with the use of AZT and other single RT inhibitors. Present treatments include at least two drugs (e.g., AZT and 3TC) and most often three, one of which is a viral protease inhibitor.

2. When anti-HIV treatment should begin remains in question, although most physicians recommend administration of drugs if viral loads of about 10,000 RNA copies/ml are present. A decreasing $CD4^+$ cell count is also a parameter considered in therapeutic approaches.

3. Other antiviral directions under study include integrase antagonists, drugs against the viral Gag protein, and therapy to prevent nucleotide incorporation into viral DNA and to inhibit HIV replication by specific gene targets.

4. An important problem encountered with antiviral therapy is drug resistance, which has been seen with most treatments. Cross-resistance to the protease inhibitors is observed regularly.

5. Antiretroviral therapies can reduce the viral load in the lymph nodes, but whether drugs can affect HIV levels in sanctuaries such as the brain or testes remains to be studied. Importantly, present treatments do not specifically target virus-infected cells, which can remain as reservoirs of HIV production.

6. Antiviral therapies may sometimes directly compromise the function of the immune system. Yet, in some studies, they appear to enhance cell-mediated immunity and may be important in helping, either directly or indirectly, the host immune system to function with anti-HIV activity.

7. Immune system-based therapies encourage the use of cytokines that may help restore cell-mediated immunity or approaches that decrease the toxic effects of cellular products, such as TNF-α.

8. Approaches to restoring the function of the immune system in individuals who are receiving antiretroviral therapy are being emphasized. Generating naive T lymphocytes through thymus-dependent or -independent activities is required.

9. Postinfection immunization studies have been conducted but have not provided promising results.

10. Passive immunotherapy and antibody-based antiviral approaches are other directions for treating HIV infection but have not yet shown any consistent beneficial effect.

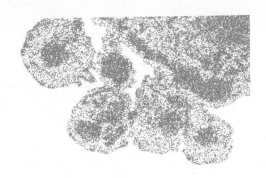

Vaccine Development

T HE PREVIOUS CHAPTER REVIEWED THE PROMISING RESULTS OBTAINED thus far in suppressing virus replication in the infected host with antiviral drugs. Most of the treatments are aimed at the virus and its de novo infection. Controlling or eliminating the reservoirs of virus-infected cells in lymphoid tissue, brain, and other sanctuaries requires further attention. Some immune system-based therapies have been considered, as well as the need to restore the immune system in individuals in whom virus replication has been controlled. Despite the promise of effective therapies, the biggest challenge is preventing HIV infection. The virus continues to spread rapidly, particularly in developing countries (see Preface). This final chapter will review the history and recent attempts to develop a vaccine against HIV. Most studies were conducted with SIV in primates, particularly rhesus macaques, but other animal models have also been evaluated. By trying past conventional vaccine approaches, a great deal has been learned about what procedures will not work. Now, new directions must be considered that are based on the knowledge that combating HIV infection requires recognition of virus-infected cells, not only free virions.

I.

Introduction

In developing a vaccine, several features of HIV infection and transmission must be considered (for reviews, see references 11, 198, 737, 929, 1069, 1249, 1489, 1824, and 2169) (Table 14.7). The approaches for conventional vaccines may not all be relevant for preventing HIV infection (Table 15.1). For example, seropositive individuals who have completely eliminated HIV infection have not been identified, and whether protection against disease is an appropriate end point for an HIV vaccine is not known. Previous vaccines have protected against viruses that do not change over time and have generally been whole-killed or live-attenuated viruses. At present, these types of agents are considered unsafe for an HIV vaccine. Moreover, the infectious virions against which effective vaccines have been directed are usually infrequently encountered and have been those that gain entry through mucosal surfaces (e.g., the respiratory and gastrointestinal tracts) aside from the genital tract. The antiviral vaccines presently in use have also been against agents that are not passed particularly by certain behavioral patterns (e.g., sexual activity) and are not cell-associated (737).

The major features challenging the development of an HIV vaccine include the appreciation of viral heterogeneity, the need for local mucosal immunity (1786), the potential for autoimmune responses, and virus transmission by infected cells (1502). The findings on the serologic cross-reacting region in the V3 loop (i.e., the principal neutralizing domain), the induction of cross-reactive cytotoxic T-lymphocyte (CTL) activity (999), and the reported broadening antiviral response in animals immunized with gp120 and the V3 loop (988, 1191) have lent encouragement to the potential development of a vaccine against HIV (see Chapters 10 and 11). Nevertheless, the question of whether the present directions would protect a host against high doses of the virus (>100 infectious particles [IP] [2974]) and virus-infected cells has not been answered.

Importantly, the correlates of protective immunity (Table 15.2) have not been

Table 15.1   Features of conventional vaccines[a]

1. Establish the state of natural immunity against reinfection similar to that observed in individuals who have recovered from the infection
2. Protect against disease and not against infection
3. Protect for years against viruses that do not change over time
4. Have generally been whole-killed or live-attenuated
5. Protect against infections that are infrequently encountered
6. Protect against infections that occur through mucosal surfaces of the respiratory or gastrointestinal tract, not the genital tract
7. Phase III efficacy trials are usually based on observations on immune responses and efficacy in appropriate animal models
8. Directed against microbes that are not predominantly related to behavioral patterns
9. Directed at free microbes, not cell-associated pathogens

[a] Reviewed in reference 737.

Table 15.2   Possible correlates of protective immunity against HIV infection[a]

1. CTL activity (CD4[+] and CD8[+] cells)
2. CD8[+] cell noncytotoxic antiviral response
3. Natural killer (NK) cell activity
4. Antibody-dependent cellular cytotoxicity (ADCC)
5. Neutralizing antibodies

[a] The presence of these responses at mucosal sites is important. If attenuated virus is used, sufficient replication of the virus must occur to induce protective immune responses.

well defined in terms of an HIV vaccine. Most noteworthy is the role of cell-mediated immune responses in the prevention of HIV infection (12). Induction of mucosal immunity also needs to be seriously considered (1762, 1786). Moreover, the most effective immunization procedure needs to be determined (Table 15.3).

A major problem in vaccine development has been finding an appropriate animal model (Table 15.4). Chimpanzees are expensive and do not generally replicate HIV to high titer or get disease. In one recent report, an HIV-infected chimpanzee developed AIDS, but that was only after several inoculations of different HIV-1 strains with perhaps the development of a recombinant pathogenic virus (1951). Studies with SIV have been very helpful, and the macaque model has thus far been the major approach for studying lentivirus vaccines. In addition, observations in our laboratory on HIV-2 infection of baboons have been encouraging (144, 375), as has been the successful infection of pig-tail monkeys (*Macaca nemestrina*) with HIV-1 (24) and HIV-2 (2830). Finally, the use of SIV:HIV (SHIV) chimeric viruses (1204, 1600, 2207, 2479), or perhaps eventually HIV-2:HIV-1 (HIV²) chimeras, might offer an approach for evaluating vaccines in convenient primate model systems (1481, 1592, 2163).

Essentially, nine different types of vaccines for preventing HIV infection have been explored (Table 15.5) (1489). Each has provided some promise for the development of a vaccine in other viral systems, including the novel use of anti-idiotypes (101, 565, 2549). In the future, plants may offer an avenue for vaccine development whereby protection is induced with plant viruses carrying HIV proteins (e.g., alfalfa

Table 15.3   Immunization procedures evaluated for an HIV vaccine

1. Parenteral (with and without adjuvant)
2. Oral administration (adenovirus, poliovirus, salmonellae, transgenic plants)
3. Intravaginal, intrarectal, or intraurethral inoculation
4. Liposomes, microspheres, microcapsules, immunostimulatory complexes (ISCOM)
5. DNA immunization
6. Use of adjuvants
7. Use of cytokines (e.g., IL-12)

Table 15.4 Potential animal models for developing an HIV vaccine

Animal	Virus
Chimpanzee	HIV-1
Rhesus macaque	SIV, SHIV
Baboon	HIV-2
Pig-tail macaques	HIV-2, SIV
Cynomolgus monkeys	HIV-2, SIV
Cat	FIV
Horse	EIAV
Mouse (SCID-hu)	HIV-1, HIV-2

or cowpea mosaic virus) (2951) or with plant products derived directly through genetic engineering techniques (568) (Table 15.6). Those vaccine approaches that have received the most attention are reviewed below.

For any attempt at vaccine development, the fact that "sterilizing immunity" has never been achieved against other viral infections must be appreciated. Thus, early infection and some replication of HIV would be expected before the subsequent immune responses against the virus would prevent spread in the host. In fact, the realization that HIV itself produces a chronic infection despite strong antiviral immune responses reflects the challenge for an effective AIDS vaccine. Perhaps protection from disease, but not infection, will be the first accomplishment. Conceivably, if a decrease in viral load is achieved by a vaccine, transmission would be equally reduced.

The most powerful mechanism for inhibiting the establishment of infection is cell-mediated immunity (12, 332, 644), particularly cytotoxic CD8$^+$ cells that show a cross-reactivity to a variety of strains (999). Moreover, in HIV infection, other humoral and cellular immune functions can play substantial roles in limiting HIV replication and spread (see Chapters 10 and 11).

Table 15.5 HIV vaccine approaches[a]

1. Whole-killed (inactivated) virus: natural or engineered
2. Live (attenuated) variants: natural or engineered (e.g., Nef-deleted)
3. Subunit vaccine (natural or engineered): envelope glycoproteins (gp120, gp160, gp41); Gag proteins: oligomerization
4. Viral proteins in live vectors (e.g., vaccinia virus, poliovirus, herpes simplex virus, adenovirus, baculovirus, Ty particle, various bacteria)
5. Viral cores with envelope proteins (pseudovirions)—virus-like particles (VLPs)
6. Sequence-derived peptides of HIV (e.g., V3 epitopes, CTL/Th epitopes)
7. Anti-idiotypes of neutralizing antibodies
8. DNA gene transfer
9. Plant-derived proteins

[a] Some of these approaches include cytokine enhancement.

Table 15.6 Potential value of transgenic plants in vaccine development

1. Economical means for scaling up production of a protein
2. Eliminates potential contamination with animal viruses
3. Can be delivered either parenterally or as an edible product

II. Inactivated and Attenuated Viruses

A. Inactivated Whole Virus

The predominant early vaccine studies with lentiviruses, initially showing some virus protection, involved the use of killed SIV in macaques (modeled after the Salk polio vaccine) (624, 1881, 2564). This approach demonstrated protection against a low-dose challenge with the homologous SIV strain. In general, delays in virus challenge after the final immunization dose (up to 12 months) gave the best results and have formed the basis for further evaluation of these types of vaccines (1881). Nevertheless, some studies showed that killed-virus vaccines cannot protect against infection or disease when the challenge virus is inoculated onto the genital mucosal lining (2618). Protection of macaques immunized with killed HIV-2 strains has also been reported (2160). Once again, the challenge was a low dose (10 to 40 IP) of a homotypic type. Protection against a heterologous HIV-2 strain or, more importantly, virus-infected cells was not evaluated.

Very disturbing was the recognition, subsequent to many early vaccine studies, that most trials with inactivated SIV strains as immunogens most probably measured anticellular and not antiviral responses (535, 1427, 2601). Both the immunizing and the challenging viruses were grown in the same human cell line. Antibodies appeared to be induced against the human cellular proteins (e.g., human leukocyte antigen [HLA] class I) associated with the virion and not against the viral proteins (89, 395). This possibility was supported by the protection of macaques from SIV infection following HLA-DR immunization (90, 394). Thus, protection occurred via anticellular protein responses. The results, however, were impressive in that they suggested complete prevention of SIV transmission. Essentially, sterilizing immunity was achieved, since any successful infection by SIV would have produced progeny lacking the human cell antigens and thus not sensitive to the immune response. Future studies should evaluate the virus-specific immune activity (e.g., $CD8^+$ cells) that might have been responsible for preventing any de novo infection.

One study with killed SIV and low-dose homologous SIV challenge did seem to reflect induction of a true antiviral state (624). In addition, an inactivated, molecularly cloned SIV vaccine induced antiviral and not anticellular antibodies and protection against homologous and heterologous strains (1207). Nevertheless, many of the aforementioned SIV studies are being reevaluated with appropriate virus preparations. Some have not shown protection even with the successful induction of antiviral antibodies (2502). However, the vaccination of two rhesus monkeys with whole inactivated HIV-1 protected the animals from an SHIV challenge (1592). Human antigens were not involved, and the results provided further encouragement for using killed virus and the SHIV model to study protection from HIV infection in nonhuman primates.

With the cat lentivirus feline immunodeficiency virus (FIV), immunization with inactivated infected cells or killed cell-free FIV protected >90% of cats against intraperitoneal infection with small amounts of homologous (1698, 2930) or heterologous (2930) strains. Neutralizing antibodies were not necessarily present (1698). In one study, only protection from the homologous FIV strain was noted in association with neutralizing antibodies (1109). Finally, a killed-virus vaccine with the equine lentivirus equine infectious anemia virus (EIAV) induced protection against infection by up to 10^5 infectious doses of the homologous virus. The vaccine did not prevent infection by a heterologous virus but protected against disease (1165). These encouraging results did not involve anticellular responses.

B.   Whole Attenuated Virus

Some investigators have demonstrted that immunization of macaques with a live, naturally attenuated SIV strain ($SIV_{mac1A11}$) prevents disease in adults and neonates by a virulent strain but does not prevent infection (1679, 1998). In addition, previous infection of macaques with the $SHIV_{89.6}$ isolate provided protection against vaginal challenge with the pathogenic SIV_{mac239} strain (1789). Moreover, infection of cynomolgus monkeys with a nonpathogenic HIV-2 strain protected the animals from subsequent SIV-induced disease (2158). Also, preinfection with a weakly pathogenic HIV-2 strain protected one of six macaques from subsequent superinfection with the pathogenic SIV_{mac251} strain given via the rectal route (2808). The protection correlated with high levels of antibodies in the SIV enzyme-linked immunosorbent assay (ELISA) and cross-reacting neutralizing antibodies. However, the difference in the ability to prevent superinfection of one animal revealed no conclusive information about the correlates of protection involved.

These limited results are not as encouraging as those of previous studies suggesting almost universal protection of animals from SIV infection after HIV-2 inoculation (2087). In the latter case, notably, the vaccine-administered virus was reactivated. Moreover, previous infection by one HIV-2 strain protected baboons from superinfection by a heterologous HIV-2 strain (1577). Other studies in animals demonstrating this apparent resistance to superinfection are reviewed in Chapter 11. The common observation from several reports is that a certain threshold of replication of the initiating (attenuated) virus should be reached with live virus immunogens to induce protective immune responses (1577, 2808). These findings could offer insights into the correlates of protection (Table 15.2).

In another approach, a *nef*-deleted mutant of SIV that does not cause disease in rhesus monkeys (1280) induced high-titer antibodies against the virus (569). Results on the cellular immune response were not reported at the time, but CTL activity has been noted in recent studies (1206a). Subsequent challenge of these animals with up to 1,000 rhesus monkey infectious doses of a wild-type virus gave protection from infection (569). Similar findings with *nef*-deleted mutants have since been reported by other groups and have involved SIV strains as well as SHIV viruses (1152, 1942, 2563). Protection in one case did not correlate with neutralizing antibodies (1942). In another study, anti-Env CTLs were considered important (1152). In one noteworthy study, protection was achieved against challenge with virus-infected cells (49). In other investigations, rhesus macaques previously infected with a *nef*-attenuated SIV strain resisted subsequent exposure to an SHIV strain (241). Since the envelope region differs between these two strains, cell-mediated immune activity must have been involved. In contrast, previous infection with a non-pathogenic SHIV strain did not protect against intravenous infection by a pathogenic SIV strain (1481). In the latter case, however, adequate replication of the SHIV strains may not have taken place. The mechanism for these results could be a strong cellular immune recognition of the *nef*-deleted mutants (1206a, 2563), perhaps as a result of somewhat better viral antigen expression (see Chapter 5). Nef can down-modulate major histocompatibility complex (MHC) class I expression by the infected cell (2428). Thus, the wild-type virus could elude the host immune system. In addition, the protective immunity may have reflected a maturation of the antibody response that has been shown to take 6 to 8 months to develop after inoculation of an attenuated strain. This increase in antibody avidity and effectiveness in neutralization was not observed with inactivated whole virus or envelope subunit vaccines (511a).

In recent trials, an SIV lacking *nef, vpr,* and the upstream sequences in U3 as well as an SIV lacking *nef* were evaluated. Protection was associated with high levels of replication of the vaccine strains in the animals. Some correlation with virus neutralizing and binding antibodies was noted (2921). Other studies with several independent or combined mutations (e.g., *vpr, vpx,* and *vif*) are in progress (879). In many of these studies with attenuated viruses, protection has been limited to high virus replication soon after the initial infection (241, 1481). This correlation was particularly observed in studies of SIV strains that varied in the extent of attenuation. As noted above, only viruses that induced a prolonged initial viremia (i.e., with the less attenuated virus) provided resistance to challenge by wild-type SIV (1578). In this regard, administration of a live attenuated SIV together with pathogenic virus did not protect against disease (1557). Evidently, a state of protective immunity must be established before challenge with a pathogenic virus can be countered.

Other studies of protection involving live virus inoculation are discussed in

PIONEERS IN AIDS RESEARCH

Donald Francis
Chief Executive Officer of Genenvax. Dr. Francis led some of the early studies on the epidemiology of AIDS. He is actively engaged in vaccine research.

Section VII, where induction of mucosal immunity is considered. As a model, the attenuated virus comes closest to resembling the replicating virion that would be infecting the host. Thus, studies with this type of virus should be continued and could indicate whether conventional vaccine approaches with virus particles would induce protective immunity against an agent such as HIV. The use of live attenuated viruses, however, has been challenged by results indicating that inoculation of some of these viruses (e.g., *nef*-deleted SIV) into neonatal macaques can give rise to AIDS (108). Moreover, some adult animals receiving these attenuated viruses have developed disease after several months of infection, and the *nef*-deleted mutants of SIV may not prevent infection by heterologous virus strains (1525a, 1525b). In addition, in the SCID-hu mouse model, the attenuated strains still showed pathogenic properties when high doses were used or observations were made over longer periods (42). Furthermore, the risk of reversion of a single deleted mutant must be appreciated (2369, 2563). Finally, integration of attenuated viruses may lead to other pathogenic processes (e.g., neoplasia). Acceptance of this approach, therefore, will be difficult unless other methods using a noninfectious virus or viral proteins are not successful.

III. Vaccines Containing Purified Envelope gp120 Alone or in Association with an Expression Vector

A. Purified Virus Envelope

Limited success has been achieved with a vaccine containing purified envelope glycoproteins expressed in the baculovirus system or in mammalian cells (e.g., Chinese hamster ovary [CHO] cells) in which close to normal glycosylation occurs (91, 186, 187, 888, 1882). In a trial using chimpanzees, immunization with purified HIV gp120 expressed in CHO cells but not a variant of gp160 (modified at the cleavage site) prevented infection after a low-dose challenge with a homologous HIV strain (186). Moreover, chimpanzees immunized with multiple booster shots of a recombinant gp120 (rgp120) of HIV-1$_{SF2}$ in MF59 adjuvant resisted challenge with homologous virus (692). Most recently, chimpanzees immunized with the HIV-1$_{MN}$ rgp120 in alum and challenged with the heterologous strain HIV-1$_{SF2}$ were not infected. Neutralizing antibodies did not correlate with this protection (189). Several vaccine trials in the SIV system have also shown some potentially positive results with native (1882) or recombinant envelope proteins (2456). Some studies suggest that immunization with a soluble CD4:gp120 complex will best induce neutralizing antibodies to a conformation-dependent epitope on gp120 (1233). This approach has not yet been evaluated.

In other animal model systems, purified EIAV envelope proteins protected horses from infection with a high-dose challenge of homologous but not heterologous viruses (1165). Noteworthy in these experiments was the apparent enhancement of disease observed in some animals immunized with the baculovirus-derived envelope protein. The finding emphasizes the potential for a detrimental response that might occur with certain vaccine strategies (see Chapter 10, Section III).

In studies of protection from challenge with infected cells, chimpanzees immunized many times with HIV-1 antigens showed resistance to intravenous injection of infected peripheral blood mononuclear cells (PBMC) (809). These results provide the first evidence that immunization can induce host responses against HIV-infected cells. Further experiments to confirm these observations are needed, including inoculation of infected cells into the anal and vaginal canals.

B. Recombinant Envelope Proteins Expressed by Live Vectors

The most promising results have come from vaccine studies with poxvirus vectors, whereby viral proteins are produced in cells of the host in association with vaccinia virus or canarypox virus infection (71, 513, 2956). This approach has elicited good humoral and cellular (i.e., CTL) immune responses in animals (2627, 2629).

Vaccinia vector vaccination (with gp120) has protected chimpanzees from low-dose HIV challenge (10 to 40 infectious doses), but only after subsequent booster immunizations with a purified baculovirus-derived gp160 and particularly a V3:KLH conjugate (888). In this case, protection could have come from the anti-V3-specific neutralizing antibodies elicited. This and other observations have led to the adoption by many groups of a prime/boost procedure for vaccination (Table 15.7). For example, a live vector expressing a viral protein is used for priming, and a subunit viral protein is used for the booster (Table 15.8). Chimpanzees immunized several times with a live vaccinia virus expressing an $rgp120_{MN}$ protein or the V3 domain of $HIV-1_{MN}$ were protected from intravenous infection with a heterologous HIV-1 strain (889). In other experiments with macaques, a vaccinia virus vector expressing gp130 of SIV_{mac} followed by a booster of gp130 oligomers elicited protection from challenge with the homologous SIV strain (1605), without a substantial antibody response. Moreover, protection from homologous virus challenge was achieved in rhesus monkeys after immunization with a vaccinia virus construct and a booster of baculovirus-produced SIV gp160 (1122). Nevertheless, studies of the CTL response suggested that the challenge virus replicated in the host but did not induce disease (1272).

Table 15.7 Vaccination procedures involving the prime-and-boost approach[a]

Virus	Prime	Boost	Animal	Reference(s)
HIV-1	Vaccinia virus (gp120)	rgp160	Chimpanzee	888, 889
SIV	Vaccinia virus (gp130)	rgp130	Rhesus monkey	1605
SIV	Vaccinia virus (gp160)	rgp160	Rhesus monkey	1122
SIV	Vaccinia virus (gp160)	rgp160	Rhesus monkey	1123
SIV	Vaccinia virus (gp160)	Gag	Rhesus monkey	1124
HIV-2	Canarypox virus (gp120)	rpg120 or V3 peptide	Cynomolgus monkey	71
HIV-2	Canarypox virus (gp120)	rgp120	Rhesus monkey	1886
HIV-2	Canarypox virus (gp120, *gag, pol*)	rgp160	Rhesus monkey	785

[a] All these trials showed some protection from infection except for that of Myagkikih et al. (1886). Only limited numbers of animals were used for all studies.

Table 15.8   Effective HIV immunization (recent approaches)

Prime	Boost
Live virus vector (vaccinia virus, canarypox virus)	Envelope subunit
DNA vaccine	Pseudovirions or envelope subunit

Countering these positive results are observations showing no protective effect of these vaccine approaches. In one study, a gp160 vaccinia virus construct derived from a molecular clone of SIV_{mne} in combination with recombinant gp160 protected immunized animals only from infection by the molecularly cloned SIV and not by the parental virus consisting of several quasi-species (1123). Similarly, monkeys immunized on three separate occasions with a vaccinia virus recombinant expressing the Gag, Pol, and Env polypeptides in an SIV pseudovirion, as well as with various vaccinia virus recombinants followed by the SIV particle booster, showed a strong immune response. Nevertheless, they were not protected from a low-dose challenge with virulent SIV_{mac} (571). More recent studies, however, have shown that envelope gp160 used for live vaccinia recombinant virus priming, followed by subunit protein (particularly Gag) boosting, protected macaques against challenge with both cloned and uncloned homologous virus (1121a, 1124).

In related studies with HIV-2 and rhesus monkeys, canarypox virus expressing the HIV envelope was used for priming in combination with the HIV-2 envelope gp125 or the V3 synthetic peptide. HIV-2-specific CTL and high antibody titers were induced with some neutralizing antibodies. Despite booster immunizations with gp125, only 4 of 10 animals showed full protection from challenge with infectious homologous HIV-2. There was no correlation between immunologic response and protection (71). In other studies, vaccine regimens employing naturally attenuated vaccinia virus or the nonreplicating canarypox vector (ALVAC) expressing HIV-2 antigens with subunit boosters were used to immunize 18 juvenile rhesus macaques. Despite several boosters and the presence of neutralizing antibodies against the virus, none of the animals was protected (1886). Thus, this immunization procedure was not sufficient to give protective immunity in this monkey model. Nevertheless, in other studies, protection from SIV infection was achieved with an HIV-2 recombinant vaccinia virus vaccine in rhesus macaques (785). In general, the data thus far indicate a lack of wide cross-reactivity after vaccination and underline further the problems in developing an effective anti-HIV vaccine based solely on the viral envelope (Section VIII). Incorporation of core proteins into the vaccine strategy may offer promise in achieving a cross-reacting response (1124). In any case, very few animals were used for the above studies, so conclusions on the approaches and correlates for any protective immunity cannot be immediately determined.

On another note, one caveat to the use of vaccinia virus-based vaccines in humans is the reduced response observed in subjects who have previously been vaccinated for smallpox (513). However, repeated boosting with gp160 did overcome this problem in the SIV model (1123), and the use of canarypox virus vectors can avoid this problem in humans.

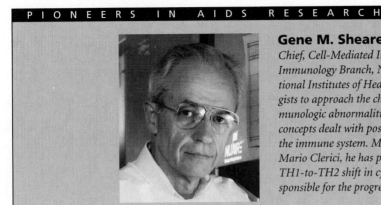

Gene M. Shearer

Chief, Cell-Mediated Immunity Section, Experimental Immunology Branch, National Cancer Institute, National Institutes of Health. One of the first immunologists to approach the challenge of defining the immunologic abnormalities in AIDS. Dr. Shearer's early concepts dealt with possible activation events within the immune system. Most recently, with his colleague, Mario Clerici, he has pioneered the potential role of a TH1-to-TH2 shift in cytokine production as being responsible for the progression to disease.

Finally, the expression of HIV envelope proteins in association with other replicating viruses (e.g., Ty particle, hepatitis B virus, adenovirus, Semliki Forest virus, rhinovirus, influenza virus, equine encephalitis virus, and poliovirus) and with bacteria (mycobacteria, bacillus Calmette-Guérin, salmonellae) is being evaluated in animals (Table 15.9) (40, 335, 403, 719, 785, 944, 1466, 1535, 1778, 2051, 2216, 2391, 2935). An adenovirus-based vaccine regimen has been effective in protecting chimpanzees from HIV-1 infection (1596a). Moreover, a recombinant Semliki Forest virus expressing the SIV PBJ14 envelope rgp160 or rgp120 protected immunized animals from lethal disease, although they became infected with the virus (1867). Some systems, like hepatitis B virus, are limited, since only small portions of the viral envelope can be inserted into the viral genome. Observations on induction of anti-HIV responses with poliovirus chimeras, particularly those involving the replacement of the VP2 and VP3 genes with HIV-1 proteins (73, 2125), have provided promising results.

A new vector being explored is *Listeria monocytogenes* (1154, 2676a). This gram-positive intracellular bacterium, by the nature of its replicative cycle, can pre-

Table 15.9   Vectors evaluated for HIV vaccines

Viruses
    Vaccinia virus
    Canarypox virus
    Hepatitis B virus
    Adenovirus
    Semliki Forest virus
    Rhinovirus
    Influenza virus
    Equine encephalitis virus
    Poliovirus
    Ty particle

Bacteria
    Mycobacterium (BCG)
    Listeria
    Salmonella

sent antigens through either MHC class I or class II molecules (Figure 15.1) (1154). Cell-mediated immune responses have been induced in mice by the use of this bacterium as a live vaccine vector for the HIV-1 Gag protein (789). Other chromosomally modified strains of *L. monocytogenes* may prove useful in primate and human studies.

C.   Summary

Most vaccine studies now suggest that priming with a vector-based vaccine (e.g., vaccinia virus or canarypox virus) followed by a protein subunit booster offers the best chance for induction of protection against virus challenge (Tables 15.7 and 15.8). The time of challenge is important. At least 6 months is required to establish protective immunity, and longer periods may work better. In studies with HIV-2 recombinant poxviruses, long-lasting protection, even to a second challenge, was achieved in rhesus macaques (785). In contrast, oral immunization with recombinants from salmonellae expressing HIV-2 Gag and gp120 did not induce protection (785). A major question is whether these promising results in the HIV-2 model can be extrapolated to HIV-1, since similar successes with SIV in protecting against infection by a virulent strain have not been achieved (Section III.B).

Using viral subunit proteins, and not complete virus, as immunogens eliminates the possibility of viral nucleic acids becoming transcribed or undergoing cellular integration and avoids the possibility of HIV-1 not being inactivated when

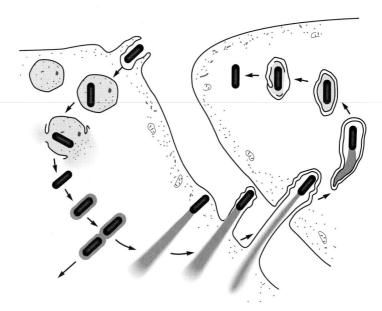

Figure 15.1   Stages in the entry, growth, movement, and spread of *L. monocytogenes*. The bacteria are endocytosed, fused with intracellular vesicles, and digested, and their antigens can be expressed with class II molecules. Alternatively, they can replicate out of the vesicles, become digested, and subsequently are expressed with class I molecules. Because of the value in expressing antigens by these two processes, this bacterium is being evaluated for use in HIV vaccine development. (From reference 2676a, with permission.)

killed virus is used. Moreover, a killed HIV-1 preparation cannot guarantee antigenic stability of the viral proteins or the lack of residual infectivity. Nevertheless, as with other agents, these vaccine procedures with purified proteins, either alone or with a replicating vector, need to protect against high-dose virus challenge, transmission by infected cells, and mucosal inoculation.

IV.   Viral Cores as Vaccines

In a related approach to vaccine development, viral cores containing HIV envelope proteins are produced through the use of the HIV or other retrovirus *gag* genetic regions (1136, 2523). For example, infection of cells with vaccinia virus constructs containing the core and envelope regions of HIV gives rise to virus-like particles (VLPs) that express gp120 on the surface and lack the HIV genome (984, 1136, 2486, 2523) (Figure 15.2). These released retrovirus-like structures can be purified in sucrose density gradients and potentially used for immunization (984, 2471). Moreover, HIV-1-like particles can be produced with unprocessed gp160 glycoproteins that can elicit neutralizing antibodies on immunization of guinea pigs. They represent alternative immunogens for a particle-based AIDS vaccine (2251). These approaches offer the advantage of a close similarity to HIV without the potential danger of an infectious virion. Thus, they could provide an immunogen that might induce an immune response best suited to recognizing the invading organism.

Vaccines with viral cores have also utilized the genetic sequences of other retroviruses or retrovirus-like agents. VLPs expressing the HIV-1 V3 loop have been made with the HIV-2 Gag protein (1607). Moreover, the yeast Ty retrotransposon was manipulated to produce VLPs expressing HIV-1 envelope epitopes (944, 1453; for a review, see reference 380). The induction of mucosal immunity (i.e., anti-SIV antibodies) in primates after vaginal or rectal immunization with a Ty VLP expressing an SIV protein has offered some hope for the successful induction of local immune responses (1466, 1468). In addition, virus-like particles have been derived using baculovirus recombinants containing the HIV-1 envelope (617a). Nevertheless, the potential problem of envelope glycosylation differences between vaccines grown in yeast and insect cells and those grown in mammalian cells must be considered.

V.   Viral DNA Inoculation

A new approach under consideration for a vaccine is the injection of DNA constructs directly into the host in vivo (for reviews see references 2251a and 2869). For effectiveness, certain issues must be considered (Table 15.10). By this procedure, the

Table 15.10 Important issues with DNA vaccines

1. Should deliver to antigen-presenting cells
2. Potential integration of plasmid DNA in the host genome must be avoided
3. Generation of anti-DNA antibodies must be avoided

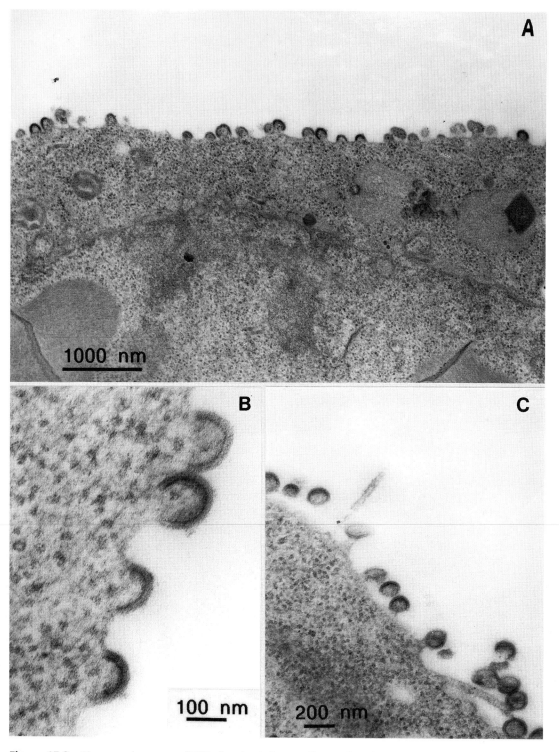

Figure 15.2 Electron microscopy of VLPs forming in insect cells transfected with a baculovirus construct expressing Gag/Pol. (A) VLPs budding from the plasma membrane. (B) A high magnification showing several intermediate stages in the budding process. (C) Extracellular VLPs. (Reprinted from reference 1138 with permission.)

antigenic epitopes of the immunizing proteins are produced in a form that would be naturally recognized in the recipient host. This procedure could be especially helpful in inducing cell-mediated immunity. It has been demonstrated as a method of gene therapy for cancer (2906) and for expression of cytokines (1894). In the early studies of this approach, intramuscular injection of mice with an HIV-1 envelope gp160 DNA construct elicited antibodies that neutralized HIV-1 and prevented virally induced syncytium formation in vitro. Some cellular antiviral immune responses were also demonstrated in these animals (2818). The most efficient induction of immune response appears to result from gene gun targeting to the skin and not the muscle (2693) (Table 15.11).

In studies involving nonhuman primates, inoculation and boosting of chimpanzees with a DNA HIV gp160 plasmid expression vector produced neutralizing and T-cell proliferative responses in all inoculated animals (2817). An HIV-1 envelope DNA vaccine given to rhesus monkeys elicited a TH1-like immune response (1474). Similarly, a plasmid DNA encoding the SIV envelope and Gag proteins elicited CTL responses in rhesus macaques (2936). Recently, chimpanzees have been protected against HIV-1 challenge by DNA immunizations with gp160 and *rev* as well as *gag* and *pol* sequences (267). This approach provides encouragement for obtaining protective immunity in humans. Moreover, most recently, macaques were primed with an HIV-1 envelope DNA (multiple doses) followed by boosting with the envelope DNA plus the HIV envelope protein. An immune response was induced which protected the monkeys from infection with the HIV-1 chimeric SHIV virus. Thus, DNA prime followed by boost with both the DNA and envelope protein could be an effective vaccine strategy (1481a).

However, negative results have also been obtained. An experimental vaccine containing five DNA plasmids expressing different combinations and forms of the SIV$_{mac}$ proteins was used for multiple inoculations of rhesus macaques. Some were inoculated intravenously, some intramuscularly, and others by gene gun procedures. CTLs were induced, and neutralizing antibodies appeared in all the vaccinated animals but were transient. Some attenuation of the acute phase of infection was noted, but no protection from infection was achieved (1589).

Another method for vaccination involves immunization with a random-sheared DNA expression library. It produces a response to a variety of antigens that could provide protection against challenge by a pathogen (148). This approach differs from the use of selected DNA regions of the virus since it provides expression of antigens that might be masked on the virion. The random DNA library may thus give a broader immune response that can be protective. Moreover, the use of a facilitating adjuvant (bupivacaine) or other compounds to increase DNA delivery is being explored to enhance this approach to immunization (2818). Because of their

Table 15.11 Advantages of the gene gun

1. Facilitates optimization of vaccine delivery
2. Intracellular delivery at epidermis (safety advantage)
3. Provides control over the number of plasmid vector copies delivered and the number of cell penetration events
4. Requires two to three times less DNA than intramuscular administration

stability, ease of preparation and delivery, and potential to induce both humoral and cellular immunity, DNA vaccines with modifications in their makeup and delivery will certainly receive increased attention in the coming years (Table 15.12).

VI.	Cytokine Enhancement

Recent studies have explored the possibility that immunization of animals together with the administration of cytokines would increase the immune response and enhance protection from virus challenge. For example, vaccination of mice with leishmanial antigens and interleukin-12 (IL-12) promoted the development of TH1 cells and resistance to subsequent infection (23). Moreover, plasmids encoding HIV-1 envelope and IL-12, when inoculated into mice, enhanced CTL activity (2722a). This TH1 type response appeared mediated by gamma interferon (IFN-γ). In experiments with primates, rhesus macaques were vaccinated with an SIV attenuated (*nef*-deleted) mutant that expressed IFN-γ. Although the animals became infected on challenge, they had a less pathogenic course and remained healthy for a longer period of time than did the naive controls (877). Work in other infectious disease systems has suggested that an IL-2-based vaccine might enhance the TH1 responses needed for good cell-mediated immunity (2923).

In attempts to preferentially induce a TH1-type response, attention has been placed on low-dose antigen exposure. These directions are derived from earlier experimental evidence suggesting that inoculation of small amounts of antigen can influence the immune response toward cell-mediated immunity rather than antibody-directed immunity (278). In one experiment focusing on this approach, rhesus monkeys inoculated with a low dose of infectious SIV did not seroconvert and did not become infected, but they showed resistance to challenge with a higher dose of SIV (471). In other studies, however, rhesus macaques exposed to low doses of SIV intravenously showed some proliferative T-cell response but not CTL production. Boosting with a second low-dose exposure did not lead to infection, but when the animals were challenged with a higher dose of SIV, no protection was observed (642). Conceivably, the absence of CTL or strong cell-mediated immunity was the determining factor in the lack of protection. This approach of low antigen dosage to direct the immune response during immunization merits further consideration.

Table 15.12 Advantages of DNA vaccines

1. Can be manufactured more easily than standard vaccines
2. All plasmids can be manufactured essentially in the same way
3. DNA is very stable at temperature extremes
4. DNA can be mutated to increase immunogenicity
5. After immunization, immune responses can be assessed without further experimental steps (e.g., preparation of recombinant protein)
6. Resembles a viral infection; induces protein expression on the cell surface in context of MHC class I and class II molecules
7. Can be used in countries that cannot support expensive strategies

VII.   **Induction of Mucosal Immunity**

In attempting to induce immune responses in the mucosa (Figure 15.3), a variety of techniques have been evaluated (for a review, see reference 1762). In one series of experiments, young mice were immunized orally with peptides of HIV-1 strains after their stomach acidity was neutralized. A high-titer secretory neutralizing antibody of IgA type was found in the bowel (311). In another group of studies using intranasal administration to mice, a DNA HIV vaccine, combined with liposomes and IL-12 and GM-CSF-expressing plasmids, induced strong levels of both humoral and cellular immune responses (1976a). Anti-HIV neutralizing antibodies were found in both feces and serum. This simple and relatively safe method of immunization, involving no infectious organism, merits further evaluation in primates to determine its potential use in humans.

Anti-HIV antibodies have been induced in primates after vaginal or rectal immunization with a Ty VLP expressing an SIV protein (1466, 1468). A targeted lymph node route of immunization has also been tried with SIV proteins, and this approach resulted in B- and T-cell proliferation and TH1 responses comparable to those obtained after administration via the vaginal, male genital, urethral, and rectal mucosal routes. The response was augmented by oral immunization. The resulting IgG antibodies in the mucosa, along with T- and B-cell immunity in the draining lymph nodes and in the circulation, prevented transmission of virus in the

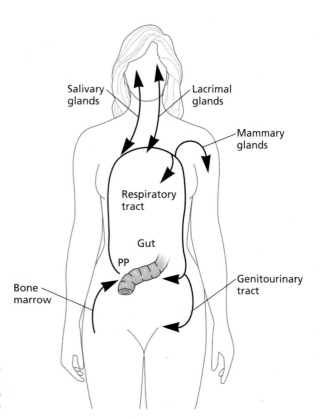

Figure 15.3 Interconnections of the mucosal immune system that involve the oral, nasal, urethral, vaginal, and rectal cavities. PP, Peyer's patches. (From a diagram provided by J. Mestecky.)

mucosa (1467). In other studies, recombinant SIV gp120 and core p27 were inoculated into the iliac lymph nodes draining the genital and rectal region. Infection by the rectal route was prevented in four of seven macaques in association with an increase in IgG antibody-secreting cells (1469).

In another group of studies, nontraumatic inoculation of the vaginas of rhesus macaques was performed with an SHIV chimera (HIV-$1_{89.6}$) that can establish a systemic infection (1592, 1789). Once this infection was controlled in the host, the monkeys were superinfected intravaginally with pathogenic SIV$_{mac239}$, and protection was achieved (1591, 1592). In similar studies using the rectal route for HIV-2 administration, monkeys were not protected from subsequent SIV challenge (2808). The result may reflect low-level replication of the HIV-2 strain (Section II). Nevertheless, macaques infected with a *nef*-deleted SHIV were protected against superinfection via the rectal mucosa of a pathogenic strain of SIV or an SHIV isolate composed of the envelope of the cytopathic HIV-1_{SF33} strain (536). In other studies, direct inoculation of live attenuated SIV into the vagina generated IgM and IgA antibodies against the virus in serum and vaginal secretions and viral-specific CTL in the peripheral blood (1579). Likewise, in an attenuated SIV$_{mac1A11}$ infection of fetal or neonatal rhesus macaques, transient viremia, anti-SIV responses, and weak or no CTL activity were observed. Some of the animals were protected from a subsequent oral challenge with pathogenic SIV$_{mac251}$ given shortly after birth. The results showed that protection can be achieved early in development and confirmed that SIV can be transmitted to newborn monkeys by the oral route (108, 1998).

Encouraging results were also obtained when three pregnant macaques were vaccinated against the SIV$_{mac}$ strain. The newborns were challenged by virus through the oral or conjunctival routes. Two of the animals were protected against SIV infection at birth. Thus, active immunization and receipt of immunoglobulin from the mother may decrease the rate of perinatal transmission by the mucosal route (2757).

In some studies involving vaginal inoculation of SIV, the virus was found in vaginal fluids several days before seroconversion and before systemic infection was noted (1454). The results suggest that a local immune response to a virus can occur without a systemic reaction. Thus, certain high-risk, presumably uninfected individuals should be examined for immune responses in the mucosa and not just in the blood (1703a) (see Chapter 13, Section VI). Finally, some studies have indicated that protection from mucosal infection can be achieved by systemic immunization (2109). Thus, depending on the strategy used with HIV, mucosal immunity could be elicited by either local or peripheral administration of the vaccine.

VIII.   Human Vaccine Trials

A.   Viral Envelope Proteins

Several phase I and phase II vaccine trials have now been conducted with vaccinia virus-expressed or purified HIV envelope glycoprotein gp160 or gp120 in humans. These studies, involving over 2,000 volunteers, have revealed no untoward clinical effects. The induction of moderate levels of neutralizing antibodies against laboratory strains of HIV-1 and some cellular immune responses have been demonstrated (7, 245, 513, 646, 686, 693, 930, 999, 1218, 1220, 1362, 1816, 1988, 2426). In one study, CTL responses and possibly CD8$^+$ cell antiviral factor production were induced in seronegative volunteers by a recombinant HIV-1$_{SF2}$ gp160 vaccine (245). Moreover, experiments with a vaccine based on muramyl tripeptide phosphatidyl-ethanolamine (MTP-PE) (Section VIII.B) containing the glycosylated gp120 from the HIV-1$_{SF2}$ strain showed encouraging results; relatively high levels of neutralizing antibodies and cellular immune responses were observed in human volunteers (1218, 1220). In studies with a different HIV-1 isolate, a low dose of ALVAC (canarypox virus), expressing the HIV-1$_{MN}$ envelope-like protein, induced CTL activity in seronegative volunteers (686). Finally, some approaches have involved immunization of antigens linked to dendritic cells for delivery as has been described in animal systems (298a). Results on these studies with HIV have not yet been reported.

Despite this progress in human vaccine trials, whether immunized subjects are truly protected is unclear because of the limitations in monitoring antiviral responses. When PBMC and primary isolates are used in neutralization assays, most vaccinated subjects show low levels of neutralizing antibodies to the vaccine strain and none to primary isolates (1005, 1690). Some groups believe that, optimally, neutralizing antibodies to primary isolates should be induced at least to the level detected in long-term asymptomatic individuals. Moreover, the question whether mucosal immunity is elicited has been evaluated only by limited antibody assays (813).

Some volunteers immunized with gp160- or gp120-based vaccines have subsequently become infected by HIV-1 (164, 1220, 1271, 1721). The lack of protection, despite the presence of neutralizing antibodies to the vaccine strain, is discouraging, and the factors involved need to be identified (Section VIII.C). Conceivably, a greater number of the vaccinees would have become infected if they had not been immunized. Alternatively, the possible role of antibodies that enhance transmission in some cases should be considered (Chapter 10, Section III) (1577b, 1815). Moreover, as noted above, whether these types of vaccines can prevent disease requires evaluation over time.

The use of the SCID-hu mouse system has offered a potential way to examine the immune response of human subjects. A sample of the immunized human PBMC can be injected into these immunosuppressed animals, and then the reconstituted SCID-hu mice can be challenged with infectious HIV. In preliminary studies, the best protection from infection was observed with PBMC from vaccinia virus vector-immunized subjects who had subsequently received a booster of baculovirus-derived gp160 protein (1858). The mechanism of protection is unknown but probably involves antiviral cell-mediated immunity. The SCID-hu mouse model could also be helpful in examining sera from HIV envelope-vaccinated volunteers, as it was in evaluating sera from immunized baboons (114).

B.   **Adjuvants**

In addition to using the appropriate antigen in a vaccine, an adjuvant can be very important for eliciting protective immune responses against the virus (for a review, see reference 48). The adjuvant should not produce unacceptable reactions at the injection sites and should have low systemic toxicity. It should induce cell-mediated immunity, including CTL, and antibodies of high affinity for vaccine antigens and of protective isotypes. Antibodies of those isotypes should activate complement and function synergistically with effector cells in antibody-dependent cellular cytotoxicity processes. The only adjuvants now approved for general human use are aluminum sulfate and aluminum phosphate (alum). Alum augments antibody formation by using most, but not all, antigens; it is ineffective with influenza virus hemagglutinin. Moreover, alum-precipitated antigens do not consistently elicit cell-mediated immunity. Hence, there is a need for adjuvants that have the potency of Freund's complete adjuvant (FCA) but do not induce granulomas at injection sites or produce other unacceptable side effects.

Some new adjuvant formulations are listed in Table 15.13. In some of these, the mycobacterial cell wall component of FCA has been replaced by a synthetic muramyl dipeptide (MDP) or tripeptide (MTP) or by adjuvant-active analogs that are nonpyrogenic and have fewer other side effects, e.g., *N*-acetylmuramyl-L-threonyl-D-isoglutamine (Thr-MDP). FCA is a water-in-mineral-oil emulsion. The bulk oil phase remains at the injection site and is infiltrated by macrophages, which is why it produces granulomas. In the new adjuvants, the mineral oil in FCA has been replaced by the naturally occurring lipid squalene, or squalene in the form of a 5% microfluidized oil-in-water emulsion. The lipids can thus be metabolized by the body. In addition, more-defined surfactants such as Tween 80 and Span-85 are used instead of the Ariacel A surfactant in FCA. Some studies indicate that large animal species (e.g., primates), in contrast to rodents and rabbits, respond best to small-droplet stable emulsions (2753). Thus, this type of adjuvant formulation is recommended for inoculation in humans.

In the Syntex Adjuvant Formulation (331), the polyoxyethylene-polyoxypropylene triblock copolymer L121 is added. By hydrogen bonding, this surface-active agent retains antigens on the surface of the lipid microspheres and activates complement. The microspheres migrate through the lymphatic system to the lymph nodes, and C3b on their surface targets them to antigen-presenting dendritic and follicular dendritic cells. The MDP analog added to the emulsion induces the production of a cascade of cytokines, elicits CTL, and can induce mucosal immunity (e.g., with herpes simplex virus in guinea pigs) (185).

Another microfluidized formulation, MF59, consists of an emulsion containing

Table 15.13 New adjuvants augmenting cell-mediated and humoral immune responses[a]

Adjuvant	Vehicle
Muramyl dipeptide analogs (e.g., Thr-MDP [*N*-acetylmuramyl-L-threonyl-D-isoglutamine])	Squalene-L121 emulsion
Muramyl tripeptide phosphatidylethanolamine (MTP-PE)	Squalene emulsion
Monophosphoryl lipid A (MPL)	Squalene emulsion, liposomes
Saponin (e.g., QS21)	Immune-stimulating complexes

[a] See Section VIII.B.

squalene and the surfactants Tween 80 and Span-85. The lipophilic muramyl peptide derivative MTP-PE (2753) is sometimes added. MF59 contains a phospholipid tail that facilitates association with the lipid phases. It has been demonstrated to be an effective adjuvant for influenza virus, herpes simplex virus, and HIV antigens in animal models and is used in clinical trials with these virus vaccines (1218, 1220).

In the Ribi adjuvant, the toxicity of the lipid A component of gram-negative bacterial lipopolysaccharide is decreased by removal of a labile phosphate group. The resulting monophosphoryl-lipid A (MPL) is added to squalene emulsions alone or in combination with trehalose dimycolate and/or cell wall skeleton from *Mycobacterium phlei* (2304). One form of the Ribi adjuvant (Detox) has been used in clinical trials for melanoma and malaria vaccines (2231). MPL has also been combined with liposomes, augmenting their efficacy as adjuvants (2225), and these formulations have also been used in clinical trials with a malaria vaccine. For cell-mediated immunity, liposomes have the potential to carry antigens to the antigen-presenting cells such as macrophages, dendritic cells, and Langerhans cells in the skin. They can also concentrate the proteins at the site of inoculation and release them gradually, thus maintaining a constant antigenic stimulation.

Yet another group of adjuvants is based on saponins, glycosylated triterpenes derived from plants, usually *Quillaia saponaria*. Saponins are highly surface active and cytolytic, so they can produce tissue damage at injection sites. Such damage is reduced by using purified fractions (e.g., QS21) (1269). This adjuvant has been used with SIV Gag and envelope proteins and has induced CTL responses (1921) but no protection from challenge. Toxic effects of adjuvants can also be avoided by decreasing the amount of residual saponin in the vaccine through the formation of immune system-stimulating complexes (or ISCOMs) (1841). These are regular, cage-like structures containing saponin and virus envelope glycoproteins. Immunostimulating complexes containing gp120 of HIV elicit neutralizing antibodies and $CD8^+$ CTL in mice (2629). SIV envelope and Gag proteins incorporated into ISCOMs were used to immunize monkeys. Despite the induction of CTL and neutralizing antibodies, no protection was achieved (1140). Highly purified saponin has also enhanced cell-mediated immune responses to HIV when used as a component in an experimental gp160 vaccine with alum (2919).

The new adjuvant formulations have been shown to induce protective responses against HIV and perhaps SIV, although in the latter case, cellular antigens could be involved (360, 624, 1881). Some have demonstrated effectiveness in inducing immunogenicity to the vaccine in chimpanzees and humans, e.g., in eliciting anti-HIV responses, with an encouraging safety profile (888, 1218). It seems likely that these adjuvants will be components of new generations of vaccines containing recombinant viral antigens and viral DNA.

Most recently, genetic adjuvants derived from small DNA sequences (with CpG motifs) were found to increase immune reactivity, particularly TH-1 type responses (2269a). In addition, the coadministration of a B7-2 expression plasmid with a DNA vaccine has enhanced cell-mediated immune responses to HIV in mice (2722b). These approaches using immunostimulatory DNA sequences (ISSs) and costimulatory molecules may provide new methods for enhancing immunologic response with HIV vaccines.

C.   Potential Problems Involved in Vaccination

Some concern has been raised about the following risks resulting from vaccination:

- antibody-dependent enhancement (ADE)
- clonal dominance
- T-cell receptor antagonism

In the first case, monkeys immunized with an SIV variable (V2) domain produced neutralizing antibodies to the homologous virus but were not protected from infection. In some cases, viral loads were higher in controls than in vaccinated animals, suggesting the presence of antibody-mediated enhancement (ADE) of virus infection (2392). In other vaccine studies, monkeys immunized against the region in the SIV gp41 transmembrane glycoprotein that is associated with ADE had enhancing antibodies and showed a more rapid progression to disease (1797). Similar observations were noted in EIAV vaccine studies with a baculovirus-derived virus envelope (1165), which lacks the normal host cell-derived glycosylation pattern. Moreover, cats immunized with three different recombinant FIV candidate vaccines, including vaccinia virus-based vectors, showed higher viral loads after challenge. Antibodies produced during the recombinant vaccinia virus immunization were transferred to naive cats, and enhancement in virus infection and replication was noted (2498). Thus, ADE could be a detrimental result of ineffective vaccination. Concern about the possibility of ADE as a result of HIV immunization has led to recommendations to evaluate this phenomenon in vaccine trials (1689). Nevertheless, some studies have indicated that as titers of neutralizing antibodies increase, the effect of enhancing antibodies can be prevented (1319a, 1819). The findings suggest that booster shots that increase antibody production could elicit more high-affinity neutralizing antibodies.

As for the concern about clonal dominance, priming of B cells for an immunologic response may induce a dominant reaction and prevent the response of other B cells to new antigens (1335) (see Chapter 10, Section II.C). This possibility of "original antigenic sin" has been observed in studies in mice receiving polyvalent mixtures of HIV immunogens (1335). In one model, adult mice were immunized with recombinant gp120 before mating. The 3-week-old offspring were subsequently immunized with the same vaccine, and an inhibition of the IgG response was noted (1198). However, various procedures for changing the sequence of administration or the administration of many components together overcame some of this suppression (1036). Moreover, masking of the antigenic domain through the addition of carbohydrates and a reduction in net positive charge has been evaluated in animals to counter the supressive effects of immunodominant epitopes in a primary immune response to HIV. A qualitative shift in antibody production was noted (848a). This approach might be helpful in eliciting a more broadly reactive response from HIV vaccines.

Finally, in related studies of immune competition, one vaccinated human volunteer who subsequently became infected by virus showed the presence only of a CTL clone that was able to recognize the vaccine strain. When the CD8$^+$ cells were exposed to a peptide based on the epitope sequence of the infecting isolate, the CTL activity against the vaccine strain was inhibited (1271). This finding possibly presents the first evidence in vivo of the T-cell receptor antagonism suggested by previous in vitro studies (196, 1318).

D.   Ideal Properties of an Effective Vaccine

Several properties besides a lack of toxicity are necessary for a successful vaccine (Table 15.14) (for reviews, see references 12, 380, 737, 1069, 1249, and 1489) (Section I). It should induce strong cellular and humoral immune responses (11, 2627, 2629). Toward this objective, the question of which antigens to use is under close study. Both envelope proteins (non-antibody-enhancing regions) and other viral proteins (e.g., Gag) should be considered. The inclusion of Gag appears to be very important, since CTL activity against this viral protein seems to correlate with an asymptomatic state (243, 2238). In this regard, vaccination studies with the full envelope protein gp160 and the core protein of SIV protected rhesus macaques from challenge with both cloned and uncloned homologous virus (1121a, 1124). Cellular immune activity appeared to be involved.

An anti-HIV vaccine should produce long-lasting responses that are present not only in the blood but also in the mucosal linings of the vagina, the rectum, and perhaps the oral cavity. This mucosal immunity might require the use of a vaccine administered orally or placed in contact with the mucosal immune system via the bowel, vagina, rectum, or nasal/oral passages (1786, 1788) (Table 15.3). In this regard, immunization by the respiratory or gastrointestinal route along with systemic immunization has protected monkeys from HIV challenge via the vagina (1684). However, results from some studies in mice suggest that immunization via the vaginal route might not be very effective (2284a). This observation should not be surprising, since a natural active immune response in this site could lead to inappropriate immune reactions to foreign antigens, some of which might induce sterility. Selective immunization at other mucosal sites might bring the effective responses, since the mucosal system appears to be interconnected throughout the body (for reviews, see references 1724 and 1762) (Figure 15.3). Alternatively, as noted above (Section VII), induction of systemic immunity could elicit protection at mucosal sites (2109).

Side effects such as autoimmune phenomena and enhancing antibodies must also be avoided in any vaccination procedure. In this regard, some studies with sera of volunteers immunized with recombinant gp160 have indicated the induction of anti-CD4, anti-idiotype antibodies (1258), anti-HLA class I antibodies (599), and,

Table 15.14 Ideal properties of an anti-HIV vaccine

1. Elicits neutralizing antibodies that react with all HIV strains and subtypes
2. Induces cellular and humoral immune responses against virus-infected cells
3. Induces immune responses that recognize latently infected cells
4. Does not induce antibodies that enhance HIV infection
5. Does not induce autoimmune responses
6. Induces local immunity at all sites of HIV entry in the host
7. Is safe, showing no toxic effects
8. Effect is long-lasting

in some cases, enhancing antibodies for certain HIV-1 strains (Section VIII.C) (1319b). In all these vaccine approaches, prevention of infection would be optimal, but protection from disease could also be a satisfactory result.

Finally, several studies suggest that vaccines that induce a strong cellular immune response rather than a humoral immune response might be most effective in HIV infection (2343) (see Chapters 11 and 13). In this case, the use of selected TH1-type cytokines or antibodies to certain TH2-type cytokines along with the vaccine could be considered. Adjuvants that preferentially induce TH1 responses (956) or a low antigen dose that has been shown to produce a TH1-type response in other systems (278, 380, 2043, 2821) could be used. Obtaining strong cell-mediated immune responses may require live virus vectors or DNA inoculations so that antigen presentation is optimal for CD8$^+$ cell responses.

A low concentration of antigen in a vaccine has been advised, based on observations on type 1 and type 2 responses in humans and monkeys (2343). Cellular immune proliferative responses of PBMC and CD8$^+$ cell antiviral activity have been noted in high-risk individuals who have no evidence of infection (see Chapter 11). Moreover, in monkeys inoculated intrarectally with low doses of SIV, cell-mediated immune responses were detected without seroconversion. When these animals were subsequently challenged with low-dose virus, they were protected from infection (471). These observations should lead to increased discussion about the amount of antigen used in a vaccine and its means of presentation. It has been said that if cell-mediated immune responses were as easy to measure as antibodies, much lower antigen doses would have been used in many of the present vaccines. Nevertheless, it seems certain that some degree of both humoral and cellular immune response mediated by a variety of cytokines will be needed in a successful vaccine.

E.   Summary

Despite a decade of research, work on an HIV vaccine is still in its early stages. A great deal of information on why vaccines will not work has been accumulated. Unfortunately, very few experiments have been conclusive in showing protection from infection, but some have provided promising results (Table 15.15). The most effective approaches thus far have involved prime-and-boost procedures in which priming is performed with a live vector, attenuated strain, or DNA and the boost is done with a subunit viral protein (Tables 15.7 and 15.8). In general, however, only ho-

Table 15.15   Examples of presumed protection against HIV or SIV infection

1. Chimpanzees immunized with recombinant gp120 and challenged with primary or laboratory HIV-1 isolates
2. Macaques protected against HIV-2 or SIV following various vaccine approaches
3. Macaques vaccinated with live attenuated (*nef*-deleted) SIV
4. Macaques exposed to low-dose rectal inoculation of SIV
5. Macques and baboons infected with attenuated SIV or HIV-2 protected from superinfection by pathogenic strains
6. Seronegative individuals with multiple exposures to HIV

mologous virus challenge has been prevented. These studies are now beginning in human volunteers (e.g., ALVAC with HIV-1 gp120$_{MN}$) and have shown induction of cross-reacting CTL activity (751, 999). DNA vaccine approaches, through inoculation of either specific viral genes or a random expression library (148), also offer encouraging results for future trials because the viral proteins can be expressed with MHC molecules on the surface of the host cells. Some DNA vaccines may involve new techniques with lipid-containing cochleates, which could induce good immune responses when administered orally (1661). Many reasons for the use of DNA vaccines in the future can be appreciated (Table 15.12).

It appears that, in general, a TH1 response is the most effective in protecting against infection, although neutralizing antibodies for blocking incoming free virus are also important. Vaccines using low-dose antigen or cytokines that will preferentially induce a TH1 response should be encouraged. New information has been provided over the last 3 years on mechanisms for inducing mucosal immunity, and new animal models have been provided that could facilitate evaluation of vaccine approaches. These approaches include the SHIV models and HIV-2 infection of pigtail macaques and baboons. In these studies, it is important to define the correlates of protective immunity that can be addressed in human trials (Table 15.2).

Despite the lack of convincing evidence that an effective vaccine for HIV is available, some human trials are being conducted, particularly in Thailand and parts of Africa. Recombinant protein vaccines are being evaluated because of some success in chimpanzee models, and eventually the prime-and-boost procedures noted above with live virus vectors and recombinant peptides will be studied. What perhaps needs further emphasis is the use of whole killed virus. While this technique carries a risk of live-virus survival, this risk should be controllable (e.g., with the use of killed attenuated strains). This method, which has not received sufficient attention, offers the advantage of presenting a similar viral structure that would be encountered by the infected host. Furthermore, subunit vaccines might be delivered as oligomers of viral envelope (1605) or polymers containing mixtures of viral proteins, as has been used in malaria (2046). Important in all these discussions is the recognition that HIV-1 transmission by the virus-infected cell can occur readily and that recognizing and destroying this cell before transmission takes place will require new ideas in vaccine development (1492) (Table 15.14).

One concern is whether weak vaccines will induce enhancing antibodies that will increase the chance of infection in some individuals. Moreover, through the induction of clonal dominance (1335), a weak immune response to one vaccine might prevent induction of a better antiviral response with a subsequent, more effective vaccine. For this reason, those conducting large-scale vaccine trials need to consider not only the correlates of immunity that might be induced but also the parameters that might be detrimental to the immunized host and that might prevent an effective immune response when a more successful vaccine is developed.

The present vaccine trials being conducted in various parts of the world should offer important information over the next few years. Moreover, the U.S. government is currently focusing on achieving effective prevention of HIV infection, since promising antiviral therapies are now available (see Chapter 14). Progress in efforts to develop an HIV vaccine should be made in the near future.

IX.   Other Anti-HIV Prevention Approaches

Some investigators have explored the possibility that passive immunotherapy with antibodies or serum from HIV-positive individuals would be helpful in preventing infection. This treatment for already-infected individuals is discussed in Chapter 14. Animal studies using chimpanzees at first showed no protection from HIV after the administration of anti-HIV antibodies followed by a high-dose virus challenge (100 chimpanzee-infectious doses for a 50% infection rate [CID_{50}]) (2146). Nevertheless, a subsequent study with 10 CID_{50} prevented infection (2147). In one animal in the first experiment, enhancement of HIV infection was suspected (2146). As noted above, immunized-baboon sera administered to SCID-hu mice have provided protection from virus challenge (114).

In one study, an anti-V3 loop monoclonal antibody was found to protect chimpanzees from infection with 75 CID given 24 h after the antibodies (701). Moreover, when 75 CID was first inoculated into chimpanzees and followed 10 min later by the antiviral antibodies, protection from infection was also observed (701). A similar finding on protection by passive immunization has been made with HIV and SIV in macaques (2159). However, the efficacy of this approach appears to be limited to just a few minutes after virus inoculation (2145a). Passive immunization of macaques with immune sera or a pool of neutralizing monoclonal antibodies did not protect against an SIV challenge (49a, 1270). This finding counters the results of an earlier study (2159), but the viruses in that earlier study were grown in human PBMC and not monkey PBMC. The application of passive immunization to prevention of infection, particularly after needlestick injuries or during childbirth, requires much further study, including the use of selected (even monoclonal) antibodies (2996).

Chapter 15 **SALIENT FEATURES**

1. Development of a vaccine for prevention of HIV infection has included approaches with inactivated virus, attenuated viruses, and purified envelope gp120, alone or in association with live expression vectors (virus or bacteria).

2. Viral cores or virus-like particles (VLPs) are being evaluated as a possible approach to an HIV vaccine.

3. DNA inoculation offers a promising new direction for a vaccine.

4. Thus far, the most safe and effective procedure for immunization has been to prime the host with a live vector expressing HIV proteins, followed by a booster of a subunit protein or the live virus vector. Inoculation of attenuated virus has induced the best protection in animal studies but is not acceptable for human trials.

5. The advantage of vaccines may be increased through the coadministration of cytokines that can influence the immune response.

6. Attention to mucosal immunity requires measurement of antibody- and cell-mediated responses in mucosal regions such as the rectum and vagina. Direct administration of a vaccine to these areas is under study.

7. Several trials in human subjects have been conducted that have involved subunit vaccines and, most recently, priming with poxvirus-based vaccines. Their evaluation in the field awaits further results.

8. All vaccine approaches require appropriate adjuvants that may selectively enhance either cell-mediated or humoral immunity.

9. Vaccines must avoid the induction of enhancing antibodies, autoantibodies, and the phenomenon of clonal dominance.

10. The ideal vaccine is one that lacks toxicity, is able to induce neutralizing but not enhancing antibodies, and can provide long-lasting immune responses at mucosal sites as well as in the blood.

11. Because of the intracellular nature of HIV, cell-mediated immune responses appear to be the most important mechanism for controlling or preventing HIV infection in the host.

12. Passive immunotherapy to prevent HIV transmission is successful in animals when antibodies are administered within a few minutes after infection. This procedure for protection from infection requires more study.

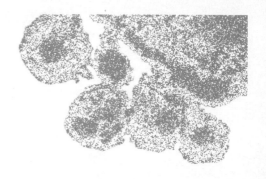

Conclusions

Encouraging progress has been made in understanding the pathogenesis of HIV infection, from the initial isolation of representative viruses in 1983 to the more recent development of effective antiviral drugs. Nevertheless, the path toward the eventual control of HIV still requires major efforts toward immune restoration and the development of an effective vaccine. While the direction appears more focused today, many avenues of study still need to be explored. Great advances continue to come from the treatment of opportunistic infections (for a review, see reference 827). Importantly, HIV represents a new type of organism arising in populations in epidemic proportions. Its characterstics define the challenges posed for its eventual control (Table A).

The exact mechanisms of CD4$^+$ cell depletion and immune deficiency are not yet clear, and its cellular latency, as well as several other features of HIV infection, remains mysterious. Moreover, whether more virulent and drug-resistant viruses are emerging in the population as a result of continual transmission merits attention. Most importantly, how the advancements made in detection and treatment of HIV infection in the United States can be shared with less economically developed countries is a vital question.

Table A How does HIV differ from other epidemic pathogens?

1. Directly attacks the immune system
2. Involves thymus incorporation into the cellular genome
3. Establishes a chronic infection before becoming pathogenic
4. Involves an agent that frequently changes or modulates itself within the host
5. Can recruit other cells by direct infection or cell-to-cell transfer

New therapeutic directions should now consider some of the other approaches described in Chapter 14, such as targeting viral integrase and other HIV proteins. Can the intracellular factor(s) determining the relative replicating abilities of HIV strains be identified, and can the knowledge gained be used therapeutically? Can the virulence gene(s) of HIV (already identified and others to be defined) be countered by direct approaches? Can the CD8$^+$ cell antiviral factor, purified and synthesized, be used as therapy? Can a treatment be developed to increase the anti-HIV response of CD8$^+$ cells? What action can be taken to increase all effective immune responses against the virus in the already infected and the treated host? Many of the experimental procedures proposed can be studied in animal model systems such as SIV and FIV. These systems provide an excellent means for evaluation, since the disease in these animal species also involves lentiviruses that replicate well in CD4$^+$ lymphocytes (Table 1.1).

In all studies, therapeutic and vaccine strategies must consider the potential danger of detrimentally affecting the immune system, leading to an increase in virus replication or onset of disease because of the loss of CD8$^+$ cell response, cytokine induction, cell toxicity, autoimmune responses, or production of enhancing antibodies. In this regard, an immunologic approach toward limiting HIV pathogenesis via specific cytokine or anti-cytokine therapies might be helpful. The ability to control HIV infection clearly requires a full understanding of the virus in all its heterogeneous forms, its genetic differences, its capacity for molecular mimicry, and its dramatic mechanisms for changing and evolving to become more virulent and to escape immune responses. Most importantly, its diverse effects on the immune sys-

Table B Common concepts to be considered for development of effective vaccines against cancer and AIDS

1. Both involve an abnormal cell.
2. The abnormal cell can exist in a latent state.
3. Both can recruit other cells into the process.
4. Both involve modulation of antigens on the abnormal cell surface.
5. Both can have compromising antibody production: blocking in cancer, enhancing in HIV infection.
6. Both produce cellular products (cytokines) that can suppress host immune response.
7. Both are affected by cytokines (directly or indirectly).
8. Both can be associated with apoptosis (directly or indirectly).
9. Both can be associated with autoimmunity.
10. Both require strong cell-mediated immunity (i.e., type 1 response).

tem must be appreciated. In other viral infections, antiviral approaches were successfully directed at cell-free agents passed through blood or other body fluids. With HIV, transmission through virus-infected cells presents a major challenge to both anti-HIV therapies and vaccine development. In this regard, the directions taken can resemble those used to attack the cancer cell.

All approaches to the control of HIV continue to require cooperation from various sectors of the population, including government officials and political activists advocating the support needed to continue adequate financial backing for research and care. Along the way, new features of virology and cell biology will be uncovered. The recognition of the Rev, Tat, Vif, and Nef proteins and their respective targets has offered insights into potential eukaryotic processes that could have widespread application. Transactivation, RNA binding proteins, and modification in RNA splicing are just a few examples of the biologic processes that have emerged from molecular studies of HIV.

Understanding further how the virus can enter a cell via its variety of receptors can be valuable, and how it can remain latent in cells may also shed light on mechanisms by which the host carries a variety of viruses for a lifetime. How the immune system reacts to HIV can also help in approaches to control autoimmune disease and infections by other intracellular pathogens, such as malaria. Importantly, as noted above, the biologic and immunologic challenges of HIV infection mimic those of cancer (Table B). Eliminating the infected cell and preventing HIV replication in the host has parallels in cancer, in which the transformed cell is also the most important culprit. Thus, approaches at solving either pathogenic process through therapy or vaccines could have relevance to both diseases. Finally, knowledge about variations in a virus and how the host responds to these changes in an infectious agent can help further our understanding of viral pathogenesis in general and of the diseases caused by human retroviruses in particular.

1993 Revised Classification System for HIV Infection and Expanded AIDS Surveillance Case Definition for Adolescents and Adults[†]

	Clinical categories[b,c]		
CD4+ T-cell categories[a]	A Asymptomatic, acute (primary) HIV or PGL[d]	B Symptomatic, not (A) or (C) conditions	C AIDS-indicator conditions[e]
1. ≥500/µl	A1	B1	C1
2. 200–499/µl	A2	B2	C2
3. 200/µl AIDS-indicator T-cell count	A3	B3	C3

[a] See Appendix IV.
[b] See Appendix II.
[c] The shaded areas illustrate the expanded AIDS surveillance case definition. Persons with AIDS-indicator conditions (category C) as well as those with CD4+ T-lymphocyte counts of <200/µl (categories A3 or B3) were reportable as AIDS cases in the United States and territories effective January 1, 1993.
[d] PGL, persistent generalized lymphadenopathy. Clinical category A includes acute (primary) HIV infection (Chapter 4).
[e] See Appendix III.

† Reprinted from reference 376.

Clinical Categories[†]

Category A

Category A consists of one or more of the conditions listed below in an adolescent or adult (≥13 years) with documented HIV infection. Conditions listed in categories B and C must not have occurred.

- Asymptomatic HIV infection
- Persistent generalized lymphadenopathy
- Acute (primary) HIV infection with accompanying illness or history of acute HIV infection

Category B

Category B consists of symptomatic conditions in an HIV-infected adolescent or adult that are not included among conditions listed in clinical category C and that meet at least one of the following criteria: (i) the conditions are attributed to HIV infection or are indicative of a defect in cell-mediated immunity, or (ii) the conditions are considered by physicians to have a clinical course or to require management that is complicated by HIV infection. Examples of conditions in clinical category B include, but are not limited to,

- Bacillary angiomatosis
- Candidiasis, oropharyngeal (thrush)

[†]Reprinted from reference 376.

- Candidiasis, vulvovaginal; persistent, frequent, or poorly responsive to therapy
- Cervical dysplasia (moderate or severe)/cervical carcinoma in situ
- Constitutional symptoms, such as fever (38.5°C) or diarrhea lasting >1 month
- Hairy leukoplakia, oral
- Herpes zoster (shingles), involving at least two distinct episodes or more than one dermatome
- Idiopathic thrombocytopenic purpura
- Listeriosis
- Pelvic inflammatory disease, particularly if complicated by tubo-ovarian abscess
- Peripheral neuropathy

For classification purposes, category B conditions take precedence over those in category A. For example, someone previously treated for oral or persistent vaginal candidiasis (and who has not developed a category C disease) but who is now asymptomatic should be classified in clinical category B.

Category C

Category C includes the clinical conditions listed in the AIDS surveillance case definition (Appendix III). For classification purposes, once a category C condition has occurred, the person will remain in category C.

Conditions Included in the 1993 AIDS Surveillance Case Definition[†]

- Candidiasis of bronchi, trachea, or lungs
- Candidiasis, esophageal
- Cervical cancer, invasive[a]
- Coccidioidomycosis, disseminated or extrapulmonary
- Cryptococcosis, extrapulmonary
- Cryptosporidiosis, chronic intestinal (>1 month's duration)
- Cytomegalovirus disease (other than liver, spleen, or nodes)
- Cytomegalovirus retinitis (with loss of vision)
- Encephalopathy, HIV-related
- Herpes simplex: chronic ulcer(s) (>1 month's duration); or bronchitis, pneumonitis, or esophagitis
- Histoplasmosis, disseminated or extrapulmonary
- Isosporiasis, chronic intestinal (>1 month's duration)
- Kaposi's sarcoma
- Lymphoma, Burkitt's (or equivalent term)
- Lymphoma, immunoblastic (or equivalent term)
- Lymphoma, primary, of brain
- *Mycobacterium avium* complex or *Mycobacterium kansasii*, disseminated or extrapulmonary
- *Mycobacterium tuberculosis*, any site (pulmonary[a] or extrapulmonary)
- *Mycobacterium*, other species or unidentified species, disseminated or extrapulmonary
- *Pneumocystis carinii* pneumonia
- Pneumonia, recurrent[a]

[†] Reprinted from reference 376.

- Progressive multifocal leukoencephalopathy
- *Salmonella* septicemia, recurrent
- Toxoplasmosis of brain
- Wasting syndrome due to HIV

[a] Added in the 1993 expansion of the AIDS surveillance case definition.

Other Definitions in HIV Infection: CD4$^+$ T-Lymphocyte Categories[†]

CD4$^+$ category	CD4$^+$ cells/μl	CD4$^+$ cell percentage
1	≥500	≥29
2	200–400	14–28
3[a]	<200	<14

[a] Diagnosis of AIDS.

† Reprinted from reference 376.

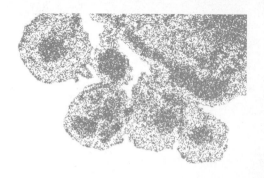

References

1. **Anonymous.** 1997. Update: trends in AIDS incidence, deaths, and prevalence—United States, 1996. *J Am Med Assoc* **277**:874–875.

2. **Aarons, E., M. Fernandez, A. Rees, M. McClure, and J. Weber.** 1997. CC-chemokine receptor 5 genotypes and *in vitro* susceptibility to HIV-1 of a cohort of British HIV-exposed uninfected homosexual men. *AIDS* **11**:688–689.

3. **Abbud, R. A., C. K. Finegan, L. A. Guay, and E. A. Rich.** 1995. Enhanced production of human immunodeficiency virus type 1 by *in vitro* infected alveolar macrophages from otherwise healthy cigarette smokers. *J Inf Dis* **172**:859–863.

4. **Abrams, D. I.** 1990. Alternative therapies in HIV infection. *AIDS* **4**:1179–1187.

5. **Abrams, D. I., S. Kuno, R. Wong, K. Jeffords, M. Nash, J. B. Molaghan, R. Gorter, and R. Ueno.** 1989. Oral dextran sulfate (UA001) in the treatment of the acquired immunodeficiency syndrome (AIDS) and AIDS-related complex. *Ann Int Med* **110**:183–188.

6. **Abrams, D. I., B. J. Lewis, J. H. Beckstead, C. A. Casavant, and W. L. Drew.** 1984. Persistent diffuse lymphadenopathy in homosexual men: endpoint or prodrome? *Ann Int Med* **100**:801–808.

7. **Abrignani, S., D. Montagna, M. Jeannet, J. Wintsch, N. L. Haigwood, J. R. Shuster, K. S. Steimer, A. Cruchaud, and T. Staehelin.** 1990. Priming of CD4+ T cells specific for conserved regions of human immunodeficiency virus glycoprotein gp120 in humans immunized with a recombinant envelope protein. *Proc Natl Acad Sci USA* **87**:6136–6140.

8. **Accornero, P., M. Radrizzani, D. Delia, F. Gerosa, R. Kurrle, and M. P. Colombo.** 1997. Differential susceptibility to HIV-gp120-sensitized apoptosis in CD4+ T-cell clones with different T-helper phenotypes: role of CD95/CD95L interactions. *Blood* **89**:558-569.

9. **Achim, C. L., M. P. Heyes, and C. A. Wiley.** 1993. Quantitation of human immunodeficiency virus, immune activation factors, and quinolinic acid in AIDS brains. *J Clin Invest* **91**:2769-2775.

10. Actor, J. K., M. Shirai, M. C. Kullberg, M. L. Buller, A. Sher, and J. A. Berzofsky. 1993. Helminth infection results in decreased virus-specific CD8+ cytotoxic T-cell and Th1 cytokine responses as well as delayed virus clearance. *Proc Natl Acad Sci USA* **90**:948–952.

11. Ada, G. 1993. Towards phase III trials for candidate vaccines. *Nature* **364**:489–490.

12. Ada, G. L., and M. J. McElrath. 1997. HIV type 1 vaccine-induced cytotoxic T cell responses: potential role in vaccine efficacy. *AIDS Res Hum Retro* **13**:205–210.

13. Adachi, A., S. Koenig, H. E. Gendelman, D. Daugherty, S. Gattoni-Celli, A. S. Fauci, and M. A. Martin. 1987. Productive, persistent infection of human colorectal cell lines with human immunodeficiency virus. *J Virol* **61**:209–213.

14. Adachi, Y., N. Oyaizu, S. Than, T. W. McCloskey, and S. Pahwa. 1996. IL-2 rescues *in vitro* lymphocyte apoptosis in patients with HIV infection. *J Immunol* **157**:4184–4193.

15. Adams, D. H., and A. R. Lloyd. 1997. Chemokines: leucocyte recruitment and activation cytokines. *Lancet* **349**:490–495.

16. Adams, L. E., R. Donovan-Brand, A. Friedman-Kien, K. el Ramahi, and E. V. Hess. 1988. Sperm and seminal plasma antibodies in acquired immune deficiency (AIDS) and other associated syndromes. *Clin Immunol Immunopathol* **46**:442–449.

17. Adams, M., L. Sharmeen, J. Kimpton, J. M. Romeo, J. V. Garcia, B. M. Peterlin, M. Gourdine, and M. Emerman. 1994. Cellular latency in human immunodeficiency virus-infected individuals with high CD4 levels can be detected by the presence of promoter-proximal transcripts. *Proc Natl Acad Sci USA* **91**:3862–3866.

18. Adamson, D. C., B. Wildemann, M. Sasaki, J. D. Glass, J. C. McArthur, V. I. Christov, T. M. Dawson, and V. L. Dawson. 1996. Immunologic NO synthase: elevation in severe AIDS dementia and induction by HIV-1 gp41. *Science* **274**:1917–1921.

19. Ades, A. E., M. L. Newell, and C. S. Peckham. 1991. Children born to women with HIV-1 infection: natural history and risk of transmission. *Lancet* **337**:253–260.

20. Ades, E. W., J. K. Nicholson, S. W. Browning, and T. W. Comans. 1992. Inability of human immunodeficiency virus to infect human microvascular endothelial cells. *Pathobiology* **60**:330–331.

21. Adjorlolo-Johnson, G., K. M. De Cock, E. Ekpini, K. M. Vetter, T. Sibailly, K. Brattegaard, D. Yavo, R. Doorly, J. P. Whitaker, L. Kestens, C.-Y. Ou, J. R. George, and H. Gayle. 1994. Prospective comparison of mother-to-child transmission of HIV-1 and HIV-2 in Abidjan, Ivory Coast. *J Am Med Assoc* **272**:462–466.

22. Adleman, L. M., and D. Wofsy. 1993. T-cell homeostasis: implications in HIV infection. *J AIDS* **6**:144–152.

23. Afonso, L. C. C., T. M. Scharton, L. Q. Vieira, M. Wysocka, G. Trinchieri, and P. Scott. 1994. The adjuvant effect of interleukin-12 in a vaccine against *Leishmania major*. *Science* **263**:235–237.

24. Agy, M. B., L. R. Frumkin, L. Corey, R. W. Coombs, S. M. Wolinsky, J. Koehler, W. R. Morton, and M. G. Katze. 1992. Infection of *Macaca nemestrina* by human immunodeficiency virus type-1. *Science* **257**:103–106.

25. Agy, M. B., M. Wambach, K. Foy, and M. G. Katze. 1990. Expression of cellular genes in CD4 positive lymphoid cells infected by the human immunodeficiency virus, HIV-1: evidence for a host protein synthesis shut-off induced by cellular mRNA degradation. *Virol* **177**:251–258.

26. Ahmad, N., R. K. Maitra, and S. Venkatesan. 1989. *Rev*-induced modulation of *nef* protein underlies temporal regulation of human immunodeficiency virus replication. *Proc Natl Acad Sci USA* **86**:6111–6115.

27. Ahmad, N., and S. Venkatesan. 1988. Nef protein of HIV-1 is a transcriptional repressor of HIV-1 LTR. *Science* **241**:1481–1485.

28. Ait-Khaled, M., J. E. McLaughlin, M. A. Johnson, and V. C. Emery. 1995. Distinct HIV-1 long terminal repeat quasispecies present in nervous tissues compared to that in lung, blood and lymphoid tissues of an AIDS patient. *AIDS* **9**:675–683.

29. Akridge, R. E., and S. G. Reed. 1996. Interleukin-12 decreases human immunodeficiency virus type 1 replication in human macrophage cultures reconstituted with autologous peripheral blood mononuclear cells. *J Inf Dis* **173**:559–564.

30. **Alaeus, A., K. Lidman, A. Sonnerborg, and J. Albert.** 1997. Subtype-specific problems with quantification of plasma HIV-1 RNA. *AIDS* **11**:859–865.

31. **Albert, J., B. Abrahamsson, K. Nagy, E. Aurelius, H. Gaines, G. Nystrom, and E. M. Fenyo.** 1990. Rapid development of isolate-specific neutralizing antibodies after primary HIV-1 infection and consequent emergence of virus variants which resist neutralization by autologous sera. *AIDS* **4**:107–112.

32. **Albert, J., U. Bredberg, F. Chiodi, B. Bottiger, E. M. Fenyo, E. Norrby, and G. Biberfeld.** 1987. A new human retrovirus isolate of West African origin (SBL-6669) and its relationship to HTLV-IV, LAV-II, and HTLV-IIIB. *AIDS Res Hum Retro* **3**:3–10.

33. **Albert, J., J. Fiore, E. M. Fenyo, C. Pedersen, J. D. Lundgren, J. Gerstoft, and C. Nielsen.** 1995. Biological phenotype of HIV-1 and transmission. *AIDS* **9**:822–823.

34. **Albert, J., P. Stalhandske, S. Marquina, J. Karis, R. A. M. Fouchier, E. Norrby, and F. Chiodi.** 1996. Biological phenotype of HIV type 2 isolates correlates with V3 genotype. *AIDS Res Hum Retro* **12**:821–828.

35. **Albert, J., J. Wahlberg, J. Lundeberg, S. Cox, E. Sandstrom, B. Wahren, and M. Uhlen.** 1992. Persistence of azidothymidine-resistant human immunodeficiency virus type 1 RNA genotypes in posttreatment sera. *J Virol* **66**:5627–5630.

36. **Albini, A., G. Barillari, R. Benelli, R. C. Gallo, and B. Ensoli.** 1995. Angiogenic properties of human immunodeficiency virus type 1 Tat protein. *Proc Natl Acad Sci USA* **92**:4838–4842.

37. **Albini, A., C. D. Mitchell, and E. W. Thompson.** 1988. Invasive activity and chemotactic response to growth factors by Kaposi's sarcoma cells. *J Cell Biochem* **36**:369–376.

38. **Albrecht, M. A., N. A. DeLuca, R. A. Byrn, P. A. Schaffer, and S. M. Hammer.** 1989. The herpes simplex virus immediate-early protein, ICP4, is required to potentiate replication of human immunodeficiency virus in CD4+ lymphocytes. *J Virol* **63**:1861–1868.

39. **Albright, A. V., J. Strizki, J. M. Harouse, E. Lavi, M. O'Connor, and F. Gonzalez-Scarano.** 1996. HIV-1 infection of cultured human adult oligodendrocytes. *Virol* **217**:211–219.

40. **Aldovini, A., and R. A. Young.** 1991. Humoral and cell-mediated immune responses to live recombinant BCG-HIV vaccines. *Nature* **351**:479–482.

41. **Aldrovandi, G. M., G. Feuer, L. Gao, B. Jamieson, M. Kristeva, I. S. Y. Chen, and J. A. Zack.** 1993. The SCID-hu mouse as a model for HIV-1 infection. *Nature* **363**:732–736.

42. **Aldrovandi, G. M., and J. A. Zack.** 1996. Replication and pathogenicity of human immunodeficiency virus type 1 accessory gene mutants in SCID-hu mice. *J Virol* **70**:1505–1511.

43. **Alexander, S., and J. H. Elder.** 1994. Carbohydrate dramatically influences immune reactivity of antisera to viral glycoprotein antigens. *Science* **226**:1328–1330.

44. **Alizon, M., P. Sonigo, F. Barre-Sinoussi, J.-C. Chermann, P. Tiollais, L. Montagnier, and S. Wain-Hobson.** 1984. Molecular cloning of lymphadenopathy-associated virus. *Nature* **312**:757–760.

45. **Alkhatib, G., C. Combadiere, C. C. Broder, Y. Feng, P. E. Kennedy, P. M. Murphy, and E. A. Berger.** 1996. CC-CKR-5: a RANTES, MIP-1α, MIP-1β receptor as a fusion cofactor for macrophage-tropic HIV-1. *Science* **272**:1955–1958.

46. **Allan, J. S., J. Strauss, and D. W. Buck.** 1990. Enhancement of SIV infection with soluble receptor molecules. *Science* **247**:1084–1088.

47. **Allan, J. S., E. M. Whitehead, K. Strout, M. Short, P. Kanda, T. K. Hart, and P. J. Bugelski.** 1992. Strong association of simian immunodeficiency virus (SIVagm) envelope glycoprotein heterodimers: possible role in receptor-mediated activation. *AIDS Res Hum Retro* **8**:2011–2020.

48. **Allison, A. C., and N. E. Byars.** 1992. Adjuvants for new generation vaccines, p. 133–141. *In* R. W. Ellis (ed.), *Vaccines: New Approaches to Immunological Problems*. Butterworths, Stoneham, Mass.

49. **Almond, N., K. Kent, M. Cranage, E. Rud, B. Clarke, and E. J. Stott.** 1995. Protection by attenuated simian immunodeficiency virus in macaques against challenge with virus-infected cells. *Lancet* **345**:1342–1344.

49a. **Almond, N., J. Rose, R. Sangster, P. Silvera, R. Stebbings, B. Walker, and E. J. Stott.** 1997.

Mechanisms of protection induced by attenuated simian immunodeficiency virus. I. Protection cannot be transferred with immune serum. *J Gen Virol* **78**:1919–1922.

50. **Aloia, R. C., H. Tian, and F. C. Jensen.** 1993. Lipid composition and fluidity of the human immunodeficiency virus envelope and host cell plasma membranes. *Proc Natl Acad Sci USA* **90**:5181–5185.

51. **Alonso, A., D. Derse, and B. M. Peterlin.** 1992. Human chromosome 12 is required for optimal interactions between Tat and TAR of human immunodeficiency virus type 1 in rodent cells. *J Virol* **66**:4617–4621.

52. **Alsip, G. R., Y. Ench, C. V. Sumaya, and R. N. Boswell.** 1988. Increased Epstein-Barr virus DNA in oropharyngeal secretions from patients with AIDS, AIDS-related complex, or asymptomatic human immunodeficiency virus infections. *J Inf Dis* **157**:1072–1076.

53. **Amadori, A., G. de Silvestro, R. Zamarchi, M. L. Veronese, M. R. Mazza, G. Schiavo, M. Panozzo, A. de Rossi, L. Ometto, J. Mous, A. Barelli, A. Borri, L. Salmaso, and L. Chieco-Bianchi.** 1992. CD4 epitope masking by gp120/anti-gp120 antibody complexes. *J Immunol* **148**:2709–2716.

54. **Amadori, A., R. Zamarchi, V. Ciminale, A. Del Mistro, S. Siervo, A. Alberti, M. Colombatti, and L. Chieco-Bianchi.** 1989. HIV-1 specific B cell activation: a major constituent of spontaneous B cell activation during HIV-1 infection. *J Immunol* **143**:2146–2152.

55. **Amadori, A., R. Zamarchi, M. L. Veronese, M. Panozzo, A. Barelli, A. Borri, M. Sironi, F. Colotta, A. Mantovani, and L. Chieco-Bianchi.** 1991. B cell activation during HIV-1 infection. II. Cell-to-cell interactions and cytokine requirement. *J Immunol* **146**:57–62.

55a. **Amara, A., S. L. Gall, O. Schwartz, J. Salamero, M. Montes, P. Loetscher, M. Baggiolini, J. L. Virelizier, and F. Arenzana-Seisdedos.** 1997. HIV co-receptor down-regulation as antiviral principle: SDF-1α-dependent internalization of the chemokine receptor CXCR4 contributes to inhibition of HIV replication. *J Exp Med* **186**:139–146.

56. **Ambroziak, J. A., D. J. Blackbourn, B. G. Herndier, R. G. Glogau, J. H. Gullett, A. R. McDonald, E. T. Lennette, and J. A. Levy.** 1995. Herpes-like sequences in HIV-infected and uninfected Kaposi's sarcoma patients. *Science* **268**:582–583.

57. **Amerongen, H. M., R. Weltzin, C. M. Farnet, P. Michetti, W. A. Haseltine, and M. R. Neutra.** 1991. Transepithelial transport of HIV-1 by intestinal M cells: a mechanism for transmission of AIDS. *J AIDS* **4**:760–765.

58. **Amirhessami-Aghili, N., and S. A. Spector.** 1991. Human immunodeficiency virus type 1 infection of human placenta: potential route for fetal infection. *J Virol* **65**:2231–2236.

59. **Ammann, A., and J. A. Levy.** 1986. Laboratory investigation of pediatric acquired immunodeficiency syndrome. *Clin Immunol Immunopathol* **40**:122–127.

60. **Ammann, A. J.** 1993. Hypothesis: absence of graft-versus-host disease in AIDS is a consequence of HIV-1 infection of CD4+ T cells. *J AIDS* **6**:1224–1227.

61. **Ammann, A. J., M. J. Cowan, D. W. Wara, P. Weintrub, S. Dritz, H. Goldman, and H. A. Perkins.** 1983. Acquired immunodeficiency in an infant: possible transmission by means of blood products. *Lancet* **i**:956–958.

62. **Ammann, A. J., G. Schiffman, D. Abrams, P. Volberding, J. Ziegler, and M. Conant.** 1984. B cell immunodeficiency in acquired immune deficiency syndrome. *J Am Med Assoc* **251**:1447–1449.

63. **Ammar, A., C. Cibert, A. M. Bertoli, V. Tsilivakos, C. Jasmin, and V. Georgoulias.** 1991. Biological and biochemical characterization of a factor produced spontaneously by adherent cells of human immunodeficiency virus-infected patients inhibiting interleukin-2 receptor alpha chain (Tac) expression on normal T cells. *J Clin Invest* **87**:2048–2055.

64. **Amory, J., N. Martin, J. A. Levy, and D. W. Wara.** 1992. The large molecular weight glycoprotein MG1, a component of human saliva, inhibits HIV-1 infectivity. *Clin Res* **40**:51A. (Abstract.)

65. **Anand, R., F. Siegal, C. Reed, T. Cheung, S. Forlenza, and J. Moore.** 1987. Non-cytocidal natural variants of human immunodeficiency virus isolated from AIDS patients with neurological disorders. *Lancet* **ii**:234–238.

66. Ancelle, R., O. Bletry, A. C. Baglin, F. Brun-Vezinet, M. A. Rey, and P. Godeau. 1987. Long incubation period for HIV-2 infection. *Lancet* i:688–689.

67. Anderson, D. J., and J. A. Hill. 1987. CD4 (T4+) lymphocytes in semen of healthy heterosexual men: implications for the transmission of AIDS. *Fert Steril* 48:703–704.

68. Anderson, D. J., T. R. O'Brien, J. A. Politch, A. Martinez, G. R. Deage, III, N. Padian, C. R. Horsburgh, and K. H. Mayer. 1992. Effects of disease stage and zidovudine therapy on the detection of human immunodeficiency virus type 1 in semen. *J Am Med Assoc* 267:2769–2774.

69. Anderson, D. J., J. A. Politch, A. Martinez, B. J. Van Voorhis, N. S. Padian, and T. R. O'Brien. 1991. White blood cells and HIV-1 in semen from vasectomised seropositive men. *Lancet* 338:573–574.

70. Anderson, S. J., M. Lenburg, N. R. Landau, and J. V. Garcia. 1994. The cytoplasmic domain of CD4 is sufficient for its down-regulation from the cell surface by human immunodeficiency virus type 1 Nef. *J Virol* 68:3092–3101.

71. Andersson, S., B. Makitalo, R. Thorstensson, G. Franchini, J. Tartaglia, K. Limbach, E. Paoletti, P. Putkonen, and G. Biberfeld. 1996. Immunogenicity and protective efficacy of a human immunodeficiency virus type 2 recombinant canarypox (ALVAC) vaccine candidate in cynomolgus monkeys. *J Inf Dis* 174:977–985.

72. Andeweg, A. C., P. Leeflang, A. D. M. E. Osterhaus, and M. L. Bosch. 1993. Both the V2 and V3 regions of the human immunodeficiency virus type 1 surface glycoprotein functionally interact with other envelope regions in syncytium formation. *J Virol* 67:3232–3239.

73. Andino, R., D. Silvera, S. D. Suggett, P. L. Achacoso, C. J. Miller, D. Baltimore, and M. B. Feinberg. 1994. Engineering poliovirus as a vaccine vector for the expression of diverse antigens. *Science* 265:1448–1451.

74. Andreasson, P. A., F. Dias, A. Naucler, S. Anderson, and G. Biberfeld. 1993. A prospective study of vertical transmission of HIV-2 in Bissau, Guinea-Bissau. *AIDS* 7:989–993.

75. Antoni, B. A., P. Sabbatini, A. B. Rabson, and E. White. 1995. Inhibition of apoptosis in human immunodeficiency virus-infected cells enhances virus production and facilitates persistent infection. *J Virol* 69:2384–2392.

76. Apolonio, E. G., D. R. Hoover, Y. He, A. J. Saah, D. W. Lyter, R. Detels, R. A. Kaslow, and J. P. Phair. 1995. Prognostic factors in human immunodeficiency virus-positive patients with a CD4+ lymphocyte count <50/μl. *J Inf Dis* 171:829–836.

76a. Aramori, I., J. Zhang, S. S. G. Ferguson, P. D. Bieniasz, B. R. Cullen, and M. G. Caron. 1997. Molecular mechanism of desensitization of the chemokine receptor CCR-5: receptor signaling and internalization are dissociable from its role as an HIV-1 co-receptor. *EMBO Journal* 16:4606–4616.

77. Aranda-Anzaldo, A., and D. Viza. 1992. Human immunodeficiency virus type 1 productive infection in staurosporine-blocked quiescent cells. *FEBS Letters* 308:170–174.

78. Archibald, D. W., and G. A. Cole. 1990. *In vitro* inhibition of HIV-1 infectivity by human salivas. *AIDS Res Hum Retro* 6:1425-1432.

79. Ardman, B., M. A. Sikorski, M. Settles, and D. E. Staunton. 1990. Human immunodeficiency virus type 1-infected individuals make autoantibodies that bind to CD43 on normal thymic lymphocytes. *J Exp Med* 172:1151–1158.

80. Arendrup, M., C. Nielsen, J.-E. S. Hansen, C. Pedersen, L. Mathiesen, and J. O. Nielsen. 1992. Autologous HIV-1 neutralizing antibodies: emergence of neutralization-resistant escape virus and subsequent development of escape virus neutralizing antibodies. *J AIDS* 5:303–307.

81. Arendrup, M., J. E. Hansen, H. Clausen, C. Nielsen, L. R. Mathiesen, and J. O. Nielsen. 1991. Antibody to histo-blood group A antigen neutralizes HIV produced by lymphocytes from blood group A donors but not from blood group B or O donors. *AIDS* 5:441–444.

82. Ariyoshi, K., M. Schim van der Loeff, S. Sabally, F. Cham, T. Corrah, and H. Whittle. 1997. Does HIV-2 infection provide cross-protection against HIV-1 infection? *AIDS* 11:1053–1054.

83. Armstrong, J. A., and R. Horne. 1984. Follicular dendritic cells and virus-like particles in AIDS related lymphadenopathy. *Lancet* ii:370–372.

84. Artenstein, A. W., C. A. Ohl, T. C. VanCott, P. A. Hegerich, and J. R. Mascola. 1996. Transmission of HIV-1 subtype E in the United States. *J Am Med Assoc* **276**:99–100.

85. Artenstein, A. W., T. C. VanCott, J. R. Mascola, J. K. Carr, P. A. Hegerich, J. Gaywee, E. Sanders-Buell, M. L. Robb, D. E. Dayhoff, S. Thitivichianlert, S. Nitayaphan, J. G. McNeil, D. L. Birx, R. A. Michael, D. S. Burke, and F. E. McCutchan. 1995. Dual infection with human immunodeficiency virus type 1 of distinct envelope subtypes in humans. *J Inf Dis* **171**:805–810.

86. Artenstein, A. W., T. C. VanCott, K. V. Sitz, M. L. Robb, K. F. Wagner, S. C. D. Veit, A. F. Rogers, R. P. Garner, J. W. Byron, P. R. Burnett, and D. L. Birx. 1997. Mucosal immune responses in four distinct compartments of women infected with human immunodeficiency virus type 1: a comparison by site and correlation with clinical information. *J Inf Dis* **175**:265–271.

87. Arthos, J., K. C. Deen, M. A. Chaikin, J. A. Fornwald, G. Sathe, Q. J. Sattentau, P. R. Clapham, R. A. Weiss, J. S. McDougal, C. Pietropaolo, R. Axel, A. Truneh, P. J. Maddon, and R. W. Sweet. 1989. Identification of the residues in human CD4 critical for the binding of HIV. *Cell* **57**:469–481.

88. Arthur, L. O., J. W. Bess, L. E. Henderson, R. Urban, D. L. Mann, and R. E. Benveniste. 1994. Evaluation of human cellular proteins as immunogens in protection from SIV challenge. *J Cell Biochem Suppl* **18B**:155.

89. Arthur, L. O., J. W. Bess, Jr., R. C. Sowder II, R. E. Benveniste, D. L. Mann, J. C. Chermann, and L. E. Henderson. 1992. Cellular proteins bound to immunodeficiency viruses: implications for pathogenesis and vaccines. *Science* **258**:1935–1938.

90. Arthur, L. O., J. W. Bess, Jr., R. G. Urban, J. L. Strominger, W. R. Morton, D. L. Mann, L. E. Henderson, and R. E. Benveniste. 1995. Macaques immunized with HLA-DR are protected from challenge with simian immunodeficiency virus. *J Virol* **69**:3117-3124.

91. Arthur, L. O., J. W. Bess, Jr., D. J. Waters, S. W. Pyle, J. C. Kelliher, P. L. Nara, K. Krohn, W. G. Robey, A. J. Langlois, R. C. Gallo, and P. J. Fischinger. 1989. Challenge of chimpanzees (*Pan troglodytes*) immunized with human immunodeficiency virus envelope glycoprotein gp120. *J Virol* **63**:5046–5053.

92. Ashida, E. R., A. R. Johnson, and P. E. Lipsky. 1981. Human endothelial cell-lymphocyte interaction. *J Clin Invest* **67**:1490-1499.

93. Ashkenazi, A., D. H. Smith, S. A. Marsters, L. Riddle, T. J. Gregory, D. D. Ho, and D. J. Capon. 1991. Resistance of primary isolates of human immunodeficiency virus type 1 to soluble CD4 is independent of CD4-rgp120 binding affinity. *Proc Natl Acad Sci USA* **88**:7056–7060.

94. Ashorn, P., B. Moss, J. N. Weinstein, V. K. Chaudhary, D. J. FitzGerald, I. Pastan, and E. A. Berger. 1990. Elimination of infectious human immunodeficiency virus from human T-cell cultures by synergistic action of CD4-*Pseudomonas* exotoxin and reverse transcriptase inhibitors. *Proc Natl Acad Sci USA* **87**:8889–8893.

95. Asjo, B., J. Albert, F. Chiodi, and E. M. Fenyo. 1988. Improved tissue culture technique for production of poorly replicating human immunodeficiency virus strains. *J Virol Meth* **19**:191–196.

96. Asjo, B., J. Albert, A. Karlsson, L. Morfeldt-Manson, G. Biberfeld, K. Lidman, and E. M. Fenyo. 1986. Replicative properties of human immunodeficiency virus from patients with varying severity of HIV infection. *Lancet* **ii**:660–662.

97. Asmuth, D. M., S. M. Hammer, and C. A. Wanke. 1994. Physiological effects of HIV infection on human intestinal epithelial cells: an in vitro model for HIV enteropathy. *AIDS* **8**:205–211.

98. Atchison, R. E., J. Gosling, F. S. Monteclaro, C. Franci, L. Digilio, I. F. Charo, and M. A. Goldsmith. 1996. Multiple extracellular elements of CCR5 and HIV-1 entry: dissociation from response to chemokines. *Science* **274**:1924–1926.

99. Atkins, M. C., E. M. Carlin, V. C. Emery, P. D. Griffiths, and F. Boag. 1996. Fluctuations of HIV load in semen of HIV positive patients with newly acquired sexually transmitted diseases. *Brit Med J* **313**:341–342.

100. Attanasio, R., J. S. Allan, S. A. Anderson, T. C. Chanh, and R. C. Kennedy. 1991. Anti-idiotypic antibody response to monoclonal anti-CD4 preparation in nonhuman primate species. *J Immunol* **146**:507–514.

101. **Attanasio, R., and R. C. Kennedy.** 1990. Idiotypic cascades associated with the CD4-HIV gp120 interaction: principles for idiotype-based vaccines. *Int Rev Immunol* 7:109–119.

102. **Aucouturier, P., L. J. Couderc, D. Gouet, F. Danon, J. Gombert, S. Matheron, A. G. Saimot, J. P. Clauvel, and J. L. Preud'homme.** 1986. Serum immunoglobulin G subclass dysbalances in the lymphadenopathy syndrome and acquired immune deficiency syndrome. *Clin Exp Immunol* 63:234–240.

103. **Auerbach, R., and Y. A. Sidky.** 1979. Nature of the stimulus leading to lymphocyte-induced angiogenesis. *J Immunol* 123:751–754.

104. **Auger, I., P. Thomas, V. De Gruttola, D. Morse, R. Williams, B. Truman, and C. E. Lawrence.** 1988. Incubation periods for paediatric AIDS patients. *Nature* 336:575–577.

105. **Aukrust, P., N.-B. Liabakk, F. Muller, E. Lien, T. Espevik, and S. S. Freland.** 1994. Serum levels of tumor necrosis factor-α (TNFα) and soluble TNF receptors in human immunodeficiency virus type 1 infection—correlations to clinical, immunologic, and virologic parameters. *J Inf Dis* 169:420–424.

105a.**Autran, B., G. Carcelain, T. S. Li, C. Blanc, D. Mathez, R. Tubiana, C. Katlama, P. Debre, and J. Liebowitch.** 1997. Positive effects of combined antiretroviral therapy on CD4+ T cell homeostasis and function in advanced HIV disease. *Science* 277:112-116.

106. **Autran, B., C. M. Mayaud, M. Raphael, F. Plata, M. Denis, A. Bourguin, J. M. Guillon, P. Debre, and G. Akoun.** 1988. Evidence for a cytotoxic T-lymphocyte alveolitis in human immunodeficiency virus-infected patients. *AIDS* 2:179–183.

107. **Baba, M., R. Pauwels, J. Balzarini, J. Arnout, J. Desmyter, and E. DeClerq.** 1988. Mechanism of inhibitory effect of dextran sulfate and heparin on replication of human immunodeficiency virus *in vitro*. *Proc Natl Acad Sci USA* 85:6132–6136.

108. **Baba, T. W., Y. S. Jeong, D. Pennick, R. Bronson, M. F. Greene, and R. M. Ruprecht.** 1995. Pathogenicity of live, attenuated SIV after mucosal infection of neonatal macaques. *Science* 267:1820–1825.

109. **Baba, T. W., A. M. Trichel, L. An, V. Liska, L. N. Martin, M. Murphey-Corb, and R. M. Ruprecht.** 1996. Infection and AIDS in adult macaques after nontraumatic oral exposure to cell-free SIV. *Science* 272:1486–1489.

110. **Bachelder, R. E., J. Bilancieri, W. Lin, and N. L. Letvin.** 1995. A human recombinant Fab identifies a human immunodeficiency virus type 1-induced conformational change in cell surface-expressed CD4. *J Virol* 69:5734–5742.

111. **Bachelerie, F., J. Alcami, U. Hazan, N. Israel, B. Goud, F. Arenzana-Seisdedos, and J.-L. Virelizier.** 1990. Constitutive expression of human immunodeficiency virus (HIV) *nef* protein in human astrocytes does not influence basal or induced HIV long terminal repeat activity. *J Virol* 64:3059–3062.

112. **Back, N. K. T., L. Smit, M. Schutten, P. L. Nara, M. Tersmette, and J. Goudsmit.** 1993. Mutations in human immunodeficiency virus type 1 gp41 affect sensitivity to neutralization by gp120 antibodies. *J Virol* 67:6897–6902.

113. **Back, N. K. T., L. Smit, J.-J. De Jong, W. Keulen, M. Schutten, J. Goudsmit, and M. Tersmette.** 1994. An N-glycan within the human immunodeficiency virus type 1 gp120 V3 loop affects virus neutralization. *Virol* 199:431–438.

113a.**Badley, A. D., J. A. McElhinny, P. J. Leibson, D. H. Lynch, M. R. Alderson, and C. V. Paya.** 1996. Upregulation of Fas ligand expression by human immunodeficiency virus in human macrophages mediates apoptosis of uninfected T lymphocytes. *J Virol* 70:199–206.

114. **Baenziger, J., D. Mosier, R. Gulizia, F. Sinangil, and K. Steimer.** 1993. The threshold level of passively transferred rgp120SF2-specific baboon antibodies required to protect hu-PBL-SCID mice from homologous HIV-SF2 challenge. *In Sixth Annual Meeting of the National Cooperative Vaccine Development Groups for AIDS*, October 30–November 4, 1993.

115. **Bagasra, O., S. E. Bachman, L. Jew, R. Tawadros, J. Cater, G. Boden, I. Ryan, and R. J. Pomerantz.** 1996. Increased human immunodeficiency virus type 1 replication in human peripheral blood mononuclear cells induced by ethanol: potential immunopathogenic mechanisms. *J Inf Dis* 173:550–558.

116. Bagasra, O., H. Farzadegan, T. Seshamma, J. W. Oakes, A. Saah, and R. J. Pomerantz. 1994. Detection of HIV-1 proviral DNA in sperm from HIV-1-infected men. *AIDS* **8**:1669–1674.

117. Bagasra, O., S. P. Hauptman, H. W. Lischner, M. Sachs, and R. J. Pomerantz. 1992. Detection of human immunodeficiency virus type 1 provirus in mononuclear cells by *in situ* polymerase chain reaction. *N Engl J Med* **326**:1385–1391.

118. Bagasra, O., A. Kajdacsy-Balla, H. W. Lischner, and R. J. Pomerantz. 1993. Alcohol intake increases human immunodeficiency virus type 1 replication in human peripheral blood mononuclear cells. *J Inf Dis* **167**:789–797.

119. Bagasra, O., E. Lavi, L. Bobroski, K. Khalili, J. P. Pestaner, R. Tawadros, and R. J. Pomerantz. 1996. Cellular reservoirs of HIV-1 in the central nervous system of infected individuals: identification by the combination of *in situ* polymerase chain reaction and immunohistochemistry. *AIDS* **10**:573–585.

120. Bagasra, O., and R. J. Pomerantz. 1993. Human immunodeficiency virus type 1 provirus is demonstrated in peripheral blood monocytes *in vivo*: a study utilizing an *in situ* polymerase chain reaction. *AIDS Res Hum Retro* **9**:69–76.

121. Bagasra, O., and R. J. Pomerantz. 1993. Human immunodeficiency virus type 1 replication in peripheral blood mononuclear cells in the presence of cocaine. *J Inf Dis* **168**:1157–1164.

122. Bagasra, O., T. Seshamma, J. W. Oakes, and R. J. Pomerantz. 1993. High percentages of CD4-positive lymphocytes harbor the HIV-1 provirus in the blood of certain infected individuals. *AIDS* **7**:1419–1425.

123. Bagetta, G., M. T. Corasaniti, L. Aloe, L. Berliocchi, N. Costa, A. Finazzi-Agro, and G. Nistico. 1996. Intracerebral injection of human immunodeficiency virus type 1 coat protein gp120 differentially affects the expression of nerve growth factor and nitric oxide synthase in the hippocampus of rat. *Proc Natl Acad Sci USA* **93**:928–933.

124. Bagnarelli, P., A. Valenza, S. Menzo, A. Manzin, G. Scalise, P. E. Varaldo, and M. Clementi. 1994. Dynamics of molecular parameters of human immunodeficiency virus type 1 activity *in vivo*. *J Virol* **68**:2495–2502.

125. Baldeweg, T., J. Catalan, E. Lovett, J. Gruzelier, M. Riccio, and D. Hawkins. 1995. Long-term zidovudine reduces neurocognitive deficits in HIV-1 infection. *AIDS* **9**:589–596.

126. Baldwin, W. M. I. 1982. The symbiosis of immunocompetent and endothelial cells. *Immunol Today* **3**:267–269.

127. Baler, M., A. Werner, N. Bannert, K. Metzner, and R. Kurth. 1995. HIV suppression by interleukin-16. *Nature* **378**:563.

128. Ballerini, P., G. Gianluca, J. Z. Gong, V. Tassi, G. Saglio, D. M. Knowles, and R. Dalla-Favera. 1993. Multiple genetic lesions in acquired immunodeficiency syndrome-related non-Hodgkin's lymphoma. *Blood* **81**:166–176.

129. Balliet, J. W., D. L. Kolson, G. Eiger, F. M. Kim, K. A. McGann, A. Srinivasan, and R. Collman. 1994. Distinct effects in primary macrophages and lymphocytes of the human immunodeficiency virus type 1 accessory genes *vpr, vpu*, and *nef*: mutational analysis of a primary HIV-1 isolate. *Virol* **200**:623–631.

130. Banda, N. K., J. Bernier, D. K. Kurahara, R. Kurrle, N. Haigwood, R.-P. Sekaly, and T. H. Finkel. 1992. Crosslinking CD4 by HIV gp120 primes T cells for activation-induced apoptosis. *J Exp Med* **176**:1099–1106.

131. Bandres, J. C., J. Trial, D. M. Musher, and R. D. Rossen. 1993. Increased phagocytosis and generation of reactive oxygen products by neutrophils and monocytes of men with stage 1 human immunodeficiency virus infection. *J Inf Dis* **168**:75–83.

132. Barbiano di Belgiojoso, G., A. Genderini, L. Vago, C. Parravicini, S. Bertoli, and N. Landriani. 1990. Absence of HIV antigens in renal tissue from patients with HIV-associated nephropathy. *Neph Dialysis Transplant* **5**:489–492.

133. Barboza, A., B. A. Castro, M. Whalen, C. C. D. Moore, J. S. Parkin, W. L. Miller, F. Gonzalez-Scarano, and J. A. Levy. 1992. Infection of cultured adrenal cells by different strains of the human immunodeficiency virus, types 1 and 2. *AIDS* **6**:1437–1444.

133a. Barboza, A., and J. A. Levy. Unpublished observations.

134. **Barker, C. F., and R. E. Billingham.** 1997. Immunologically privileged sites. *Adv Immunol* **25**:1–54.

134a.**Barker, E., S. Barnett, and J. A. Levy.** Unpublished observations.

135. **Barker, E., S. W. Barnett, L. Stamatatos, and J. A. Levy.** 1995. The human immunodeficiency viruses, p. 1–96. *In* J. A. Levy (ed.), *The Retroviridae*, vol. 4. Plenum Press, New York.

136. **Barker, E., K. N. Bossart, S. H. Fujimura, and J. A. Levy.** 1997. CD28-costimulation increases the ability of CD8+ cells to suppress HIV replication. *J Immunol*, in press.

136a.**Barker, E., K. N. Bossart, and J. A. Levy.** Primary CD8+ cells from HIV-infected individuals can suppress productive infection of macrophages independent of β-chemokines. *Proc Nat Acad Sci USA.* Submitted.

137. **Barker, E., K. N. Bossart, C. P. Locher, B. K. Patterson, and J. A. Levy.** 1996. CD8+ cells from asymptomatic human immunodeficiency virus-infected individuals suppress superinfection of their peripheral blood mononuclear cells. *J Gen Virol* **77**:2953-2962.

137a.**Barker, E., and J. A. Levy.** Unpublished observations.

138. **Barker, E., C. E. Mackewicz, and J. A. Levy.** 1995. Effects of TH1 and TH2 cytokines on CD8+ cell response against human immunodeficiency virus: implications for long-term survival. *Proc Natl Acad Sci USA* **92**:11135–11139.

139. **Barker, T. D., D. Weissman, J. A. Daucher, K. M. Roche, and A. S. Fauci.** 1996. Identification of multiple and distinct CD8+ T cell suppressor activities. *J Immunol* **156**:4476–4483.

140. **Barnes, P. J., and M. Karin.** 1997. Nuclear factor-κB—a pivotal transcription factor in chronic inflammatory diseases. *N Engl J Med* **336**:1066–1071.

141. **Barnett, S., A. Barboza, C. M. Wilcox, C. E. Forsmark, and J. A. Levy.** 1991. Characterization of human immunodeficiency virus type 1 strains recovered from the bowel of infected individuals. *Virol* **182**:802–809.

142. **Barnett, S. W., and J. A. Levy.** 1991. Human immunodeficiency viruses, p. 1011–1023. *In* A. Balows et al. (ed.), *Manual of Clinical Microbiology*, 5th ed. American Society for Microbiology, Washington, D.C.

144. **Barnett, S. W., K. K. Murthy, B. G. Herndier, and J. A. Levy.** 1994. An AIDS-like condition induced in baboons by HIV-2. *Science* **266**:642–646.

145. **Barnett, S. W., M. Quiroga, A. Werner, D. Dina, and J. A. Levy.** 1993. Distinguishing features of an infectious molecular clone of the highly divergent and non-cytopathic HIV-2$_{UCI}$ strain. *J Virol* **67**:1006–1014.

146. **Barre-Sinoussi, F., J.-C. Chermann, F. Rey, M. T. Nugeyre, S. Chamaret, J. Gruest, C. Dauguet, C. Axler-Blin, F. Vezinet-Brun, C. Rouzioux, W. Rozenbaum, and L. Montagnier.** 1983. Isolation of a T-lymphotropic retrovirus from a patient at risk for acquired immune deficiency syndrome (AIDS). *Science* **220**:868–871.

147. **Barrett, A. D. T., and E. A. Gould.** 1986. Antibody-mediated early death *in vivo* after infection with yellow fever virus. *J Gen Virol* **67**:2539–2542.

148. **Barry, M. A., W. C. Lai, and S. A. Johnston.** 1995. Protection against mycoplasma infection using expression-library immunization. *Nature* **377**:632–635.

149. **Bartholomew, C., W. Blattner, and F. Cleghorn.** 1987. Progression to AIDS in homosexual men co-infected with HIV-1 and HTLV-1 in Trinidad. *Lancet* **ii**:1469.

150. **Bartz, S. R., M. E. Rogel, and M. Emerman.** 1996. Human immunodeficiency virus type 1 cell cycle control: Vpr is cytostatic and mediates G_2 accumulation by a mechanism which differs from DNA damage checkpoint control. *J Virol* **70**:2324–2331.

151. **Batman, P. A., S. C. Fleming, P. M. Sedgwick, T. T. MacDonald, and G. E. Griffin.** 1994. HIV infection of human fetal intestinal explant cultures induces epithelial cell proliferation. *AIDS* **8**:161–167.

152. **Baucke, R. B., and P. B. Spear.** 1979. Membrane proteins specified by herpes simplex viruses. V. Identification of an Fc-binding glycoprotein. *J Virol* **32**:779–789.

153. **Bauer, F. A., D. J. Wear, P. Angritt, and S.-C. Lo.** 1991. *Mycoplasma fermentans* (incognitus strain) infection in the kidneys of patients with acquired immunodeficiency syndrome and

associated nephropathy: a light microscopic, immunohistochemical, and ultrastructural study. *Human Path* 22:63–69.

154. Baum, L. L., K. J. Cassutt, K. Knigge, R. Khattri, J. Margolick, C. Rinaldo, C. A. Kleeberger, P. Nishanian, D. R. Henrard, and J. Phair. 1996. HIV-1 gp120-specific antibody-dependent cell-mediated cytotoxicity correlates with rate of disease progression. *J Immunol* 157:2168–2173.

155. Baum, M. K., G. Shor-Posner, Y. Lu, B. Rosner, H. E. Sauberlich, M. A. Fletcher, J. Szapocznik, C. Eisdorfer, J. E. Buring, and C. H. Hennekens. 1995. Micronutrients and HIV-1 disease progression. *AIDS* 9:1051–1056.

156. Baur, A. S., E. T. Sawai, P. Dazin, W. J. Fantl, C. Cheng-Mayer, and B. M. Peterlin. 1994. HIV-1 Nef leads to inhibition or activation of T cells depending on its intracellular localization. *Immunity* 1:373–384.

157. Bayley, A. C. 1991. Occurrence, clinical behavior and management of Kaposi's sarcoma. *Cancer Survey* 10:53–71.

158. Becherer, P. R., M. L. Smiley, T. J. Matthews, K. J. Weinhold, C. W. McMillan, and G. C. White II. 1990. Human immunodeficiency virus-1 disease progresison in hemophiliacs. *Am J Hematol* 34:204–209.

159. Beckstead, J. H., G. S. Wood, and V. Fletcher. 1985. Evidence for the origin of Kaposi's sarcoma from lymphatic endothelium. *Am J Path* 119:294–300.

160. Bednarik, D. P., J. D. Mosca, and N. B. Raj. 1987. Methylation as a modulator of expression of human immunodeficiency virus. *J Virol* 61:1253–1257.

161. Behets, F., M. Kashamuka, M. Pappaioanou, T. A. Green, R. W. Ryder, V. Batter, J. R. George, W. H. Hannon, and T. C. Quinn. 1992. Stability of human immunodeficiency virus type 1 antibodies in whole blood dried on filter paper and stored under various tropical conditions in Kinshasa. *J Clin Micro* 30:1179–1182.

162. Belec, L., M. Matta, C. Payan, G. Gresenguet, C. Tevi-Benissan, and J. Pillot. 1995. Human immunodeficiency virus type 1 p24 antigen in cervicovaginal secretions. *J Inf Dis* 171:1615-1618.

163. Beljan, J. R., G. M. Bohigian, W. D. Dolan, E. H. Estes, I. R. Friedlander, R. W. Gifford, J. H. Moxley III, P. H. Sayre, W. C. Scott, J. H. Skom, R. J. Smith, and J. B. Snow. 1985. Status report on the acquired immunodeficiency syndrome. *J Am Med Assoc* 254:1342–1345.

164. Belshe, R. B., D. P. Bolognesi, M. L. Clements, L. Corey, R. Dolin, J. Mestecky, M. Mulligan, D. Stablein, and P. Wright. 1994. HIV infection in vaccinated volunteers. *J Am Med Assoc* 272:431.

165. Belsito, D. V., M. R. Sanchez, R. L. Baer, F. Valentine, and G. J. Thorbecke. 1984. Reduced Langerhans' cell Ia antigen and ATPase activity in patients with the acquired immunodeficiency syndrome. *N Engl J Med* 310:1279–1282.

166. Benito, J. M., J. M. Zabay, J. Gil, M. Bermejo, A. Escudero, E. Sanchez, and E. Fernandez-Cruz. 1997. Quantitative alterations of the functionally distinct subsets of CD4 and CD8 T lymphocytes in asymptomatic HIV infection: changes in the expression of CD45RO, CD45RA, CD11b, CD38, HLA-DR, and CD25 antigens. *J AIDS Hum Retrovirol* 14:128–135.

167. Benjouad, A., J.-C. Gluckman, H. Rochat, L. Montagnier, and E. Bahraoui. 1992. Influence of carbohydrate moieties on the immunogenicity of human immunodeficiency virus type 1 recombinant gp160. *J Virol* 66:2473–2483.

168. Benkirane, M., D. Blanc-Zouaoui, M. Hirn, and C. Devaux. 1994. Involvement of human leukocyte antigen class I molecules in human immunodeficiency virus infection of CD4-positive cells. *J Virol* 68:6332–6339.

169. Benn, S., R. Rutledge, T. Folks, J. Gold, L. Baker, J. McCormick, P. Feorino, P. Piot, T. Quinn, and M. Martin. 1985. Genomic heterogeneity of AIDS retroviral isolates from North America and Zaire. *Science* 230:949–951.

170. Benos, D. J., B. H. Hahn, J. K. Bubien, S. K. Ghosh, N. A. Mashburn, M. A. Chaikin, G. M. Shaw, and E. N. Benveniste. 1994. Envelope glycoprotein gp120 of human immunodeficiency virus type 1 alters ion transport in astrocytes: implications for AIDS dementia complex. *Proc Natl Acad Sci USA* 91:494–498.

171. Bentwich, Z., Z. Weisman, C. Moroz, S. Bar-Yehuda, and A. Kalinkovich. 1996. Immune dysregulation in Ethiopian immigrants in Israel: relevance to helminth infections? *Clin Exp Immunol* **103**:239–243.

172. Benveniste, E. N., P. Shrikant, H. K. Patton, and D. J. Benos. Neuroimmunological mechanisms for disease: the role of the astrocyte in the regulation of neural injury. *In* H. E. Gendelman, S. Lipton, L. Epstein, and S. Swindells (ed.), *Neurological Complications of HIV Infection.* Chapman and Hall, New York, in press.

173. Beral, V., T. Peterman, R. Berkelman, and H. Jaffe. 1991. AIDS-associated non-Hodgkin lymphoma. *Lancet* **337**:805–809.

174. Beral, V., T. A. Peterman, R. L. Berkelman, and H. W. Jaffe. 1990. Kaposi's sarcoma among persons with AIDS: a sexually transmitted infection? *Lancet* **335**:123–128.

175. Berberian, L., L. Goodglick, T. J. Kipps, and J. Braun. 1993. Immunoglobulin V_H3 gene products: natural ligands for HIV gp120. *Science* **261**:1588–1590.

176. Beretta, A., S. H. Weiss, G. Rappocciolo, R. Mayur, C. De Santis, J. Quirinale, A. Cosma, P. Robbioni, G. M. Shearer, J. A. Berzofsky, M. L. Villa, A. G. Siccardi, and M. Clerici. 1996. Human immunodeficiency virus type 1 (HIV-1)-seronegative infection drug users at risk for HIV exposure have antibodies to HLA class I antigens and T cells specific for HIV envelope. *J Inf Dis* **173**:472-476.

177. Bergamini, A., L. Dini, M. Capozzi, L. Ghibelli, R. Placido, E. Faggioli, A. Salanitro, E. Buonanno, L. Cappannoli, L. Ventura, M. Cepparulo, L. Falasca, and G. Rocchi. 1996. Human immunodeficiency virus-induced cell death in cytokine-treated macrophages can be prevented by compounds that inhibit late stages of viral replication. *J Inf Dis* **173**:1367–1378.

177a. Berger, E. A. 1997. HIV entry and tropism: the chemokine receptor connection. *AIDS* **11**:s3-s16.

177b. Berger, E. A., R. W. Doms, E. M. Fenyo, B. T. M. Korber, D. R. Littman, M. J.P., Q. J. Sattentau, H. Schuitemaker, J. Sodroski, and R. A. Weiss. HIV-1 phenotypes classified by coreceptor usage. *Nature* in press.

178. Berger, E. A., J. D. Lifson, and L. E. Eiden. 1991. Stimulation of glycoprotein gp120 dissociation from the envelope glycoprotein complex of human immunodeficiency virus type 1 by soluble CD4 and CD4 peptide derivatives: implications for the role of the complementarity-determining region 3-like region in membrane fusion. *Proc Natl Acad Sci USA* **88**:8082–8086.

179. Berger, E. A., J. R. Sisler, and P. L. Earl. 1992. Human immunodeficiency virus type 1 envelope glycoprotein molecules containing membrane fusion-impairing mutations in the V3 region efficiently undergo soluble CD4-stimulated gp120 release. *J Virol* **66**:6208–6212.

180. Berger, J., and J. A. Levy. 1992. The human immunodeficiency virus, type 1: the virus and its role in neurologic disease. *Semin Neurol* **12**:1–9.

181. Bergeron, L., and J. Sodroski. 1992. Dissociation of unintegrated viral DNA accumulation from single-cell lysis induced by human immunodeficiency virus type 1. *J Virol* **66**:5777–5787.

182. Bergeron, L., N. Sullivan, and J. Sodroski. 1992. Target cell-specific determinants of membrane fusion within the human immunodeficiency virus type 1 gp120 third variable region and gp41 animo terminus. *J Virol* **66**:2389–2397.

183. Bergey, E. J., M.-I. Cho, B. M. Blumberg, M.-L. Hammarskjold, D. Rekosh, L. G. Epstein, and M. J. Levine. 1994. Interaction of HIV-1 and human salivary mucins. *J AIDS* **7**:995–1002.

184. Berke, G. 1991. Lymphocyte-triggered internal target disintegration. *Immunol Today* **12**:396–403.

184a. Berkowitz, R. D., A. Ohagen, S. Hoglund, and S. P. Goff. 1995. Retroviral nucleocapsid domains mediate the specific recognition of genomic viral RNAs by chimeric gag polyproteins during packaging *in vivo. J Virol* **69**:6445–6456.

185. Berman, P. W., T. Gregory, P. Crase, and L. A. Lasky. 1985. Protection from genital herpes simplex type 2 infection by vaccination with cloned glycoprotein D. *Science* **227**:1490–1492.

186. Berman, P. W., T. J. Gregory, L. Riddle, G. R. Nakamura, M. A. Champe, J. P. Porter, F. M. Wurm, R. D. Hershberg, E. K. Cobb, and J. W. Eichberg. 1990. Protection of chimpanzees

from infection by HIV-1 after vaccination with recombinant glycoprotein gp120 but not gp160. *Nature* **345**:622–625.

187. **Berman, P. W., J. E. Groopman, T. Gregory, P. Clapham, R. A. Weiss, R. Ferriani, L. Riddle, C. Shimasaki, C. Lucas, L. A. Lasky, and J. W. Eichberg.** 1988. HIV-1 challenge of chimpanzees immunized with recombinant gp120. *Proc Natl Acad Sci USA* **85**:5200-5204.

188. **Berman, P. W., T. J. Matthews, L. Riddle, M. Champe, M. R. Hobbs, G. R. Nakamura, J. Mercer, D. J. Eastman, C. Lucas, A. J. Langlois, F. M. Wurm, and T. J. Gregory.** 1992. Neutralization of multiple laboratory and clinical isolates of human immunodeficiency virus type 1 (HIV-1) by antisera raised against gp120 from the NM isolate of HIV-1. *J Virol* **66**:4464–4469.

189. **Berman, P. W., K. K. Murthy, T. Wrin, J. C. Vennari, E. K. Cobb, D. J. Eastman, M. Champe, G. R. Nakamura, D. Davison, M. F. Powell, J. Bussiere, D. P. Francis, T. Matthews, T. J. Gregory, and J. F. Obijeski.** 1996. Protection of MN-rgp120-immunized chimpanzees from heterologous infection with a primary isolate of human immunodeficiency virus type 1. *J Inf Dis* **173**:52–59.

190. **Bernier, R., and M. Tremblay.** 1995. Homologous interference resulting from the presence of defective particles of human immunodeficiency virus type 1. *J Virol* **69**:291–300.

191. **Bernstein, M. S., S. E. Tong-Starksen, and R. M. Locksley.** 1991. Activation of human monocyte-derived macrophages with lipopolysaccharide decreases human immunodeficiency virus replication in vitro at the level of gene expression. *J Clin Invest* **88**:540–545.

192. **Berrada, F., D. Ma, J. Michaud, G. Doucet, L. Giroux, and A. Kessous-Elbaz.** 1995. Neuronal expression of human immunodeficiency virus type 1 Env proteins in transgenic mice: distribution in the central nervous system and pathological alterations. *J Virol* **69**:6770–6778.

193. **Berrios, D. C., A. L. Avins, K. Haynes-Sanstad, R. Eversley, and W. J. Woods.** 1995. Screening for human immunodeficiency virus antibody in urine. *Arch Pathol Lab Med* **119**:139–141.

194. **Berson, J. F., D. Long, B. J. Doranz, J. Rucker, F. R. Jirik, and R. W. Doms.** 1996. A seven-transmembrane domain receptor involved in fusion and entry of T-cell-tropic human immunodeficiency virus type 1 strains. *J Virol* **70**:6288–6295.

195. **Berthier, A., S. Chamaret, R. Fauchet, J. Fonlupt, N. Genetet, M. Gueguen, M. Pommereuil, A. Ruffault, and L. Montagnier.** 1986. Transmissibility of human immunodeficiency virus in haemophilic and non-haemophilic children living in a private school in France. *Lancet* **ii**:598–601.

196. **Bertoletti, A., A. Sette, F. V. Chisari, A. Penna, M. Levrero, M. De Carli, F. Fiaccadori, and C. Ferrari.** 1994. Natural variants of cytotoxic epitopes are T-cell receptor antagonists for antiviral cytotoxic T cells. *Nature* **369**:407–410.

197. **Bertram, S., F. T. Hufert, J. van Lunzen, and D. von Laer.** 1996. Coinfection of individual leukocytes with human cytomegalovirus and human immunodeficiency virus is a rare event *in vivo. J Med Virol* **49**:283–288.

198. **Berzofsky, J. A., and I. J. Berkower.** 1995. Novel approaches to peptide and engineered protein vaccines for HIV using defined epitopes: advances in 1994–1995. *AIDS* **9**:S143–S157.

199. **Besansky, N. J., S. T. Butera, S. Sinha, and T. M. Folks.** 1991. Unintegrated human immunodeficiency virus type 1 DNA in chronically infected cell lines is not correlated with surface CD4 expression. *J Virol* **65**:2695–2698.

200. **Bettaieb, A., P. Fromont, F. Louache, E. Oksenhendler, W. Vainchenker, N. Duedari, and P. Bierling.** 1992. Presence of cross-reactive antibody between human immunodeficiency virus (HIV) and platelet glycoproteins in HIV-related immune thrombocytopenic purpura. *Blood* **80**:162–169.

201. **Bettinardi, A., L. Imberti, A. Sottini, E. Quiros-Roldan, M. Puoti, F. Castelli, G. P. Cadeo, R. Gorla, and D. Primi.** 1997. Detection of clonal T cell populations with closely related T cell receptor junctional sequences in persons at high risk for human immunodeficiency virus (HIV) infection and in patients acutely infected with HIV. *J Inf Dis* **175**:272–282.

202. **Bevan, M. J., and T. J. Braciale.** 1995. Why can't cytotoxic T cells handle HIV? *Proc Natl Acad Sci USA* **92**:5765–5767.

202a.**Bhardwaj, N.** 1997. Interactions of viruses with dendritic cells: a double-edged sword. *J Exp Med* **186**:795–799.

203. Bhat, S., R. V. Mettus, E. P. Reddy, K. E. Ugen, V. Srikanthan, W. V. Williams, and D. B. Weiner. 1993. The galactosyl ceramide/sulfatide receptor binding region of HIV-1 gp120 maps to amino acids 206–275. *AIDS Res Hum Retro* **9**:175–181.

204. Bhat, S., S. L. Spitalnik, F. Gonzalez-Scarano, and D. H. Silberberg. 1991. Galactosyl ceramide or a derivative is an essential component of the neural receptor for human immunodeficiency virus type 1 envelope glycoprotein gp120. *Proc Natl Acad Sci USA* **88**:7131–7134.

205. Bienzle, D., F. M. Smaill, and K. L. Rosenthal. 1996. Cytotoxic T-lymphocytes from HIV-infected individuals recognize an activation-dependent, non-polymorphic molecule on uninfected CD4+ lymphocytes. *AIDS* **10**:247–254.

206. Biggar, R. J., N. Dunsmore, and R. J. Kurman. 1992. Failure to detect human papillomavirus in Kaposi's sarcoma. *Lancet* **339**:1604–1605.

207. Biggar, R. J., J. Horm, J. F. Farumeni, Jr., M. H. Greene, and J. J. Goedert. 1984. Incidence of Kaposi's sarcoma and mycosis fungoides in the United States including Puerto Rico, 1973-81. *JNCI* **73**:89–94.

208. Biggar, R. J., P. G. Miotti, T. E. Taha, L. Mtimavalye, R. Broadhead, A. Justesen, F. Yellin, G. Liomba, W. Miley, D. Waters, J. D. Chiphangwi, and J. J. Goedert. 1996. Perinatal intervention trial in Africa: effect of a birth canal cleansing intervention to prevent HIV transmission. *Lancet* **347**:1647–1650.

209. Biggs, B.-A., M. Hewish, S. Kent, K. Hayes, and S. M. Crowe. 1995. HIV-1 infection of human macrophages impairs phagocytosis and killing of Toxoplasma gondii. *J Immunol* **154**:6132–6139.

210. Bilello, J. A., K. Stellrecht, G. L. Drusano, and D. S. Stein. 1996. Soluble tumor necrosis factor-alpha receptor type II (sTNF-alphaRII) correlates with human immunodeficiency virus (HIV) RNA copy number in HIV-infected patients. *J Inf Dis* **173**:464–467.

211. Billich, A., F. Hammerschmid, P. Peichl, R. Wenger, G. Zenke, V. Quesniaux, and B. Rosenwirth. 1995. Mode of action of SDZ NIM 811, a nonimmunosuppressive cyclosporin A analog with activity against human immunodeficiency virus (HIV) type 1: interference with HIV protein-cyclophilin A interactions. *J Virol* **69**:2451–2461.

212. Binninger, D., J. Ennen, D. Bonn, S. G. Norley, and R. Kurth. 1991. Mutational analysis of the simian immunodeficiency virus SIVmac *nef* gene. *J Virol* **65**:5237–5243.

213. Birdsall, H. H., J. Trial, H. J. Lin, D. M. Green, G. W. Sorrentino, E. B. Siwak, A. L. de Jong, and R. D. Rossen. 1997. Transendothelial migration of lymphocytes from HIV-1-infected donors. *J Immunol* **158**:5968–5977.

214. Biron, C. A. 1997. Activation and function of natural killer cell responses during viral infections. *Curr Opin Immunol* **9**:24–34.

215. Birx, D. L., M. G. Lewis, M. Vahey, K. Tencer, P. M. Zack, C. R. Brown, P. B. Jahrling, G. Tosato, D. Burke, and R. Redfield. 1993. Association of interleukin-6 in the pathogenesis of acutely fatal SIVsmm/PBj-14 in pigtailed macaques. *AIDS Res Hum Retro* **9**:1123–1129.

216. Birx, D. L., R. R. Redfield, and G. Tosato. 1986. Defective regulation of Epstein-Barr virus infection in patients with acquired immunodeficiency syndrome (AIDS) or AIDS-related disorders. *N Engl J Med* **314**:874–879.

217. Bisaccia, E., C. Berger, and A. S. Klainer. 1990. Extracorporeal photopheresis in the treatment of AIDS-related complex: a pilot study. *Ann Int Med* **113**:270–275.

218. Biti, R., R. Ffrench, J. Young, B. Bennetts, G. Stewart, and T. Liang. 1997. HIV-1 infection in an individual homozygous for the CCR5 deletion allele. *Nature Med* **3**:252–253.

219. Bjork, R. L., Jr. 1991. HIV-1: seven facets of functional molecular mimicry. *Immunol Let* **28**:91–96.

220. Bjorling, E., K. Broliden, D. Bernardi, G. Utter, R. Thorstensson, F. Chiodi, and E. Norrby. 1991. Hyperimmune antisera against synthetic peptides representing the glycoprotein of human immunodeficiency virus type 2 can mediate neutralization and antibody-dependent cytotoxic activity. *Proc Natl Acad Sci USA* **88**:6082–6086.

221. Bjorling, E., G. Scarlatti, A. Von Gegerfelt, J. Albert, G. Biberfeld, F. Chiodi, E. Norrby, and E. M. Fenyo. 1993. Autologous neutralizing antibodies prevail in HIV-2 but not in HIV-1 infection. *Virol* **193**:528–530.

221a. Bjorndal, A., H. Deng, M. Jansson, J. R. Fiore, C. Colognesi, A. Karlsson, J. Albert, G. Scarlatti, D. R. Littman, and E. M. Fenyo. 1997. Coreceptor usage of primary human immunodeficiency virus type 1 isolates varies according to biological phenotype. *J Virol* 71:7478–7487.

222. Blackbourn, D. J., J. Ambroziak, E. Lennette, M. Adams, B. Ramachandran, and J. A. Levy. 1997. Infectious HHV-8 in a healthy North American blood donor. *Lancet* 349:609–611.

223. Blackbourn, D. J., E. T. Lennette, J. Ambroziak, D. V. Mourich, and J. A. Levy. HHV-8 detection in nasal secretions and saliva. *J. Inf Dis*, in press.

224. Blackbourn, D. J., and J. A. Levy. 1997. Human herpesvirus 8 in semen and prostate. *AIDS* 11:249–250.

224a. Blackbourn, D. J., and J. A. Levy. Unpublished observations.

225. Blackbourn, D. J., C. P. Locher, B. Ramachandran, S. W. Barnett, K. K. Murthy, K. D. Carey, K. M. Brasky, and J. A. Levy. 1997. CD8+ cells from HIV-2-infected baboons control HIV replication. *AIDS* 11:737–746.

226. Blackbourn, D. J., C. E. Mackewicz, E. Barker, T. K. Hunt, B. Herndier, A. T. Haase, and J. A. Levy. 1996. Suppression of HIV replication by lymphoid tissue CD8+ cells correlates with the clinical state of HIV-infected individuals. *Proc Natl Acad Sci USA* 93:13125–13130.

227. Blackburn, R., M. Clerici, D. Mann, D. R. Lucey, J. Goedert, B. Golding, G. M. Shearer, and H. Golding. 1991. Common sequence in HIV-1 gp41 and HLA class II beta chains can generate crossreactive autoantibodies with immunosuppressive potential early in the course of HIV-1 infection. *Immunobiol Proteins Peptides* 6:63–69.

228. Blanche, S., C. Rouzioux, M.-L. G. Moscato, F. Veber, M.-J. Mayaux, C. Jacomet, J. Tricoire, A. Deville, M. Vial, G. Firtion, A. de Crepy, D. Douard, M. Robin, C. Courpotin, N. Ciraru-Vigneron, F. Le Deist, and C. Griscelli. 1989. A prospective study of infants born to women seropositive for human immunodeficiency virus type 1. *N Engl J Med* 320:1643–1648.

229. Blanche, S., M. Tardieu, A. Duliege, C. Rouzioux, F. Le Deist, K. Fukunaga, M. Caniglia, C. Jacomet, A. Messiah, and C. Griscelli. 1990. Longitudinal study of 94 symptomatic infants with perinatally acquired human immunodeficiency virus infection. *Am J Dis Children* 144:1210–1215.

229a. Blasig, C., C. Zietz, B. Haar, F. Neipel, S. Esser, N. H. Brockmeyer, E. Tschachler, S. Colombini, B. Ensoli, and M. Sturzl. 1997. Monocytes in Kaposi's sarcoma lesions are productively infected by human herpesvirus 8. *J Virol* 71:7963–7968.

230. Blauvelt, A., C. Chougnet, G. M. Shearer, and S. I. Katz. 1996. Modulation of T cell responses to recall antigens presented by Langerhans cells in HIV-discordant identical twins by anti-interleukin (IL)-10 antibodies and IL-12. *J Clin Invest* 97:1550-1555.

231. Blazevic, V., M. Heino, A. Ranki, T. Jussila, and K. J. E. Krohn. 1996. RANTES, MIP and interleukin-16 in HIV infection. *AIDS* 10:1435–1436.

232. Blazquez, M. V., J. A. Madueno, R. Gonzalez, R. Jurado, W. W. Bachovchin, J. Pena, and E. Munoz. 1992. Selective decrease of CD26 expression in T cells from HIV-1-infected individuals. *J Immunol* 149:3073–3077.

233. Bleul, C. C., M. Farzan, H. Choe, C. Parolin, I. Clark-Lewis, J. Sodroski, and T. A. Springer. 1996. The lymphocyte chemoattractant SDF-1 is a ligand for LESTR/Fusin and blocks HIV-1 entry. *Nature* 382:829–832.

234. Bleul, C. C., L. Wu, J. A. Hoxie, T. A. Springer, and C. R. Mackay. 1997. The HIV coreceptors CXCR4 and CCR5 are differentially expressed and regulated on human T lymphocytes. *Proc Natl Acad Sci USA* 94:1925–1930.

235. Blomberg, R. S., and R. T. Schooley. 1985. Lymphocyte markers in infectious diseases. *Semin Hematol* 22:81–114.

236. Bloom, E. J., D. I. Abrams, and G. Rodgers. 1986. Lupus anticoagulant in the acquired immunodeficiency syndrome. *J Am Med Assoc* 256:491–493.

237. Bobkov, A., R. Cheingsong-Popov, M. Garaev, A. Rzhaninova, P. Kaleebu, S. Beddows, M. H. Bachmann, J. I. Mullins, W. Louwagie, W. Janssens, G. van der Groen, F. McCutchan, and J. Weber. 1994. Identification of an Env G subtype and heterogeneity of HIV-1 strains in the Russian Federation and Belarus. *AIDS* 8:1649–1655.

238. Boeri, E., A. Giri, F. Lillo, G. Ferrari, O. E. Varnier, A. Ferro, S. Sabbatani, W. C. Saxinger,

and G. Franchini. 1992. *In vivo* genetic variability of the human immunodeficiency virus type 2 V3 region. *J Virol* **66**:4546–4550.

239. Boettiger, D. 1979. Animal virus pseudotypes. *Prog Med Virol* **25**:37–68.

240. Bofill, M., W. Gombert, N. J. Borthwick, A. N. Akbar, J. E. McLaughlin, C. A. Lee, M. A. Johnson, A. J. Pinching, and G. Janossy. 1995. Presence of CD3+CD8+Bcl-2^low lymphocytes undergoing apoptosis and activated macrophages in lymph nodes of HIV-1+ patients. *Am J Path* **146**:1542–1555.

241. Bogers, W. M., H. Niphuis, P. ten Haaft, J. D. Laman, W. Koornstra, and J. L. Heeney. 1995. Protection from HIV-1 envelope-bearing chimeric simian immunodeficiency virus (SHIV) in rhesus macaques infected with attenuated SIV: consequences of challenge. *AIDS* **9**:F13-F18.

242. Boldogh, I., P. Szaniszlo, W. A. Bresnahan, C. M. Flaitz, M. C. Nichols, and T. Albrecht. 1996. Kaposi's sarcoma herpesvirus-like DNA sequences in the saliva of individuals infected with human immunodeficiency virus. *Clin Infect Dis* **23**:406–407.

243. Bollinger, R. C., M. A. Egan, T.-W. Chun, B. Mathieson, and R. F. Siliciano. 1996. Cellular immune responses to HIV-1 in progressive and non-progressive infections. *AIDS* **10**:S85-S96.

244. Bollinger, R. C., Jr., R. L. Kline, H. L. Francis, M. W. Moss, J. G. Bartlett, and T. C. Quinn. 1992. Acid dissociation increases the sensitivity of p24 antigen detection for the evaluation of antiviral therapy and disease progression in asymptomatic human immunodeficiency virus-infected persons. *J Inf Dis* **165**:913–916.

245. Bollinger, R. C., T. C. Quinn, A. Y. Liu, P. E. Stanhope, S. A. Hammond, R. Viveen, M. L. Clements, and R. F. Siliciano. 1993. Cytokines from vaccine-induced HIV-1 specific cytotoxic T lymphocytes: effects on viral replication. *AIDS Res Hum Retro* **9**:1067–1077.

246. Bomsel, M. 1997. Transcytosis of infectious human immunodeficiency virus across a tight human epithelial cell line barrier. *Nature Med* **3**:42–47.

247. Bonavida, B., J. Katz, and M. Gottlieb. 1986. Mechanism of defective NK cell activity in patients with acquired immunodeficiency syndrome (AIDS) and AIDS-related complex. I. Defective trigger on NK cells for NKCF production by target cells, and partial restoration by IL-2. *J Immunol* **137**:1157–1163.

248. Bonyhadi, M. L., L. Rabin, S. Salimi, D. A. Brown, J. Kosek, J. N. McCune, and H. Kaneshima. 1993. HIV induces thymus depletion in vivo. *Nature* **363**:728–736.

249. Borkow, G., J. Barnard, T. M. Nguyen, A. Belmonte, M. A. Wainberg, and M. A. Parniak. 1997. Chemical barriers to human immunodeficiency virus type 1 (HIV-1) infection: retrovirucidal activity of UC781, a thiocarboxanilide nonnucleoside inhibitor of HIV-1 reverse transcriptase. *J Virol* **71**:3023–3030.

250. Borkowsky, W., and K. Krasinski. 1992. Perinatal human immunodeficiency virus infection: ruminations on mechanisms of transmission and methods of intervention. *Pediatrics* **90**:133–136.

251. Born, J., T. Lange, K. Hansen, M. Molle, and H. L. Fehm. 1997. Effects of sleep and circadian rhythm on human circulating immune cells. *J Immunol* **158**:4454–4464.

252. Borrow, P., C. F. Evans, and M. B. A. Oldstone. 1995. Virus-induced immunosuppression: immune system-mediated destruction of virus-infected dendritic cells results in generalized immune suppression. *J Virol* **69**:1059–1070.

253. Borrow, P., H. Lewicki, B. H. Hahn, G. M. Shaw, and M. B. A. Oldstone. 1994. Virus-specific CD8+ cytotoxic T-lymphocyte activity associated with control of viremia in primary human immunodeficiency virus type 1 infection. *J Virol* **68**:6103–6110.

254. Borrow, P., H. Lewicki, X. Wei, M. S. Horwitz, N. Peffer, H. Meyers, J. A. Nelson, J. E. Gairin, B. H. Hahn, M. B. A. Oldstone, and G. M. Shaw. 1997. Antiviral pressure exerted by HIV-1-specific cytotoxic T lymphocytes (CTLs) during primary infection demonstrated by rapid selection of CTL escape virus. *Nature Med* **3**:205–211.

255. Borthwick, N. J., M. Bofill, W. M. Gombert, A. N. Akbar, E. Medina, K. Sagawa, M. C. Lipman, M. A. Johnson, and G. Janossy. 1994. Lymphocyte activation in HIV-1 infection. II. Functional defects of CD28-T cells. *AIDS* **8**:431–441.

256. Borzy, M. S., R. S. Connell, and A. A. Kiessling. 1988. Detection of human immunodeficiency virus in cell-free seminal fluid. *J AIDS* **1**:419–424.

257. Bosch, V., and T. Pfeiffer. 1992. HIV-1-induced cytopathogenicity in cell culture despite very decreased amounts of fusion-competent viral glycoprotein. *AIDS Res Hum Retro* **8**:1815-1821.

258. Boshoff, C., T. F. Schutz, M. M. Kennedy, A. K. Graham, C. Fisher, A. Thomas, J. O. D. McGee, R. A. Weiss, and J. J. O'Leary. 1995. Kaposi's sarcoma-associated herpesvirus infects endothelial and spindle cells. *Nature Med* **1**:1274–1278.

259. Bottiger, B., K. Ljunggren, A. Karlsson, K. Krohn, E. M. Fenyo, and G. Biberfeld. 1988. Neutralizing antibodies in relation to antibody dependent cellular cytotoxicity inducing antibodies against human immunodeficiency virus type 1. *Clin Exp Immunol* **73**:339–342.

260. Bottiger, D., N.-G. Johansson, B. Samuelsson, H. Zhang, P. Putkonen, L. Vrang, and B. Oberg. 1997. Prevention of simian immunodeficiency virus, SIV_{sm}, or HIV-2 infection in cynomolgus monkeys by pre- and postexposure administration of BEA-005. *AIDS* **11**:157–162.

261. Boue, F., C. Wallon, C. Goujard, F. Barre-Sinoussi, P. Galanud, and J.-F. Delfraissy. 1992. HIV induces IL-6 production by human B lymphocytes. *J Immunol* **148**:3761–3767.

262. Bourinbaiar, A. S. 1991. HIV and gag. *Nature* **349**:111.

263. Bourinbaiar, A. S., and R. Nagorny. 1992. Effect of human chorionic gonadotropin (hCG) on HIV-1 transmission from lymphocytes to trophoblasts. *FEBS Letters* **309**:82–84.

264. Bourinbaiar, A. S., and D. M. Phillips. 1991. Transmission of human immunodeficiency virus from monocytes to epithelia. *J AIDS* **4**:56–63.

265. Bowman, M. R., K. D. MacFerrin, S. L. Schreiber, and S. J. Burakoff. 1990. Identification and structural analysis of residues in the V1 region of CD4 involved in interaction with human immunodeficiency virus envelope glycoprotein gp120 and class II major histocompatibility complex molecules. *Proc Natl Acad Sci USA* **87**:9052–9056.

266. Boyer, J., K. Bebenek, and T. A. Kunkel. 1992. Unequal human immunodeficiency virus type 1 reverse transcriptase error rates with RNA and DNA templates. *Proc Natl Acad Sci USA* **89**:6919- 6923.

267. Boyer, J. D., K. E. Ugen, B. Wang, M. Agadjanyan, L. Gilbert, M. L. Bagarazzi, M. Chattergoon, P. Frost, A. Javadian, W. V. Williams, Y. Refaeli, R. B. Ciccarelli, D. McCallus, L. Coney, and D. B. Weiner. 1997. Protection of chimpanzees from high-dose heterologous HIV-1 challenge by DNA vaccination. *Nature Med* **3**:526-532.

268. Boyer, V., C. Delibrais, N. Noraz, F. Fischer, M. D. Kazatchkine, and C. Desgranges. 1992. Complement receptor type 2 mediates infection of the human CD4-negative Raji B-cell line with opsonized HIV. *Scand J Immunol* **36**:879–883.

269. Boyer, V., C. Desgranges, M. A. Trabaud, E. Fischer, and M. Kazatchkine. 1991. Complement mediates human immunodeficiency virus type 1 infection of a human T cell line in a CD4- and antibody-independent fashion. *J Exp Med* **173**:1151–1158.

270. Braaten, D., E. K. Franke, and J. Luban. 1996. Cyclophilin A is required for the replication of group M human immunodeficiency virus type 1 (HIV-1) and simian immunodeficiency virus SIV_{CPZ}GAB but not group O HIV-1 or other primate immunodeficiency viruses. *J Virol* **70**:4220–4227.

271. Brack-Werner, R., A. Kleinschmidt, A. Ludvigsen, W. Mellert, M. Neumann, R. Herrmann, M. C. L. Khim, A. Burny, N. Muller-Lantzsch, D. Stavrou, and V. Erfle. 1992. Infection of human brain cells by HIV-1: restricted virus production in chronically infected human glial cell lines. *AIDS* **6**:273–285.

272. Bradac, J. A., and B. J. Mathieson. An epitope map of immunity to HIV-1: a roadmap for vaccine development. Submitted for publication.

273. Bradding, P., I. H. Feather, P. H. Howarth, R. Mueller, J. A. Roberts, K. Britten, J. P. A. Bews, T. C. Hunt, Y. Okayama, C. H. Heusser, G. R. Bullock, M. K. Church, and S. T. Holgate. 1992. Interleukin 4 is localized to and released by human mast cells. *J Exp Med* **176**:1381–1386.

274. Bravo, R., M. Gutierrez, V. Soriano, M. J. Mellado, M. L. Perez-Labad, A. Mas, J. Gonzalez-Lahoz, and P. Martin-Fontelas. 1996. Lack of evidence for viral clearance in children born to HIV-infected mothers. *AIDS* **10**:1744–1745.

275. Breen, E. C., A. R. Rezai, K. Nakajima, G. N. Beall, R. T. Mitsuyasu, T. Hirano, T. Kishimoto, and O. Martinez-Maza. 1990. Infection with HIV is associated with elevated IL-6 levels and production. *J Immunol* **144**:480–484.

276. Brenneman, D. E., G. L. Westbrook, S. P. Fitzgerald, D. L. Ennist, K. L. Elkins, M. R. Ruff, and C. B. Pert. 1988. Neuronal cell killing by the envelope protein of HIV and its prevention by vasoactive intestinal peptide. *Nature* **335**:639–642.

277. Brenner, B. G., C. Gryllis, and M. A. Wainberg. 1991. Role of antibody-dependent cellular cytotoxicity and lymphokine-activated killer cells in AIDS and related diseases. *J Leukoc Biol* **50**:628–640.

278. Bretscher, P. A., G. Wei, J. N. Menon, and H. Bielefeldt-Ohmann. 1992. Establishment of stable, cell-mediated immunity that makes "susceptible" mice resistant to *Leishmania major*. *Science* **257**:539–542.

279. Brew, B. J., N. Dunbar, L. Pemberton, and J. Kaldor. 1996. Predictive markers of AIDS dementia complex: CD4 cell count and cerebrospinal fluid concentrations of β_2-microglobulin and neopterin. *J Inf Dis* **174**:294–298.

280. Briant, L., C. M. Wade, J. Puel, A. J. Leigh Brown, and M. Guyader. 1995. Analysis of envelope sequence variants suggests multiple mechanisms of mother-to-child transmission of human immunodeficiency virus type 1. *J Virol* **69**:3778–3788.

281. Brichacek, B., S. Swindells, E. N. Janoff, S. Pirruccello, and M. Stevenson. 1996. Increased plasma human immunodeficiency virus type 1 burden following antigenic challenge with pneumococcal vaccine. *J Inf Dis* **174**:1191–1199.

282. Bridges, S. H., and N. Sarver. 1995. Gene therapy and immune restoration for HIV disease. *Lancet* **345**:427–432.

283. Brighty, D. W., M. Rosenberg, I. S. Y. Chen, and M. Ivey-Hoyle. 1991. Envelope proteins from clinical isolates of human immunodeficiency virus type 1 that are refractory to neutralization by soluble CD4 possess high affinity for the CD4 receptor. *Proc Natl Acad Sci USA* **88**:7802–7805.

284. Brigino, E., S. Haraguchi, A. Koutsonikolis, G. J. Cianciolo, U. Owens, R. A. Good, and N. K. Day. 1997. Interleukin 10 is induced by recombinant HIV-1 Nef protein involving the calcium/calmodulin-dependent phosphodiesterase signal transduction pathway. *Proc Natl Acad Sci USA* **94**:3178–3182.

285. Brinchmann, J. E., J. Albert, and F. Vartdal. 1991. Few infected CD4+ T cells but a high proportion of replication-competent provirus copies in asymptomatic human immunodeficiency virus type 1 infection. *J Virol* **65**:2019–2023.

286. Brinchmann, J. E., J. H. Dobloug, B. H. Heger, L. L. Haaheim, M. Sannes, and T. Egeland. 1994. Expression of costimulatory molecule CD28 on T cells in human immunodeficiency virus type 1 infection: functional and clinical correlations. *J Inf Dis* **169**:730–738.

287. Brinchmann, J. E., G. Gaudernack, and F. Vartdal. 1990. CD8+ T cells inhibit HIV replication in naturally infected CD4+ T cells: evidence for a soluble inhibitor. *J Immunol* **144**:2961–2966.

288. Brinchmann, J. E., G. Gaudernack, and F. Vartdal. 1991. *In vitro* replication of HIV-1 in naturally infected CD4+ T cells is inhibited by rIFN alpha2 and by a soluble factor secreted by activated CD8+ T cells, but not by rIFN beta, rIFN gamma, or recombinant tumor necrosis factor-alpha. *J AIDS* **4**:480–488.

289. Brinkmann, R., A. Schwinn, O. Narayan, C. Zink, H. W. Kreth, W. Roggendorf, R. Dorries, S. Schwender, H. Imrich, and V. ter Meulen. 1992. Human immunodeficiency virus infection in microglia: correlation between cells infected in the brain and cells cultured from infectious brain tissue. *Ann Neurol* **31**:361–365.

290. Broder, C. C., and E. A. Berger. 1995. Fusogenic selectivity of the envelope glycoprotein is a major determinant of human immunodeficiency virus type 1 tropism for CD4+ T-cell lines vs. primary macrophages. *Proc Natl Acad Sci USA* **92**:9004–9008.

291. Broder, C. C., and E. A. Berger. 1993. CD4 molecules with a diversity of mutations encompassing the CDR3 region efficiently support human immunodeficiency virus type 1 envelope glycoprotein-mediated cell fusion. *J Virol* **67**:913–926.

292. Broder, C. C., D. S. Dimitrov, R. Blumenthal, and E. A. Berger. 1993. The block to HIV-1 envelope glycoprotein-mediated membrane fusion in animal cells expressing human CD4 can be overcome by a human cell component(s). *Virol* **193**:483–491.

293. Brodine, S. K., J. R. Mascola, P. J. Weiss, S. I. Ito, K. R. Porter, A. W. Artenstein, F. C. Garland, F. E. McCutchan, and D. S. Burke. 1995. Detection of diverse HIV-1 genetic subtypes in the USA. *Lancet* **346**:1198–1199.

294. Brogi, A., R. Presentini, D. Solazzo, P. Piomboni, and E. Constantino-Ceccarini. 1996. Interaction of human immunodeficiency virus type 1 envelope glycoprotein gp120 with a galactoglycerolipid associated with human sperm. *AIDS Res Hum Retro* **12**:483–489.

295. Broliden, P.-A., A. von Gegerfelt, P. Clapham, J. Rosen, E.-M. Fenyo, B. Wahren, and K. Broliden. 1992. Identification of human neutralization-inducing regions of the human immunodeficiency virus type 1 envelope glycoproteins. *Proc Natl Acad Sci USA* **89**:461–465.

296. Broliden, P. A., B. Makitalo, L. Akerblom, J. Rosen, K. Broliden, G. Utter, M. Jondal, E. Norrby, and B. Wahren. 1991. Identification of amino acids in the V3 region of gp120 critical for virus neutralization by human HIV-1-specific antibodies. *Immunol* **73**:371–376.

296a. Brooke, S., R. Chan, S. Howard, and R. Sapolsky. 1997. Endocrine modulation of the neurotoxicity of gp120: implications for AIDS-related dementia complex. *Proc Natl Acad Sci USA* **94**:9457-9462.

297. Brookmeyer, R. 1991. Reconstruction and future trends of the AIDS epidemic in the United States. *Science* **253**:37–42.

298. Brossard, Y., J. T. Aubin, L. Mandelbrot, C. Bignozzi, D. Brand, A. Chaput, J. Roume, N. Mulliez, F. Mallet, H. Agut, F. Barin, A. Brechot, A. Goudeau, J. M. Huraux, J. Barrat, P. Blot, J. Chavinie, N. Ciraru-Vigneron, P. Engelman, F. Herve, E. Papiernik, and R. Henrion. 1995. Frequency of early *in utero* HIV-1 infection: a blind DNA polymerase chain reaction study on 100 fetal thymuses. *AIDS* **9**:359–366.

298a. Brossart, P., A. W. Goldrath, E. A. Butz, S. Martin, and M. J. Bevan. 1997. Virus-mediated delivery of antigenic epitopes into dendritic cells as a means to induce CTL. *J Immunol* **158**:3270-3276.

299. Brouwers, P., M. P. Heyes, H. A. Moss, P. L. Wolters, D. G. Poplack, S. P. Markey, and P. A. Pizzo. 1993. Quinolinic acid in the cerebrospinal fluid of children with symptomatic human immunodeficiency virus type 1 disease: relationships to clinical status and therapeutic response. *J Inf Dis* **168**:1380–1386.

300. Browne, M. J., K. H. Mayer, S. B. D. Chafee, M. N. Dudley, M. R. Posner, S. M. Steinberg, K. K. Graham, S. M. Geletko, S. H. Zinner, S. L. Denman, L. M. Dunkle, S. Kaul, C. McLaren, G. Skowron, N. M. Kouttab, T. A. Kennedy, A. B. Weitberg, and G. A. Curt. 1993. 2′,3′-didehydro-3′-deoxythymidine (d4T) in patients with AIDS or AIDS-related complex: a phase I trial. *J Inf Dis* **167**:21–29.

301. Browning, P. J., J. M. G. Sechler, M. Kaplan, R. H. Washington, R. Gendelman, R. Yarchoan, B. Ensoli, and R. C. Gallo. 1994. Identification and culture of Kaposi's sarcoma-like spindle cells from the peripheral blood of human immunodeficiency virus-1-infected individuals and normal controls. *Blood* **84**:2711–2720.

302. Bruhl, P., A. Kerschbaum, K. Zimmermann, M. M. Eibl, and J. W. Mannhalter. 1996. Allostimulated lymphocytes inhibit replication of HIV type 1. *AIDS Res Hum Retro* **12**:31–37.

303. Brutkiewicz, R. R., and R. M. Welsh. 1995. Major histocompatibility complex class I antigens and the control of viral infections by natural killer cells. *J Virol* **69**:3967–3971.

304. Bryant, M. L., L. Ratner, R. J. Duronio, N. S. Kishore, B. Devadas, S. P. Adams, and J. I. Gordon. 1991. Incorporation of 12-methoxydodecanoate into the human immunodeficiency virus 1 gag polyprotein precursor inhibits its proteolytic processing and virus production in a chronically infected human lymphoid cell line. *Proc Natl Acad Sci USA* **88**:2055–2059.

305. Bryant, M. L., J. Yamamoto, P. Luciw, R. Munn, P. Marx, J. Higgins, N. Pedersen, A. Levine, and M. B. Gardner. 1985. Molecular comparison of retroviruses associated with human and simian AIDS. *Hematol Oncol* **3**:187–197.

306. Bryson, Y. J., K. Luzuriaga, J. L. Sullivan, and D. W. Wara. 1992. Proposed definitions for *in utero* versus intrapartum transmission of HIV-1. *N Engl J Med* 327:1246–1247.

307. Bryson, Y. J., S. Pang, L. S. Wei, R. Dickover, A. Diagne, and I. S. Y. Chen. 1995. Clearance of HIV infection in a perinatally infected infant. *N Engl J Med* 332:833–838.

307a. Buchbinder, S. Personal communication.

308. Buchbinder, S. P., M. H. Katz, N. A. Hessol, P. M. O'Malley, and S. D. Holmberg. 1994. Long-term HIV-1 infection without immunologic progression. *AIDS* 8:1123–1128.

309. Budhraja, M., H. Levendoglu, F. Kocka, M. Mangkornkanok, and R. Sherer. 1987. Duodenal mucosal T cell subpopulation and bacterial cultures in acquired immune deficiency syndrome. *Am J Gastro* 82:427–431.

310. Budka, H., C. A. Wiley, P. Kleihues, J. Artigas, A. K. Asbury, E. S. Cho, D. R. Cornblath, M. C. Dal Canto, U. DeGirolami, D. Dickson, L. G. Epstein, M. M. Esiri, F. Giangaspero, G. Gosztonyi, F. Gray, J. W. Griffin, D. Henin, Y. Iwasaki, R. S. Janssen, R. T. Johnson, P. L. Lantos, W. D. Lyman, J. C. McArthur, K. Nagashima, N. Peress, C. K. Petito, R. W. Price, R. H. Rhodes, M. Rosenblum, G. Said, F. Scaravilli, L. R. Sharer, and H. V. Vinters. 1991. HIV-associated disease of the nervous system: review of nomenclature and proposal for neuropathology-based terminology. *Brain Path* 1:143–152.

311. Bukawa, H., J. I. Sekigawa, K. Hamajima, J. Fukushima, Y. Yamada, H. Kiyono, and K. Okuda. 1995. Neutralization of HIV-1 by secretory IgA induced by oral immunization with a new macromolecular multicomponent peptide vaccine candidate. *Nature Med* 1:681–685.

312. Bukrinsky, M. I., S. Haggerty, M. P. Dempsey, N. Sharova, A. Adzhubel, L. Spitz, P. Lewis, D. Goldfarb, M. Emerman, and M. Stevenson. 1993. A nuclear localization signal within HIV-1 matrix protein that governs infection of non-dividing cells. *Nature* 365:666–669.

313. Bukrinsky, M. I., N. Sharova, M. P. Dempsey, T. L. Stanwick, A. G. Bukrinskaya, S. Haggerty, and M. Stevenson. 1992. Active nuclear import of human immunodeficiency virus type 1 preintegration complexes. *Proc Natl Acad Sci USA* 89:6580–6584.

314. Bukrinsky, M. I., T. L. Stanwick, M. P. Dempsey, and M. Stevenson. 1991. Quiescent T lymphocytes as an inducible virus reservoir in HIV-1 infection. *Science* 254:423–427.

315. Buonaguro, L., G. Barillari, H. K. Chang, C. A. Bohan, V. Kao, R. Morgan, R. C. Gallo, and B. Ensoli. 1992. Effects of the human immunodeficiency virus type 1 *tat* protein on the expression of inflammatory cytokines. *J Virol* 66:7159–7167.

316. Burack, J. H., D. C. Barrett, R. D. Stall, M. A. Chesney, M. L. Ekstrand, and T. J. Coates. 1993. Depressive symptoms and CD4 lymphocyte decline among HIV-infected men. *J Am Med Assoc* 270:2568-2573.

317. Burack, J. H., M. R. Cohen, J. A. Hahn, and D. I. Abrams. 1996. Pilot randomized controlled trial of Chinese herbal treatment of HIV-associated symptoms. *J AIDS Hum Retrovirol* 12:386–393.

318. Buratti, E., S. G. Tisminetzky, P. D'Agaro, and F. E. Baralle. 1997. A neutralizing monoclonal antibody previously mapped exclusively on human immunodeficiency virus type 1 gp41 recognizes an epitope in p17 sharing the core sequence IEEE. *J Virol* 71:2457–2462.

319. Burgard, M., M. J. Mayaux, S. Blanche, A. Ferroni, M. L. Guihard-Moscato, M. C. Allemon, N. Ciraru-Vigneron, G. Firtion, C. Floch, F. Guillot, E. Lachassine, M. Vial, C. Griscelli, and C. Rouzioux. 1992. The use of viral culture and p24 antigen testing to diagnose human immunodeficiency virus infection in neonates. *N Engl J Med* 327:1192–1197.

320. Burgdorf, W. H. C., K. Mukai, and J. Rsai. 1981. Immunohistochemical identification of factor VIII-related antigen in endothelial cells of cutaneous lesions of alleged vascular nature. *Am J Clin Path* 75:167–171.

321. Burger, H., B. Weiser, K. Flaherty, J. Gulla, P. N. Nguyen, and R. A. Gibbs. 1991. Evolution of human immunodeficiency virus type 1 nucleotide sequence diversity among close contacts. *Proc Natl Acad Sci USA* 88:11236–11240.

322. Burke, A. P., D. Anderson, P. Mannan, J. L. Ribas, Y.-H. Liang, J. Smialek, and R. Virmani. 1994. Systemic lymphadenopathic histology in human immunodeficiency virus-1-seropositive drug addicts without apparent acquired immunodeficiency syndrome. *Human Path* 25:248–256.

322a. Burke, D. S. 1997. Recombination in HIV: an important viral evolutionary strategy. *Emerg Infect Dis* 3:253–260.

323. Burns, B. F., G. S. Wood, and R. F. Dorfman. 1991. The varied histopathology of lymphadenopathy in the homosexual male. *Am J Surg Path* 9:287–296.

323a. Burton, D. R., and D. C. Montefiori. 1997. The antibody response in HIV-1 infection. *AIDS* 11(Suppl A):S87-S98.

324. Busch, M. P., E. A. Operskalski, J. W. Mosley, T. H. Lee, D. Henrard, S. Herman, D. H. Sachs, M. Harms, W. Huang, and D. O. Stram. 1996. Factors influencing HIV-1 transmission by blood transfusion. *J Inf Dis* 174:26–33.

325. Buseyne, F., M. Fevrier, S. Garcia, M. L. Gougeon, and Y. Riviere. 1996. Dual function of a human immunodeficiency virus (HIV)-specific cytotoxic T-lymphocyte clone: inhibition of HIV replication by noncytolytic mechanisms and lysis of HIV-infected CD4+ cells. *Virol* 225:248–253.

326. Buseyne, F., M. McChesney, F. Porrot, S. Kovarik, B. Guy, and Y. Riviere. 1993. Gag-specific cytotoxic T lymphocytes from human immunodeficiency virus type 1-infected individuals: Gag epitopes are clustered in three regions of the p24 gag protein. *J Virol* 67:694–702.

327. Butera, S. T., V. L. Perez, B. Y. Wu, G. J. Nabel, and T. M. Folks. 1991. Oscillation of the human immunodeficiency virus surface receptor is regulated by the state of viral activation in a CD4+ cell model of chronic infection. *J Virol* 65:4645–4653.

328. Butler, K. M., R. N. Husson, F. M. Balis, P. Brouwers, J. Eddy, D. el-Amin, J. Gress, M. Hawkins, P. Jarosinski, H. Moss, D. Poplack, S. Santacroce, D. Venzon, L. Wiener, P. Wolters, and P. A. Pizzo. 1991. Dideoxyinosine in children with symptomatic human immunodeficiency virus infection. *N Engl J Med* 324:137–144.

329. Buzy, J. M., L. M. Lindstrom, M. C. Zink, and J. E. Clements. 1995. HIV-1 in the developing CNS: developmental differences in gene expression. *Virol* 210:361–371.

330. Bwayo, J. J., N. J. D. Nagelkerke, S. Moses, J. Embree, E. N. Ngugi, A. Mwatha, J. Kimani, A. Anzala, S. Choudhri, J. O. Ndinya-Achola, and F. A. Plummer. 1995. Comparison of the declines in CD4 counts in HIV-1 seropositive female sex workers and women from the general population in Nairobi, Kenya. *J AIDS Hum Retrovirol* 10:457–461.

331. Byars, N. E., and A. Allison. 1987. Adjuvant formulation for use in vaccines to elicit both cell-mediated immunity and humoral immunity. *Vaccine* 5:223–228.

332. Byrne, J. A., and M. B. A. Oldstone. 1984. Biology of cloned cytotoxic T lymphocytes specific for lymphocytic choriomeningitis virus: clearance of virus *in vivo*. *J Virol* 51:682–686.

333. Cai, Q., X.-L. Huang, G. Rappocciolo, and C. R. Rinaldo, Jr. 1990. Natural killer cell responses in homosexual men with early HIV infection. *J AIDS* 3:669–676.

334. Calabrese, L. H., D. M. Kelley, A. Myers, M. O'Connell, and K. Easley. 1991. Rheumatic symptoms and human immunodeficiency virus infection. *Arth Rheum* 34:257–263.

335. Caley, I. J., M. R. Betts, D. M. Irlbeck, N. L. Davis, R. Swanstrom, J. A. Frelinger, and R. E. Johnston. 1997. Humoral, mucosal, and cellular immunity in response to a human immunodeficiency virus type 1 immunogen expressed by a Venezuelan equine encephalitis virus vaccine vector. *J Virol* 71:3031–3038.

336. Callebaut, C., B. Krust, E. Jacotot, and A. G. Hovanessian. 1994. T cell activation antigen, CD26, as a cofactor for entry of HIV in CD4+ cells. *Science* 262:2045–2050.

337. Camaur, D., and D. Trono. 1996. Characterization of human immunodeficiency virus type 1 Vif particle incorporation. *J Virol* 70:6106–6111.

338. Camerini, D., B. D. Jamieson, J. A. Zack, and I. S. Y. Chen. 1994. Pathogenesis of syncytium-inducing and non-syncytium inducing HIV-1 isolates and molecular clones in SCID-hu mice. *Keystone Symp Mol Cell Biol Suppl* 18B:155.

339. Camerini, D., and B. Seed. 1990. A CD4 domain important for HIV-mediated syncytium formation lies outside the virus binding site. *Cell* 60:747–754.

340. Cameron, D. W., J. N. Simonsen, L. J. D'Costa, A. R. Ronald, G. M. Maitha, M. N. Gakinya, M. Cheang, J. O. Ndinya-Achola, P. Piot, R. C. Brunham, and F. A. Plummer. 1989. Female to male transmission of human immunodeficiency virus type 1: risk factors for seroconversion in men. *Lancet* ii:403–407.

341. Cameron, M. L., D. L. Granger, T. J. Matthews, and J. B. Weinberg. 1994. Human immunodeficiency virus (HIV)-infected human blood monocytes and peritoneal macrophages have reduced anticryptococcal activity whereas HIV-infected alveolar macrophages retain normal activity. *J Inf Dis* **170**:60–67.

342. Cameron, P., M. Pope, A. Granelli-Piperno, and R. M. Steinman. 1996. Dendritic cells and the replication of HIV-1. *J Leukoc Biol* **59**:158–171.

343. Cameron, P. U., P. S. Freudenthal, J. M. Barker, S. Gezelter, K. Inaba, and R. M. Steinman. 1992. Dendritic cells exposed to human immunodeficiency virus type-1 transmit a vigorous cytopathic infection to CD4+ T cells. *Science* **257**:383–387.

344. Campbell, I. L., C. R. Abraham, E. Masliah, P. Kemper, J. D. Inglis, M. B. A. Oldstone, and L. Mucke. 1993. Neurologic disease induced in transgenic mice by cerebral overexpression of interleukin 6. *Proc Natl Acad Sci USA* **90**:10061–10065.

344a.Campbell, P. J., S. Aurelius, G. Blowes, and D. Harvey. 1997. Decrease in CD4 lymphocyte counts with rest: implications for the monitoring of HIV infection. *Int J STD and AIDS* **8**:423–426.

345. Canivet, M., A. D. Hoffman, D. Hardy, J. Sernatinger, and J. A. Levy. 1990. Replication of HIV-1 in a wide variety of animal cells following phenotypic mixing with murine retroviruses. *Virol* **178**:543–551.

346. Cann, A. J., M. J. Churcher, M. Boyd, W. O'Brien, J.-Q. Zhao, J. Zack, and I. S. Y. Chen. 1992. The region of the envelope gene of human immunodeficiency virus type 1 responsible for determination of cell tropism. *J Virol* **66**:305–309.

347. Cann, A. J., J. A. Zack, A. S. Go, S. J. Arrigo, Y. Koyanagi, P. L. Green, Y. Koyanagi, S. Pang, and I. S. Y. Chen. 1990. Human immunodeficiency virus type 1 T-cell tropism is determined by events prior to provirus formation. *J Virol* **64**:4735–4742.

348. Cantin, R., J.-F. Fortin, G. Lamontagne, and M. Tremblay. 1997. The presence of host-derived HLA-DR1 on human immunodeficiency virus type 1 increases viral infectivity. *J Virol* **71**:1922–1930.

349. Cantin, R., J.-F. Fortin, and M. Tremblay. 1996. The amount of host HLA-DR proteins acquired by HIV-1 is virus strain- and cell type-specific. *Virol* **218**:372–381.

350. Cantrill, H. L., K. Henry, B. Jackson, A. Erice, F. M. Ussery, and H. H. Balfour, Jr. 1988. Recovery of human immunodeficiency virus from ocular tissues in patients with acquired immune deficiency syndrome. *Ophthalmol* **95**:1458–1462.

351. Cao, J., I. W. Park, A. Cooper, and J. Sodroski. 1996. Molecular determinants of acute single-cell lysis by human immunodeficiency virus type 1. *J Virol* **70**:1340–1354.

352. Cao, Y., D. Dieterich, P. A. Thomas, Y. Huang, M. Mirabile, and D. D. Ho. 1992. Identification and quantitation of HIV-1 in the liver of patients with AIDS. *AIDS* **6**:65–70.

353. Cao, Y., D. D. Ho, J. Todd, R. Kokka, M. Urdea, J. D. Lifson, M. Piatak, Jr., S. Chen, B. H. Hahn, M. S. Saag, and G. M. Shaw. 1995. Clinical evaluation of branched DNA signal amplification for quantifying HIV type 1 in human plasma. *AIDS Res Hum Retro* **11**:353–361.

354. Cao, Y., L. Qin, L. Zhang, J. Safrit, and D. D. Ho. 1995. Virologic and immunologic characterization of long-term survivors of human immunodeficiency virus type 1 infection. *N Engl J Med* **332**:201–208.

355. Cao, Y. Z., A. E. Friedman-Kien, Y. X. Huang, X. L. Li, M. Mirabile, T. Moudgil, D. Zucker-Franklin, and D. D. Ho. 1990. CD4-independent, productive human immunodeficiency virus type 1 infection of hepatoma cell lines *in vitro*. *J Virol* **64**:2553–2559.

356. Capobianchi, M. R., C. Barresi, P. Borghi, S. Gessani, L. Fantuzzi, F. Ameglio, F. Belardelli, S. Papadia, and F. Dianzani. 1997. Human immunodeficiency virus type 1 gp120 stimulates cytomegalovirus replication in monocytes: possible role of endogenous interleukin-8. *J Virol* **71**:1591–1597.

357. Capon, D. J., and R. H. Ward. 1991. The CD4-gp120 interaction and AIDS pathogenesis. *Annu Rev Immunol* **9**:649–678.

358. Cara, A., F. Guarnaccia, M. S. Reitz, Jr., R. C. Gallo, and F. Lori. 1995. Self-limiting, cell type dependent replication of an integrase-defective human immunodeficiency virus type 1 in human primary macrophages but not T lymphocytes. *Virol* **208**:242–248.

359. Carlson, J. R. 1988. Serological diagnosis of human immunodeficiency virus infection by Western blot testing. *J Am Med Assoc* **260**:674–679.

360. Carlson, J. R., T. P. McGraw, E. Keddie, J. L. Yee, A. Rosenthal, A. J. Langlois, R. Dickover, R. Donovan, P. A. Luciw, M. B. Jennings, and M. B. Gardner. 1990. Vaccine protection of rhesus macaques against simian immunodeficiency virus infection. *AIDS Res Hum Retro* **6**:1239–1246.

361. Carmichael, A., X. Jin, P. Sissons, and L. Borysiewicz. 1993. Quantitative analysis of the human immunodeficiency virus type (HIV-1)-specific cytotoxic T lymphocytes (CTL) response at different stages of HIV-1 infection: differential CTL responses to HIV-1 and Epstein-Barr virus in late disease. *J Exp Med* **177**:249–256.

362. Carne, C. A., R. S. Tedder, A. Smith, S. Sutherland, S. G. Elkington, H. M. Daly, F. E. Preston, and J. Craske. 1985. Acute encephalopathy coincident with seroconversion for anti-HTLV-III. *Lancet* ii:1206–1208.

363. Carpenter, C. C. J., M. A. Fischl, S. M. Hammer, M. S. Hirsch, D. M. Jacobsen, D. A. Katzenstein, J. S. G. Montaner, D. D. Richman, M. S. Saag, R. T. Schooley, M. A. Thompson, S. Vella, P. G. Yeni, and P. A. Volberding. 1997. Antiretroviral therapy for HIV infection in 1997. *J Am Med Assoc* **277**:1962–1969.

364. Carre, N., C. Deveau, F. Belanger, F. Boufassa, A. Persoz, C. Jadand, C. Rouzioux, J.-F. Delfraissy, and D. Bucquet. 1994. Effect of age and exposure group on the onset of AIDS in heterosexual and homosexual HIV-infected patients. *AIDS* **8**:797–802.

365. Carrigan, D. R., K. K. Knox, and M. A. Tapper. 1990. Suppression of human immunodeficiency virus type 1 replication by human herpesvirus-6. *J Inf Dis* **162**:844–851.

366. Carrillo, A., and L. Ratner. 1996. Cooperative effects of the human immunodeficiency virus type 1 envelope variable loops V1 and V3 in mediating infectivity for T cells. *J Virol* **70**:1310–1316.

367. Carrillo, A., and L. Ratner. 1996. Human immunodeficiency virus type 1 tropism for T-lymphoid cell lines: role of the V3 loop and C4 envelope determinants. *J Virol* **70**:1301–1309.

368. Carrillo, A., D. B. Trowbridge, P. Westervelt, and L. Ratner. 1993. Identification of HIV-1 determinants for T lymphoid cell line infection. *Virol* **197**:817–824.

369. Carroll, R. G., J. L. Riley, B. L. Levine, Y. Feng, S. Kaushal, D. W. Ritchey, W. Bernstein, O. S. Weislow, C. R. Brown, E. A. Berger, C. H. June, and D. C. St. Louis. 1997. Activation of CD4+ T lymphocytes by CD28 costimulation modulates human immunodeficiency virus type 1 (HIV-1) entry cofactor expression and susceptibility to HIV-1 infection. *Science* **276**:273–276.

370. Casareale, D., M. Fiala, C. M. Chang, L. A. Cone, and E. S. Mocarski. 1989. Cytomegalovirus enhances lysis of HIV-infected T lymphoblasts. *Int J Cancer* **44**:124–130.

371. Castro, B. A., S. W. Barnett, L. A. Evans, J. Moreau, K. Odehouri, and J. A. Levy. 1990. Biologic heterogeneity of human immunodeficiency virus type 2 (HIV-2). *Virol* **178**:527–534.

372. Castro, B. A., C. Cheng-Mayer, L. A. Evans, and J. A. Levy. 1988. HIV heterogeneity and viral pathogenesis. *AIDS '88* **2**:s17–s28.

373. Castro, B. A., J. W. Eichberg, N. W. Lerche, and J. A. Levy. 1989. HIV from experimentally infected chimpanzees: isolation and characterization. *J Med Primatol* **18**:337–342.

374. Castro, B. A., J. Homsy, E. Lennette, K. K. Murthy, J. W. Eichberg, and J. A. Levy. 1992. HIV-1 expression in chimpanzees can be activated by CD8+ cell depletion or CMV infection. *Clin Immunol Immunopathol* **65**:227–233.

374a. Castro, B. A., and J. A. Levy. Unpublished observations.

375. Castro, B. A., M. Nepomuceno, N. W. Lerche, J. W. Eichberg, and J. A. Levy. 1991. Persistent infection of baboon and rhesus monkeys with different strains of HIV-2. *Virol* **184**:219–226.

376. Castro, K. G., J. W. Ward, L. Slutsker, J. W. Buehler, H. W. Jaffe, R. L. Berkelman, and J. W. Curran. 1992. 1993 revised classification system for HIV infection and expanded surveillance case definition for AIDS among adolescents and adults. *Morbid Mortal Weekly Rep* **41**:1–19.

377. Cauda, R., M. Tumbarello, L. Ortona, P. Kanda, R. C. Kennedy, and T. C. Chanh. 1988. In-

hibition of normal human natural killer cell activity by human immunodeficiency virus synthetic transmembrane peptides. *Cell Immunol* **115**:57–65.

378. Cavard, C., A. Zider, M. Vernet, M. Bennoun, S. Saragosti, G. Grimber, and P. Briand. 1990. *In vivo* activation by ultraviolet rays of the human immunodeficiency virus type 1 long terminal repeat. *J Clin Invest* **86**:1369–1374.

379. Cavert, W., D. W. Notermans, K. Staskus, S. W. Wietgrefe, M. Zupancic, K. Gebhard, K. Henry, Z. Q. Zhang, R. Mills, H. McDade, J. Goudsmit, S. A. Danner, and A. T. Haase. 1997. Kinetics of response in lymphoid tissues to antiretroviral therapy of HIV-1 infection. *Science* **276**:960–964.

380. Cease, K. B., and J. A. Berzofsky. 1994. Toward a vaccine for AIDS: the emergence of immunobiology-based vaccine development. *Annu Rev Immunol* **12**:923–989.

381. Celada, F., C. Cambiaggi, J. Maccari, S. Burastero, T. Gregory, E. Patzer, J. Porter, C. McDanal, and T. Matthews. 1990. Antibody raised against soluble CD4-rgp120 complex recognizes the CD4 moiety and blocks membrane fusion without inhibiting CD4-gp120 binding. *J Exp Med* **172**:1143–1150.

382. Centers for Disease Control. 1982. *Pneumocystis carinii* pneumonia among persons with hemophilia A. *Morbid Mortal Weekly Rep* **31**:365–367.

383. Centers for Disease Control. 1981. Pneumocystis pneumonia—Los Angeles. *Morbid Mortal Weekly Rep* **30**:250–252.

384. Centers for Disease Control. 1992. 1993 revised classification system for HIV infection and expanded surveillance case definition for AIDS among adolescents and adults. *Morbid Mortal Weekly Rep* **41**:1–19.

385. Centers for Disease Control. 1985. Revision of the case definition of acquired immunodeficiency syndrome for national reporting—United States. *Ann Int Med* **103**:402.

386. Centers for Disease Control. 1994. Zidovudine for the prevention of HIV transmission from mother to infant. *Morbid Mortal Weekly Rep* **43**:285–287.

386a. Centers for Disease Control. 1997. Update: trends in AIDS incidence, deaths, and prevalence—United States, 1996. *Morbid Mortal Weekly Rep* **46**:167–173.

387. Cerdan, C., Y. Martin, M. Courcoul, H. Brailly, C. Mawas, F. Birg, and D. Olive. 1992. Prolonged IL2 receptor-alpha/CD25 expression after T cell activation via the adhesion molecule CD2 and CD28. *J Immunol* **149**:2255–2261.

388. Cesarman, E., Y. Chang, P. S. Moore, J. W. Said, and D. M. Knowles. 1995. Kaposi's sarcoma-associated herpesvirus-like DNA sequences in AIDS-related body-cavity-based lymphomas. *N Engl J Med* **332**:1186–1191.

389. Chackerian, B., E. M. Long, P. A. Luciw, and J. Overbaugh. 1997. Human immunodeficiency virus type 1 coreceptors participate in postentry stages in the virus replication cycle and function in simian immunodeficiency virus infection. *J Virol* **71**:3932–3939.

390. Chad, D. A., T. W. Smith, A. Blumenfeld, P. G. Fairchild, and U. DeGirolami. 1990. Human immunodeficiency virus (HIV)-associated myopathy: immunocytochemical identification of an HIV antigen (gp 41) in muscle macrophages. *Ann Neurol* **28**:579–582.

391. Chadwick, E. G., E. J. Connor, C. G. Hanson, V. V. Joshi, H. Abu-Farsakh, R. Yogev, G. McSherry, K. McClain, and S. B. Murphy. 1990. Tumors of smooth-muscle origin in HIV-infected children. *J Am Med Assoc* **263**:3182–3184.

392. Chams, V., T. Jouault, E. Fenouillet, J.-C. Gluckman, and D. Klatzmann. 1988. Detection of anti-CD4 autoantibodies in the sera of HIV-infected patients using recombinant soluble CD4 molecules. *AIDS* **2**:353–361.

393. Chan, D. C., D. Fass, J. M. Berger, and P. S. Kim. 1997. Core structure of gp41 from the HIV envelope glycoprotein. *Cell* **89**:263–273.

394. Chan, W. L., A. Rodgers, C. Grief, N. Almond, S. Ellis, B. Flanagan, P. Silvera, J. Bootman, J. Stott, K. Kent, and R. Bomford. 1995. Immunization with class I human histocompatibility leukocyte antigen can protect macaques against challenge infection with SIV$_{mac-32H}$. *AIDS* **9**:223–228.

395. Chan, W. L., A. Rodgers, R. D. Hancock, F. Taffs, P. Kitchin, G. Farrar, and F. Y. Liew. 1992.

Protection in simian immunodeficiency virus-vaccinated monkeys correlates with anti-HLA class I antibody response. *J Exp Med* **176**:1203–1207.

396. Chandwani, S., M. A. Greco, K. Mittal, C. Antoine, K. Krasinski, and W. Borkowsky. 1991. Pathology and human immunodeficiency virus expression in placentas of seropositive women. *J Inf Dis* **163**:1134–1138.

397. Chang, S.-Y. P., B. H. Bowman, J. B. Weiss, R. E. Garcia, and T. J. White. 1993. The origin of HIV-1 isolate HTLV-IIIB. *Nature* **363**:466–469.

398. Chang, Y., E. Cesarman, M. S. Pessin, F. Lee, J. Culpepper, D. M. Knowles, and P. S. Moore. 1994. Identification of herpesvirus-like DNA sequences in AIDS-associated Kaposi's sarcoma. *Science* **266**:1865–1869.

399. Chang, Y., P. S. Moore, S. J. Talbot, C. H. Boshoff, T. Zarkowska, D. Godden-Kent, H. Paterson, R. A. Weiss, and S. Mittnacht. 1996. Cyclin encoded by KS herpesvirus. *Nature* **382**:410.

400. Chanh, T. C., G. R. Dreesman, P. Kanda, G. P. Linette, J. T. Sparrow, D. D. Ho, and R. C. Kennedy. 1986. Induction of anti-HIV neutralizing antibodies by synthetic peptides. *EMBO J* **5**:3065–3071.

401. Chanh, T. C., R. C. Kennedy, and P. Kanda. 1988. Synthetic peptides homologous to HIV transmembrane glycoprotein suppress normal human lymphocyte blastogenic response. *Cell Immunol* **111**:77–86.

402. Chapel, A., A. Bensussan, E. Vilmer, and D. Dormont. 1992. Differential human immunodeficiency virus expression in CD4+ cloned lymphocytes: from viral latency to replication. *J Virol* **66**:3966–3970.

403. Charbit, A., A. Molla, J. Ronco, J. M. Clement, V. Favier, E. Bahraoui, L. Montagnier, A. Leguern, and M. Hofnung. 1990. Immunogenicity and antigenicity of conserved peptides from the envelope of HIV-1 expressed at the surface of recombinant bacteria. *AIDS* **4**:545–551.

404. Chargelegue, D., C. M. Stanley, C. M. O'Toole, B. T. Colvin, and M. W. Steward. 1995. The affinity of IgG antibodies to gag p24 and p17 in HIV-1-infected patients correlates with disease progression. *Clin Exp Immunol* **99**:175–181.

405. Charman, H. P., S. Bladen, R. V. Gilden, and L. Coggins. 1976. Equine infectious anemia virus: evidence favoring classification as a retrovirus. *J Virol* **19**:1073–1079.

406. Charpentier, B., C. Hiesse, O. Lantz, C. Ferran, S. Stephens, D. O'Shaugnessy, M. Bodmer, G. Benoit, J. F. Bach, and L. Chatenoud. 1992. Evidence that antihuman tumor necrosis factor monoclonal antibody prevents OKT3-induced acute syndrome. *Transplantation* **54**:997–1002.

407. Chaturvedi, S., P. Frame, and S. L. Newman. 1995. Macrophages from human immunodeficiency virus-positive persons are defective in host defense against *Histoplasma capsulatum*. *J Inf Dis* **171**:320–327.

408. Chayt, K. J., M. E. Harper, L. M. Marselle, E. B. Lewin, R. M. Rose, J. M. Oleske, L. G. Epstein, F. Wong-Staal, and R. C. Gallo. 1986. Detection of HTLV-III RNA in lungs of patients with AIDS and pulmonary involvement. *J Am Med Assoc* **256**:2356–2359.

409. Cheevers, W. P., and T. C. McGuire. 1988. The lentiviruses: maedi/visna, caprine arthritis-encephalitis, and equine infectious anemia. *Adv Virus Res* **34**:189–215.

410. Chehimi, J., S. Bandyopadhyay, K. Prakash, B. Perussia, N. F. Hassan, H. Kawashima, D. Campbell, J. Kornbluth, and S. E. Starr. 1991. In vitro infection of natural killer cells with different human immunodeficiency virus type 1 isolates. *J Virol* **65**:1812–1822.

411. Chehimi, J., K. Prakash, V. Shanmugam, S. J. Jackson, S. Bandyopadhyay, and S. E. Starr. 1993. In vitro infection of peripheral blood dendritic cells with human immunodeficiency virus-1 causes impairment of accessory functions. *Adv Exp Med Biol* **329**:521–526.

412. Chehimi, J., S. E. Starr, I. Frank, M. Rengaraju, S. J. Jackson, C. Llanes, M. Kobayashi, B. Perussia, D. Young, E. Nickbarg, S. F. Wolf, and G. Trinchieri. 1992. Natural killer (NK) cell stimulatory factor increases the cytotoxic activity of NK cells from both healthy donors and human immunodeficiency virus-infected patients. *J Exp Med* **175**:789–796.

413. Chelucci, C., H. J. Hannsan, C. Locardi, D. Bulgarini, E. Pelosi, G. Mariani, U. Testa, M.

Federico, M. Valtieri, and C. Peschle. 1995. In vitro human immunodeficiency virus-1 infection of purified hematopoietic progenitors in single-cell culture. *Blood* **85**:1181–1187.

414. Chen, B. K., J. T. Gandhi, and D. Baltimore. 1996. CD4 down-modulation during infection of human T cells with human immunodeficiency virus type 1 involves independent activities of *vpu, env,* and *nef. J Virol* **70**:6044–6053.

415. Chen, C. H., K. J. Weinhold, J. A. Bartlett, D. P. Bolognesi, and M. L. Greenberg. 1993. CD8+ T lymphocyte-mediated inhibition of HIV-1 long terminal repeat transcription: a novel antiviral mechanism. *AIDS Res Hum Retro* **9**:1079–1086.

416. Chen, Y., and P. Gupta. 1996. CD8+ T-cell-mediated suppression of HIV-1 infection may not be due to chemokines RANTES, MIP-1α, and MIP-1β. *AIDS* **10**:1434–1435.

416a.Chen, Z., A. Luckay, D. L. Sodora, P. Telfer, P. Reed, A. Gettie, J. M. Kanu, R. F. Sadek, J. Yee, D. D. Ho, L. Zhang, and P. A. Marx. 1997. Human immunodeficiency virus type 2 (HIV-2) seroprevalence and characterization of a distinct HIV-2 genetic subtype from the natural range of simian immunodeficiency virus-infected sooty mangabeys. *J Virol* **71**:3953–3960.

417. Chen, Z., P. Zhou, D. D. Ho, N. R. Landau, and P. A. Marx. 1997. Genetically divergent strains of simian immunodeficiency virus use CCR5 as a coreceptor for entry. *J Virol* **71**:2705–2714.

418. Chen, Z. W., Z.-C. Kou, L. Shen, K. A. Reimann, and N. L. Letvin. 1993. Conserved T-cell receptor repertoire in simian immunodeficiency virus-infetced rhesus monkeys. *J Immunol* **151**:2177–2187.

419. Chen, Z. W., S. Shen, M. D. Miller, S. H. Ghim, A. L. Hughes, and N. L. Letvin. 1992. Cytotoxic T lymphocytes do not appear to select for mutations in an immunodominant epitope of simian immunodeficiency virus gag. *J Immunol* **149**:4060–4066.

420. Cheng-Mayer, C. 1993. Unpublished observations.

421. Cheng-Mayer, C., J. M. Homsy, L. A. Evans, and J. A. Levy. 1988. Identification of HIV subtypes with distinct patterns of sensitivity to serum neutralization. *Proc Natl Acad Sci USA* **85**:2815–2819.

422. Cheng-Mayer, C., P. Ianello, K. Shaw, P. A. Luciw, and J. A. Levy. 1989. Differential effects of *nef* on HIV replication: implications for viral pathogenesis in the host. *Science* **246**:1629-1632.

423. Cheng-Mayer, C., and J. A. Levy. 1988. Distinct biologic and serologic properties of HIV isolates from the brain. *Ann Neurol* **23**:s58-s61.

424. Cheng-Mayer, C., and J. A. Levy. 1990. Human immunodeficiency virus infection of the CNS: Characterization of "neurotropic" strains. *Curr Top Micro Immunol* **160**:145–156.

424a.Cheng-Mayer, C., and J. A. Levy. Unpublished observations.

425. Cheng-Mayer, C., R. Liu, N. R. Landau, and L. Stamatatos. 1997. Macrophage tropism of human immunodeficiency virus type 1 and utilization of the CC-CKR5 coreceptor. *J Virol* **71**:1657–1661.

426. Cheng-Mayer, C., M. Quiroga, J. W. Tung, D. Dina, and J. A. Levy. 1990. Viral determinants of HIV-1 T-cell/macrophage tropism, cytopathicity, and CD4 antigen modulation. *J Virol* **64**:4390–4398.

427. Cheng-Mayer, C., J. T. Rutka, M. L. Rosenblum, T. McHugh, D. P. Stites, and J. A. Levy. 1987. The human immunodeficiency virus (HIV) can productively infect cultured human glial cells. *Proc Natl Acad Sci USA* **84**:3526–3530.

428. Cheng-Mayer, C., D. Seto, and J. A. Levy. 1991. Altered host range of HIV-1 after passage through various human cell types. *Virol* **181**:288–294.

429. Cheng-Mayer, C., D. Seto, M. Tateno, and J. A. Levy. 1988. Biologic features of HIV that correlate with virulence in the host. *Science* **240**:80–82.

430. Cheng-Mayer, C., T. Shioda, and J. A. Levy. 1991. Host range, replicative, and cytopathic properties of human immunodeficiency virus type 1 are determined by very few amino acid changes in *tat* and gp120. *J Virol* **65**:6931–6941.

431. Cheng-Mayer, C., T. Shioda, and J. A. Levy. 1992. Small regions of the *env* and *tat* genes control cellular tropism, cytopathology and replicative properties of HIV-1, p. 188–195. *In* G. B. Rossi, E. Beth-Giraldo, L. Chieco-Bianchi, F. Dianzani, G. Giraldo, and P. Verani (ed.), *Science Challenging AIDS*. S. Karger, Basel.

432. Cheng-Mayer, C., C. Weiss, D. Seto, and J. A. Levy. 1989. Isolates of human immunodeficiency virus type 1 from the brain may constitute a special group of the AIDS virus. *Proc Natl Acad Sci USA* **80:**8575–8579.

433. Chermann, J. C., G. Donker, N. Yahi, D. Salaun, N. Guettari, O. Gayet, and I. Hirsh. 1991. Discrepancies in AIDS virus data. *Nature* **351:**277–278.

434. Chesebro, B., R. Buller, J. Portis, and K. Wehrly. 1990. Failure of human immunodeficiency virus entry and infection in CD4-positive human brain and skin cells. *J Virol* **64:**215–221.

435. Chesebro, B., J. Nishio, S. Perryman, A. Cann, W. O'Brien, I. S. Y. Chen, and K. Wehrly. 1991. Identification of human immunodeficiency virus envelope gene sequences influencing viral entry into CD4-positive HeLa cells, T-leukemia cells, and macrophages. *J Virol* **65:**5782–5789.

436. Cheynier, R., S. Henrichwark, F. Hadida, E. Pelletier, E. Oksenhendler, B. Autran, and S. Wain-Hobson. 1994. HIV and T cell expansion in splenic white pulps is accompanied by infiltration of HIV-specific cytotoxic T lymphocytes. *Cell* **78:**373–387.

437. Cheynier, R., P. Langlade-Demoyen, M.-R. Marescot, S. Blanche, G. Blondin, S. Wain-Hobson, C. Griscelli, E. Vilmer, and F. Plata. 1992. Cytotoxic T lymphocyte responses in the peripheral blood of children born to human immunodeficiency virus-1-infected mothers. *Eur J Immunol* **22:**2211–2217.

438. Cheingsong-Popov, R., D. Callow, S. Beddows, S. Shaunak, C. Wasi, P. Kaleebu, C. Gilks, I. V. Petrascu, M. M. Garaev, D. M. Watts, N. T. Constantine, and J. N. Weber. 1992. Geographic diversity of human immunodeficiency virus type 1: serologic reactivity to *env* epitopes and relationship to neutralization. *J Inf Dis* **165:**256–261.

439. Chirmule, N., V. S. Kalyanaraman, C. Saxinger, F. Wong-Staal, J. Ghrayeb, and S. Pahwa. 1990. Localization of B-cell stimulatory activity of HIV-1 to the carboxyl terminus of gp41. *AIDS Res Hum Retro* **6:**299–305.

440. Chirmule, N., M. Lesser, A. Gupta, M. Ravipati, N. Kohn, and S. Pahwa. 1995. Immunological characteristics of HIV-infected children: relationship to age, CD4 counts, disease progression, and survival. *AIDS Res Hum Retro* **11:**1209–1219.

440a. Chirmule, N., T. W. McCloskey, R. Hu, V. S. Kalyanaraman, and S. Pahwa. 1995. HIV gp120 inhibits T cell activation by interfering with expression of costimulatory molecules CD40 ligand and CD80 (B71). *J Immunol* **155:**917–924.

441. Chirmule, N., N. Oyaizu, V. S. Kalyanaraman, and S. Pahwa. 1992. Inhibition of normal B-cell function by human immunodeficiency virus envelope glycoprotein, gp120. *Blood* **79:**1245–1254.

442. Chiu, I. M., A. Yaniv, J. E. Dahlberg, A. Gazit, S. F. Skuntz, S. R. Tronick, and S. A. Aaronson. 1985. Nucleotide sequence evidence for relationship of AIDS retrovirus to lentiviruses. *Nature* **317:**366–368.

443. Chlebowski, R. T., M. B. Grosvenor, and N. H. Bernhard. 1989. Nutritional status, gastrointestinal dysfunction, and survival in patients with AIDS. *Am J Gastro* **84:**1288–1293.

444. Choe, H., M. Farzan, Y. Sun, N. Sullivan, B. Rollins, P. D. Ponath, L. Wu, C. R. Mackay, G. LaRosa, W. Newman, N. Gerard, C. Gerard, and J. Sodroski. 1996. The β-chemokine receptors CCR3 and CCR5 facilitate infection by primary HIV-1 isolates. *Cell* **85:**1135–1148.

445. Chou, C. S., O. Ramilo, and E. S. Vitetta. 1997. Highly purified CD25− resting T cells cannot be infected *de novo* with HIV-1. *Proc Natl Acad Sci USA* **94:**1361–1365.

446. Chougnet, C., T. A. Wynn, M. Clerici, A. L. Landay, H. A. Kessler, J. Rusnak, G. P. Melcher, A. Sher, and G. M. Shearer. 1996. Molecular analysis of decreased interleukin-12 production in persons infected with human immunodeficiency virus. *J Inf Dis* **174:**46–53.

447. Chowers, M. Y., C. A. Spina, T. J. Kwoh, N. J. S. Fitch, D. D. Richman, and J. C. Guitelli. 1994. Optimal infectivity in vitro of human immunodeficiency virus type 1 requires and intact Nef gene. *J Virol* **68:**2906–2914.

448. Chuang, L. F., K. F. Killam, Jr., and R. Y. Chuang. 1993. Increased replication of simian immunodeficiency virus in CEM x174 cells by morphine sulfate. *Biochem Biophys Res Comm* **195:**1165–1173.

449. Chuang, R. Y., D. J. Blackbourn, L. F. Chuang, Y. Liu, and K. F. Killam, Jr. 1993. Modulation of simian AIDS by opioids. *Adv Biosci* **86:**573–583.

450. Chun, T.-W., L. Carruth, D. Finzi, X. Shen, J. A. DiGiuseppe, H. Taylor, M. Hermankova, K. Chadwick, J. Margolick, T. C. Quinn, Y. H. Kuo, R. Brookmeyer, M. A. Zeiger, P. Barditch-Crovo, and R. F. Siliciano. 1997. Quantification of latent tissue reservoirs and total body viral load in HIV-1 infection. *Nature* **387**:183–188.

451. Chun, T.-W., K. Chadwick, J. Margolick, and R. F. Siliciano. 1997. Differential susceptibility of naive and memory CD4+ T cells to the cytopathic effects of infection with human immunodeficiency virus type 1 strain LAI. *J Virol* **71**:4436–4444.

452. Chun, T. W., D. Finzi, J. Margolick, K. Chadwick, D. Schwartz, and R. F. Siliciano. 1995. *In vivo* fate of HIV-1-infected T cells: quantitative analysis of the transition to stable latency. *Nature Med* **1**:1284–1290.

453. Cianciolo, G. J., T. D. Copeland, S. Oroszlan, and R. Snyderman. 1985. Inhibition of lymphocyte proliferation by a synthetic peptide homologous to retroviral envelope proteins. *Science* **230**:453–455.

454. Cichutek, K., H. Merget, S. Norley, R. Linde, W. Kreuz, M. Gahr, and R. Kurth. 1992. Development of a quasispecies of human immunodeficiency virus type 1 *in vivo*. *Proc Natl Acad Sci USA* **89**:7365–7369.

455. Cichutek, K., S. Norley, R. Linde, W. Kreuz, M. Gahr, J. Lower, G. Von Wangenheim, and R. Kurth. 1991. Lack of HIV-1 V3 region sequence diversity in two haemophiliac patients infected with a putative biologic clone of HIV-1. *AIDS* **5**:1185–1187.

456. Cimarelli, A., G. Zambruno, A. Marconi, G. Girolomoni, U. Bertazzoni, and A. Giannetti. 1994. Quantitation by competitive PCR of HIV-1 proviral DNA in epidermal Langerhans cells of HIV-infected patients. *J AIDS* **7**:230–235.

457. Clapham, P. R., D. Blanc, and R. A. Weiss. 1991. Specific cell surface requirements for the infection of CD4-positive cells by human immunodeficiency virus types 1 and 2 and by simian immunodeficiency virus. *Virol* **181**:703–715.

458. Clapham, P. R., A. McKnight, and R. A. Weiss. 1992. Human immunodeficiency virus type 2 infection and fusion of CD4-negative human cell lines: induction and enhancement by soluble CD4. *J Virol* **66**:3531–3537.

459. Clapham, P. R., J. N. Weber, D. Whitby, K. McIntosh, A. G. Dalgleish, P. J. Maddon, K. C. Deen, R. W. Sweet, and R. A. Weiss. 1989. Soluble CD4 blocks the infectivity of diverse strains of HIV and SIV for T cells and monocytes but not for brain and muscle cells. *Nature* **337**:368–370.

460. Clark, A. G. B., M. Holodniy, D. G. Schwartz, D. A. Katzenstein, and T. C. Merigan. 1992. Decrease in HIV provirus in peripheral blood mononuclear cells during zidovudine and human rIL-2 administration. *J AIDS* **5**:52–59.

461. Clark, S. J., M. S. Saag, W. D. Decker, S. Campbell-Hill, J. L. Roberson, P. J. Veldkamp, J. C. Kappes, B. H. Hahn, and G. M. Shaw. 1991. High titers of cytopathic virus in plasma of patients with symptomatic primary HIV-1 infection. *N Engl J Med* **324**:954–960.

462. Clavel, F., D. Guetard, F. Brun-Vezinet, S. Chamaret, M.-A. Rey, M. O. Santos-Ferreira, A. G. Laurent, C. Dauguet, C. Katlama, C. Rouzioux, D. Klatzmann, J. L. Champalimaud, and L. Montagnier. 1986. Isolation of a new human retrovirus from West African patients with AIDS. *Science* **233**:343–346.

463. Clavel, F., K. Mansinho, S. Chamaret, D. Guetard, V. Favier, J. Nina, M.-O. Santos-Ferreira, J.-L. Champalimaud, and L. Montagnier. 1987. Human immunodeficiency virus type 2 infection associated with AIDS in West Africa. *N Engl J Med* **316**:1180–1185.

464. Clayton, L. K., R. E. Hussey, R. Steinbrich, H. Ramachandran, Y. Husain, and E. L. Reinherz. 1988. Substitution of murine for human CD4 residues identifies amino acids critical for HIV-gp120 binding. *Nature* **335**:363–366.

465. Clegg, C. H., J. T. Rulffes, P. M. Wallace, and H. S. Haugen. 1996. Regulation of an extrathymic T-cell development pathway by oncostatin M. *Nature* **384**:261–263.

466. Clements, G. J., M. J. Price-Jones, P. E. Stephens, C. Sutton, T. F. Schultz, P. R. Clapham, J. A. McKeating, M. O. McClure, S. Thomson, M. Marsh, J. Kay, R. A. Weiss, and J. P. Moore. 1991. The V3 loops of the HIV-1 and HIV-2 surface glycoproteins contain proteolytic cleavage sites: a possible function in viral fusion? *AIDS Res Hum Retro* **7**:3–16.

467. Clemetson, D. B. A., G. B. Moss, D. M. Willerford, M. Hensel, P. L. Emonyi, S. Hillier, and J. K. Kreiss. 1993. Detection of HIV DNA in cervical and vaginal secretions. *J Am Med Assoc* **269**:2860–2864.

468. Clerici, M., C. Balotta, L. Meroni, E. Ferrario, C. Riva, D. Trabattoni, A. Ridolfo, M. Villa, G. M. Shearer, M. Moroni, and M. Galli. 1996. Type 1 cytokine production and low prevalence of viral isolation correlate with long-term nonprogression in HIV infection. *AIDS Res Hum Retro* **12**:1053–1061.

469. Clerici, M., C. Balotta, A. Salvaggio, C. Riva, D. Trabattoni, L. Papagno, A. Berlusconi, S. Rusconi, M. L. Villa, M. Moroni, and M. Galli. 1996. Human immunodeficiency virus (HIV) phenotype and interleukin-2/interleukin-10 ratio are associated markers of protection and progression in HIV infection. *Blood* **88**:574–579.

470. Clerici, M., C. Balotta, D. Trabattoni, L. Papagno, S. Ruzzante, S. Rusconi, M. L. Fusi, M. C. Colombo, and M. Galli. 1996. Chemokine production in HIV-seropositive long-term asymptomatic individuals. *AIDS* **10**:1432–1433.

471. Clerici, M., E. A. Clark, P. Polacino, I. Axberg, L. Kuller, N. I. Casey, W. R. Morton, G. M. Shearer, and R. E. Benveniste. 1994. T-cell proliferation to subinfectious SIV correlates with lack of infection after challenge of macaques. *AIDS* **8**:1391–1395.

472. Clerici, M., J. V. Giorgi, C. C. Chou, V. K. Gudeman, J. A. Zack, P. Gupta, H. N. Ho, P. G. Nishanian, J. A. Berzofsky, and G. M. Shearer. 1992. Cell-mediated immune response to human immunodeficiency virus (HIV) type 1 in seronegative homosexual men with recent sexual exposure to HIV-1. *J Inf Dis* **165**:1012–1019.

473. Clerici, M., F. T. Hakim, D. J. Venzon, S. Blatt, C. W. Hendrix, T. A. Wynn, and G. M. Shearer. 1993. Changes in interleukin-2 and interleukin-4 production in asymptomatic, human immunodeficiency virus-seropositive individuals. *J Clin Invest* **91**:759–765.

474. Clerici, M., A. L. Landay, H. A. Kessler, J. P. Phair, D. J. Venzon, C. W. Hendrix, D. R. Lucey, and G. M. Shearer. 1992. Reconstitution of long-term T helper cell function after zidovudine therapy in human immunodeficiency virus-infected patients. *J Inf Dis* **166**:723–730.

475. Clerici, M., J. M. Levin, H. A. Kessler, A. Harris, J. A. Berzofsky, A. L. Landay, and G. M. Shearer. 1994. HIV-specific T-helper activity in seronegative health care workers exposed to contaminated blood. *J Am Med Assoc* **271**:42–46.

476. Clerici, M., D. R. Lucey, J. A. Berzofsky, L. A. Pinto, T. A. Wynn, S. P. Blatt, M. J. Dolan, C. W. Hendrix, S. F. Wolf, and G. M. Shearer. 1993. Restoration of HIV-specific cell-mediated immune responses by interleukin-12 in vitro. *Science* **262**:1721–1724.

477. Clerici, M., E. Roilides, C. S. Via, P. A. Pizzo, and G. M. Shearer. 1992. A factor from CD8 cells of human immunodeficiency virus-infected patients suppresses HLA self-restricted T helper cell responses. *Proc Natl Acad Sci USA* **89**:8424–8428.

478. Clerici, M., A. Sarin, J. A. Berzofsky, A. L. Landay, H. A. Kessler, F. Hashemi, C. W. Hendrix, S. P. Blatt, J. Rusnak, M. J. Dolan, R. L. Coffman, P. A. Henkart, and G. M. Shearer. 1996. Antigen-stimulated apoptotic T-cell death in HIV infection is selective for CD4+ T cells, modulated by cytokines and effected by lymphotoxin. *AIDS* **10**:603–611.

479. Clerici, M., A. Sarin, R. L. Coffman, T. A. Wynn, S. P. Blatt, C. W. Hendrix, S. F. Wolf, G. M. Shearer, and P. A. Henkart. 1994. Type 1/type 2 cytokine modulation of T cell programmed cell death as a model for HIV pathogenesis. *Proc Natl Acad Sci USA* **91**:11811–11815.

480. Clerici, M., and G. M. Shearer. 1993. A TH1 to TH2 switch is a critical step in the etiology of HIV infection. *Immunol Today* **14**:107–111.

481. Clerici, M., and G. M. Shearer. 1994. The Th1-Th2 hypothesis of HIV infection: new insights. *Immunol Today* **15**:575–581.

482. Clerici, M., A. V. Sison, J. A. Berzofsky, T. A. Rakusan, C. D. Brandt, M. Ellaurie, M. L. Villa, C. Colie, D. J. Venzon, J. L. Sever, and G. M. Shearer. 1993. Cellular immune factors associated with mother-to-infant transmission of HIV. *AIDS* **7**:1427–1433.

483. Clerici, M., N. I. Stocks, R. A. Zajac, R. N. Boswell, D. R. Lucey, C. S. Via, and G. M. Shearer. 1989. Detection of three distinct patterns of T helper cell dysfunction in asymptomatic, human immunodeficiency virus-positive patients. Independence of CD4+ cell numbers and clinical staging. *J Clin Invest* **84**:1892–1899.

484. Clerici, M., T. A. Wynn, J. A. Berzofsky, S. P. Blatt, C. W. Hendrix, A. Sher, R. L. Coffman, and G. M. Shearer. 1994. Role of interleukin-10 in T helper cell dysfunction in asymptomatic individuals infected with the human immunodeficiency virus. *J Clin Invest* **93**:768–775.

485. Cloyd, M. W., and W. S. Lynn. 1991. Perturbation of host-cell membrane is a primary mechanism of HIV cytopathology. *Virol* **181**:500–511.

486. Cloyd, M. W., and B. E. Moore. 1990. Spectrum of biological properties of human immunodeficiency virus (HIV-1) isolates. *Virol* **174**:103–116.

487. Cocchi, F., A. L. DeVico, A. Garzino-Demo, S. K. Arya, R. C. Gallo, and P. Lusso. 1995. Identification of RANTES, MIP-1alpha, and MIP-1beta as the major HIV-suppressive factors produced by CD8+ T cells. *Science* **270**:1811–1815.

488. Cocchi, F., A. L. DeVico, A. Garzino-Demo, A. Cara, R. C. Gallo, and P. Lusso. 1996. The V3 domain of the HIV-1 gp120 envelope glycoprotein is critical for chemokine-mediated blockade of infection. *Nature Med* **2**:1244–1247.

489. Coffin, J., A. Haase, J. A. Levy, L. Montagnier, S. Oroszlan, N. Teich, H. Temin, K. Toyoshima, H. Varmus, P. Vogt, and R. Weiss. 1986. Human immunodeficiency viruses. *Science* **232**:697. (Letter.)

490. Coffin, J. M. 1992. Structure and classification of retroviruses, p. 19–50. *In* J. A. Levy (ed.), *The Retroviridae*, volume 1. Plenum Press, New York.

491. Coffin, J. M. 1992. Superantigens and endogenous retroviruses: a confluence of puzzles. *Science* **255**:411–413.

492. Cohen, A. H., N. C. J. Sun, P. Shapshak, and D. T. Imagawa. 1989. Demonstration of human immunodeficiency virus in renal epithelium in HIV-associated nephropathy. *Mod Path* **2**:125–128.

493. Cohen, D. I., Y. Tani, H. Tian, E. Boone, L. W. Samelson, and E. C. Lane. 1992. Participation of tyrosine phosphorylation in the cytopathic effect of human immunodeficiency virus-1. *Science* **256**:542–545.

494. Cohen, J. H. M., C. Geffriaud, V. Caudwell, and M. D. Kazatchkine. 1989. Genetic analysis of CR1 (the C3b complement receptor, CD35) expression on erythrocytes of HIV-infected individuals. *AIDS* **3**:397–399.

495. Cohen, J. J., R. C. Duke, V. A. Fadok, and K. S. Sellins. 1992. Apoptosis and programmed cell death in immunity. *Annu Rev Immunol* **10**:267–293.

496. Cohen, O. J., G. Pantaleo, M. Holodniy, C. H. Fox, J. M. Orenstein, S. Schnittman, M. Niu, C. Graziosi, G. N. Pavlakis, J. Lalezari, J. A. Bartlett, R. T. Steigbigel, J. Cohn, R. Novak, D. McMahon, J. Bilello, and A. S. Fauci. 1996. Antiretroviral monotherapy in early stage human immunodeficiency virus disease has no detectable effect on virus load in peripheral blood and lymph nodes. *J Inf Dis* **173**:849–856.

497. Cohen, O. J., G. Pantaleo, M. Holodniy, S. Schnittman, M. Niu, C. Graziosi, G. N. Pavlakis, J. Lalezari, J. A. Bartlett, R. T. Steigbigel, J. Cohn, R. Novak, D. McMahon, and A. S. Fauci. 1995. Decreased human immunodeficiency virus type 1 plasma viremia during antiretroviral therapy reflects downregulation of viral replication in lymphoid tissue. *Proc Nat Acad Sci USA* **92**:6017–6021.

497a.Cohen, O. J., G. Pantaleo, D. J. Schwartzentruber, C. Graziosi, M. Vaccarezza, and A. S. Fauci. 1995. Pathogenic insights from studies of lymphoid tissue from HIV-infected individuals. *J AIDS Hum Retrovirol* **10**(SI):S6–S14.

498. Cohen, S., and G. M. Williamson. 1991. Stress and infectious disease in humans. *Psychol Bull* **109**:5–24.

499. Collette, Y., H.-L. Chang, C. Cerdan, H. Chambost, M. Algarte, C. Mawas, J. Imbert, A. Burny, and D. Olive. 1996. Specific Th1 cytokine down-regulation associated with primary clinically derived human immunodeficiency virus type 1 *nef* gene-induced expression. *J Immunol* **156**:360–370.

500. Collier, A. C., S. Bozzette, R. W. Coombs, D. M. Causey, D. A. Schoenfeld, S. A. Spector, C. B. Pettinelli, G. Davies, D. D. Richman, J. M. Leedom, P. Kidd, and L. Corey. 1990. A pilot study of low-dose zidovudine in human immunodeficiency virus infection. *N Engl J Med* **323**:1015–1021.

501. Collier, A. C., R. W. Coombs, D. A. Schoenfeld, R. L. Bassett, J. Timpone, A. Baruch, M. Jones, K. Facey, C. Whitacre, V. J. McAuliffe, H. M. Friedman, T. C. Merigan, R. C. Reichman, C. Hooper, and L. Corey. 1996. Treatment of human immunodeficiency virus infection with saquinavir, zidovudine, and zalcitabine. *N Engl J Med* **334**:1011–1018.

502. Collman, R., B. Godfrey, J. Cutilli, A. Rhodes, N. F. Hassan, R. Sweet, S. D. Douglas, H. Friedman, N. Nathanson, and F. Gonzalez-Scarano. 1990. Macrophage-tropic strains of human immunodeficiency virus type 1 utilize the CD4 receptor. *J Virol* **64**:4468–4476.

503. Conant, M., D. Hardy, J. Sernatinger, D. Spicer, and J. A. Levy. 1986. Condoms prevent transmission of the AIDS-asosciated retrovirus by oral-genital contact. *J Am Med Assoc* **225**:1706.

504. Condra, J. H., W. A. Schleif, O. M. Blahy, L. J. Gabryelski, D. J. Graham, J. C. Quintero, A. Rhodes, H. L. Robbins, E. Roth, M. Shivaprakash, D. Titus, T. Yang, H. Teppler, K. E. Squires, P. J. Deutsch, and E. A. Emini. 1995. *In vivo* emergence of HIV-1 variants resistant to multiple protease inhibitors. *Nature* **374**:569–571.

505. Conlon, K., A. Lloyd, U. Chattopadhyay, N. Lukacs, S. Kunkel, T. Schall, D. Taub, C. Morimoto, J. Osborne, J. Oppenheim, H. Young, D. Kelvin, and J. Ortaldo. 1995. CD8+ and CD45RA+ human peripheral blood lymphocytes are potent sources of macrophage inflammatory protein 1*a*, interleukin-8 and RANTES. *Eur J Immunol* **25**:751–756.

507. Connor, R. I., and D. D. Ho. 1994. Human immunodeficiency virus type 1 variants with increased replicative capacity develop during the asymptomatic stage before disease progression. *J Virol* **68**:4400–4408.

508. Connor, R. I., W. A. Paxton, K. E. Sheridan, and R. A. Koup. 1996. Macrophages and CD4+ T lymphocytes from two multiply exposed, uninfected individuals resist infection with primary non-syncytium-inducing isolates of human immunodeficiency virus type 1. *J Virol* **70**:8758–8764.

509. Connor, R. I., K. E. Sheridan, D. Ceradini, S. Choe, and N. R. Landau. 1997. Change in co-receptor use correlates with disease progression in HIV-1-infected individuals. *J Exp Med* **185**:621–628.

510. Connors, M., J. A. Kovacs, S. Krevat, J. C. Gea-Banacloche, M. C. Sneller, M. Flanigan, J. A. Metcalf, R. E. Walker, J. Falloon, M. Baseler, R. Stevens, I. Feuerstein, H. Masur, and H. C. Lane. 1997. HIV infection induces changes in CD4+ T-cell phenotype and depletions within the CD4+ T-cell repertoire that are not immediately restored by antiviral or immune-based therapies. *Nature Med* **3**:533–540.

511. **Centers for Disease Control and Prevention.** 1995. Case-control of HIV seroconversion in health-care workers after percutaneous exposure to HIV-infected blood—France, United Kingdom, and United States, January 1988–August 1994. *Morbid Mortal Weekly Rep* **44**:949–953.

511a.Cole, K. S., J. L. Rowles, B. A. Jagerski, M. Murphey-Corb, T. Unangst, J. E. Clements, J. Robinson, M. S. Wyand, R. C. Desrosiers, and R. C. Montelaro. 1997. Evolution of envelope-specific antibody responses in monkeys experimentally infected or immunized with simian immunodeficiency virus and its association with the development of protective immunity. *J Virol* **71**:5069–5079.

512. Coombs, R. W., A. C. Collier, J.-P. Allain, B. Nikora, M. Leuther, G. F. Gjerset, and L. Corey. 1989. Plasma viremia in human immunodeficiency virus infection. *N Engl J Med* **321**:1626–1631.

513. Cooney, E. L., M. J. McElrath, L. Corey, S.-L. Hu, A. C. Collier, D. Arditti, M. Hoffman, G. E. Smith, and P. D. Greenberg. 1993. Enhanced immunity to human immunodeficiency virus (HIV) envelope elicited by a combined vaccine regimen consisting of priming with a vaccinia recombinant expressing HIV envelope and boosting with gp160 protein. *Proc Natl Acad Sci USA* **90**:1882–1886.

513a.Cooper, D. Personal communication.

514. Cooper, D. A., J. Gold, P. Maclean, B. Donovan, R. Finlayson, T. G. Barnes, H. M. Michelmore, P. Brooke, and R. Penny. 1985. Acute AIDS retrovirus infection: definition of a clinical illness associated with seroconversion. *Lancet* **i**:537–540.

515. Cooper, D. A., B. Tindall, E. J. Wilson, A. A. Imrie, and R. Penny. 1988. Characterization of

T lymphocyte responses during primary infection with human immunodeficiency virus. *J Inf Dis* **157**:889–896.

516. **Copeland, K. F. T., P. J. McKay, and K. L. Rosenthal.** 1995. Suppression of activation of the human immunodeficiency virus long terminal repeat by CD8+ T cells is not lentivirus specific. *AIDS Res Hum Retro* **11**:1321–1326.

517. **Copeland, K. F. T., P. J. McKay, and K. L. Rosenthal.** 1996. Suppression of the human immunodeficiency virus long terminal repeat by CD8+ T cells is dependent on the NFAT-1 element. *AIDS Res Hum Retro* **12**:143–148.

518. **Coppenhaver, D. H., P. Sriyuktasuth-Woo, S. Baron, C. E. Barr, and M. N. Qureshi.** 1994. Correlation of nonspecific antiviral activity with the ability to isolate infectious HIV-1 from saliva. *N Engl J Med* **330**:1314–1315.

519. **Corallini, A., G. Altavilla, L. Pozzi, F. Bignozzi, M. Negrini, P. Rimessi, F. Gualandi, and G. Barbanti-Brodano.** 1993. Systemic expression of HIV-1 *tat* gene in transgenic mice induces endothelial proliferation and tumors of different histotypes. *Cancer Res* **53**:5569–5575.

520. **Corapi, W. V., C. W. Olsen, and F. W. Scott.** 1992. Monoclonal antibody analysis of neutralization and antibody-dependent enhancement of feline infectious peritonitis virus. *J Virol* **66**:6695–6705.

521. **Corbeil, J., L. A. Evans, E. Vasak, D. A. Cooper, and R. Penny.** 1991. Culture and properties of cells derived from Kaposi's sarcoma. *J Immunol* **146**:2972–2976.

522. **Corbeil, J., M. Tremblay, and D. D. Richman.** 1996. HIV-induced apoptosis requires the CD4 receptor cytoplasmic tail and is accelerated by interaction of CD4 with p56lck. *J Exp Med* **183**:39–48.

523. **Corbellino, M., G. Bestetti, M. Galli, and C. Parravicini.** 1996. Absence of HHV-8 in prostate and semen. *N Engl J Med* **335**:1237.

524. **Corbellino, M., C. Parravicini, J. T. Aubin, and E. Berti.** 1996. Kaposi's sarcoma and herpesvirus-like DNA sequences in sensory ganglia. *N Engl J Med* **334**:1341–1342.

525. **Corboy, J. R., J. M. Buzy, M. C. Zink, and J. E. Clements.** 1992. Expression directed from HIV long terminal repeats in the central nervous system of transgenic mice. *Science* **258**:1804–1808.

526. **Cordonnier, A., L. Montagnier, and M. Emerman.** 1989. Single amino-acid changes in HIV envelope affect viral tropism and receptor binding. *Nature* **340**:571–574.

527. **Cordonnier, A., Y. Riviere, L. Montagnier, and M. Emerman.** 1989. Effects of mutations in hyperconserved regions of the extracellular glycoprotein of human immunodeficiency virus type 1 on receptor binding. *J Virol* **63**:4464–4468.

528. **Cornelissen, M., G. Kampinga, F. Zorgdrager, and J. Goudsmit.** 1996. Human immunodeficiency virus type 1 subtypes defined by *env* show high frequency of recombinant *gag* genes. *J Virol* **70**:8209–8212.

529. **Cornelissen, M., C. Kuiken, F. Zorgdrager, S. Hartman, and J. Goudsmit.** 1997. Gross defects in the *vpr* and *vpu* genes of HIV type 1 cannot explain the differences in RNA copy number between long-term asymptomatics and progressors. *AIDS Res Hum Retro* **13**:247–252.

530. **Cornelissen, M., G. Mulder-Kampinga, J. Veenstra, F. Zorgdrager, C. Kuiken, S. Hartman, J. Dekker, L. van der Hoek, C. Sol, R. Coutinho, and J. Goudsmit.** 1995. Syncytium-inducing (SI) phenotype suppression at seroconversion after intramuscular inoculation of a non-syncytium-inducing/SI phenotypically mixed human immunodeficiency virus population. *J Virol* **69**:1810–1818.

531. **Cossarizza, A.** 1997. T cell repertoire and HIV infection: facts and perspectives. *AIDS* **11**:1075–1088.

532. **Cossarizza, A., C. Ortolani, C. Mussini, G. Guaraldi, N. Mongiardo, V. Borghi, D. Barbieri, E. Bellesia, M. G. Franceschini, B. De Rienzo, and C. Franceschi.** 1995. Lack of selective Vβ deletion in CD4+ or CD8+ T lymphocytes and functional integrity of T-cell repertoire during acute HIV syndrome. *AIDS* **9**:547–553.

533. **Costa, J., and A. S. Rabson.** 1983. Generalised Kaposi's sarcoma is not a neoplasm. *Lancet* **i**:58.

534. Courgnaud, V., F. Laure, A. Brossard, A. Goudeau, F. Barin, and C. Brechot. 1991. Frequent and early *in utero* HIV-1 infection. *AIDS Res Hum Retro* **7**:337–341.

535. Cranage, M. P., N. Polyanskaya, B. McBride, N. Cook, L. A. E. Ashworth, M. Dennis, A. Baskerville, P. J. Greenaway, T. Corcoran, P. Kitchin, J. Rose, M. Murphy-Corb, R. C. Desrosiers, E. J. Stott, and G. H. Farrar. 1993. Studies on the specificity of the vaccine effect elicited by inactivated simian immunodeficiency virus. *AIDS Res Hum Retro* **9**:13–22.

536. Cranage, M. P., A. M. Whatmore, S. A. Sharpe, N. Polyanskaya, S. Leech, J. D. Smith, E. W. Rud, M. J. Dennis, and G. A. Hall. 1997. Macaques infected with live attenuated SIVmac are protected against superinfection via the rectal mucosa. *Virol* **229**:143–154.

537. Crawford, T. B., D. S. Adams, W. P. Cheevers, and L. C. Cork. 1980. Chronic arthritis in goats caused by a retrovirus. *Science* **207**:997–999.

538. Cremer, K. J., S. B. Spring, and J. Gruber. 1990. Role of human immunodeficiency virus type 1 and other viruses in malignancies associated with acquired immunodeficiency disease syndrome. *JNCI* **82**:1016–1024.

539. Cremoni, L., L. L. Vaira, P. D'Amico, M. G. Grassi, and F. Milazzo. 1993. Does zidovudine reduce tumor necrosis factor-alpha in HIV-positive patients? *AIDS* **7**:128–129.

540. Crise, B., L. Buonocore, and J. K. Rose. 1990. CD4 is retained in the endoplasmic reticulum by the human immunodeficiency virus type 1 glycoprotein precursor. *J Virol* **64**:5585–5593.

541. Crise, B., and J. K. Rose. 1992. Human immunodeficiency virus type 1 glycoprotein precursor retains a CD4-p56^{lck} complex in the endoplasmic reticulum. *J Virol* **66**:2296–2301.

542. Crook, T., D. Wrede, J. Tidy, J. Scholefield, L. Crawford, and K. H. Vousden. 1991. Status of c-myc, p53 and retinoblastoma genes in human papillomavirus positive and negative squamous cell carcinomas of the anus. *Oncogene* **6**:1251–1257.

543. Crowe, S., J. Mills, and M. S. McGrath. 1987. Quantitative immunocytofluorographic analysis of CD4 surface antigen expression and HIV infection of human peripheral blood monocyte-macrophages. *AIDS Res Hum Retro* **3**:135–145.

544. Crowley, R. W., P. Secchiero, D. Zella, A. Cara, R. C. Gallo, and P. Lusso. 1996. Interference between human herpesvirus 7 and HIV-1 in mononuclear phagocytes. *J Immunol* **156**:2004–2008.

545. Cruikshank, W. W., D. M. Center, N. Nisar, M. Wu, B. Natke, A. C. Theodore, and H. Kornfeld. 1994. Molecular and functional analysis of a lymphocyte chemoattractant factor: association of biologic function with CD4 expression. *Proc Nat Acad Sci USA* **91**:5109–5113.

546. Cullen, B. R. 1994. The role of Nef in the replication cycle of the human and simian immunodeficiency viruses. *Virol* **205**:1–6.

547. Cullen, B. R., and W. C. Greene. 1990. Functions of the auxiliary gene products of the human immunodeficiency virus type 1. *Virol* **178**:1–5.

548. Cunningham, A. L., D. E. Dwyer, J. Mills, and L. Montagnier. 1997. Structure and function of HIV, p. 17–21. *In* G. Stewart (ed.), *Managing HIV*. **164**:17–21.

549. Curtis, B. M., S. Scharnowske, and A. J. Watson. 1992. Sequence and expression of a membrane-associated C-type lectin that exhibits CD4-independent binding of human immunodeficiency virus envelope glycoprotein gp120. *Proc Natl Acad Sci USA* **89**:8356–8360.

550. Cvetkovich, T. A., E. Lazar, B. M. Blumberg, Y. Saito, T. A. Eskin, R. Reichman, D. A. Baram, C. del Cerro, H. E. Gendelman, M. del Cerro, and L. G. Epstein. 1992. Human immunodeficiency virus type 1 infection of neural xenografts. *Proc Natl Acad Sci USA* **89**:5162–5166.

551. D'Andrea, A., M. Aste-Amezaga, N. M. Valiante, X. Ma, M. Kubin, and G. Trinchieri. 1993. Interleukin 10 (IL-10) inhibits human lymphocyte interferon gamma-production by suppressing natural killer cell stimulatory factor/IL-12 synthesis in accessory cells. *J Exp Med* **178**:1041–1048.

552. d'Cruz-Grote, D. 1996. Prevention of HIV infection in developing countries. *Lancet* **348**:1071–1074.

553. D'Souza, M. P., P. Durda, C. V. Hanson, and G. Milman. 1991. Evaluation of monoclonal antibodies to HIV-1 by neutralization and serological assays: an international collaboration. *AIDS* **5**:1061–1070.

554. da Silva, M., M. M. Shevchuck, W. J. Cronin, N. A. Armenakas, M. Tannenbaum, J. A. Fracchia, and H. L. Ioachim. 1989. Detection of HIV-related protein in testes and prostates of patients with AIDS. *Am J Clin Path* **93**:196–201.

555. Daar, E. S., T. Chernyavskiy, J.-Q. Zhao, P. Krogstad, I. S. Y. Chen, and J. A. Zack. 1995. Sequential determination of viral load and phenotype in human immunodeficiency virus type 1 infection. *AIDS Res Hum Retro* **11**:3–9.

556. Daar, E. S., and D. D. Ho. 1991. Relative resistance of primary HIV-1 isolates to neutralization by soluble CD4. *Am J Med* **90**:22s-26s.

557. Daar, E. S., T. Moudgil, R. D. Meyer, and D. D. Ho. 1991. Transient high levels of viremia in patients with primary human immunodeficiency virus type 1 infection. *N Engl J Med* **324**:961–964.

558. Dadaglio, G., S. Garcia, L. Montagnier, and M. L. Gougeon. 1994. Selective anergy of V beta 8+ T cells in human immunodeficiency virus-infected individuals. *J Exp Med* **179**:413–424.

559. Dadaglio, G., F. Michel, P. Langlade-Demoyen, P. Sansonetti, D. Chevrier, F. Vuillier, F. Plata, and A. Hoffenbach. 1992. Enhancement of HIV-specific cytotoxic T lymphocyte responses by zidovudine (AZT) treatment. *Clin Exp Immunol* **87**:7–14.

560. Dahl, K., K. Martin, and G. Miller. 1987. Differences among human immunodeficiency virus strains in their capacities to induce cytolysis of persistent infection or a lymphoblastoid cell line immortalized by Epstein-Barr virus. *J Virol* **61**:1602–1608.

561. Dahl, K. E., T. Burrage, F. Jones, and G. Miller. 1990. Persistent nonproductive infection of Epstein-Barr virus-transformed human B lymphocytes by human immunodeficiency virus type 1. *J Virol* **64**:1771–1783.

562. Dai, L.-C., K. West, R. Littaua, K. Takahashi, and F. A. Ennis. 1992. Mutation of human immunodeficiency virus type 1 at amino acid 585 on gp41 results in loss of killing by CD8+ A24-restricted cytotoxic T lymphocytes. *J Virol* **66**:3151–3154.

563. Dalgleish, A. G., P. C. Beverley, P. R. Clapham, D. H. Crawford, M. F. Greaves, and R. A. Weiss. 1984. The CD4 (T4) antigen is an essential component of the receptor for the AIDS retrovirus. *Nature* **312**:763–767.

564. Dalgleish, A. G., T. C. Chahn, R. C. Kennedy, P. Kanda, P. R. Clapham, and R. A. Weiss. 1988. Neutralization of diverse HIV-1 strains by monoclonal antibodies raised against a gp41 synthetic peptide. *Virol* **165**:209–215.

565. Dalgleish, A. G., B. J. Thomson, T. C. Chanh, M. Malkovsky, and R. C. Kennedy. 1987. Neutralisation of HIV isolates by anti-idiotypic antibodies which mimic the T4 (CD4) epitope: a potential AIDS vaccine. *Lancet* **ii**:1047–1049.

566. Dalgleish, A. G., S. Wilson, M. Gompels, C. Ludlam, B. Gazzard, A. M. Coates, and J. Habeshaw. 1992. T-cell receptor variable gene products and early HIV-1 infection. *Lancet* **339**:824–828.

567. Daling, J. R., N. S. Weiss, L. L. Klopfenstein, L. E. Cochran, W. H. Chow, and R. Daifuku. 1982. Correlates of homosexual behavior and the incidence of anal cancer. *J Am Med Assoc* **247**:1988–1990.

568. Dalsgaard, K., A. Uttenthal, T. D. Jones, F. Xu, A. Merryweather, W. D. O. Hamilton, J. P. M. Langeveld, R. S. Boshuizen, S. Kamstrup, G. P. Lomonossoff, C. Porta, C. Vela, J. I. Casal, R. H. Meloen, and P. B. Rodgers. 1997. Plant-derived vaccine protects target animals against a viral disease. *Nature Biotechnol* **15**:248–252.

568a. Daluge, S. M., S. S. Good, M. B. Faletto, W. H. Miller, M. H. St. Clair, L. R. Boone, M. Tisdale, N. R. Parry, J. E. Reardon, R. E. Dornsife, D. R. Averett, and T. A. Krenitsky. 1997. 1592U89, a novel carbocyclic nucleoside analog with potent, selective anti-human immunodeficiency virus activity. *Antimicrob Agents Chemo* **41**:1082–1093.

569. Daniel, M. D., F. Kirchhoff, P. K. Czajak, P. K. Sehgal, and R. C. Desrosiers. 1992. Protective effects of a live attenuated SIV vaccine with a deletion in the *nef* gene. *Science* **258**:1938–1941.

570. Daniel, M. D., N. L. Letvin, N. W. King, M. Kannagi, P. K. Sehgal, R. D. Hunt, P. J. Kanki, M. Essex, and R. C. Desrosiers. 1985. Isolation of T-cell tropic HTLV-III-like retrovirus from macaques. *Science* **228**:1201–1204.

571. Daniel, M. D., G. P. Mazzara, M. A. Simon, P. K. Sehgal, T. Kodama, D. L. Panicali, and R. C. Desrosiers. 1994. High-titer immune respones elicted by recombinant vaccinia virus priming and particle boosting are ineffective in preventing virulent SIV infection. *AIDS Res Hum Retro* **10**:839–851.

572. Dantzer, R., and K. W. Kelley. 1989. Stress and immunity: an integrated view of relationships between the brain and the immune system. *Life Sci* **44**:1995–2008.

573. Darby, S. C., D. W. Ewart, P. L. F. Giangrande, R. J. D. Spooner, and C. R. Rizza. 1996. Importance of age at infection with HIV-1 for survival and development of AIDS in UK haemophilia population. *Lancet* **347**:1573–1579.

574. Darko, D. F., J. C. Miller, C. Gallen, J. White, J. Koziol, S. J. Brown, R. Hayduk, J. H. Atkinson, J. Assmus, D. T. Munnell, P. Naitoh, J. A. McCutchan, and M. M. Mitler. 1995. Sleep electroencephalogram delta-frequency amplitude, night plasma levels of tumor necrosis factor-alpha, and human immunodeficiency virus infection. *Proc Natl Acad Sci USA* **92**:12080–12084.

575. Davey, R. T., Jr., D. G. Chaitt, S. C. Piscitelli, M. Wells, J. A. Kovacs, R. E. Walker, J. Falloon, M. A. Polis, J. A. Metcalf, H. Masur, G. Fyfe, and H. C. Lane. 1997. Subcutaneous administration of interleukin-2 in human immunodeficiency virus type 1-infected persons. *J Inf Dis* **175**:781–789.

576. Davis, B. R., D. H. Schwartz, J. C. Marx, C. E. Johnson, J. M. Berry, J. Lyding, T. C. Merigan, and A. Zander. 1991. Absent or rare human immunodeficiency virus infection of bone marrow stem/progenitor cells *in vivo*. *J Virol* **65**:1985–1990.

577. Davis, D., D. M. Stephens, C. Willers, and P. J. Lachmann. 1990. Glycosylation governs the binding of antipeptide antibodies to regions of hypervariable amino acid sequence within recombinant gp120 of human immunodeficiency virus type 1. *J Gen Virol* **71**:2889–2898.

578. Davis, D. A., R. W. Humphrey, F. M. Newcomb, T. R. O'Brien, J. J. Goedert, S. E. Straus, and R. Yarchoan. 1997. Detection of serum antibodies to a Kaposi's sarcoma-associated herpesvirus-specific peptide. *J Inf Dis* **175**:1071–1079.

579. Davis, L. E., B. L. Hjelle, V. E. Miller, D. L. Palmer, A. L. Llewellyn, T. L. Merlin, S. A. Young, R. G. Mills, W. Wachsman, and C. A. Wiley. 1992. Early viral brain invasion in iatrogenic human immunodeficiency virus infection. *Neurol* **42**:1736–1739.

580. Davis, M. G., S. C. Kenney, J. Kamine, J. S. Pagano, and E.-S. Huang. 1987. Immediate-early gene region of human cytomegalovirus trans-activates the promoter of human immunodeficiency virus. *Proc Natl Acad Sci USA* **84**:8642–8646.

581. Dawson, V. L., T. M. Dawson, G. R. Uhl, and S. H. Snyder. 1993. Human immunodeficiency virus type 1 coat protein neurotoxicity mediated by nitric oxide in primary cortical cultures. *Proc Natl Acad Sci USA* **90**:3256–3259.

582. Dayton, A. J., J. G. Sodroski, and C. A. Rosen. 1986. The *trans*-activator gene of the human T-cell lymphotropic virus type III is required for replication. *Cell* **4**:941–947.

583. De Andreis, C., G. Simoni, C. Castagna, L. Sacchi, S. M. Sirchia, I. Garagiola, T. Persico, P. Serafini, G. Pardi, and A. E. Semprini. 1997. Absence of detectable maternal DNA and identification of proviral HIV in the cord blood of two infants who became HIV-infected. *AIDS* **11**:840–841.

584. De Andreis, C., G. Simoni, F. Rossella, C. Castagna, E. Pesenti, G. Porta, G. Colucci, S. Giuntelli, G. Pardi, and A. E. Semprini. 1996. HIV-1 proviral DNA polymerase chain reaction detection in chorionic villi after exclusion of maternal contamination by variable number of tandem repeats analysis. *AIDS* **10**:711–715.

585. De Cock, K. M., G. Adjoriolo, E. Ekpini, T. Sibailly, J. Kouadio, M. Maran, K. Brattegaard, K. M. Vetter, R. Doorly, and H. D. Gayle. 1993. Epidemiology and transmission of HIV-2: why there is no HIV-2 pandemic. *J Am Med Assoc* **270**:2083–2086.

586. de Gast, G. C., L. F. Verdonck, J. M. Middeldorp, T. H. The, A. Hekker, J. A. van den Linden, H. A. J. G. Kreeft, and B. J. E. G. Bast. 1985. Recovery of T cell subsets after autologous bone marrow transplantation is mainly due to proliferation of mature T cells in the graft. *Blood* **66**:428–431.

587. de Jong, A. L., D. M. Green, J. A. Trial, and H. H. Birdsall. 1996. Focal effects of mononu-

clear leukocyte transendothelial migration: TNF-α production by migrating monocytes promotes subsequent migration of lymphocytes. *J Leukoc Biol* **60**:129–136.

588. de Jong, J.-J., A. de Ronde, W. Keulen, M. Tersmette, and J. Goudsmit. 1992. Minimal requirements for the human immunodeficiency virus type 1 V3 domain to support the syncytium-inducing phenotype: analysis by single amino acid substitution. *J Virol* **66**:6777–6780.

589. de Jong, J.-J., J. Goudsmit, W. Keulen, B. Klaver, W. Krone, M. Tersmette, and A. De Ronde. 1992. Human immunodeficiency virus type 1 clones chimeric for the envelope V3 domain differ in syncytium formation and replication capacity. *J Virol* **66**:757–765.

590. de la Monte, S. M., D. H. Gabuzda, D. D. Ho, R. H. Brown, Jr., E. T. Hedley-Whyte, R. T. Schooley, M. S. Hirsch, and A. K. Bhan. 1988. Peripheral neuropathy in the acquired immunodeficiency syndrome. *Ann Neurol* **23**:485–492.

591. De Luca, A., L. Teofile, A. Antinori, M. S. Iovino, P. Mencarini, E. Visconti, E. Tamburrini, G. Leone, and L. Ortona. 1993. Haemopoietic CD34+ progenitor cells are not infected by HIV-1 *in vivo* but show impaired clonogenesis. *Br J Haematol* **85**:20–24.

592. de Maria, A., C. Cirillo, and L. Moretta. 1994. Occurrence of human immunodeficiency virus type 1 (HIV-1)-specific cytolytic T cell activity in apparently uninfected children born to HIV-1-infected mothers. *J Inf Dis* **170**:1296–1299.

593. de Maria, A., G. Pantaleo, S. M. Schnittman, J. J. Greenhouse, M. Baseler, J. M. Orenstein, and A. S. Fauci. 1991. Infection of CD8+ T lymphocytes with HIV. Requirement for interaction with infected CD4+ cells and induction of infectious virus from chronically infected CD8+ cells. *J Immunol* **146**:2220–2226.

594. de Martino, M., P. A. Tovo, L. Galli, and C. Gabiano. 1994. Features of children perinatally infected with HIV-1 surviving longer than 5 years. *Lancet* **343**:191–195.

595. de Ronde, A., B. Kalver, W. Keulen, L. Smit, and J. Goudsmit. 1992. Natural HIV-1 *nef* accelerates virus replication in primary human lymphocytes. *Virol* **188**:391–395.

596. De Rossi, A., S. Masiero, C. Giaquinto, E. Ruga, M. Comar, M. Giacca, and L. Chieco-Bianchi. 1996. Dynamics of viral replication in infants with vertically acquired human immunodeficiency virus type 1 infection. *J Clin Invest* **97**:323–330.

597. De Rossi, A., L. Ometto, F. Mammano, C. Zanotto, C. Giaquinto, and L. Chieco-Bianchi. 1992. Vertical transmission of human immunodeficiency virus type 1 (HIV-1): lack of detectable virus in peripheral blood cells of infected children at birth. *AIDS* **6**:1117–1120.

598. De Rossi, A., M. Pasti, F. Mammano, L. Ometto, C. Giaquinto, and L. Chieco-Bianchi. 1991. Perinatal infection by human immunodeficiency virus type 1 (HIV-1): relationship between proviral copy number *in vivo*, viral properties *in vitro*, and clinical outcome. *J Med Virol* **35**:283–289.

599. De Santis, C., P. Robbioni, R. Longhi, L. Lopalco, A. G. Siccardi, A. Beretta, and N. J. Roberts, Jr. 1993. Cross-reactive response to human immunodeficiency virus type 1 (HIV-1) gp120 and HLA class I heavy chains induced by receipt of HIV-1-derived envelope vaccines. *J Inf Dis* **168**:1396–1403.

600. De Vincenzi, I. 1994. A longitudinal study of human immunodeficiency virus transmission by heterosexual partners. *N Engl J Med* **331**:341–346.

601. De Vincenzi, I., R. A. Ancell-Park, J. B. Brunet, P. Costigliola, E. Ricchi, F. Chiodo, A. Roumeliotou, G. Papaevengelou, R. A. Coutinhi, and H. J. A. van Haastrecht. 1992. Comparison of female to male and male to female transmission of HIV in 563 stable couples. *Brit Med J* **304**:809–813.

602. de Vreese, K., V. Kofler-Mongold, C. Leutgeb, V. Weber, K. Vermeire, S. Schacht, J. Anne, E. de Clercq, R. Datema, and G. Werner. 1996. The molecular target of bicyclams, potent inhibitors of human immunodeficiency virus replication. *J Virol* **70**:689–696.

603. de Waal Malefyt, R., H. Yssel, M.-G. Roncarolo, H. Spits, and J. E. de Vries. 1992. Interleukin-10. *Curr Opin Immunol* **4**:314–320.

604. de Wolf, F., R. H. Meloen, M. Bakker, F. Barin, and J. Goudsmit. 1991. Characterization of human antibody-binding sites on the external envelope of human immunodeficiency virus type 2. *J Gen Virol* **72**:1261–1267.

604a. de Wolf, F. J., M. A. Lange, and T. M. Houweling. 1988. Numbers of CD4$^+$ cells and the levels of core antigens and of antibodies to the human immunodeficiency virus as predictors of AIDS among seropositive homosexual men. *J Inf Dis* **158**:615–622.

605. Deacon, N. J., A. Tsykin, A. Solomon, K. Smith, M. Ludford-Menting, D. J. Hooker, D. A. McPhee, A. L. Greenway, A. Ellett, C. Chatfield, V. A. Lawson, S. Crowe, A. Maerz, S. Sonza, J. Learmont, J. S. Sullivan, A. Cunningham, D. Dwyer, D. Dowton, and J. Mills. 1995. Genomic structure of an attenuated quasi species of HIV-1 from a blood transfusion donor and recipients. *Science* **270**:988–991.

606. Dean, G. A., G. H. Reubel, and N. C. Pedersen. 1996. Simian immunodeficiency virus infection of CD8$^+$ lymphocytes in vivo. *J Virol* **70**:5646–5650.

607. Dean, M., M. Carrington, C. Winkler, G. A. Huttley, M. W. Smith, R. Allikmets, J. J. Goedert, S. P. Buchbinder, E. Vittinghoff, E. Gomperts, S. Donfield, D. Vlahov, R. Kaslow, A. Saah, C. Rinaldo, R. Detels, and S. J. O'Brien. 1996. Genetic restriction of HIV-1 infection and progression to AIDS by a deletion allele of the CKR5 structural gene. *Science* **273**:1856–1862.

608. Dean, N. C., J. A. Golden, L. Evans, M. L. Warnock, T. E. Addison, P. C. Hopewell, and J. A. Levy. 1988. Human immunodeficiency virus recovery from bronchoaveolar lavage fluid in patients with AIDS. *Chest* **93**:1176–1179.

609. DeCarli, C., L. Fugate, J. Falloon, J. Eddy, D. A. Katz, R. P. Friedland, S. I. Rapoport, P. Brouwers, and P. A. Pizzo. 1991. Brain growth and cognitive improvement in children with human immunodeficiency virus-induced encephalopathy after 6 months of continuous infusion zidovudine therapy. *J AIDS* **4**:585–592.

610. Deeks, S. G., A. Collier, J. Lalezari, A. Pavia, D. Rodrigue, W. L. Drew, J. Toole, H. S. Jaffe, A. S. Mulato, P. D. Lamy, W. Li, J. M. Cherrington, N. Hellmann, and J. Kahn. The safety and efficacy of adefovir dipivoxil, a novel anti-HIV therapy, in HIV infected adults. *J Inf Dis* in press.

610a. Deeks, S. G., R. L. Coleman, R. White, C. Pachl, M. Schambelan, D. N. Chernoff, and M. B. Feinberg. 1997. Variance of plasma human immunodeficiency virus type 1 RNA levels measured by branched DNA within and between days. *J Inf Dis* **176**:514–517.

610b. Deeks, S. G., R. Loftus, P. Cohen, S. Chin, and R. Grant. 1997. Incidence and predictors of virologic failure of indinavir and/or ritonavir in an urban health clinic., abstr. LB-02. *37th Interscience Conference on Antimicrobial Agents and Chemotherapy,*

611. Deeks, S. G., M. Smith, M. Holodniy, and J. O. Kahn. 1997. HIV-1 protease inhibitors. *J Am Med Assoc* **277**:145–153.

612. Del Prete, G., M. De Carli, F. Almerigogna, M. G. Giudizi, R. Biagiotti, and S. Romagnani. 1993. Human IL-10 is produced by both type 1 helper (Th1) and type 2 helper (Th2) T cell clones and inhibits their antigen-specific proliferation and cytokine production. *J Immunol* **150**:353–360.

613. Del Prete, G. F., M. De Carli, M. Ricci, and S. Romagnani. 1991. Helper activity for immunoglobulin synthesis of T helper type 1 (Th1) and Th2 human T cell clones: the help of Th1 clones is limited by their cytolytic capacity. *J Exp Med* **174**:809–813.

613a. Delamare, C., M. Burgard, M. J. Mayaux, S. Blanche, A. Doussin, S. Ivanoff, M. L. Chaix, C. Khan, and C. Rouzioux. 1997. HIV-1 RNA detection in plasma for the diagnosis of infection in neonates. *J AIDS Hum Retrovirol* **15**:121–125.

614. Delassus, S., R. Cheynier, and S. Wain-Hobson. 1991. Evolution of human immunodeficiency virus type 1 *nef* and long terminal repeat sequences over 4 years in vivo and in vitro. *J Virol* **65**:225–231.

615. Delezay, O., N. Koch, N. Yahi, D. Hammache, C. Tourres, C. Tamalet, and J. Fantini. 1997. Co-expression of CXCR4/fusin and galactosyl ceramide in the human intestinal epithelial cell line HT-29. *AIDS* **11**:1311–1318.

616. Delwart, E. L., H. W. Sheppard, B. D. Walker, J. Goudsmit, and J. I. Mullins. 1994. Human immunodeficiency virus type 1 evolution in vivo tracked by DNA heteroduplex mobility assays. *J Virol* **68**:6672–6683.

617. Delwart, E. L., E. G. Shpaer, J. Louwagie, F. E. McCutchan, M. Grez, H. Rubsamen-Waig-

mann, and J. I. Mullins. 1993. Genetic relationships determined by a DNA heteroduplex mobility assay: analysis of HIV-1 env genes. *Science* **262**:1257–1261.

617a. Deml, L. G. Kratochwil, N. Osterrieder, R. Knuchel, H. Wolf, and R. Wagner. 1997. Increased incorporation of chimeric human immunodeficiency virus type 1 gp 320 proteins into Pr55^{gag} virus-like particles by an Epstein-Barr gp220/350-derived transmembrane domain. *Virol* **235**:10–25.

618. Deng, H., R. Liu, W. Ellmeier, S. Choe, D. Unutmaz, M. Burkhart, P. Di Marzio, S. Marmon, R. E. Sutton, C. M. Hill, C. B. Davis, S. C. Peiper, T. J. Schall, D. R. Littman, and N. R. Landau. 1996. Identification of a major co-receptor for primary isolates of HIV-1. *Nature* **381**:661–666.

618a. Deng, H., D. Unutmaz, V. N. KewalRamani, and D. R. Littman. 1997. Expression cloning of new receptors used by simian and human immunodeficiency viruses. *Nature* **388**:296–300.

619. deRossi, A., G. Franchini, A. Aldovini, A. del Mistro, L. Chieco-Bianchi, R. C. Gallo, and F. Wong-Staal. 1986. Differential response to the cytopathic effects of human T-cell lymphotropic virus type III (HTLV-III) superinfection in T4+ (helper) and T8+ (suppressor) T-cell clones transformed by HTLV-I. *Proc Natl Acad Sci USA* **83**:4297–4301.

620. Des Jarlais, D. C., S. R. Friedman, and W. Hopkins. 1985. Risk reduction for the acquired immunodeficiency syndrome among intravenous drug users. *Ann Int Med* **103**:755–759.

621. Des Jarlais, D. C., S. R. Friedman, D. M. Novick, J. L. Sotheran, P. Thomas, S. R. Yancovitz, D. Mildvan, J. Weber, M. J. Kreek, R. Maslansky, S. Bartelme, T. Spira, and M. Marmor. 1989. HIV-1 infection among intravenous drug users in Manhattan, New York City, from 1977 through 1987. *J Am Med Assoc* **261**:1008–1012.

622. Des Jarlais, D. C., M. Marmor, D. Paone, S. Titus, Q. Shi, T. Perlis, B. Jose, and S. R. Friedman. 1996. HIV incidence among injecting drug users in New York City syringe-exchange programmes. *Lancet* **148**:987–991.

623. Desai, K., P. M. Loewenstein, and M. Green. 1991. Isolation of a cellular protein that binds to the human immunodeficiency virus *tat* protein and can potentiate transactivation of the viral promoter. *Proc Natl Acad Sci USA* **88**:8875–8879.

623a. Desrosiers, R. Personal communication.

624. Desrosiers, R. C., M. S. Wyand, T. Kodama, D. J. Ringler, L. O. Arthur, P. K. Sehgal, N. L. Letvin, N. W. King, and M. D. Daniel. 1989. Vaccine protection against simian immunodeficiency virus infection. *Proc Natl Acad Sci USA* **86**:6353–6357.

625. Dewar, R. L., H. C. Highbarger, M. D. Sarmiento, J. A. Todd, M. B. Vasudevachari, R. T. Davey, Jr., J. A. Kovacs, N. P. Salzman, H. C. Lane, and M. S. Urdea. 1994. Application of branched DNA signal amplification to monitor human immunodeficiency virus type 1 burden in human plasma. *J Inf Dis* **170**:1172–1179.

626. Dezube, B. J., A. B. Pardee, B. Chapman, L. A. Beckett, J. A. Korvick, W. J. Novick, J. Chiurco, P. Kasdan, C. M. Ahlers, L. T. Ecto, and C. S. Crumpacker. 1993. Pentoxifylline decreases tumor necrosis factor expression and serum triglycerides in people with AIDS. *J AIDS* **6**:787–794.

627. Dhawan, S., B. S. Weeks, C. Soderland, H. W. Schnaper, L. A. Toro, S. P. Asthana, I. K. Hewlett, W. G. Stetler-Stevenson, S. S. Yamada, K. M. Yamada, and M. S. Meltzer. 1995. HIV-1 infection alters monocyte interactions with human microvascular endothelial cells. *J Immunol* **154**:422–432.

628. Di Alberti, L., S. L. Ngui, S. R. Porter, P. M. Speight, C. M. Scully, J. M. Zakrewska, I. G. Williams, L. Artese, A. Piattelli, and C. G. Teo. 1997. Presence of human herpesvirus 8 variants in the oral tissues of human immunodeficiency virus-infected persons. *J Inf Dis* **175**:703–707.

629. Di Stefano, M., F. Sabri, T. Leitner, B. Svennerholm, L. Hagberg, G. Norkrans, and F. Chiodi. 1995. Reverse transcriptase sequence of paired isolates of cerebrospinal fluid and blood from patients infected with human immunodeficiency virus type 1 during zidovudine treatment. *J Clin Micro* **33**:352–355.

630. Diamond, D. C., B. P. Sleckman, T. Gregory, L. A. Lasky, J. L. Greenstein, and S. J. Burakoff. 1988. Inhibition of CD4+ T cell function by the HIV envelope protein, gp120. *J Immunol* **141**:3715–3717.

630a. Diaz, R. S., L. Zhang, M. P. Busch, J. W. Mosley, and A. Mayer. 1997. Divergence of HIV-1 quasispecies in an epidemiologic cluster. *AIDS* 11:415–422.

631. Diaz, R. S., E. C. Sabino, A. Mayer, C. F. deOliveira, J. W. Mosley, and M. P. Busch. 1996. Lack of dual HIV infection in a transfusion recipient exposed to two seropositive blood components. *AIDS Res Hum Retro* 12:1291–1295.

632. Dickover, R. E., E. M. Garratty, S. A. Herman, M.-S. Sim, S. Plaeger, P. J. Boyer, M. Keller, A. Deveikis, E. R. Stiehm, and Y. J. Bryson. 1996. Identification of levels of maternal HIV-1 RNA associated with risk of perinatal transmission. *J Am Med Assoc* 275:599–605.

633. Diegel, M. L., P. A. Moran, L. K. Gilliland, N. K. Damle, M. S. Hayden, J. M. Zarling, and J. A. Ledbetter. 1993. Regulation of HIV production by blood mononuclear cells from HIV-infected donors II. HIV-1 production depends on T cell-monocyte interaction. *AIDS Res Hum Retro* 9:465–473.

634. Digiovanna, J. J., and B. Safai. 1981. Kaposi's sarcoma. Retrospective study of 90 cases with particular reference to the familial occurrence, ethnic background, and prevalence of other diseases. *Am J Med* 71:779–783.

635. Dikeacou, T., A. Katsambas, W. Lowenstein, C. Romana, A. Balamotis, P. Tsianakas, A. Carabinis, N. Renieri, N. Metaxotos, E. Fragouli, and J. Stratigos. 1992. Clinical manifestations of allergy and their relation to HIV infection. *Int Arch Allergy Immunol* 102:408–413.

636. Dimitrov, D. S., H. Golding, and R. Blumenthal. 1991. Initial stages of HIV-1 envelope glycoprotein-mediated cell fusion monitored by a new assay based on redistribution of fluorescent dyes. *AIDS Res Hum Retro* 7:799–805.

637. Dimitrov, D. S., R. L. Willey, M. A. Martin, and R. Blumenthal. 1992. Kinetics of HIV-1 interactions with sCD4 and CD4+ cells: implications for inhibition of virus infection and initial steps of virus entry into cells. *Virol* 187:398–406.

638. Dimitrov, D. S., R. L. Willey, H. Sato, L.-J. Chang, R. Blumenthal, and M. A. Martin. 1993. Quantitation of human immunodeficiency virus type 1 infection kinetics. *J Virol* 67:2182–2190.

639. Dimmock, N. J. 1982. Initial stages in infection with animal viruses. *J Gen Virol* 59:1–22.

640. Dimmock, N. J. 1995. Update on the neutralization of animal viruses. *Rev Med Virol* 5:163–179.

641. Dittmar, M. T., A. McNight, G. Simmons, P. R. Clapham, R. A. Weiss, and P. Simmonds. 1997. HIV-1 tropism and co-receptor use. *Nature* 385:495–496.

641a. Dittmar, M. T., G. Simmons, S. Hibbitts, M. O'Hare, S. Louisirirotchanakul, S. Beddows, J. Weber, P. R. Clapham, and R. A. Weiss. 1997. Langerhans cell tropism of human immunodeficiency virus type 1 subtype A through F isolates derived from different transmission groups. *J Virol* 71:8008–8013.

642. Dittmer, U., C. Stahl-Hennig, C. Coulibaly, T. Nisslein, W. Luke, D. Fuchs, W. Bodemer, H. Petry, and G. Hunsmann. 1995. Repeated exposure of rhesus macaques to low doses of simian immunodeficiency virus (SIV) did not protect them against the consequences of a high-dose SIV challenge. *J Gen Virol* 76:1307–1315.

643. Dobrescu, D., S. Kabak, K. Mehta, C. H. Suh, A. Asch, P. U. Cameron, A. S. Hodtsev, and D. N. Posnett. 1995. Human immunodeficiency virus 1 reservoir in CD4+ T cells is restricted to certain Vβ subsets. *Proc Natl Acad Sci USA* 92:5563–3367.

644. Doherty, P. C., B. B. Knowles, and P. J. Wettstein. 1984. Immunological surveillance of tumors in the context of major histocompatibility complex restriction of T cell function. *Adv Cancer Res* 42:1–65.

645. Dolei, A., C. Serra, M. V. Arca, and A. Toiolo. 1992. Acute HIV-1 infection of CD4+ human lung fibroblasts. *AIDS* 6:232–233.

646. Dolin, R., B. S. Graham, S. B. Greenberg, C. O. Tacket, R. B. Belshe, K. Midthun, M. L. Clements, G. J. Gorse, B. W. Horgan, R. L. Atmar, D. T. Larzon, W. Bonnez, B. F. Fernie, D. C. Montefiore, D. M. Stablein, G. E. Smith, and W. C. Koff. 1991. The safety and immunogenicity of a human immunodeficiency virus type 1 (HIV-1) recombinant gp160 candidate vaccine in humans. *Ann Int Med* 114:119–127.

647. Donahue, R. E., M. M. Johnson, L. I. Zon, S. C. Clark, and J. E. Groopman. 1987. Suppression of *in vitro* haematopoiesis following human immunodeficiency virus infection. *Nature* **326**:200–203.

648. Donaldson, Y. K., J. E. Bell, E. C. Holmes, E. S. Hughes, H. K. Brown, and P. Simmonds. 1994. In vivo distribution and cytopathology of variants of human immunodeficiency virus type 1 showing restricted sequence variability in the V3 loop. *J Virol* **68**:5991–6005.

649. Donegan, E., M. Stuart, J. C. Niland, H. S. Sacks, S. P. Azen, S. L. Dietrich, C. Faucett, M. A. Fletcher, S. H. Kleinman, and E. A. Operskalski. 1990. Infection with human immunodeficiency virus type 1 (HIV-1) among recipients of antibody-positive blood donations. *Ann Int Med* **113**:733–739.

649a. Donnelly, C., W. Leisenring, P. Kanki, T. Awerbuch, and S. Sandberg. 1993. Comparison of transmission rates of HIV-1 and HIV-2 in a cohort of prostitutes in Senegal. *Bull Math Biol* **55**:731–743.

650. Donovan, B. 1996. HIV-1 infection and the female genital tract. *Lancet* **348**:59–60.

651. Donovan, R. M., R. E. Dickover, E. Goldstein, R. G. Huth, and J. R. Carlson. 1991. HIV-1 proviral copy number in blood mononuclear cells from AIDS patients on zidovudine therapy. *J AIDS* **4**:766–769.

652. Doranz, B. J., J. Rucker, Y. Yi, R. J. Smyth, M. Samsom, S. C. Peiper, M. Parmentier, R. G. Collman, and R. W. Doms. 1996. A dual-tropic primary HIV-1 isolate that uses fusin and the β-chemokine receptors CKR-5, CKR-3, and CKR-2b as fusion cofactors. *Cell* **85**:1149–1158.

653. Dorrucci, M., G. Rezza, D. Vlahov, P. Pezzotti, A. Sinicco, A. Nicolosi, A. Lazzarins, N. Galai, S. Gafa, R. Pristera, and G. Angarano. 1995. Clinical characteristics and prognostic value of acute retroviral syndrome among injecting drug users. *AIDS* **9**:597–604.

654. Dorsett, B. H., W. Cronin, and H. L. Ioachim. 1990. Presence and prognostic significance of antilymphocyte antibodies in symptomatic and asymptomatic human immunodeficiency virus infection. *Arch Int Med* **150**:1025–1028.

655. Douglas, G. C., G. N. Fry, T. Thirkill, E. Holmes, H. Hakim, M. Jennings, and B. F. King. 1991. Cell-mediated infection of human placental trophoblast with HIV *in vitro*. *AIDS Res Hum Retro* **7**:735–740.

656. Dournon, E., S. Matheron, W. Rozenbaum, S. Gharakhanian, C. Michon, P. M. Girard, C. Perronne, D. Salmon, P. De Truchis, C. Leport, E. Bouvet, M. C. Dazza, M. Levacher, and B. Regnier. 1988. Effects of zidovudine in 365 consecutive patients with AIDS or AIDS-related complex. *Lancet* **ii**:1297–1302.

657. Douvas, A., Y. Takehana, G. Ehresmann, T. Chernyovskiy, and E. S. Daar. 1996. Neutralization of HIV type 1 infectivity by serum antibodies from a subset of autoimmune patients with mixed connective tissue disease. *AIDS Res Hum Retro* **12**:1509–1517.

658. Downs, A. M., and I. De Vincenzi. 1996. Probability of heterosexual transmission of HIV: relationship to the number of unprotected sexual contacts. *J AIDS Hum Retrovirol* **11**:388–395.

659. Dragic, T., and M. Alizon. 1993. Different requirements for membrane fusion mediated by the envelopes of human immunodeficiency virus types 1 and 2. *J Virol* **67**:2355–2359.

660. Dragic, T., P. Charneau, F. Clavel, and M. Alizon. 1992. Complementation of murine cells for human immunodeficiency virus envelope/CD4-mediated fusion in human/murine heterokaryons. *J Virol* **66**:4794–4802.

661. Dragic, T., V. Litwin, G. P. Allaway, S. R. Martin, Y. Huang, K. A. Nagashima, C. Cayanan, P. J. Maddon, R. A. M. Koup, J. P. Moore, and W. A. Paxton. 1996. HIV-1 entry into CD4+ cells is mediated by the chemokine receptor CC-CKR-5. *Nature* **381**:667–673.

662. Dragic, T., L. Picard, and M. Alizon. 1995. Proteinase-resistant factors in human erythrocyte membranes mediate CD4-dependent fusion with cells expressing human immunodeficiency virus type 1 envelope glycoproteins. *J Virol* **69**:1013–1018.

663. Dreesman, G. R., and R. C. Kennedy. 1985. Anti-idiotypic antibodies: Implications of internal image-based vaccines for infectious diseases. *J Inf Dis* **151**:761–765.

664. Dreyer, E. B., P. K. Kaiser, J. T. Offermann, and S. A. Lipton. 1990. HIV-1 coat protein neurotoxicity prevented by calcium channel antagonists. *Science* **248**:364–367.

665. Drummond, J. E., P. Mounts, R. J. Gorelick, J. R. Casas-Finet, W. J. Bosche, L. E. Henderson, D. J. Waters, and L. O. Arthur. 1997. Wild-type and mutant HIV type 1 nucleocapsid proteins increase the proportion of long cDNA transcripts by viral reverse transcriptase. *AIDS Res Hum Retro* **13**:533–543.

666. Drysdale, C. M., and G. N. Pavlakis. 1991. Rapid activation and subsequent down-regulation of the human immunodeficiency virus type 1 promoter in the presence of *tat*: possible mechanisms contributing to latency. *J Virol* **65**:3044–3051.

667. DuPont, H. L., and G. D. Marshall. 1995. HIV-associated diarrhea and wasting. *Lancet* **346**:352–356.

668. Duan, L., J. W. Oakes, A. Ferraro, O. Bagasra, and R. J. Pomerantz. 1994. Tat and Rev differentially affect restricted replication of human immunodeficiency virus type 1 in various cells. *Virol* **199**:474–478.

669. Dudhane, A., B. Conti, T. Orlikowsky, Z. Q. Wang, N. Mangla, A. Gupta, G. P. Wormser, and M. K. Hoffmann. 1996. Monocytes in HIV type 1-infected individuals lose expression of costimulatory B7 molecules and acquire cytotoxic activity. *AIDS Res Hum Retro* **12**:885–892.

670. Duesberg, P. H. 1992. AIDS acquired by drug consumption and other noncontagious risk factors. *Pharmacol Ther* **55**:201–277.

671. Duh, E. J., W. J. Maury, T. M. Folks, A. S. Fauci, and A. B. Rabson. 1989. Tumor necrosis factor alpha activates human immunodeficiency virus type 1 through induction of nuclear factor binding to the NF-kappa B sites in the long terminal repeat. *Proc Natl Acad Sci USA* **86**:5794–5978.

672. Duke, R. C., and J. J. Cohen. 1986. IL-2 addiction: withdrawal of growth factor activates a suicide program in dependent T cells. *Lymphokine Res* **5**:289–299.

673. Dukes, C. S., Y. Yu, E. D. Rivadeneira, D. L. Sauls, H.-X. Liao, B. F. Haynes, and J. B. Weinberg. 1995. Cellular CD44S as a determinant of human immunodeficiency virus type 1 infection and cellular tropism. *J Virol* **69**:4000–4005.

674. Dumitrescu, O., M. Kalish, S. C. Kliks, C. I. Bandea, and J. A. Levy. 1994. Characterization of HIV-1 strains isolated from children in Romania: identification of a new envelope subtype. *J Inf Dis* **169**:281–288.

675. Dunn, D. T., M. L. Newell, A. E. Ades, and C. S. Peckham. 1992. Risk of human immunodeficiency virus type 1 transmission through breastfeeding. *Lancet* **340**:585–588.

676. Dyda, F., A. B. Hickman, T. M. Jenkins, A. Engelman, R. Craigie, and D. R. Davies. 1994. Crystal structure of the catalytic domain of HIV-1 integrase: similarity to other polynucleotidyl transferases. *Science* **266**:1981–1986.

677. Dyson, N., P. M. Howley, K. Munger, and E. Harlow. 1989. The human papilloma virus-16 E7 oncoprotein is able to bind to the retinoblastoma gene product. *Science* **243**:934–937.

678. Earl, P. L., R. W. Doms, and B. Moss. 1992. Multimeric CD4 binding exhibited by human and simian immunodeficiency virus envelope protein dimers. *J Virol* **66**:5610–5614.

679. Earl, P. L., R. W. Doms, and B. Moss. 1990. Oligomeric structure of the human immunodeficiency virus type 1 envelope glycoprotein. *Proc Natl Acad Sci USA* **87**:648–652.

680. Eaton, A. M., T. Wildes, and J. A. Levy. 1994. An anti-gp41 human monoclonal antibody which enhances HIV-1 infection in the absence of complement. *AIDS Res Hum Retro* **10**:13–18.

681. Ebenbichler, C., P. Westervelt, A. Carrillo, T. Henkel, D. Johnson, and L. Ratner. 1993. Structure-function relationships of the HIV-1 envelope V3 loop tropism determinant: evidence for two distinct conformations. *AIDS* **7**:639–646.

682. Ebenbichler, C. F., C. Roder, R. Vornhagen, L. Ratner, and M. P. Dierich. 1993. Cell surface proteins binding to recombinant soluble HIV-1 and HIV-2 transmembrane proteins. *AIDS* **7**:489–495.

683. Ebenbichler, C. F., N. M. Thielens, R. Vornhagen, P. Marschang, G. J. Arlaud, and M. P. Dierich. 1991. Human immunodeficiency virus type 1 activates the classical pathway of complement by direct C1 binding through specific sites in the transmembrane glycoprotein gp41. *J Exp Med* **174**:1417–1424.

684. Edwards, J. R., P. P. Ulrich, P. S. Weintrub, M. J. Cowan, J. A. Levy, D. W. Wara, and G. N. Vyas. 1989. Polymerase chain reaction compared with concurrent viral cultures for rapid identification of human immunodeficiency virus infection among high-risk infants and children. *J Peds* 115:200–203.

685. Effros, R. B., R. Allsopp, C. P. Chiu, M. A. Hausner, K. Hirji, L. Wang, C. B. Harley, B. Villeponteau, M. D. West, and J. V. Giorgi. 1996. Shortened telomeres in the expanded CD28−CD8+ cell subset in HIV disease implicate replicative senescence in HIV pathogenesis. *AIDS* 10:F17-F22.

686. Egan, M. A., W. A. Pavlat, J. Tartaglia, E. Paoletti, K. J. Weinhold, M. L. Clements, and R. F. Siliciano. 1995. Induction of human immunodeficiency virus type 1 (HIV-1)-specific cytolytic T lymphocyte responses in seronegative adults by a nonreplicating, host-range-restricted canarypox vector (ALVAC) carrying the HIV-1$_{MN}$ env gene. *J Inf Dis* 171:1623–1627.

687. Ehrenreich, H., P. Rieckmann, F. Sinowatz, K. A. Weih, L. O. Arthur, F. D. Goebel, P. R. Burd, J. E. Coligan, and K. A. Clouse. 1993. Potent stimulation of monocytic endothelin-1 production by HIV-1 glycoprotein 120. *J Immunol* 150:4601–4609.

688. Ehret, A., M. O. Westendorp, I. Herr, K. M. Debatin, J. L. Heeney, R. Frank, and P. H. Krammer. 1996. Resistance of chimpanzee T cells to human immunodeficiency virus type 1 Tat-enhanced oxidative stress and apoptosis. *J Virol* 70:6502–6507.

689. Ehrnst, A., S. Lindgren, M. Dictor, B. Johansson, A. Sonnerborg, J. Czajkowski, G. Sundin, and A.-B. Bohlin. 1991. HIV in pregnant women and their offspring: evidence for late transmission. *Lancet* 338:203–207.

690. Ehrnst, A., A. Sonnerborg, S. Bergdahl, and O. Strannegard. 1988. Efficient isolation of HIV from plasma during different stages of HIV infection. *J Med Virol* 26:23–32.

691. Eigen, M., and K. Nieselt-Struwe. 1990. How old is the immunodeficiency virus? *AIDS* 4:S85-S93.

692. El-Amad, Z., K. K. Murthy, K. Higgins, E. K. Cobb, N. L. Haigwood, J. A. Levy, and K. S. Steimer. 1995. Resistance of chimpanzees immunized with recombinant gp120$_{SF2}$ to challenge by HIV-1$_{SF2}$. *AIDS* 9:1313–1322.

693. El-Daher, N., M. C. Keefer, R. C. Reichman, R. Dolin, and N. J. Roberts, Jr. 1993. Persisting human immunodeficiency virus type 1 gp160-specific human T lymphocyte responses including CD8+ cytotoxic activity after receipt of envelope vaccines. *J Inf Dis* 168:306–313.

694. Emau, P., H. M. McClure, M. Isahakia, J. G. Else, and P. N. Fultz. 1991. Isolation from African Sykes' monkeys (*Cercopithecus mitis*) of a lentivirus related to human and simian immunodeficiency viruses. *J Virol* 65:2135–2140.

695. Embretson, J., M. Zupancic, J. Beneke, M. Till, S. Wolinsky, J. L. Ribas, A. Burke, and A. T. Haase. 1993. Analysis of human immunodeficiency virus-infected tissues by amplification and *in situ* hybridization reveals latent and permissive infections at single-cell resolution. *Proc Natl Acad Sci USA* 90:357–361.

696. Embretson, J., M. Zupancic, J. L. Ribas, A. Burke, P. Racz, K. Tenner-Racz, and A. T. Haase. 1993. Massive covert infection of helper T lymphocytes and macrophages by HIV during the incubation period of AIDS. *Nature* 362:359–362.

697. Emerman, M. Personal communication.

698. Emery, S., and H. C. Lane. Immune reconstitution in HIV infection. *Curr Opin Immunol,* in press.

699. Emiliani, S., C. Van Lint, W. Fischle, P. Paras, Jr., M. Ott, J. Brady, and E. Verdin. 1996. A point mutation in the HIV-1 Tat responsive element is associated with postintegration latency. *Proc Natl Acad Sci USA* 93:6377–6381.

700. Emilie, D., M. Peuchmaur, M. C. Mailott, M. C. Crevon, N. Brousse, J. F. Delfraissy, J. Dormont, and P. Galanaud. 1990. Production of interleukins in human immunodeficiency virus-1-replicating lymph nodes. *J Clin Invest* 86:148–159.

701. Emini, E. A., W. A. Schleif, J. H. Nunberg, A. J. Conley, Y. Eda, S. Tokiyoshi, S. D. Putney, S. Matsushita, K. E. Cobb, C. M. Jett, J. W. Eichberg, and K. K. Murthy. 1992. Prevention of HIV-1 infection in chimpanzees by gp120 V3 domain-specific monoclonal antibody. *Nature* 355:728–730.

702. Endres, M. J., P. R. Clapham, M. Marsh, M. Ahuja, J. D. Turner, A. McKnight, J. F. Thomas, B. Stoebenau-Haggarty, S. Choe, P. J. Vance, T. N. C. Wells, C. A. Power, S. S. Sutterwala, R. W. Doms, N. R. Landau, and J. A. Hoxie. 1996. CD4-independent infection by HIV-2 is mediated by fusin/CXCR4. *Cell* **87**:745–756.

703. Engelman, A., G. Englund, J. M. Orenstein, M. A. Martin, and R. Craigie. 1995. Multiple effects of mutations in human immunodeficiency virus type 1 integrase on viral replication. *J Virol* **69**:2729–2736.

704. Ennen, J., I. Seipp, S. G. Norley, and R. Kurth. 1990. Decreased accessory cell function of macrophages after infection with human immunodeficiency virus type 1 *in vitro*. *Eur J Immunol* **20**:2451–2456.

705. Ensoli, B., G. Barillari, and S. K. Salahuddin. 1990. Tat protein of HIV-1 stimulates growth of cells derived from Kaposi's sarcoma-lesions of AIDS patients. *Nature* **345**:84–86.

706. Ensoli, B., R. Gendelman, P. Markham, V. Fiorelli, S. Colombini, M. Raffeld, A. Cafaro, H. K. Chang, J. N. Brady, and R. C. Gallo. 1994. Synergy between basic fibroblast growth factor and HIV-1 Tat protein in induction of Kaposi's sarcoma. *Nature* **371**:674–680.

707. Ensoli, B., S. Nakamura, and S. Z. Salahuddin. 1989. AIDS-Kaposi's sarcoma-derived cells express cytokines with autocrine and paracrine growth effects. *Science* **243**:223–226.

708. Ensoli, F., A. Cafaro, V. Fiorelli, B. Vannelli, B. Ensoli, and C. J. Thiele. 1995. HIV-1 infection of primary human neuroblasts. *Virol* **210**:221–225.

709. Epstein, L. G., C. Kuiken, B. M. Blumberg, S. Hartman, L. R. Sharer, M. Clement, and J. Goudsmit. 1991. HIV-1 V3 domain variation in brain and spleen of children with AIDS: tissue-specific evolution within host-determined quasispecies. *Virol* **180**:583–590.

710. Epstein, L. G., and L. R. Sharer. 1988. Neurology of human immunodeficiency virus infection in children, p. 70–101. *In* M. L. Rosenblum, R. M. Levy, and D. E. Bredesen (ed.), *AIDS and the Nervous System*. Raven Press, New York.

711. Epstein, M. A., and B. G. Achong. 1979. The relationship of the virus to Burkitt's lymphoma, p. 321–338. *In* M. A. Epstein and B. G. Achong (ed.), *The Epstein-Barr Virus*. Springer-Verlag, New York.

712. Erickson, J., D. J. Neidhart, J. VanDrie, D. J. Kempf, X.-C. Wang, D. W. Norbeck, J. J. Plattner, J. W. Rittenhouse, M. Turon, N. Wideburg, W. E. Kohlbrenner, R. Simmer, R. Helfrich, D. A. Paul, and M. Knigge. 1990. Design, activity, and 2.8 angstrom crystal structure of a C2 symmetric inhibitor complexed to HIV-1 protease. *Science* **249**:527–533.

713. Eron, J. J., Jr., M. A. Ashby, M. F. Giordano, M. Chernow, W. M. Reiter, S. G. Deeks, J. P. Lavelle, M. A. Conant, B. G. Yangco, P. G. Pate, R. A. Torres, R. T. Mitsuyasu, and T. Twaddell. 1996. Randomised trial of MNrgp120 HIV-1 vaccine in symptomless HIV-1 infection. *Lancet* **348**:1547–1551.

714. Eron, J. J., S. L. Benoit, J. Jemsek, R. D. MacArthur, J. Santana, J. B. Quinn, D. R. Kuritzkes, M. A. Fallon, and M. Rubin. 1995. Treatment with lamivudine, zidovudine, or both in HIV-positive patients with 200 to 500 CD4+ cells per cubic millimeter. *N Engl J Med* **333**:1662–1669.

715. Escaich, S., J. Ritter, P. Rougier, D. Lepot, J.-P. Lamelin, M. Sepetjan, and C. Trepo. 1991. Plasma viraemia as a marker of viral replication in HIV-infected individuals. *AIDS* **5**:1189–1194.

716. Espinoza, L. R., J. L. Aguilar, C. G. Espinoza, A. Berman, F. Gutierrez, F. B. Vasey, and B. F. Germain. 1990. HIV associated arthropathy: HIV antigen demonstration in the synovial membrane. *J Rheumatol* **17**:1195–1201.

717. Estaquier, J., T. Idziorek, F. de Bels, F. Barre-Sinoussi, B. Hurtrel, A. M. Aubertin, A. Venet, M. Mehtali, E. Muchmore, P. Michel, Y. Mouton, M. Girard, and J. C. Ameisen. 1994. Programmed cell death and AIDS: significance of T-cell apoptosis in pathogenic and non-pathogenic primate lentiviral infections. *Proc Natl Acad Sci USA* **91**:9431–9435.

718. Estaquier, J., M. Tanaka, T. Suda, S. Nagata, P. Golstein, and J. C. Ameisen. 1996. Fas-mediated apoptosis of CD4+ and CD8+ T cells from human immunodeficiency virus-infected persons: differential *in vitro* preventive effect of cytokines and protease antagonists. *Blood* **87**:4959–4966.

719. Evans, D. J., J. McKeating, J. M. Meredith, K. L. Burke, K. Katrak, A. John, M. Ferguson, P. D. Minor, R. A. Weiss, and J. W. Almond. 1989. An engineered poliovirus chimaera elicits broadly reactive HIV-1 neutralizing antibodies. *Nature* **339**:385–388.

720. Evans, L. A., T. M. McHugh, D. P. Stites, and J. A. Levy. 1987. Differential ability of human immunodeficiency virus isolates to productively infect human cells. *J Immunol* **138**:3415–3418.

721. Evans, L. A., J. Moreau, K. Odehouri, H. Legg, A. Barboza, C. Cheng-Mayer, and J. A. Levy. 1988. Characterization of a noncytopathic HIV-2 strain with unusual effects on CD4 expression. *Science* **240**:1522–1525.

722. Evans, L. A., J. Moreau, K. Odehouri, D. Seto, G. Thomson-Honnebier, H. Legg, A. Barboza, C. Cheng-Mayer, and J. A. Levy. 1988. Simultaneous isolation of HIV-1 and HIV-2 from an AIDS patient. *Lancet* **ii**:1389–1391.

723. Evans, L. A., G. Thomson-Honnebier, K. Steimer, E. Paoletti, M. Perkus, H. Hollander, and J. A. Levy. 1989. Antibody-dependent cellular cytotoxicity is directed against both the gp120 and gp41 envelope proteins of the human immunodeficiency virus. *AIDS* **3**:1357–1360.

724. Evatt, B. L., R. B. Ramsey, D. N. Lawrence, L. D. Zyla, and J. W. Curran. 1984. The acquired immunodeficiency syndrome in patients with hemophilia. *Ann Int Med* **100**:499–504.

725. Everall, I. P., P. J. Luthert, and P. L. Lantos. 1991. Neuronal loss in the frontal cortex in HIV infection. *Lancet* **337**:1119–1121.

726. Eyster, M. E., M. H. Gail, J. O. Ballard, H. Al-Mondhiry, and J. J. Goedert. 1987. Natural history of human immunodeficiency virus infections in hemophiliacs: effects of T-cell subsets, platelet counts, and age. *Ann Int Med* **107**:1–6.

727. Eyster, M. E., C. S. Rabkin, M. W. Hilgartner, L. M. Aledort, M. V. Ragni, J. Sprandio, G. C. White, S. Eichinger, P. de Moerloose, W. A. Andes, A. R. Cohen, M. Manco-Johnson, G. L. Bray, W. Schramm, A. Hatzakis, M. M. Lederman, C. M. Kessler, and J. J. Goedert. 1993. Human immunodeficiency virus-related conditions in children and adults with hemophilia: rates, relationship to CD4 counts, and predictive value. *Blood* **81**:828–834.

728. Ezekowitz, A. B., M. Kuhlman, J. E. Groopman, and R. A. Byrn. 1989. A human serum mannose-binding protein inhibits *in vitro* infection by the human immunodeficiency virus. *J Exp Med* **169**:185–196.

728a. Fahey, J. L., J. M. G. Taylor, R. Detels, B. Hofmann, R. Melmed, P. Nishanian, and J. V. Giorgi. 1990. The prognostic value of cellular and serologic markers in infection with human immunodeficiency virus type 1. *N Engl J Med* **322**:166–172.

729. Falk, L. A., Jr., D. A. Paul, A. Landay, and H. Kessler. 1987. HIV isolation from plasma of HIV-infected persons. *N Engl J Med* **316**:1547–1548.

730. Fantini, J., N. Yahi, S. Baghdiguian, and J.-C. Chermann. 1992. Human colon epithelial cells productively infected with human immunodeficiency virus show impaired differentiation and altered secretion. *J Virol* **66**:580–585.

731. Fantini, J., N. Yahi, and J.-C. Chermann. 1991. Human immunodeficiency virus can infect the apical and basolateral surfaces of human colonic epithelial cells. *Proc Natl Acad Sci USA* **88**:9297–9301.

732. Faraci, F. M. 1989. Effects of endothelin and vasopressin on cerebral blood vessels. *Am J Physiol* **257**:H799–H803.

733. Farrell, H. E., H. Vally, D. M. Lynch, P. Fleming, G. R. Shellam, A. A. Scalzo, and N. J. Davis-Poynter. 1997. Inhibition of natural killer cells by a cytomegalovirus MHC class I homologue *in vivo*. *Nature* **386**:510–514.

734. Farzadegan, H., M. A. Polis, S. M. Wolinsky, C. R. Rinaldo, Jr., J. J. Sninsky, S. Kwok, R. L. Griffith, R. A. Kaslow, J. P. Phair, B. F. Polk, and A. J. Saah. 1988. Loss of human immunodeficiency virus type 1 (HIV-1) antibodies with evidence of viral infection in asymptomatic homosexual men. *Ann Int Med* **108**:785–790.

735. Farzadegan, H., D. Vlahov, L. Solomon, A. Munoz, J. Astemborski, E. Taylor, A. Burnley, and K. E. Nelson. 1993. Detection of human immunodeficiency virus type 1 infection by polymerase chain reaction in a cohort of seronegative intravenous drug users. *J Inf Dis* **168**:327–331.

735a.Fatkenheuer, G., A. Theisen, J. Rockstroh, T. Grabow, C. Wicke, K. Becker, U. Wieland, H. Pfister, M. Reiser, P. Hegener, C. Franzen, A. Schwenk, and B. Salzberger. Virological treatment failures of protease inhibitor therapy in an unselected cohort of HIV infected patients. *AIDS* in press.

736. Fauci, A. S. 1993. CD4+ T-lymphocytopenia without HIV infection—no lights, no camera, just facts. *N Engl J Med* **328**:429-431.

737. Fauci, A. S. 1996. An HIV vaccine: breaking the paradigms. *Proc Assoc Am Physicians* **108**:6–13.

738. Fauci, A. S. 1993. Multifactorial nature of human immunodeficiency virus disease: implications for therapy. *Science* **262**:1011–1018.

738a.Fauci, A. S. Personal communication.

739. Feinberg, M. B., R. F. Jarrett, A. Aldovini, R. C. Gallo, and F. Wong-Staal. 1986. HTLV-III expression and production involve complex regulation at the levels of splicing and translation of viral RNA. *Cell* **46**:807–817.

740. Feinberg, M. B., and D. Trono. 1992. Intracellular immunization: trans-dominant mutants of HIV gene products as tools for the study and interruption of viral replication. *AIDS Res Hum Retro* **8**:1013–1022.

741. Feizi, T., and M. Larkin. 1990. AIDS and glycosylation. *Glycobiol* **1**:17–23.

742. Feldmann, H., H. Bugany, F. Mahner, H. D. Klenk, D. Drenckhahn, and H. J. Schnittler. 1996. Filovirus-induced endothelial leakage triggered by infected monocytes/macrophages. *J Virol* **70**:2208–2214.

743. Feng, Y., C. C. Broder, P. E. Kennedy, and E. A. Berger. 1996. HIV-1 entry cofactor: functional cDNA cloning of a seven-transmembrane, G protein-coupled receptor. *Science* **272**:872–877.

744. Feng, Y. X., T. D. Copeland, L. E. Henderson, R. J. Gorelick, W. J. Bosche, J. G. Levin, and A. Rein. 1996. HIV-1 nucleocapsid protein induces "maturation" of dimeric retroviral RNA *in vitro*. *Proc Nat Acad Sci USA* **93**:7577–7581.

745. Fenouillet, E., B. Clerget-Raslain, J. C. Gluckman, D. Guetard, L. Montagnier, and E. Bahraoui. 1989. Role of N-linked glycans in the interaction between the envelope glycoprotein of human immunodeficiency virus and its CD4 cellular receptor. *J Exp Med* **169**:807–822.

746. Fenyo, E. M., L. Morfeldt-Manson, F. Chiodi, B. Lind, A. von Gegerfelt, J. Albert, E. Olausson, and B. Asjo. 1988. Distinct replicative and cytopathic characteristics of human immunodeficiency virus isolates. *J Virol* **62**:4414–4419.

747. Ferbas, J., E. S. Daar, K. Grovit-Ferbas, W. J. Lech, R. Detels, J. V. Giorgi, and A. H. Kaplan. 1996. Rapid evolution of human immunodeficiency virus strains with increased replicative capacity during the seronegative window of primary infection. *J Virol* **70**:7285–7289.

748. Ferbas, J., A. H. Kaplan, M. A. Hausner, L. E. Hultin, J. L. Matud, Z. Liu, D. L. Panicali, H. Nerng-Ho, R. Detels, and J. V. Giorgi. 1995. Virus burden in long-term survivors of human immunodeficiency virus (HIV) infection is a determinant of anti-HIV CD8+ lymphocyte activity. *J Inf Dis* **172**:329–339.

749. Fermin, C. D., and R. F. Garry. 1992. Membrane alterations linked to early interactions of HIV with the cell surface. *Virol* **191**:941–946.

750. Fernandez-Larsson, R., K. K. Srivastava, S. Lu, and H. L. Robinson. 1992. Replication of patient isolates of human immunodeficiency virus type 1 in T cells: a spectrum of rates and efficiencies of entry. *Proc Natl Acad Sci USA* **89**:2223–2226.

751. Ferrari, G., W. Humphrey, M. J. McElrath, J. L. Excler, A. M. Duliege, M. L. Clements, L. C. Corey, D. P. Bolognesi, and K. J. Weinhold. 1997. Clade B-based HIV-1 vaccines elicit crossclade cytotoxic T lymphocyte reactivities in uninfected volunteers. *Proc Natl Acad Sci USA* **94**:1396–1401.

752. Fields, A. P., D. P. Bednarik, A. Hess, and W. S. May. 1988. Human immunodeficiency virus induces phosphorylation of its cell surface receptor. *Nature* **333**:278–280.

753. Finkel, T. H., G. Tudor-Williams, N. K. Banda, M. F. Cotton, T. Curiel, C. Monks, T. W.

Baba, R. M. Ruprecht, and A. Kupfer. 1995. Apoptosis occurs predominantly in bystander cells and not in productively infected cells of HIV- and SIV-infected lymph nodes. *Nature Med* 1:129–134.

754. Finnegan, A., K. A. Roebuck, B. E. Nakai, D. S. Gu, M. F. Rabbi, S. Song, and A. L. Landay. 1996. IL-10 cooperates with TNF-alpha to activate HIV-1 from latently and acutely infected cells of monocyte/macrophage lineage. *J Immunol* 156:841–851.

755. Fiore, J. R., A. Bjorndal, K. A. Peipke, M. Di Stefano, G. Angarano, G. Pastore, H. Gaines, E. M. Fenyo, and J. Albert. 1994. The biological phenotype of HIV-1 is usually retained during and after sexual transmission. *Virol* 204:297–303.

755a. Fiore, J. R., Y. J. Zhang, A. Bjorndal, M. Di Stefano, G. Angarano, G. Pastore, and E. M. Fenyo. 1997. Biological correlates of HIV-1 heterosexual transmission. *AIDS* 11:1089–1094.

756. Fiorelli, V., R. Gendelman, F. Samaniego, P. D. Markham, and B. Ensoli. 1995. Cytokines from activated T cells induce normal endothelial cells to acquire the phenotypic and functional features of AIDS-Kaposi's sarcoma spindle cells. *J Clin Invest* 95:1723–1734.

757. Fiorentino, S., M. Dalod, D. Olive, J. G. Guillet, and E. Gomard. 1996. Predominant involvement of CD8$^+$CD28$^-$ lymphocytes in human immunodeficiency virus-specific cytotoxic activity. *J Virol* 70:2022–2026.

758. Fischl, M. A., D. D. Richman, M. H. Grieco, M. S. Gottlieb, P. A. Volberding, O. L. Laskin, J. M. Leedom, J. E. Groopman, D. Mildvan, R. T. Schooley, G. G. Jackson, D. T. Durack, and D. King. 1987. The efficacy of azidothymidine (AZT) in the treatment of patients with AIDS and AIDS-related complex. A double blind placebo controlled trial. *N Engl J Med* 317:185–191.

759. Fiscus, S. A., A. A. Adimora, V. J. Schoenbach, W. Lim, R. McKinney, D. Rupar, J. Kenny, C. Woods, and C. Wilfert. 1996. Perinatal HIV infection and the effect of zidovudine therapy on transmission in rural and urban counties. *J Am Med Assoc* 275:1483–1488.

760. Fisher, A. G., B. Ensoli, D. Looney, A. Rose, R. C. Gallo, M. S. Saag, G. M. Shaw, B. H. Hahn, and F. Wong-Staal. 1988. Biologically diverse molecular variants within a single HIV-1 isolate. *Nature* 334:444–447.

761. Fisher, A. G., M. B. Feinberg, and S. F. Josephs. 1986. The *trans*-activator gene of HTLV-III is essential for virus replication. *Nature* 320:2367–2371.

762. Fisher, A. G., L. Ratner, H. Mitsuya, L. M. Marselle, M. E. Harper, S. Broder, R. C. Gallo, and F. Wong-Staal. 1986. Infectious mutants of HTLV-III with changes in the 3′ region and markedly reduced cytopathic effects. *Science* 233:655–659.

763. Fitzgibbon, J. E., A. E. Farnham, S. J. Sperber, H. Kim, and D. T. Dubin. 1993. Human immunodeficiency virus type 1 *pol* gene mutations in an AIDS patient treated with multiple antiretroviral drugs. *J Virol* 67:7271–7275.

764. Fitzgibbon, J. E., R. M. Howell, C. A. Haberzettl, S. J. Sperber, D. J. Gocke, and D. T. Dubin. 1992. Human immunodeficiency virus type 1 *pol* gene mutations which cause decreased susceptibility to 2′,3′-dideoxycytidine. *Antimicrob Agents Chemo* 36:153–157.

765. Flamand, L., J. Gosselin, M. D'Addario, J. Hiscott, D. V. Ablashi, R. C. Gallo, and J. Menezes. 1991. Human herpesvirus 6 induces interleukin-1-beta and tumor necrosis factor alpha, but not interleukin-6, in peripheral blood mononuclear cell cultures. *J Virol* 65:5105–5110.

766. Flamand, L., R. A. Zeman, J. L. Bryant, Y. Lunardi-Iskandar, and R. C. Gallo. 1996. Absence of human herpesvirus 8 DNA sequences in neoplastic Kaposi's sarcoma cell lines. *J AIDS Hum Retrovirol* 13:194–197.

767. Fleming, S. C., M. S. Kapembwa, T. T. MacDonald, and G. E. Griffin. 1992. Direct *in vitro* infection of human intestine with HIV-1. *AIDS* 6:1099–1104.

768. Fleury, S., D. Lamarre, S. Meloche, S. E. Ryu, C. Cantin, W. A. Hendrickson, and R. P. Sekaly. 1991. Mutational analysis of the interaction between CD4 and class II MHC: class II antigens contact CD4 on a surface opposite the gp120-binding site. *Cell* 66:1037–1049.

769. Folks, T., D. M. Powell, M. M. Lightfoote, S. Benn, M. A. Martin, and A. S. Fauci. 1986. Induction of HTLV-III/LAV from a nonvirus-producing T-cell line: implications for latency. *Science* 231:600–602.

770. Folks, T. M., and D. P. Bednarik. 1992. Mechanisms of HIV-1 latency. *AIDS* 6:3–16.

771. Folks, T. M., K. A. Clouse, J. Justement, A. Rabson, E. Duh, J. H. Kehrl, and A. S. Fauci. 1989. Tumor necrosis factor alpha induces expression of human immunodeficiency virus in a chronically infected T-cell clone. *Proc Natl Acad Sci USA* 86:2365–2368.

772. Folks, T. M., J. Justement, A. Kinter, C. A. Dinarello, and A. S. Fauci. 1987. Cytokine-induced expression of HIV-1 in a chronically infected promonocyte cell line. *Science* 238:800–802.

773. Folks, T. M., S. W. Kessler, J. M. Orenstein, J. S. Justement, E. S. Jaffe, and A. S. Fauci. 1988. Infection and replication of HIV-1 in purified progenitor cells of normal human bone marrow. *Science* 242:919–922.

774. Fomsgaard, A., V. M. Hirsch, J. S. Allan, and P. R. Johnson. 1991. A highly divergent proviral DNA clone of SIV from a distinct species of African green monkey. *Virol* 182:397–402.

775. Fontana, A., W. Fierz, and H. Wekerle. 1984. Astrocytes present myelin basic protein to encephalitogenic T-cell lines. *Nature* 307:273–276.

776. Fontana, L., M. C. Sirianni, G. De Sanctis, M. Carbonari, B. Ensoli, and F. Aiuti. 1986. Deficiency of natural killer activity, but not of natural killer binding, in patients with lymphadenopathy syndrome positive for antibodies to HTLV-III. *Immunobiol* 171:425–435.

777. Foreman, K. E., J. Friborg, Jr., W. P. Kong, C. Woffendin, P. J. Polverini, B. J. Nickoloff, and G. J. Nabel. 1997. Propagation of a human herpesvirus from AIDS-associated Kaposi's sarcoma. *N Engl J Med* 336:163–171.

777a. Forster, S. M., L. M. Osborne, R. Cheingsong-Popov, C. Kenny, R. Burnell, D. J. Jeffries, A. J. Pinching, J. R. W. Harris, and J. N. Weber. 1987. Decline of anti-p24 antibody precedes antigenaemia as correlate of prognosis in HIV-1 infection. *AIDS* 1:235–240.

778. Fouchier, R. A. M., M. Brouwer, S. M. Broersen, and H. Schuitemaker. 1995. Simple determination of human immunodeficiency virus type 1 syncytium-inducing V3 genotype by PCR. *J Clin Micro* 33:906–911.

779. Fouchier, R. A. M., M. Groenink, N. A. Kootstra, M. Tersmette, H. G. Huisman, F. Miedema, and H. Schuitemaker. 1992. Phenotype-associated sequence variation in the third variable domain of the human immunodeficiency virus type 1 gp120 molecule. *J Virol* 66:3183–3187.

780. Fouchier, R. A. M., L. Meyaard, M. Brouwer, E. Hovenkamp, and H. Schuitemaker. 1996. Broader tropism and higher cytopathicity for CD4+ T cells of a syncytium-inducing compared to a non-syncytium-inducing HIV-1 isolate as a mechanism for accelerated CD4+ T cell decline *in vivo*. *Virol* 219:87–96.

781. Fowke, K. R., N. J. D. Nagelkerke, J. Kimani, J. N. Simonsen, A. O. Anzala, J. J. Bwayo, K. S. MacDonald, E. N. Ngugi, and F. A. Plummer. 1996. Resistance to HIV-1 among persistently seronegative prostitutes in Nairobi, Kenya. *Lancet* 348:1347–1351.

782. Fox, C. H., D. Kotler, A. Tierney, C. S. Wilson, and A. S. Fauci. 1989. Detection of HIV-1 RNA in the lamina propria of patients with AIDS and gastrointestinal disease. *J Inf Dis* 159:467–471.

783. Fox, C. H., K. Tenner-Racz, P. Racz, A. Firpo, P. A. Pizzo, and A. S. Fauci. 1991. Lymphoid germinal centers are reservoirs of human immunodeficiency virus type 1 RNA. *J Inf Dis* 164:1051–1057.

784. Fox, R., L. J. Eldren, E. J. Fuchs, R. A. Kaslow, B. R. Visscher, M. Ho, J. P. Phair, and B. F. Polk. 1987. Clinical manifestations of acute infection with human immunodeficiency virus in a cohort of gay men. *AIDS* 1:35–38.

784a. Frade, J. M. R., M. Llorente, M. Mellado, J. Alcami, J. C. Gutierrez-Ramos, A. Zaballos, G. del Real, and C. Martinez-A. 1997. The amino-terminal domain of the CCR2 chemokine receptor acts as a coreceptor for HIV-1 infection. *J Clin Invest* 100:497–502.

785. Franchini, G., M. Robert-Guroff, J. Tartaglia, A. Aggarwal, A. Abimiku, J. Benson, P. Markham, K. Limbach, G. Hurteau, J. Fullen, K. Aldrich, N. Miller, J. Sadoff, E. Paoletti, and R. C. Gallo. 1995. Highly attenuated HIV type 2 recombinant poxviruses, but not HIV-2 recombinant *Salmonella* vaccines, induce long-lasting protection in rhesus macaques. *AIDS Res Hum Retro* 11:909–920.

786. Francis, T., Jr. 1953. Influenza: new acquaintance. *Ann Int Med* **39**:203–221.

787. Franke, E. K., and J. Luban. 1996. Inhibition of HIV-replication by cyclosporine A or related compounds correlates with the ability to disrupt the Gag-cyclophilin A interaction. *Virol* **222**:279–282.

788. Franke, E. K., H. E. Yuan, and J. Luban. 1994. Specific incorporation of cyclosporin A into HIV-1 virions. *Nature* **372**:359–362.

789. Frankel, F. R., S. Hegde, J. Lieberman, and Y. Paterson. 1995. Induction of cell-mediated immune responses to human immunodeficiency virus type 1 gag protein by using *Listeria monocytogenes* as a live vaccine vector. *J Immunol* **155**:4775–4782.

790. Franza, B. R., Jr., S. F. Josephs, M. Z. Gilman, W. Ryan, and B. Clarkson. 1987. Characterization of cellular proteins recognizing the HIV enhancer using a microscale DNA-affinity precipitation assay. *Nature* **330**:391–395.

790a.Fraser, J. D., B. A. Irving, G. R. Crabtree, and A. Weiss. 1991. Regulation of interleukin-2 gene enhancer activity by the T cell accessory molecule CD28. *Science* **251**:313–316.

791. Frederick, T., L. Mascola, A. Eller, L. O'Neil, and B. Byers. 1994. Progression of human immunodeficiency virus disease among infants and children infected perinatally with human immunodeficiency virus or through neonatal blood transfusion. *Pediatr Infect Dis J* **13**:1091–1097.

792. Freed, E. O., E. L. Delwart, G. L. Buchschacher, Jr., and A. T. Panganiban. 1992. A mutation in the human immunodeficiency virus type 1 transmembrane glycoprotein gp41 dominantly interferes with fusion and infectivity. *Proc Natl Acad Sci USA* **89**:70–74.

793. Freed, E. O., and M. A. Martin. 1994. Evidence for a functional interaction between the V1/V2 and C4 domains of human immunodeficiency virus type 1 envelope glycoprotein gp120. *J Virol* **68**:2503–2512.

794. Freed, E. O., and D. J. Myers. 1992. Identification and characterization of fusion and processing domains of the human immunodeficiency virus type 2 envelope glycoprotein. *J Virol* **66**:5472–5478.

795. Freed, E. O., D. J. Myers, and R. Risser. 1991. Identification of the principal neutralizing determinant of human immunodeficiency virus type 1 as a fusion domain. *J Virol* **65**:190–194.

796. Freedman, A. R., F. M. Gibson, S. C. Fleming, C. J. Spry, and G. E. Griffin. 1991. Human immunodeficiency virus infection of eosinophils in human bone marrow cultures. *J Exp Med* **174**:1661–1664.

797. Freitas, A. A., and B. B. Rocha. 1993. Lymphocyte lifespans: homeostasis, selection and competition. *Immunol Today* **14**:25–29.

798. Frey, S., M. Marsh, S. Gunther, A. Pelchen-Matthews, P. Stephens, S. Ortlepp, and T. Stegmann. 1995. Temperature dependence of cell-cell fusion induced by the envelope glycoprotein of human immunodeficiency virus type 1. *J Virol* **69**:1462–1472.

799. Friedland, G., P. Kahl, B. Saltzman, M. Rogers, C. Feiner, M. Mayers, C. Schable, and R. S. Klein. 1990. Additional evidence for lack of transmission of HIV infection by close interpersonal (casual) contact. *AIDS* **4**:639–644.

800. Friedman-Kien, A. E., L. J. Laubenstein, P. Rubinstein, E. Buimovici-Klein, M. Marmor, R. Stahl, I. Spigland, K. S. Kim, and S. Zolla-Pazner. 1982. Disseminated Kaposi's sarcoma in homosexual men. *Ann Int Med* **96**:693–700.

801. Fu, Y. K., T. K. Hart, Z. L. Jonak, and P. J. Bugelski. 1993. Physiochemical dissociation of CD4-mediated syncytium formation and shedding of human immunodeficiency virus type 1 gp120. *J Virol* **67**:3818–3825.

802. Fujii, Y., K. Otake, M. Tashiro, and A. Adachi. 1996. In vitro cytocidal effects of human immunodeficiency virus type 1 Nef on unprimed human CD4+ T cells without MHC restriction. *J Gen Virol* **77**:2943–2951.

803. Fujii, Y., K. Otake, M. Tashiro, and A. Adachi. 1996. Soluble Nef antigen of HIV-1 is cytotoxic for human CD4+ T cells. *FEBS Letters* **393**:93–96.

804. Fujikawa, L. S., S. Z. Salahuddin, A. G. Palestine, R. B. Nussenblatt, and R. C. Gallo. 1985. Isolation of human T-lymphotropic virus type III from the tears of a patient with acquired immunodeficiency syndrome. *Lancet* **ii**:529–530.

805. Fujino, T., T. Fujiyoshi, S. Yashiki, S. Sonoda, H. Otsuka, and Y. Nagata. 1992. HTLV-I transmission from mother to fetus via placenta. *Lancet* **340**:1157.

806. Fultz, P., H. M. McClure, H. Daugharty, A. Brodie, C. R. McGrath, B. Swenson, and D. P. Francis. 1986. Vaginal transmission of human immunodeficiency virus (HIV) to a chimpanzee. *J Inf Dis* **5**:896–900.

807. Fultz, P. N., J.-C. Gluckman, E. Muchmore, and M. Girard. 1992. Transient increases in numbers of infectious cells in an HIV-infected chimpanzee following immune stimulation. *AIDS Res Hum Retro* **8**:313–317.

808. Fultz, P. N., H. M. McClure, D. C. Anderson, and W. M. Switzer. 1989. Identification and biologic characterization of an acutely lethal variant of simian immunodeficiency virus from sooty mangabeys (SIV/SMM). *AIDS Res Hum Retro* **5**:397–409.

809. Fultz, P. N., P. Nara, F. Barre-Sinoussi, A. Chaput, M. L. Greenberg, E. Muchmore, M.-P. Kieny, and M. Girard. 1992. Vaccine protection of chimpanzees against challenge with HIV-1-infected peripheral blood mononuclear cells. *Science* **256**:1687–1690.

810. Fultz, P. N., A. Srinivasan, C. R. Greene, D. Butler, R. B. Swenson, and H. M. McClure. 1987. Superinfection of a chimpanzee with a second strain of human immunodeficiency virus. *J Virol* **61**:4026–4029.

811. Fung, M. S. C., C. R. Y. Sun, W. L. Gordon, R.-S. Liou, T. W. Chang, W. N. C. Sun, E. S. Daar, and D. D. Ho. 1992. Identification and characterization of a neutralization site within the second variable region of human immunodeficiency virus type 1 gp120. *J Virol* **66**:848–856.

812. Funke, I., A. Hahn, E. P. Rieber, E. Weiss, and G. Riethmuller. 1987. The cellular receptor (CD4) of the human immunodeficiency virus is expressed on neurons and glial cells in human brain. *J Exp Med* **165**:1230–1235.

813. Funkhouser, A., M. L. Clements, S. Slome, B. Clayman, and R. Viscidi. 1993. Antibodies to recombinant gp160 in mucosal secretions and sera of persons infected with HIV-1 and seronegative vaccine recipients. *AIDS Res Hum Retro* **9**:627–632.

814. Furuta, Y., K. Eriksson, B. Svennerholm, P. Fredman, P. Horal, S. Jeansson, A. Vahlne, J. Holmgren, and C. Czerkinsky. 1994. Infection of vaginal and colonic epithelial cells by the human immunodeficiency virus type 1 is neutralized by antibodies raised against conserved epitopes in the envelope glycoprotein gp120. *Proc Natl Acad Sci USA* **91**:12559–12563.

815. Fust, G., E. Ujhelyi, T. Hidvegi, K. Paloczi, R. Mihalik, S. Hollan, K. Nagy, and M. Kirschfink. 1991. The complement system in HIV disease. *Immunol Investig* **20**:231–241.

816. Gabuzda, D. H., A. Lever, E. Terwilliger, and J. Sodroski. 1992. Effects of deletions in the cytoplasmic domain on biological functions of human immunodeficiency virus type 1 envelope glycoproteins. *J Virol* **66**:3306–3315.

817. Gaidano, G., P. Ballerini, J. Z. Gong, G. Inghirami, A. Neri, E. Q. Mewcomb, I. T. Magrath, D. M. Knowles, and R. Dalla-Favera. 1991. p53 mutations in human lymphoid malignancies: association with Burkitt lymphoma and chronic lymphocytic leukemia. *Proc Natl Acad Sci USA* **88**:5413–5417.

818. Gaidano, G., D. Capello, C. Pastore, A. Antinori, A. Gloghini, A. Carbone, L. M. Larocca, and G. Saglio. 1997. Analysis of human herpesvirus type 8 infection in AIDS-related and AIDS-unrelated primary central nervous system lymphoma. *J Inf Dis* **175**:1193–1197.

819. Gaidano, G., C. Pastore, C. Lanza, U. Mazza, and G. Saglio. 1994. Molecular pathology of AIDS-related lymphomas. Biologic aspects and clinicopathologic heterogeneity. *Ann Hematol* **69**:281–290.

820. Gail, M. H., J. M. Pluda, C. S. Rabkin, R. J. Biggar, J. J. Goedert, J. W. Horm, E. J. Sondik, R. Yarchoan, and S. Broder. 1991. Projections of the incidence of non-Hodgkin's lymphoma related to acquired immunodeficiency syndrome. *JNCI* **83**:695–701.

821. Gaines, H., J. Albert, M. von Sydow, A. Sonnerborg, F. Chiodi, A. Ehrnst, O. Strannegard, and B. Asjo. 1987. HIV antigenaemia and virus isolation from plasma during primary HIV infection. *Lancet* **i**:1317–1318.

822. Gaines, H., M. von Sydow, J. V. Parry, M. Forsgren, P. O. Pehrson, A. Sonnerborg, P. P. Mortimer, and O. Strannegard. 1988. Detection of immunoglobulin M antibody in primary human immunodeficiency virus infection. *AIDS* **2**:11–15.

823. Gaines, H., M. von Sydow, A. Sonnerborg, J. Albert, J. Czajkowski, P. O. Pehrson, F. Chiodi, L. Moberg, E.-M. Fenyo, B. Asjo, and M. Forsgren. 1987. Antibody response in primary human immunodeficiency virus infection. *Lancet* **i**:1249–1253.

824. Gajewski, T. F., J. Joyce, and F. W. Fitch. 1989. Antiproliferative effect of IFN-gamma in murine regulation. III. Differential selection of TH1 and TH2 murine helper T lymphocyte clones using recombinant IL-2 and recombinant IFN-gamma. *J Immunol* **143**:15–22.

825. Galetto-Lacour, A., S. Yerly, T. V. Perneger, C. Baumberger, B. Hirschel, and L. Perrin. 1996. Prognostic value of viremia in patients with long-standing human immunodeficiency virus infection. *J Inf Dis* **173**:1388–1393.

826. Gallaher, W. R. 1987. Detection of a fusion peptide sequence in the transmembrane protein of human immunodeficiency virus. *Cell* **50**:327–328.

826a. Gallaher, W. R., J. M. Ball, R. F. Garry, M. C. Grinnin, and R. C. Montelaro. 1989. A general model for the transmembrane proteins of HIV and other retroviruses. *AIDS Res Hum Retro* **5**:431–440.

827. Gallant, J. E., R. D. Moore, and R. E. Chaisson. 1994. Prophylaxis for opportunistic infections in patients with HIV infection. *Ann Int Med* **120**:932–944.

828. Gallarda, J. L., D. R. Henrard, D. Liu, S. Harrington, S. L. Stramer, J. E. Valinsky, and P. Wu. 1992. Early detection of antibody to human immunodeficiency virus type 1 by using an antigen conjugate immunoassay correlates with the presence of immunoglobulin M antibody. *J Clin Micro* **30**:2379–2384.

828a. Gallay, P., T. Hope, D. Chin, and D. Trono. 1997. HIV-1 infection of nondividing cells through the recognition of integrase by the importin/karyopherin pathway. *Proc Natl Acad Sci USA* **94**:9825–9830.

829. Gallay, P., V. Stitt, C. Mundy, M. Oettinger, and D. Trono. 1996. Role of the karyopherin pathway in human immunodeficiency virus type 1 nuclear import. *J Virol* **70**:1027–1032.

830. Gallay, P., S. Swingler, J. Song, F. Bushman, and D. Trono. 1995. HIV nuclear import is governed by the phosphotyrosine-mediated binding of matrix to the core domain of integrase. *Cell* **83**:569–576.

831. Galli, L., M. de Martino, P.-A. Tovo, C. Gabiano, M. Zappa, C. Giaquinto, S. Tulisso, A. Vierucci, M. Guerra, P. Marchisio, P. Dallacasa, and M. Stegagno. 1995. Onset of clinical signs in children with HIV-1 perinatal infection. *AIDS* **9**:455–461.

832. Gallo, D., J. R. George, J. H. Fitchen, A. S. Goldstein, and M. S. Hindahl. 1997. Evaluation of a system using oral mucosal transudate for HIV-1 antibody screening and confirmatory testing. *J Am Med Assoc* **277**:254–258.

833. Gallo, P., K. Frei, C. Rordorf, J. Lazdins, B. Tavolato, and A. Fontana. 1989. Human immunodeficiency virus type 1 (HIV-1) infection of the central nervous sytem: an evaluation of cytokines in cerebrospinal fluid. *J Neuroimmunol* **23**:109–116.

834. Gallo, R. C., S. Z. Salahuddin, M. Popovic, G. M. Shearer, M. Kaplan, B. F. Haynes, T. J. Palker, R. Redfield, J. Oleske, and B. Safai. 1984. Frequent detection and isolation of cytopathic retroviruses (HTLV-III) from patients with AIDS and at risk for AIDS. *Science* **224**:500–503.

835. Gallo, R. C., P. S. Sarin, E. P. Gelmann, M. Robert-Guroff, E. Richardson, V. S. Kalyanaraman, D. Mann, G. D. Sidhu, R. E. Stahl, S. Zolla-Pazner, J. Leibowitch, and M. Popovic. 1983. Isolation of human T-cell leukemia virus in acquired immune deficiency syndrome (AIDS). *Science* **220**:865–867.

836. Galloway, D. A., and J. K. McDougall. 1983. The oncogenic potential of herpes simplex virus: evidence for a "hit and run" mechanism. *Nature* **302**:21–24.

837. Gao, F., L. Yue, D. L. Robertson, S. C. Hill, H. Hui, R. J. Biggar, A. E. Neequaye, T. M. Whelan, D. D. Ho, G. M. Shaw, P. M. Sharp, and B. H. Hahn. 1994. Genetic diversity of human immunodeficiency virus type 2: evidence for distinct sequence subtypes with differences in virus biology. *J Virol* **68**:7433–7447.

838. Gao, F., L. Yue, A. T. White, P. G. Pappas, J. Barchue, A. P. Hanson, B. M. Greene, P. M. Sharp, G. M. Shaw, and B. H. Hahn. 1992. Human infection by genetically diverse SIV$_{sm}$-related HIV-2 in West Africa. *Nature* **358**:495–499.

839. **Gao, Q., Z. X. Gu, M. A. Parniak, X. G. Li, and M. A. Wainberg.** 1992. *In vitro* selection of variants of human immunodeficiency virus type 1 resistant to 3′-azido-3′-deoxythymidine and 2′,3′-dideoxyinosine. *J Virol* **66:**12–19.

840. **Gao, S. J., L. Kingsley, M. Li, W. Zheng, C. Parravicini, J. Ziegler, R. Newton, C. R. Rinaldo, A. Saah, J. Phair, R. Detels, Y. Chang, and P. S. Moore.** 1996. KSHV antibodies among Americans, Italians and Ugandans with and without Kaposi's sarcoma. *Nature Med* **2:**925–928.

841. **Gao, S. J., L. Kingsley, D. R. Hoover, T. J. Spira, C. R. Rinaldo, A. Saah, J. Phair, R. Detels, P. Parry, Y. Chang, and P. S. Moore.** 1996. Seroconversion to antibodies against Kaposi's sarcoma-associated herpesvirus-related latent nuclear antigens before the development of Kaposi's sarcoma. *N Engl J Med* **335:**233–241.

842. **Gao, W. Y., A. Cara, R. C. Gallo, and F. Lori.** 1993. Low levels of deoxynucleotides in peripheral blood lymphocytes: a strategy to inhibit human immunodeficiency virus type 1 replication. *Proc Natl Acad Sci USA* **90:**8925–8928.

843. **Garcia, F., C. Vidal, J. M. Gatell, J. M. Miro, A. Soriano, and T. Pumarola.** 1997. Viral load in asymptomatic patients with CD4+ lymphocyte counts above 500 × 10^6/l. *AIDS* **11:**53–57.

844. **Garcia, J. V., J. Alfano, and A. D. Miller.** 1993. The negative effect of human immunodeficiency virus type 1 Nef on cell surface CD4 expression is not species specific and requires the cytoplasmic domain of CD4. *J Virol* **67:**1511–1516.

845. **Garcia, J. V., and A. D. Miller.** 1991. Serine phosphorylation-independent downregulation of cell-surface CD4 by *nef. Nature* **350:**508–511.

846. **Gardner, M., A. Rosenthal, M. Jennings, J. Yee, L. Antipa, and E. Robinson, Jr.** 1995. Passive immunization of rhesus macaques against SIV infection and disease. *AIDS Res Hum Retro* **11:**843–854.

847. **Gardner, M. B.** 1996. The history of simian AIDS. *J Med Primatol* **25:**148–157.

848. **Garred, P., J. Eugen-Olsen, A. K. N. Iversen, T. L. Benfield, A. Svejgaard, and B. Hofmann.** 1997. Dual effect of CCR5 delta 32 gene deletion in HIV-1-infected patients. *Lancet* **349:**1884.

848a. **Garrity, R. R., G. Rimmelzwaan, A. Minassian, W. P. Tsai, G. Lin, J. J. deJong, J. Goudsmit, and P. L. Nara.** 1997. Refocusing neutralizing antibody response by targeted dampening of an immunodominant epitope. *J Immunol* **159:**279–289.

849. **Garry, R. F.** 1990. Extensive antigenic mimicry by retrovirus capsid proteins. *AIDS Res Hum Retro* **6:**1361–1362.

850. **Garry, R. F.** 1989. Potential mechanisms for the cytopathic properties of HIV. *AIDS* **3:**683–694.

851. **Garry, R. F., and G. Koch.** 1992. Tat contains a sequence related to snake neurotoxins. *AIDS* **6:**1541–1542.

852. **Garry, R. F., J. J. Kort, F. Koch-Nolte, and G. Koch.** 1991. Similarities of viral proteins to toxins that interact with monovalent cation channels. *AIDS* **5:**1381–1384.

853. **Gartner, S., P. Markovits, D. M. Markovitz, M. H. Kaplan, R. C. Gallo, and M. Popovic.** 1986. The role of mononuclear phagocytes in HTLV-III/LAV infection. *Science* **233:**215–219.

854. **Gates, A., R. Coker, R. Miller, D. Mitchell, J. Williamson, and J. Clarke.** 1997. Zidovudine-resistant variants of HIV-1 in lung. *AIDS* **11:**702–703.

855. **Gattegno, R., A. Ramdani, and T. Jouault.** 1992. Lectin-carbohydrate interactions and infectivity of human immunodeficiency virus type 1 (HIV-1). *AIDS Res Hum Retro* **8:**27–37.

856. **Gaulton, G. N., J. V. Scobie, and M. Rosenzweig.** 1997. HIV-1 and the thymus. *AIDS* **11:**403–414.

856a. **Gaynor, R.** Personal communication.

857. **Gazzard, B. G., G. J. Moyle, J. Weber, M. Johnson, J. S. Bingham, R. Brettle, D. Churchill, M. Fisher, G. Griffin, D. Jefferies, E. King, R. Gormer, C. Lee, A. Pozniak, J. R. Smith, G. Tudor-Williams, and I. Williams.** 1997. British HIV Association guidelines for antiretroviral treatment of HIV seropositive individuals. *Lancet* **349:**1086–1092.

858. **Gazzinelli, R. T., M. Makino, S. K. Chattopadhyay, C. M. Snapper, A. Sher, A. W. Hugin, and H. C. Morse III.** 1992. CD4+ subset regulation in viral infection. *J Immunol* **148:**182–188.

859. Gelbard, H. A., K. A. Dzenko, D. DiLoreto, C. del Cerro, M. del Cerro, and L. G. Epstein. 1993. Neurotoxic effects of tumor necrosis factor alpha in primary human neuronal cultures are mediated by activation of the glutamate AMPA receptor subtype: implications for AIDS neuropathogenesis. *Dev Neurosci* **15**:417–422.

860. Gelbard, H. A., H. S. L. M. Nottet, S. Swindells, M. Jett, K. A. Dzenko, P. Genis, R. White, L. Wang, Y.-B. Choi, D. Zhang, S. A. Lipton, W. W. Tourtellotte, L. G. Epstein, and H. E. Gendelman. 1994. Platelet-activating factor: a candidate human immunodeficiency virus type-1-induced neurotoxin. *J Virol* **68**:4628–4635.

861. Gelderblom, H. R., M. Ozel, E. H. S. Hausmann, T. Winkel, G. Pauli, and M. A. Koch. 1988. Fine structure of human immunodeficiency virus (HIV), immunolocalization of structural proteins and virus-cell relation. *Micron Microscop* **19**:41–60.

862. Gelderblom, H. R., M. Ozel, and G. Pauli. 1989. Morphogenesis and morphology of HIV. Structure-function relations. *Arch Virol* **106**:1–13.

863. Gendelman, H. E., J. M. Orenstein, L. M. Baca, B. Weiser, H. Burger, D. C. Kalter, and M. S. Meltzer. 1989. The macrophage in the persistence and pathogenesis of HIV infection. *AIDS* **3**:475–495.

864. Gendelman, H. E., J. M. Orenstein, M. A. Martin, C. Ferruca, R. Mitra, T. Phipps, L. A. Wahl, H. C. Lane, A. S. Fauci, and D. S. Burke. 1988. Efficient isolation and propagation of human immunodeficiency virus on recombinant colony-stimulating factor 1-treated monocytes. *J Exp Med* **167**:1428–1441.

865. Gendelman, H. E., W. Phelps, L. Feigenbaum, J. M. Ostrove, A. Adachi, P. M. Howley, G. Khoury, H. S. Ginsberg, and M. A. Martin. 1986. Trans-activation of the human immunodeficiency virus long terminal repeat sequence by DNA viruses. *Proc Natl Acad Sci USA* **83**:9759–9763.

866. Genesca, J., R. Y.-H. Wang, H. J. Alter, and J. W.-K. Shih. 1990. Clinical correlation and genetic polymorphism of the human immunodeficiency virus proviral DNA obtained after polymerase chain reaction amplification. *J Inf Dis* **162**:1025–1030.

867. Genis, P., M. Jett, E. W. Bernton, T. Boyle, H. A. Gelbard, K. Dzenko, R. W. Keane, L. Resnick, Y. Mizrachi, D. J. Volsky, L. G. Epstein, and H. E. Gendelman. 1992. Cytokines and arachidonic metabolites produced during human immunodeficiency virus (HIV)-infected macrophage-astroglia interactions: implications for the neuropathogenesis of HIV disease. *J Exp Med* **176**:1703–1718.

868. Gentric, A., M. Blaschek, C. Julien, J. Jouquan, Y. Pennec, J.-M. Berthelot, D. Mottier, R. Casburn-Budd, and P. Youinou. 1991. Nonorgan-specific autoantibodies in individuals infected with type 1 human immunodeficiency virus. *Clin Immunol Immunopathol* **59**:487–494.

869. George, J. R., C. Y. Ou, B. Parekh, K. Brattegaard, V. Brown, E. Boateng, and K. M. De Cock. 1992. Prevalence of HIV-1 and HIV-2 mixed infections in Cote d'Ivoire. *Lancet* **340**:337–339.

870. Gerberding, J. L. 1995. Management of occupational exposures to blood-borne viruses. *N Engl J Med* **332**:444–451.

871. Geretti, A. M., M. E. M. Dings, C. A. C. M. van Els, C. A. van Baalen, F. Wijnholds, J. C. C. Borleffs, and A. D. M. E. Osterhaus. 1996. Human immunodeficiency virus type 1 (HIV-1)- and Epstein-Barr virus-specific cytotoxic T lymphocyte precursors exhibit different kinetics in HIV-1-infected persons. *J Inf Dis* **174**:34–45.

872. Gerschenson, L. E., and R. J. Rotello. 1992. Apoptosis: a different type of cell death. *FASEB J* **6**:2450–2455.

873. Gershon, R. R. M., D. Vlahov, and K. E. Nelson. 1990. The risk of transmission of HIV-1 through non-percutaneous, non-sexual modes—a review. *AIDS* **4**:645–650.

874. Ghanekar, S., L. Zheng, A. Logar, J. Navratil, L. Borowski, P. Gupta, and C. Rinaldo. 1996. Cytokine expression by human peripheral blood dendritic cells stimulated in vitro with HIV-1 and herpes simplex virus. *J Immunol* **157**:4028–4036.

875. Ghazal, P., J. Young, E. Giulietti, C. DeMattei, J. Garcia, R. Gaynor, R. M. Stenberg, and J. A. Nelson. 1991. A discrete *cis* element in the human immunodeficiency virus long terminal repeat mediates synergistic *trans* activation by cytomegalovirus immediate-early proteins. *J Virol* **65**:6735–6742.

876. **Ghosh, D.** 1992. Glucocorticoid receptor-binding site in the human immunodeficiency virus long terminal repeat. *J Virol* **66**:586–590.

877. **Giavedoni, L., S. Ahmad, L. Jones, and T. Yilma.** 1997. Expression of gamma interferon by simian immunodeficiency virus increases attenuation and reduces postchallenge virus load in vaccinated rhesus macaques. *J Virol* **71**:866–872.

878. **Gibbons, J., J. M. Cory, I. K. Hewlett, J. S. Epstein, and M. E. Eyster.** 1990. Silent infections with human immunodeficiency virus type 1 are highly unlikely in multitransfused seronegative hemophiliacs. *Blood* **76**:1924–1926.

879. **Gibbs, J., D. Regier, M. Daniel, and R. Desrosiers.** 1992. *In vivo* and *in vitro* effects of SIV mutants deleted in the "non-essential" genes, abstract 23. *In Tenth Annual Symposium on Nonhuman Primate Models for AIDS.*

880. **Gilbert, J. M., D. Mason, and J. M. White.** 1990. Fusion of Rous sarcoma virus with host cells does not require exposure to low pH. *J Virol* **64**:5106–5113.

881. **Gilbert, M., J. Kirihara, and J. Mills.** 1991. Enzyme-linked immunoassay for human immunodeficiency virus type 1 envelope glycoprotein 120. *J Clin Micro* **29**:142–147.

882. **Gill, M. J., L. R. Sutherland, and D. L. Church.** 1992. Gastrointestinal tissue cultures for HIV in HIV-infected/AIDS patients. *AIDS* **6**:553–556.

882a. **Gilliam, B. L., J. R. Dyer, S. A. Fiscus, C. Marcus, S. Zhou, L. Wathen, W. W. Freimuth, M. S. Cohen, and J. J. Eron, Jr.** 1997. Effects of reverse transcriptase inhibitor therapy on the HIV-1 viral burden in semen. *J AIDS Hum Retrovirol* **15**:54–60.

883. **Gilson, R. J. C., A. E. Hawkins, M. R. Beecham, E. Ross, J. Waite, M. Briggs, T. McNally, G. E. Kelly, R. S. Tedder, and I. V. D. Weller.** 1997. Interactions between HIV and hepatitis B virus in homosexual men: effects on the natural history of infection. *AIDS* **11**:597–606.

884. **Gimble, J. M., E. Duh, J. M. Ostrove, H. E. Gendelman, E. E. Max, and A. B. Rabson.** 1988. Activation of the human immunodeficiency virus long terminal repeat by herpes simplex virus type 1 is associated with induction of a nuclear factor that binds to the NF-kappaB/core enhancer sequence. *J Virol* **62**:4104–4112.

885. **Giorgi, J. V.** 1996. Phenotype and function of T cells in HIV disease, p. 181–199. *In* S. Gupta (ed.), *Immunology of HIV Infection.* Plenum Press, New York.

886. **Giorgi, J. V., Z. Liu, L. E. Hultin, W. G. Cumberland, K. Hennessey, and R. Detels.** 1993. Elevated levels of CD38+ CD8+ T cells in HIV infection add to the prognostic value of low CD4+ T cell levels: results of 6 years of follow-up. *J AIDS* **6**:904–912.

887. **Giraldo, G., E. Beth, and F. Haguenau.** 1972. Herpes-type virus particles in tissue culture of Kaposi's sarcoma from different geographic regions. *JNCI* **49**:1509–1526.

887a. **Giraldo, G., E. Beth, and E. S. Huang.** 1980. Kaposi's sarcoma and its relationship to cytomegalovirus (CMV). III. CMV DNA and CMV early antigens in Kaposi's sarcoma. *Int J Cancer* **26**:23–29.

888. **Girard, M., M.-P. Kieny, A. Pinter, F. Barre-Sinoussi, P. Nara, H. Kobe, K. Kusumi, A. Chaput, T. Reinhart, E. Muchmore, J. Ronco, M. Kaczonek, E. Garrard, J.-C. Gluckman, and P. N. Fultz.** 1991. Immunization of chimpanzees confers protection against challenge with human immunodeficiency virus. *Proc Natl Acad Sci USA* **88**:542–546.

889. **Girard, M., B. Meignier, F. Barre-Sinoussi, M. P. Kieny, T. Matthews, E. Muchmore, P. L. Nara, Q. Wei, L. Rimsky, K. Weinhold, and P. N. Fultz.** 1995. Vaccine-induced protection of chimpanzees against infection by a heterologous human immunodeficiency virus type 1. *J Virol* **69**:6239–6248.

890. **Giulian, D., K. Vaca, and C. A. Noonan.** 1990. Secretion of neurotoxins by mononuclear phagocytes infected with HIV-1. *Science* **250**:1593–1596.

891. **Giulian, D., E. Wendt, K. Vaca, and C. A. Noonan.** 1993. The envelope glycoprotein of human immunodeficiency virus type 1 stimulates release of neurotoxins from monocytes. *Proc Natl Acad Sci USA* **90**:2769–2773.

892. **Glesby, M. J., D. R. Hoover, H. Farzadegan, J. B. Margolick, and A. J. Saah.** 1996. The effect of influenza vaccination on human immunodeficiency virus type 1 load: a randomized, double-blind, placebo-controlled study. *J Inf Dis* **174**:1332–1336.

893. **Glick, M., M. Trope, O. Bagasra, and M. E. Pliskin.** 1991. Human immunodeficiency virus

infection of fibroblasts in dental pulp in seropositive patients. *Oral Surg Oral Med Oral Pathol* 71:733–736.

893a. Glushakova, S., B. Baibakov, J. Zimmerberg, and L. B. Margolis. 1997. Experimental HIV infection of human lymphoid tissue: correlation of CD4+ T cell depletion and virus syncytium-inducing/non-syncytium-inducing phenotype in histocultures inoculated with laboratory strains and patient isolates of HIV type 1. *AIDS Res Hum Retro* 13:461–471.

894. Gnann, J. W., Jr., J. B. McCormick, S. Mitchell, J. A. Nelson, and M. B. A. Oldstone. 1987. Synthetic peptide immunoassay distinguishes HIV type 1 and HIV type 2 infections. *Science* 237:1346–1349.

894a. Godfried, M. H., T. van der Poll, J. Jansen, J. A. Romijn, J. K. M. Eeftink Schattenkerk, E. Endert, S. J. H. van Deventer, and H. P. Sauerwein. 1993. Soluble receptors for tumour necrosis factor: a putative marker of disease progression in HIV infection. *AIDS* 7:33–36.

895. Goedert, J. J., A. R. Cohen, C. M. Kessler, S. Eichinger, S. V. Seremetis, C. S. Rabkin, F. J. Yellin, P. S. Rosenberg, and L. M. Aledort. 1994. Risks of immunodeficiency, AIDS, and death related to purity of factor VIII concentrate. *Lancet* 344:791–792.

896. Goedert, J. J., A.-M. Duliege, C. I. Amos, S. Felton, and R. J. Biggar. 1991. High risk of HIV-1 infection for first-born twins. *Lancet* 338:1471–1475.

897. Goedert, J. J., C. M. Kessler, L. M. Aledort, R. J. Biggar, W. A. Andes, G. C. White, J. E. Drummond, K. Vaidya, D. L. Mann, M. E. Eyster, M. V. Ragni, M. M. Lederman, A. R. Cohen, G. L. Bray, P. S. Rosenberg, R. M. Friedman, M. W. Hilgartner, W. A. Blattner, B. Kroner, and M. Gail. 1989. A prospective study of human immunodeficiency virus type 1 infection and the development of AIDS in subjects with hemophilia. *N Engl J Med* 321:1141–1148.

898. Goedert, J. J., H. Mendez, J. E. Drummond, M. Robert-Guroff, A. L. Minkoff, S. Holman, R. Stevens, A. Rubinstein, W. A. Blattner, and A. Willoughby. 1989. Mother-to-infant transmission of human immunodeficiency virus type 1. Association with prematurity or low anti-gp120. *Lancet* 11:1351–1354.

899. Golden, M. P., S. Kim, S. M. Hammer, E. Z. Ladd, P. A. Schaffer, N. DeLuca, and M. A. Albrecht. 1992. Activation of human immunodeficiency virus by herpes simplex virus. *J Inf Dis* 166:494–499.

900. Golding, H., R. Blumenthal, J. Manischewitz, D. R. Littman, and D. S. Dimitrov. 1993. Cell fusion mediated by interaction of a hybrid CD4.CD8 molecule with the human immunodeficiency virus type 1 envelope glycoprotein does occur after a long lag time. *J Virol* 67:6469–6475.

901. Golding, H., F. A. Robey, F. T. Gates III, W. Linder, P. R. Beining, T. Hoffman, and B. Golding. 1988. Identification of homologous regions in human immunodeficiency virus I gp41 and human MHC class II beta 1 domain. I. Monoclonal antibodies against the gp41-derived peptide and patients' sera react with native HLA class II antigens, suggesting a role for autoimmunity in the pathogenesis of acquired immune deficiency syndrome. *J Exp Med* 167:914–923.

902. Goldsmith, M. A., M. T. Warmerdam, R. E. Atchison, M. D. Miller, and W. C. Greene. 1995. Dissociation of the CD4 downregulation and viral infectivity enhancement functions of human immunodeficiency virus type 1 Nef. *J Virol* 69:4112–4121.

903. Gollub, E. L., and Z. A. Stein. 1993. The new female condom—item 1 on a women's AIDS prevention agenda. *Am J Pub Health* 83:498–500.

904. Gomatos, P. J., N. M. Stamatos, H. E. Gendelman, A. Fowler, D. L. Hoover, D. C. Kalter, D. S. Burke, E. C. Tramont, and M. S. Meltzer. 1990. Relative inefficiency of soluble recombinant CD4 for inhibition of infection by monocyte-tropic HIV in monocytes and T cells. *J Immunol* 144:4183–4188.

905. Gomez, A. M., F. M. Smaill, and K. L. Rosenthal. 1994. Inhibition of HIV replication by CD8+ T cells correlates with CD4 counts and clinical stage of disease. *Clin Exp Immunol* 97:68–75.

906. Gomez, M. B., and J. E. K. Hildreth. 1995. Antibody to adhesion molecule LFA-1 enhances plasma neutralization of human immunodeficiency virus type 1. *J Virol* 69:4628–4632.

907. Gonda, M., F. Wong-Staal, R. C. Gallo, J. E. Clements, O. Narayan, and R. V. Gilden. 1985.

Sequence homology and morphologic similarity of HTLV-III and visna virus, a pathogenic lentivirus. *Science* 227:173–177.

908. **Gonda, M. A.** 1992. Bovine immunodeficiency virus. *AIDS* 6:759–776.

909. **Gonzalez-Scarano, F., M. N. Waxham, A. M. Ross, and J. A. Hoxie.** 1987. Sequence similarities between human immunodeficiency virus gp41 and paramyxovirus fusion proteins. *AIDS Res Hum Retro* 3:245–252.

910. **Gorny, M. K., A. J. Conley, S. Karwowska, A. Buchbinder, J. Y. Xu, E. A. Emini, S. Koenig, and S. Zolla-Pazner.** 1992. Neutralization of diverse human immunodeficiency virus type 1 variants by an anti-V3 human monoclonal antibody. *J Virol* 66:7538–7542.

911. **Gorny, M. K., J. P. Moore, A. J. Conley, S. Karwowska, J. Sodroski, C. Williams, S. Burda, L. J. Boots, and S. Zolla-Pazner.** 1994. Human anti-V2 monoclonal antibody that neutralizes primary but not laboratory isolates of human immunodeficiency virus type 1. *J Virol* 68:8312–8320.

912. **Gorny, M. K., J. Y. Xu, S. Karwowska, A. Buchbinder, and S. Zolla-Pazner.** 1993. Repertoire of neutralizing human monoclonal antibodies specific for the V3 domain of HIV-1 gp120. *J Immunol* 150:635–643.

913. **Gosling, J., F. S. Monteclaro, R. E. Atchison, H. Arai, C. L. Tsou, M. A. Goldsmith, and I. F. Charo.** 1997. Molecular uncoupling of C-C chemokine receptor 5-induced chemotaxis and signal transduction from HIV-1 coreceptor activity. *Proc Natl Acad Sci USA* 94:5061–5066.

914. **Gotch, F., S. Rowland-Jones, and D. Nixon.** 1992. Longitudinal study of HIV-*gag* specific cytotoxic T lymphocyte responses over time in several patients, p. 60–65. *In* P. Racz, N. L. Letvin, and J. C. Gluckman (ed.), *Cytotoxic T Cells in HIV and Other Retroviral Infections*. Karger, Basel.

915. **Goto, T., S. Harada, M. Yamomoto, and M. Nakai.** 1988. Entry of human immunodeficiency virus (HIV) into MT-2, human T cell leukemic virus carrier cell line. *Arch Virol* 102:29–38.

916. **Goto, T., C. K. Yet, A. L. Notkins, and B. S. Prabhakar.** 1991. Detection of proviral sequences in saliva of patients infected with human immunodeficiency virus type 1. *AIDS Res Hum Retro* 7:343–347.

917. **Gottlieb, G. J., and A. B. Ackerman.** 1982. Kaposi's sarcoma: pathogenesis, clinical course, and treatment. *Human Path* 13:882–892.

918. **Gottlieb, M. D., R. Schroff, H. M. Schanker, J. D. Weisman, P. T. Fan, R. A. Wolf, and A. Saxon.** 1981. Pneumocystis carinii pneumonia and mucosal candidiasis in previously healthy homosexual men. *N Engl J Med* 305:1425–1431.

919. **Goudsmit, J.** 1995. The role of viral diversity in HIV pathogenesis. *J AIDS Hum Retrovirol* 10:S15-S19.

920. **Goudsmit, J., F. deWolf, D. A. Paul, L. G. Epstein, J. M. A. Lange, W. J. A. Krone, H. Speelman, E. C. Wolters, J. Van der Noordaa, J. M. Oleske, Y. J. van der Helm, and R. A. Coutinho.** 1986. Expression of human immunodeficiency virus antigen (HIV-Ag) in serum and cerebrospinal fluid during acute and chronic infection. *Lancet* ii:177–180.

921. **Goudsmit, J., J. M. A. Lange, D. A. Paul, and G. J. Dawson.** 1987. Antigenemia and antibody titers to core and envelope antigens in AIDS, AIDS-related complex and subclinical human immunodeficiency virus infection. *J Inf Dis* 155:558–560.

922. **Gougeon, M.-L., S. Garcia, J. Heeney, R. Tschopp, H. Lecoeur, D. Guetard, V. Rame, C. Dauguet, and L. Montagnier.** 1993. Programmed cell death in AIDS-related HIV and SIV infections. *AIDS Res Hum Retro* 9:553–563.

923. **Gougeon, M.-L., S. Garcia, H. Jonathan, and L. Montagnier.** 1992. Programmed cell death of T cells in HIV infection and its enhancement by superantigens, abstr. WeA1044. *In VIII International AIDS Conference, Amsterdam.*

924. **Gougeon, M.-L., H. Lecoeur, F. Boudet, E. Ledru, S. Marzabal, S. Boullier, R. Roue, S. Nagata, and J. Heeney.** 1997. Lack of chronic immune activation in HIV-infected chimpanzees correlates with the resistance of T cells to Fas/Apo-1 (CD95)-induced apoptosis and reservation of a T helper 1 phenotype. *J Immunol* 158:2964–2976.

925. **Gougeon, M.-L., H. Lecoeur, A. Dulioust, M.-G. Enouf, M. Crouvoiser, C. Goujard, T. Debord, and L. Montagnier.** 1996. Programmed cell death in peripheral lymphocytes from HIV-infected persons. *J Immunol* 156:3509–3520.

926. Goulden, M. G., N. Cammack, P. L. Hopewell, C. R. Penn, and J. M. Cameron. 1996. Selection *in vitro* of an HIV-1 variant resistant to both lamivudine (3TC) and zidovudine. *AIDS* 10:101–102.

927. Goulder, P. J. R., R. E. Phillips, R. A. Colbert, S. McAdam, G. Ogg, M. A. Nowak, P. Giangrande, G. Luzzi, B. Morgan, A. Edwards, A. J. McMichael, and S. Rowland-Jones. 1997. Late escape from an immunodominant cytotoxic T-lymphocyte response associated with progression to AIDS. *Nature Med* 3:212–217.

928. Gowda, S. D., B. S. Stein, N. Mohagheghpour, C. J. Benike, and E. G. Engleman. 1989. Evidence that T cell activation is required for HIV-1 entry in CD4+ lymphocytes. *J Immunol* 142:773-780.

929. Graham, B. S., and P. F. Wright. 1995. Candidate AIDS vaccines. *N Engl J Med* 333:1331–1339.

930. Graham, N. M. H., S. L. Zeger, L. P. Park, S. H. Vermund, R. Detels, C. R. Rinaldo, and J. P. Phair. 1992. The effects on survival of early treatment of human immunodeficiency virus infection. *N Engl J Med* 326:1037–1042.

931. Grant, M. D., F. M. Smaill, and K. L. Rosenthal. 1994. Cytotoxic T-lymphocytes that kill autologous CD4+ lymphocytes are associated with CD4+ lymphocyte depletion in HIV-1 infection. *J AIDS* 7:571–579.

932. Grant, M. D., F. M. Smaill, K. Laurie, and K. L. Rosenthal. 1993. Changes in the cytotoxic T-cell repertoire of HIV-1-infected individuals: relationship to disease progression. *Viral Immunol* 6:85–95.

933. Grant, M. D., F. M. Smaill, D. P. Singal, and K. L. Rosenthal. 1992. The influence of lymphocyte counts and disease progression on circulating and inducible anti-HIV-1 cytotoxic T-cell activity in HIV-1-infected subjects. *AIDS* 6:1085–1094.

934. Grant, M. D., M. S. Weaver, C. Tsoukas, and G. W. Hoffmann. 1990. Distribution of antibodies against denatured collagen in AIDS risk groups and homosexual AIDS patients suggests a link between autoimmunity and the immunopathogenesis of AIDS. *J Immunol* 144:1241–1250.

935. Grant, R. M., J. A. Wiley, and W. Winkelstein. 1987. Infectivity of the human immunodeficiency virus: estimates from a prospective study of homosexual men. *J Inf Dis* 156:189–193.

936. Gras, G. S., and D. Dormont. 1991. Antibody-dependent and antibody-independent complement-mediated enhancement of human immunodeficiency virus type 1 infection in a human, Epstein-Barr virus-transformed B-lymphocytic cell line. *J Virol* 65:541–545.

937. Graziosi, C., K. R. Gantt, M. Vaccarezza, J. F. Demarest, M. Daucher, M. S. Saag, G. M. Shaw, T. C. Quinn, O. J. Cohen, C. C. Welbon, G. Pantaleo, and A. S. Fauci. 1996. Kinetics of cytokine expression during primary human immunodeficiency virus type 1 infection. *Proc Natl Acad Sci USA* 93:4386–4391.

938. Green, D. F., L. Resnick, and J. J. Bourgoignie. 1992. HIV infects glomerular endothelial and mesangial but not epithelial cells in vitro. *Kidney Int* 41:956–960.

938a. Greco, G. and J.A. Levy. Unpublished observations.

939. Greenberg, R. N. 1984. Overview of patient compliance with medication dosing: a literature review. *Clin Ther* 6:592–599.

940. Greene, L. W., W. Cole, J. B. Greene, and B. Levy. 1984. Adrenal insufficiency as a complication of the acquired immunodeficiency syndrome. *Ann Int Med* 101:497–498.

941. Greene, W. C. 1990. Regulation of HIV-1 gene expression. *Annu Rev Immunol* 8:453–475.

942. Greene, W. C. 1991. The molecular biology of human immunodeficiency virus type 1 infection. *N Engl J Med* 324:308–317.

943. Greenspan, D., J. S. Greenspan, M. Conant, V. Petersen, S. Silverman, Jr., and Y. deSouza. 1984. Oral "hairy" leucoplakia in male homosexuals: evidence of association with both papillomavirus and a herpes-group virus. *Lancet* ii:831–834.

944. Griffiths, J. C., E. L. Berrie, L. N. Holdsworth, J. P. Moore, S. J. Harris, J. M. Senior, S. M. Kingsman, A. J. Kingsman, and S. E. Adams. 1991. Induction of high-titer neutralizing antibodies, using hybrid human immunodeficiency virus V3-Ty virus-like particles in a clinically relevant adjuvant. *J Virol* 65:450–456.

945. Grimaila, R. J., B. A. Fuller, P. D. Rennert, M. B. Nelson, M.-L. Hammarskjold, B. Potts, M. Murray, S. D. Putney, and G. Gray. 1992. Mutations in the principal neutralization determinant of human immunodeficiency virus type affect syncytium formation, virus infectivity, growth kinetics, and neutralization. *J Virol* **66**:1875–1883.

946. Grimaldi, L. M. E., G. V. Martino, D. M. Franciotta, R. Brustia, A. Castagna, R. Pristera, and A. Lazzarin. 1991. Elevated alpha-tumor necrosis factor levels in spinal fluid from HIV-1-infected patients with central nervous system involvement. *Ann Neurol* **29**:21–25.

947. Grinspoon, S. K., and J. P. Bilezikian. 1992. HIV disease and the endocrine system. *N Engl J Med* **327**:1360–1365.

948. Grody, W. W., L. Cheng, and W. Lewis. 1990. Infection of the heart by the human immunodeficiency virus. *Am J Cardiol* **66**:203–206.

949. Groenink, M., A. C. Andeweg, R. A. M. Fouchier, S. Broersen, R. C. M. van der Jagt, H. Schuitemaker, R. E. Y. de Goede, M. L. Bosch, H. G. Huisman, and M. Tersmette. 1992. Phenotype-associated *env* gene variation among eight related human immunodeficiency virus type 1 clones: evidence for in vivo recombination and determinants of cytotropism outside the V3 domain. *J Virol* **66**:6175–6180.

950. Groenink, M., R. A. M. Fouchier, S. Broersen, C. H. Baker, M. Koot, A. B. van't Wout, H. G. Huisman, F. Miedema, M. Tersmette, and H. Schuitemaker. 1993. Relation of phenotype evolution of HIV-1 to envelope V2 configuration. *Science* **260**:1513–1516.

951. Groenink, M., R. A. M. Fouchier, R. E. Y. de Goede, F. de Wolf, R. A. Gruters, H. T. M. Cuypers, H. G. Huisman, and M. Tersmette. 1991. Phenotypical heterogeneity in a panel of infectious molecular human immunodeficiency virus type 1 clones derived from a single individual. *J Virol* **65**:1968–1975.

952a. Grossman, Z., and R. B. Herberman. 1997. T-cell homeostasis in HIV infection is neither failing nor blind: modified cell counts reflect an adaptive response of the host. *Nature Med* **3**:486–490.

952. Groopman, J. E., S. Z. Salahuddin, M. G. Sarngadharan, P. D. Markham, M. Gonda, A. Sliski, and R. C. Gallo. 1984. HTLV-III in saliva of people with AIDS-related complex and healthy homosexual men at risk for AIDS. *Science* **226**:447–449.

953. Groux, H., G. Torpier, D. Monte, Y. Mouton, A. Capron, and J. C. Ameisen. 1992. Activation-induced death by apoptosis in CD4+ T cells from human immunodeficiency virus-infected asymptomatic individuals. *J Exp Med* **175**:331–340.

954. Gruber, M. F., K. A. Weih, E. J. Boone, P. D. Smith, and K. A. Clouse. 1995. Endogenous macrophage CSF production is associated with viral replication in HIV-1-infected human monocyte-derived macrophages. *J Immunol* **154**:5528–5535.

955. Grulich, A. E., and J. M. Kaldor. 1996. The sex ratio of AIDS-associated Kaposi's sarcoma does not provide evidence that sex hormones play a role in pathogenesis. *AIDS* **10**:1595–1609.

956. Grun, J. L., and P. H. Maurer. 1989. Different T helper cell subsets elicited in mice utilizing two different adjuvant vehicles: the role of endogenous interleukin 1 in proliferative responses. *Cell Immunol* **121**:134–145.

957. Grunfeld, C., D. P. Kotler, and R. Hamadeh. 1992. Hypertriglyceridemia in the acquired immunodeficiency syndrome. *Am J Med* **86**:27–31.

958. Grunfeld, C., M. Pang, and W. Doerrier. 1992. Lipids, lipoproteins, triglyceride clearance and cytokines in HIV infection and AIDS. *J Clin Endocrin Metabol* **74**:1045–1052.

959. Gruters, R. A., J. J. Neefjes, M. Tersmette, R. E. Y. de Goede, A. Tulp, H. G. Huisman, F. Miedema, and H. L. Ploegh. 1987. Interference with HIV-induced syncytium formation and viral infectivity by inhibitors of trimming glucosadase. *Nature* **330**:74–77.

960. Gruters, R. A., F. G. Terpstra, R. E. Y. De Goede, J. W. Mulder, F. De Wolf, P. T. A. Schellekens, R. A. W. Van Lier, M. Tersmette, and F. Miedema. 1991. Immunological and virological markers in individuals progressing from seroconversion to AIDS. *AIDS* **5**:837–844.

961. Gruters, R. A., F. G. Terpstra, R. De Jong, C. J. M. Van Noesel, R. A. W. Van Lier, and F. Miedema. 1990. Selective loss of T cell function in different stages of HIV infection. Early loss of anti-CD3-induced T cell proliferation followed by decreased anti-CD3-induced cytotoxic T lymphocyte generation in AIDS-related complex and AIDS. *Eur J Immunol* **20**:1039–1044.

962. **Gu, R., P. Westervelt, and L. Ratner.** 1993. Role of HIV-1 envelope V3 loop cleavage in cell tropism. *AIDS Res Hum Retro* **9**:1007–1015.

963. **Guarda, L. A., J. J. Butler, P. Mansell, E. M. Hersh, J. Reuben, and G. R. Newell.** 1983. Lymphadenopathy in homosexual men: morbid anatomy with clinical and immunologic correlations. *Am J Clin Path* **79**:559–568.

964. **Guidotti, L. G., P. Borrow, M. V. Hobbs, B. Matzke, I. Gresser, M. B. A. Oldstone, and F. V. Chisari.** 1996. Viral cross talk: intracellular inactivation of the hepatitis B virus during an unrelated viral infection of the liver. *Proc Natl Acad Sci USA* **93**:4589–4594.

965. **Gulizia, R. J., R. G. Collman, J. A. Levy, D. Trono, and D. E. Mosier.** 1997. Deletion of *nef* slows but does not prevent CD4-positive T-cell depletion in human immunodeficiency virus type 1-infected human-PBL-SCID mice. *J Virol* **71**:4161–4164.

966. **Guo, H. G., J. C. Chermann, D. Waters, L. Hall, A. Louie, R. C. Gallo, H. Streicher, M. S. Reitz, M. Popovic, and W. Blattner.** 1991. Sequence analysis of original HIV-1. *Nature* **349**:745–746.

967. **Guo, M. M. L., and J. E. K. Hildreth.** 1995. HIV acquires functional adhesion receptors from host cells. *AIDS Res Hum Retro* **11**:1007–1013.

968. **Gupta, P., R. Balachandran, M. Ho, A. Enrico, and C. Rinaldo.** 1989. Cell-to-cell transmission of human immunodeficiency virus type 1 in the presence of azidothymidine and neutralizing antibody. *J Virol* **63**:2361–2365.

969. **Gupta, P., L. Kingsley, J. Armstrong, M. Ding, M. Cottrill, and C. Rinaldo.** 1993. Enhanced expression of human immunodeficiency virus type 1 correlates with development of AIDS. *Virol* **196**:586–595.

969a.**Gupta, P., J. Mellors, L. Kingsley, S. Riddler, M. K. Singh, S. Schreiber, M. Cronin, and C. R. Rinaldo.** 1997. High viral load in semen of human immunodeficiency virus type 1-infected men at all stages of disease and its reduction by therapy with protease and nonnocleoside reverse transcriptase inhibitors. *J Virol* **71**:6271–6275.

970. **Gupta, P., M. K. Singh, C. Rinaldo, M. Ding, H. Farzadegan, A. Saah, D. Hoover, P. Moore, and L. Kingsley.** 1996. Detection of Kaposi's sarcoma herpesvirus DNA in semen of homosexual men with Kaposi's sarcoma. *AIDS* **10**:1596–1598.

971. **Gupta, S., and B. Vayuvegula.** 1987. Human immunodeficiency virus-associated changes in signal transduction. *J Clin Immunol* **7**:486–489.

972. **Gutierrez-Ortega, P., S. Hierro-Orozco, R. Sanchez-Cisneros, and L. F. Montano.** 1988. Kaposi's sarcoma in a 6-day-old infant with human immunodeficiency virus. *Peds Path* **125**:432–433. (Letter.)

973. **Guy, B., M. P. Kieny, Y. Riviere, C. Le Peuch, K. Dott, M. Girard, L. Montagnier, and J. P. Lecocq.** 1987. HIV F/3' *orf* encodes a phosphorylated GTP-binding protein resembling an oncogene product. *Nature* **330**:266–269.

974. **Guy, B., Y. Riviere, K. Dott, A. Regnault, and M. P. Kieny.** 1990. Mutational analysis of the HIV *nef* protein. *Virol* **176**:413–425.

975. **Guyader, M., M. Emerman, P. Sonigo, F. Clavel, L. Montagnier, and M. Alizon.** 1987. Genome organization and transactivation of the human immunodeficiency virus type 2. *Nature* **326**:662–669.

976. **Gyorkey, F., J. L. Melnick, and P. Gyorkey.** 1987. Human immunodeficiency virus in brain biopsies of patients with AIDS and progressive encephalopathy. *J Inf Dis* **155**:870–876.

977. **Gyorkey, F., J. G. Sinkovics, J. L. Melnick, and P. Gyorkey.** 1984. Retroviruses in Kaposi-sarcoma cells in AIDS. *N Engl J Med* **311**:1183–1184.

978. **Haas, G., U. Plikat, P. Debre, M. Lucchiari, C. Katlama, Y. Dudoit, O. Bonduelle, M. Bauer, H.-G. Ihlenfeldt, G. Jing, B. Maier, A. Meyerhans, and B. Autran.** 1996. Dynamics of viral variants in HIV-1 Nef and specific cytotoxic T lymphocytes in vivo. *J Immunol* **157**:4212–4221.

979. **Haase, A.** 1975. The slow infection caused by visna virus. *Curr Top Micro Immunol* **72**:101–156.

979a.**Haase, A.** Personal communication.

980. Haase, A. T. 1986. Pathogenesis of lentivirus infections. *Nature* 322:130–136.

981. Haase, A. T., K. Henry, M. Zupancic, G. Sedgewick, R. A. Faust, H. Melroe, W. Cavert, K. Gebhard, K. Staskus, Z. Q. Zhang, P. J. Dailey, H. H. Balfour, Jr., A. Erice, and A. S. Perelson. 1996. Quantitative image analysis of HIV-1 infection in lymphoid tissue. *Science* 274:985–989.

982. Habeshaw, J. A., A. G. Dalgleish, L. Bountiff, A. L. Newell, D. Wilks, L. C. Walker, and F. Manca. 1990. AIDS pathogenesis: HIV envelope and its interaction with cell proteins. *Immunol Today* 11:418–425.

983. Hadler, S. C., F. N. Judson, P. M. O'Malley, N. L. Altman, K. Penley, S. Buchbinder, C. A. Schable, P. J. Coleman, D. N. Ostrow, and D. P. Francis. 1991. Outcome of hepatitis B virus infection in homosexual men and its relation to prior human immunodeficiency virus infection. *J Inf Dis* 163:454–459.

984. Haffar, O., J. Garrigues, B. Travis, P. Moran, J. Zarling, and S.-L. Hu. 1990. Human immunodeficiency virus-like, nonreplicating, gag-env particles assemble in a recombinant vaccinia virus expression system. *J Virol* 64:2653–2659.

985. Haggerty, S., and M. Stevenson. 1991. Predominance of distinct viral genotypes in brain and lymph node compartments of HIV-1-infected individuals. *Viral Immunol* 4:123–131.

985a. Hahn, B. Personal communication.

986. Hahn, B. H., G. M. Shaw, S. K. Arya, M. Popovic, R. C. Gallo, and F. Wong-Staal. 1984. Molecular cloning and characterization of the HTLV-III virus associated with AIDS. *Nature* 312:166–169.

987. Hahn, B. H., G. M. Shaw, M. E. Taylor, R. R. Redfield, P. D. Markham, S. Z. Salahuddin, F. Wong-Staal, R. C. Gallo, E. S. Parks, and W. P. Parks. 1986. Genetic variation in HTLV-III/LAV over time in patients with AIDS or at risk for AIDS. *Science* 232:1548-1553.

988. Haigwood, N. L., P. L. Nara, E. Brooks, G. A. Van Nest, G. Ott, K. W. Higgins, N. Dunlop, C. J. Scandella, J. W. Eichberg, and K. S. Steimer. 1992. Native but not denatured recombinant human immunodeficiency virus type 1 gp120 generates broad-spectrum neutralizing antibodies in baboons. *J Virol* 66:172–182.

989. Haigwood, N. L., A. Watson, W. F. Sutton, J. McClure, A. Lewis, J. Ranchalis, B. Travis, G. Voss, N. L. Letvin, S. L. Hu, V. M. Hirsch, and P. R. Johnson. 1996. Passive immune globulin therapy in the SIV/macaque model: early intervention can alter disease profile. *Immunol Let* 51:107–114.

990. Haigwood, N. S., J. R. Shuster, G. K. Moore, H. Lee, P. V. Skiles, K. W. Higgins, P. J. Barr, C. George-Nascimento, and K. S. Steimer. 1990. Importance of hypervariable regions of HIV-1 gp120 in the generation of virus-neutralizing antibodies. *AIDS Res Hum Retro* 6:855–869.

991. Halapi, E., D. Gigliotti, V. Hodara, G. Scarlatti, P. A. Tovo, A. DeMaria, H. Wigzell, and P. Rossi. 1996. Detection of CD8 T-cell expansions with restricted T-cell receptor V gene usage in infants vertically infected by HIV-1. *AIDS* 10:1621–1626.

992. Hall, W. W., T. Kubo, S. Ijichi, H. Takahashi, and S. W. Zhu. 1994. Human T cell leukemia lymphoma virus, type II (HTLV-II): emergence of an important newly recognized pathogen. *Sem Virol* 5:165–178.

993. Halstead, S. B. 1979. *In vivo* enhancement of dengue virus infection in rhesus monkeys by passively transferred antibody. *J Inf Dis* 140:527–533.

994. Hamed, K. A., M. A. Winters, M. Holodniy, D. A. Katzenstein, and T. C. Merigan. 1993. Detection of human immunodeficiency virus type 1 in semen: effects of disease stage and nucleoside therapy. *J Inf Dis* 167:798–802.

995. Hamilton, D. P. 1991. What next in the Gallo case? *Science* 254:944–945.

996. Hamilton-Dutoit, S. F., G. Pallesen, and M. B. Franzman. 1991. Histopathology, immunophenotype and association with Epstein-Barr virus as demonstrated by *in situ* nucleic acid hybridization. *Am J Path* 138:149–163.

996a. Hammer, S. M. 1996. Advances in antiretroviral therapy and viral load monitoring. *AIDS* 10(Suppl. 3):S1–S11.

997. Hammer, S. M., D. A. Katzenstein, M. D. Hughes, H. Gundacker, R. T. Schooley, R. H. Haubrich, W. K. Henry, M. M. Lederman, J. P. Phair, M. Niu, M. S. Hirsch, and T. C. Merigan. 1996. A trial comparing nucleoside monotherapy with combination therapy in HIV-in-

fected adults with CD4 cell counts from 200 to 500 per cubic millimeter. *N Engl J Med* 335:1081–1090.

998. Hammes, S. R., E. P. Dixon, M. H. Malim, B. R. Cullen, and W. C. Greene. 1989. *Nef* protein of human immunodeficiency virus type 1: evidence against its role as a transcriptional inhibitor. *Proc Natl Acad Sci USA* 86:9549–9553.

999. Hammond, S. A., R. C. Bollinger, P. E. Stanhope, T. C. Quinn, D. Schwartz, M. L. Clements, and R. F. Siliciano. 1993. Comparative clonal analysis of human immunodeficiency virus type 1 (HIV-1)-specific CD4+ and CD8+ cytolytic T lymphocytes isolated from seronegative humans immunized with candidate HIV-1 vaccines. *J Exp Med* 176:1531–1542.

1000. Han, X.-M., A. Laras, M. P. Rounseville, A. Kumar, and P. R. Shank. 1992. Human immunodeficiency virus type 1 Tat-mediated *trans* activation correlates with the phosphorylation state of a cellular TAR RNA stem-binding factor. *J Virol* 66:4065–4072.

1001. Hansen, J.-E. S., H. Clausen, C. Nielsen, L. S. Teglbjaerg, L. L. Hansen, C. M. Nielsen, E. Dabelsteen, L. Mathiesen, S.-I. Hakomori, and J. O. Nielsen. 1990. Inhibition of human immunodeficiency virus (HIV) infection in vitro by anticarbohydrate monoclonal antibodies: peripheral glycosylation of HIV envelope glycoprotein gp120 may be a target for virus neutralization. *J Virol* 64:2833–2840.

1002. Hansen, J. E. S., C. Nielsen, M. Arendrup, S. Olofsson, L. Mathiesen, J. O. Nielsen, and H. Clausen. 1991. Broadly neutralizing antibodies targeted to mucin-type carbohydrate epitopes of human immunodeficiency virus. *J Virol* 65:6461–6467.

1003. Hansen, J. E. S., C. Nielsen, L. R. Mathiesen, and J. O. Nielsen. 1991. Involvement of lymphocyte function-associated antigen-1 (LFA-1) in HIV infection: inhibition by monoclonal antibody. *Scand J Infect Dis* 23:31–36.

1004. Hansen, J. E. S., C. M. Nielsen, C. Nielsen, P. Heegaard, L. R. Mathiesen, and J. O. Nielsen. 1989. Correlation between carbohydrate structures on the envelope glycoprotein gp120 of HIV-1 and HIV-2 and syncytium inhibition with lectins. *AIDS* 3:635–641.

1005. Hanson, C. V. 1994. Measuring vaccine-induced HIV neutralization: report of a workshop. *AIDS Res Hum Retro* 10:645-648.

1006. Hanto, D. W., K. J. Gajl-Peczalkska, and G. Frizzera. 1983. Epstein-Barr virus induced polyclonal and monoclonal B-cell lymphoproliferative disease occurring after renal transplantation. *Ann Surg* 198:356–369.

1007. Harada, S., Y. Koyanagi, H. Nakashima, N. Kobayashi, and N. Yamamoto. 1986. Tumor promoter, TPA, enhances replication of HTLV-III/LAV. *Virol* 154:249–258.

1008. Harada, S., Y. Koyanagi, and N. Yamamoto. 1985. Infection of HTLV-III/LAV in HTLV-I-carrying cells MT-2 and MT-4 and application in a plaque assay. *Science* 229:563–566.

1009. Harhaj, E. W., S. B. Maggirwar, L. Good, and S.-C. Sun. 1996. CD28 mediates a potent costimulatory signal for rapid degradtion of IκBβ which is associated with accelerated activation of various NF-κB/Rel heterodimers. *Mol Cell Biol* 16:6736–6743.

1010. Harouse, J. M., S. Bhat, S. L. Spitalnik, M. Laughlin, K. Stefano, D. H. Silberberg, and F. Gonzalez-Scarano. 1991. Inhibition of entry of HIV-1 in neural cell lines by antibodies against galactosyl ceramide. *Science* 253:320–323.

1011. Harouse, J. M., R. G. Collman, and F. Gonzalez-Scarano. 1995. Human immunodeficiency virus type 1 infection of SK-N-MC cells: domains of gp120 involved in entry into a CD4-negative, galactosyl ceramide/3' sulfogalactosyl ceramide-positive cell line. *J Virol* 69:7383–7390.

1012. Harouse, J. M., C. Kunsch, H. T. Hartle, M. A. Laughlin, J. A. Hoxie, B. Wigdahl, and F. Gonzalez-Scarano. 1989. CD4-independent infection of human neural cells by human immunodeficiency virus type 1. *J Virol* 63:2527–2533.

1013. Harouse, J. M., Z. Wroblewska, M. A. Laughlin, W. F. Hickey, B. S. Schonwetter, and F. Gonzalez-Scarano. 1989. Human choroid plexus cells can be latently infected with human immunodeficiency virus. *Ann Neurol* 25:406–411.

1014. Harper, D. R., R. L. Gilbert, T. J. O'Connor, D. Kinchington, N. Mahmood, R. A. J. McIlhinney, and D. J. Jeffries. 1996. Antiviral activity of 2-hydroxy fatty acids. *Antivir Chem Chemother* 7:138–141.

1015. Harper, M. E., L. M. Marselle, R. C. Gallo, and F. Wong-Staal. 1986. Detection of lympho-cytes expressing human T-lymphotropic virus type III in lymph nodes and peripheral blood from infected individuals by *in situ* hybridization. *Proc Natl Acad Sci USA* 83:772–776.

1016. Harrer, T., E. Harrer, S. A. Kalams, P. Barbosa, A. Trocha, R. P. Johnson, T. Elbeik, M. B. Feinberg, S. P. Buchbinder, and B. D. Walker. 1996. Cytotoxic T lymphocytes in asymp-tomatic long-term nonprogressing HIV-1 infection. *J Immunol* 156:2616–2623.

1017. Harrer, T., E. Harrer, S. A. Kalams, T. Elbeik, S. I. Staprans, M. B. Feinberg, Y. Cao, D. D. Ho, T. Yilma, A. M. Caliendo, R. P. Johnson, S. P. Buchbinder, and B. D. Walker. 1996. Strong cytotoxic T cell and weak neutralizing antibody responses in a subset of persons with stable nonprogressing HIV type 1 infection. *AIDS Res Hum Retro* 12:585–592.

1018. Harrington, R. D., and A. P. Geballe. 1993. Cofactor requirement for human immunodefi-ciency virus type 1 entry into a CD4-expressing human cell line. *J Virol* 67:5939–5947.

1019. Harrington, W., Jr., L. Sieczkowski, C. Sosa, S. Chan-a-Sue, J. P. Cai, L. Cabral, and C. Wood. 1997. Activation of HHV-8 by HIV-1 tat. *Lancet* 349:774–775.

1020. Harris, C., C. B. Small, R. S. Klein, G. H. Friedland, B. Moll, E. E. Emeson, I. Spigland, and N. H. Steigbigel. 1983. Immunodeficiency in female sexual partners of men with the ac-quired immunodeficiency syndrome. *N Engl J Med* 308:1181–1184.

1021. Harris, J. D., H. Blum, J. Scott, B. Traynor, P. Ventura, and A. Haase. 1984. Slow virus visna: reproduction *in vitro* of virus from extrachromosomal DNA. *Proc Natl Acad Sci USA* 81:7212–7215.

1021a. Harrison, T. S., and S. M. Levitz. 1997. Mechanisms of impaired anticryptococcal activity of monocytes from donors infected with human immunodeficiency virus. *J Inf Dis* 176:537–540.

1022. Harrowe, G., and C. Cheng-Mayer. 1995. Amino acid substitutions in the V3 loop are re-sponsible for adaptation to growth in transformed T-cell lines of a primary human im-munodeficiency virus type 1. *Virol* 210:490–494.

1023. Hart, A. R., and M. W. Cloyd. 1990. Interference patterns of human immunodeficiency viruses HIV-1 and HIV-2. *Virol* 177:1–10.

1024. Hart, C. E., C.-Y. Ou, J. C. Galphin, J. Moore, L. T. Bacheler, J. J. Wasmuth, S. R. Petteway, Jr., and G. Schochetman. 1989. Human chromosome 12 is required for elevated HIV-1 ex-pression in human-hamster hybrid cells. *Science* 246:488–491.

1025. Hart, C. E., M. J. Saltrelli, J. C. Galphin, and G. Schochetman. 1995. A human chromosome 12-associated 83-kilodalton cellular protein specifically binds to the loop region of human immunodeficiency virus type 1 *trans*-activation response element RNA. *J Virol* 69:6593–6599.

1027. Hart, T. K., R. Kirsh, H. Ellens, R. W. Sweet, D. M. Lambert, S. R. Petteway, Jr., J. Leary, and P. J. Bugelski. 1991. Binding of soluble CD4 proteins to human immunodeficiency virus type 1 and infected cells induces release of envelope glycoprotein gp120. *Proc Natl Acad Sci USA* 88:2189–2193.

1028. Hartley, C. A., M. J. Gilbert, L. Brigido, T. Elbeik, J. A. Levy, S. M. Crowe, and J. Mills. 1996. Human immunodeficiency virus grown in CD4-expressing cells is associated with CD4. *J Gen Virol* 77:2015–2023.

1029. Harwood, A. R., D. Osoba, and S. L. Hofstader. 1979. Kaposi's sarcoma in recipients of re-nal transplants. *Am J Med* 67:759–765.

1030. Haseltine, W. A. 1988. Replication and pathogenesis of the AIDS virus. *J AIDS* 1:217–240.

1031. Hasunuma, T., H. Tsubota, M. Watanabe, Z. W. Chen, C. I. Lord, L. C. Burkly, J. F. Daley, and N. L. Letvin. 1992. Regions of the CD4 molecule not involved in virus binding or syn-cytia formation are required for HIV-1 infection of lymphocytes. *J Immunol* 148:1841–1846.

1032. Hatakeyama, M., T. Koni, N. Kobyashi, A. Kawahara, S. D. Levin, R. M. Perlmuther, and T. Taniguichi. 1991. Interaction of the IL-2 receptor with the src-family kinase p56 lck: identification of novel intermolecular association. *Science* 252:1523–1528.

1033. Hattori, T., A. Koito, K. Takatsuki, H. Kido, and N. Katunuma. 1989. Involvement of tryptase-related cellular protease(s) in human immunodeficiency virus type 1 infection. *FEBS Letters* 248:48–52.

1034. Haverkos, J. W., P. F. Pinsky, P. Drotman, and D. J. Bregman. 1985. Disease manifestations among homosexual men with acquired immunodeficiency syndrome: a possible role of nitrites in Kaposi's sarcoma. *STD* **12**:203–208.

1035. Hawkins, R. E., L. S. Rickman, S. H. Vermund, and M. Carl. 1992. Association of mycoplasma and human immunodeficiency virus infection: detection of amplified *Mycoplasma fermentans* DNA in blood. *J Inf Dis* **165**:581–585.

1036. Haynes, B. F., M. A. Moody, C. S. Heinley, B. Korber, W. A. Millard, and R. M. Scearce. 1995. HIV type 1 V3 region primer-induced antibody suppression is overcome by administration of C4-V3 peptides as a polyvalent immunogen. *AIDS Res Hum Retro* **11**:211–221.

1037. Haynes, B. F., G. Pantaleo, and A. S. Fauci. 1996. Toward an understanding of the correlates of protective immunity to HIV infection. *Science* **271**:324–328.

1038. Hays, E. F., C. H. Uittenbogaart, J. C. Brewer, L. W. Vollger, and J. A. Zack. 1991. In vitro studies of HIV-1 expression in thymocytes from infants and children. *AIDS* **6**:265–272.

1039. He, J., Y. Chen, M. Farzan, H. Choe, A. Ohagen, S. Gartner, J. Busciglio, X. Yang, W. Hofmann, W. Newman, C. R. Mackay, J. Sodroski, and D. Gabuzda. 1997. CCR3 and CCR5 are co-receptors for HIV-1 infection of microglia. *Nature* **385**:645–649.

1040. He, J., S. Choe, R. Walker, P. De Marzio, D. O. Morgan, and N. R. Landau. 1995. Human immunodeficiency virus type 1 viral protein R (vpr) arrests cells in the G_2 phase of the cell cycle by inhibiting p34^{cdc2} activity. *J Virol* **69**:6705–6711.

1041. Heagy, W., C. Crumpacker, P. A. Lopez, and R. W. Finberg. 1991. Inhibition of immune functions by antiviral drugs. *J Clin Invest* **87**:1916–1924.

1042. Healey, D., L. Dianda, J. P. Moore, J. S. McDougal, M. J. Moore, P. Estess, D. Buck, P. D. Kwong, P. C. L. Beverley, and Q. J. Sattentau. 1990. Novel anti-CD4 monoclonal antibodies separate human immunodeficiency virus infection and fusion of CD4+ cells from virus binding. *J Exp Med* **172**:1233–1242.

1043. Heath, S. L., J. G. Tew, J. G. Tew, A. K. Szakal, and G. F. Burton. 1995. Follicular dendritic cells and human immunodeficiency virus infectivity. *Nature* **377**:740–744.

1044. Heinkelein, M., S. Sopper, and C. Jassoy. 1995. Contact of human immunodeficiency virus type 1-infected and uninfected CD4+ T lymphocytes is highly cytolytic for both cells. *J Virol* **69**:6925–6931.

1045. Heinzinger, N., L. Baca-Regen, M. Stevenson, and H. Gendelman. 1995. Efficient synthesis of viral nucleic acids following monocyte infection by HIV-1. *Virol* **206**:731–735.

1046. Heinzinger, N. K., M. I. Bukinsky, S. A. Haggerty, A. M. Ragland, V. Kewalramani, M. A. Lee, H. E. Gendelman, L. Ratner, M. Stevenson, and M. Emerman. 1994. The Vpr protein of human immunodeficiency virus type 1 influences nuclear localization of viral nucleic acids in nondividing host cells. *Proc Natl Acad Sci USA* **91**:7311–7315.

1047. Heise, C., S. Dandekar, P. Kumar, R. Duplantier, R. M. Donovan, and C. H. Halsted. 1991. Human immunodeficiency virus infection of enterocytes and mononuclear cells in human jejunal mucosa. *Gastroenterology* **100**:1521–1527.

1048. Heise, C., C. J. Miller, A. Lackner, and S. Dandekar. 1994. Primary acute simian immunodeficiency virus infection of intestinal lymphoid tissue is associated with gastrointestinal dsyfunction. *J Inf Dis* **169**:1116–1120.

1049. Helbert, M. R., J. L'age-Stehr, and N. A. Mitchison. 1993. Antigen presentation, loss of immunological memory and AIDS. *Immunol Today* **14**:340–344.

1050. Helseth, E., U. Olshevsky, C. Furman, and J. Sodroski. 1991. Human immunodeficiency virus type 1 gp120 envelope glycoprotein regions important for association with the gp41 transmembrane glycoprotein. *J Virol* **65**:2119–2123.

1051. Henderson, E. E., J.-Y. Yang, R.-D. Zhang, and M. Bealer. 1991. Altered HIV expression and EBV-induced transformation in coinfected PBLs and PBL subpopulations. *Virol* **182**:186–198.

1052. Henderson, L. A., and M. N. Qureshi. 1993. A peptide inhibitor of human immunodeficiency virus infection binds to novel human cell surface polypeptides. *J Biol Chem* **268**:15291–15297.

1053. Henderson, L. A., N. M. Qureshi, S. Rasheed, and R. Garry. 1988. Human immunodeficiency virus-induced cytotoxicity for CD8 cells from some normal donors and virus-specific induction of a suppressor factor. *Clin Immunol Immunopathol* 48:174–186.

1054. Henderson, S., M. Rowe, C. Gregory, D. Croom-Carter, F. Wang, R. Longnecker, E. Kieff, and A. Rickinson. 1991. Induction of bcl-2 expression by Epstein-Barr virus latent membrane protein 1 protects infected B cells from programmed cell death. *Cell* 65:1107–1115.

1055. Heng, M. C. Y., S. Y. Heng, and S. G. Allen. 1994. Co-infection and synergy of human immunodeficiency virus-1 and herpes simplex virus-1. *Lancet* 343:255–258.

1056. Henin, Y., L. Mandelbrot, R. Henrion, R. Pradinaud, J. P. Coulaud, and L. Montagnier. 1993. Virus excretion in the cervicovaginal secretions of pregnant and nonpregnant HIV-infected women. *J AIDS* 6:72–75.

1057. Henle, G., and W. Henle. 1979. The virus as the etiologic agent of infectious mononucleosis, p. 297–320. *In* M. A. Epstein and B. G. Achong (ed.), *The Epstein-Barr Virus.* Springer-Verlag, Berlin.

1058. Henrard, D. R., J. F. Phillips, L. R. Muenz, W. A. Blattner, D. Wiesner, M. E. Eyster, and J. J. Goedert. 1995. Natural history of HIV-1 cell-free viremia. *J Am Med Assoc* 274:554–558.

1059. Herbein, G., L. J. Montaner, and S. Gordon. 1996. Tumor necrosis factor alpha inhibits entry of human immunodeficiency virus type 1 into primary human macrophages: a selective role for the 75-kilodalton receptor. *J Virol* 70:7388–7397.

1060. Herndier, B. G., L. Kaplan, and M. McGrath. 1994. Pathogenesis of AIDS lymphomas. *AIDS* 8:1025–1049.

1061. Herndier, B. G., H. C. Sanchez, K. L. Chang, Y. Y. Chen, and L. M. Weiss. 1993. High prevalence of Epstein-Barr virus in the Reed-Sternberg cells of HIV-associated Hodgkin's disease. *Am J Path* 142:1073–1079.

1062. Herndier, B. G., B. T. Shiramizu, N. E. Jewett, K. D. Aldape, G. R. Reyes, and M. S. McGrath. 1992. AIDS-associated T-cell lymphoma: evidence for human immunodeficiency virus type 1-associated T-cell transformation. *Blood* 79:1768–1774.

1063. Herndier, B. G., A. Werner, P. Arnstein, N. W. Abbey, F. Demartis, R. L. Cohen, M. A. Shuman, and J. A. Levy. 1994. Characterization of a human Kaposi's sarcoma cell line that induces angiogenic tumors in animals. *AIDS* 8:575–581.

1064. Herrmann, C. H., and A. P. Rice. 1993. Specific interaction of the human immunodeficiency virus Tat proteins with a cellular protein kinase. *Virol* 197:601–608.

1065. Heyes, M. P., B. J. Brew, A. Martin, R. W. Price, A. M. Salazar, J. J. Sidfis, J. A. Vergey, M. M. Mouradian, A. E. Sadler, and J. Keilp. 1991. Quinolinic acid in cerebrospinal fluid and serum in HIV-1 infection: relationship to clinical and neurological status. *Ann Neurol* 29:202–209.

1066. Heyes, M. P., K. Saito, D. Jacobowitz, S. P. Markey, O. Takikawa, and J. H. Vickers. 1992. Poliovirus induces indoleamine-2,3-dioxygenase and quinolinic acid synthesis in macaque brain. *FASEB J* 6:2977–2989.

1066a. Hickey, W. Personal communication.

1067. Hickey, W. F., B. L. Hsu, and H. Kimura. 1991. T-lymphocyte entry into the central nervous system. *J Neurosci Res* 28:254–260.

1068. Hildreth, J. E., and R. J. Orentas. 1989. Involvement of a leukocyte adhesion receptor (LFA-1) in HIV-induced syncytium formation. *Science* 244:1075–1078.

1068a. Hill, J. M., R. F. Mervis, R. Avidor, T. W. Moddy, and D. E. Brenneman. 1993. HIV envelope protein-induced neuronal damage and retardation of behavioral development in rat neonates. *Brain Res* 603:222–233.

1069. Hilleman, M. R. 1994. Comparative biology and pathogenesis of AIDS and hepatitis B viruses: related but different. *AIDS Res Hum Retro* 10:1409–1419.

1070. Hillemanns, P., T. V. Ellerbrock, S. McPhillips, P. Dole, S. Alperstein, D. Johnson, X. W. Sun, M. A. Chiasson, and T. C. Wright, Jr. 1996. Prevalence of anal human papillomavirus infection and anal cytologic abnormalities in HIV-seropositive women. *AIDS* 10:1641–1647.

1071. Himathongkham, S., and P. A. Luciw. 1996. Restriction of HIV-1 (subtype B) replication at the entry step in rhesus macaque cells. *Virol* **219**:485–488.

1072. Hino, S., K. Yamaguchi, S. Katamine, H. Sugiyama, T. Amagasaki, K. Kinoshita, Y. Yoshida, H. Doi, Y. Tsuji, and T. Miyamoto. 1985. Mother-to-child transmission of human T-cell leukemia virus type-I. *Jpn J Cancer Res* **76**:474–480.

1073. Hira, S. K., J. Kamanga, R. Macuacua, N. Mwansa, D. F. Cruess, and P. L. Perine. 1990. Genital ulcers and male circumcision as risk factors for acquiring HIV-1 in Zambia. *J Inf Dis* **161**:584–585.

1074. Hira, S. K., U. G. Mangrola, C. Mwale, C. Chintu, G. Tembo, W. E. Brady, and P. L. Perine. 1990. Apparent vertical transmission of human immunodeficiency virus type 1 by breast-feeding in Zambia. *J Peds* **117**:421–424.

1075. Hirsch, I., J. de Mareuil, D. Salaun, and J.-C. Chermann. 1996. Genetic control of infection of primary macrophages with T-cell-tropic strains of HIV-1. *Virol* **219**:257–261.

1076. Hirsch, V. M., R. A. Olmsted, M. Murphey-Corb, R. H. Purcell, and P. R. Johnson. 1989. An African primate lentivirus (SIVsm) closely related to HIV-2. *Nature* **339**:389–392.

1077. Ho, D. D., R. E. Byington, R. T. Schooley, T. Flynn, T. R. Rota, and M. S. Hirsch. 1985. Infrequency of isolation of HTLV-III virus from saliva in AIDS. *N Engl J Med* **313**:1606.

1078. Ho, D. D., M. S. C. Fung, Y. Cao, X. L. Li, C. Sun, T. W. Chang, and N. C. Sun. 1991. Another discontinuous epitope on gp120 that is important in human immunodeficiency virus type 1 neutralization is identified by a monoclonal antibody. *Proc Natl Acad Sci USA* **88**:8949–8952.

1079. Ho, D. D., J. C. Kaplan, I. E. Rackauskas, and M. E. Gurney. 1988. Second conserved domain of gp120 is important for HIV infectivity and antibody neutralization. *Science* **239**:1021–1023.

1080. Ho, D. D., J. A. McKeating, X. L. Li, T. Moudgil, E. S. Daar, N. C. Sun, and J. E. Robinson. 1991. Conformational epitope on gp120 important in CD4 binding and human immunodeficiency virus type 1 neutralization identified by a human monoclonal antibody. *J Virol* **65**:489–493.

1081. Ho, D. D., T. Moudgil, and M. Alam. 1989. Quantitation of human immunodeficiency virus type 1 in the blood of infected persons. *N Engl J Med* **321**:1621–1625.

1082. Ho, D. D., A. U. Neumann, A. S. Perelson, W. Chen, J. M. Leonard, and M. Markowitz. 1995. Rapid turnover of plasma virions and CD4 lymphocytes in HIV-1 infection. *Nature* **373**:123–126.

1083. Ho, D. D., T. R. Rota, and M. S. Hirsch. 1986. Infection of monocyte/macrophages by human T lymphotropic virus type III. *J Clin Invest* **77**:1712–1715.

1084. Ho, D. D., T. R. Rota, R. T. Schooley, J. C. Kaplan, J. D. Allan, J. E. Groopman, L. Resnick, D. Felsenstein, C. A. Andrews, and M. S. Hirsch. 1985. Isolation of HTLV-III from cerebrospinal fluid and neural tissues of patients with neurologic syndromes related to the acquired immunodeficiency syndrome. *N Engl J Med* **313**:1493–1497.

1085. Ho, D. D., M. G. Sarngadharan, M. S. Hirsch, R. T. Schooley, T. R. Rota, R. C. Kennedy, T. C. Chanh, and V. L. Sato. 1987. Human immunodeficiency virus neutralizing antibodies recognize several conserved domains on the envelope glycoproteins. *J Virol* **61**:2024–2028.

1086. Ho, D. D., R. T. Schooley, T. R. Rota, J. C. Kaplan, T. Flynn, S. Z. Salahuddin, M. A. Gonda, and M. S. Hirsch. 1984. HTLV-III in the semen and blood of a healthy homosexual man. *Science* **226**:451–453.

1087. Ho, H. N., L. E. Hultin, R. T. Mitsuyasu, J. L. Matud, M. A. Hausner, D. Bockstoce, C. C. Chou, S. O'Rourke, J. M. G. Taylor, and J. V. Giorgi. 1993. Circulating HIV-specific CD8+ cytotoxic T cells express CD38 and HLA-DR antigens. *J Immunol* **150**:3070–3079.

1088. Ho, M., J. Armstrong, D. McMahon, G. Pazin, X.-L. Huang, C. Rinaldo, T. Whiteside, T. Tripoli, G. Levine, D. Moody, T. Okarma, E. Elder, P. Gupta, N. Tauxe, D. Torpey, and R. Herberman. 1993. A phase I study of adoptive transfer of autologous CD8+ T lymphocytes in patients with acquired immunodeficiency syndrome (AIDS)-related complex or AIDS. *Blood* **81**:2093–2101.

1089. Ho, W.-Z., V. Ayyavoo, A. Srinivasan, M. F. Stinski, S. A. Plotkin, and E. Gonczol. 1991. Human immunodeficiency virus type 1 *tat* gene enhances human cytomegalovirus gene expression and viral replication. *AIDS Res Hum Retro* **7**:689–695.

1090. Hodora, V. L., M. Jeddi-Tehrani, J. Grunewald, R. Andersson, G. Scarlatti, S. Esin, V. Holmberg, O. Libonatti, and H. Wigzell. 1993. HIV infection leads to differential expression of T-cell receptor Vβ genes in CD4⁺ and CD8⁺ T cells. *AIDS* **7**:633–638.

1091. Hoffenbach, A., P. Langlade-Demoyen, G. Dadaglio, E. Vilmer, F. Michel, C. Mayaud, B. Autran, and F. Plata. 1989. Unusually high frequencies of HIV-specific cytotoxic T lymphocytes in humans. *J Immunol* **142**:452–462.

1092. Hofman, F. M., M. M. Dohadwala, A. D. Wright, D. R. Hinton, and S. M. Walker. 1994. Exogenous tat protein activates central nervous system-derived endothelial cells. *J Neuroimmunol* **54**:19–28.

1093. Hofmann, B., P. Nishanian, R. L. Baldwin, P. Insixiengmay, A. Nel, and J. L. Fahey. 1990. HIV inhibits the early steps of lymphocyte activation, including initiation of inositol phospholipid metabolism. *J Immunol* **145**:3699–3705.

1094. Hogervorst, E., S. Jurriaans, F. de Wolf, A. van Wijk, A. Wiersma, M. Valk, M. Roos, B. van Gemen, R. Coutinho, F. Miedema, and J. Goudsmit. 1995. Predictors for non- and slow progression in human immunodeficiency virus (HIV) type 1 infection: low viral RNA copy numbers in serum and maintenance of high HIV-1 p24-specific but not V3-specific antibody levels. *J Inf Dis* **171**:811–821.

1095. Hogg, R. S., M. V. O'Shaughnessy, N. Gataric, B. Yip, K. Craib, M. T. Schechter, and J. S. G. Montaner. 1997. Decline in deaths from AIDS due to new antiretrovirals. *Lancet* **349**:1294.

1096. Hohdatsu, T., R. Pu, B. A. Torres, S. Trujillo, M. B. Gardner, and J. K. Yamamoto. 1993. Passive antibody protection of cats against feline immunodeficiency virus infection. *J Virol* **67**:2344–2348.

1097. Hohmann, A. W., K. Booth, V. Peters, D. L. Gordon, and R. M. Comacchio. 1993. Common epitope on HIV p24 and human platelets. *Lancet* **342**:1274–1275.

1098. Hollander, H., and J. A. Levy. 1987. Neurologic abnormalities and recovery of human immunodeficiency virus from cerebrospinal fluid. *Ann Int Med* **106**:692–695.

1099. Holmes, E. C., L. Q. Zhang, P. Simmonds, C. A. Lundlam, and A. J. Leigh Brown. 1992. Convergent and divergent sequence evolution in the surface envelope glycoprotein of human immunodeficiency virus type 1 within a single infected patient. *Proc Natl Acad Sci USA* **89**:4835–4839.

1100. Holodniy, M., D. A. Katzenstein, S. Sengupta, A. M. Wang, C. Casipit, D. H. Schwartz, M. Konrad, E. Groves, and T. C. Merigan. 1991. Detection and quantification of human immunodeficiency virus RNA in patient serum by use of the polymerase chain reaction. *J Inf Dis* **163**:862–866.

1101. Holodniy, M., L. Mole, D. Margolis, J. Moss, H. Dong, E. Boyer, M. Urdea, J. Kolberg, and S. Eastman. 1995. Determination of human immunodeficiency virus RNA in plasma and cellular viral DNA genotypic zidovudine resistance and viral load during zidovudine-didanosine combination therapy. *J Virol* **69**:3510–3516.

1102. Homsy, J., M. Meyer, and J. A. Levy. 1990. Serum enhancement of human immunodeficiency virus (HIV) correlates with disease in HIV infected individuals. *J Virol* **64**:1437–1440.

1103. Homsy, J., M. Meyer, M. Tateno, S. Clarkson, and J. A. Levy. 1989. The Fc and not the CD4 receptor mediates antibody enhancement of HIV infection in human cells. *Science* **244**:1357–1360.

1104. Homsy, J., M. Tateno, and J. A. Levy. 1988. Antibody-dependent enhancement of HIV infection. *Lancet* **i**:1285–1286.

1105. Hook, E. W., III, R. O. Cannon, A. J. Nahmias, F. F. Lee, C. H. Campbell, Jr., D. Glasser, and T. C. Quinn. 1992. Herpes simplex virus infection as a risk factor for human immunodeficiency virus infection in heterosexuals. *J Inf Dis* **165**:251–255.

1106. Hoover, D. R., C. Rinaldo, Y. He, J. Phair, J. Fahey, and N. M. H. Graham. 1995. Long-term survival without clinical AIDS after CD4+ cell counts fall below 200 × 10^6/l. *AIDS* **9**:145–152.

1107. Horsburgh, C. R., Jr., C.-Y. Ou, J. Jason, S. D. Holmberg, I. M. Longini, Jr., C. Schable, K. H. Mayer, A. R. Lifson, G. Schochetman, J. W. Ward, G. W. Rutherford, B. L. Evatt, G. R. Seage III, and H. W. Jaffe. 1989. Duration of human immunodeficiency virus infection before detection of antibody. *Lancet* **ii**:637–640.

1108. Horvat, R. T., C. Wood, and N. Balachandran. 1989. Transactivation of human immunodeficiency virus promoter by human herpesvirus 6. *J Virol* **63**:970–973.

1109. Hosie, M. J., R. Osborne, J. K. Yamamoto, J. C. Neil, and O. Jarrett. 1995. Protection against homologous but not heterologous challenge induced by inactivated feline immunodeficiency virus vaccines. *J Virol* **69**:1253–1255.

1110. Housset, C., E. Lamas, B. Courgnaud, O. Boucher, P. M. Girard, C. Marche, and C. Brechot. 1993. Presence of HIV-1 in human parenchymal and non-parenchymal liver cells in vivo. *J Hepatol* **19**:252–258.

1111. Howard, M. R., D. Whitby, G. Bahadur, F. Suggett, C. Boshoff, M. Tenant-Flowers, T. F. Schulz, S. Kirk, S. Matthews, I. V. D. Weller, R. S. Tedder, and R. A. Weiss. 1996. Detection of human herpesvirus 8 DNA in semen from HIV-infected individuals but not healthy semen donors. *AIDS* **11**:F15–F19.

1112. Howcroft, T. K., K. Strebel, M. A. Martin, and D. S. Singer. 1993. Repression of MHC class I gene promoter activity by two-exon Tat of HIV. *Science* **260**:1320–1323.

1112a. Howell, A. L., R. D. Edkins, S. E. Rier, G. R. Yeaman, J. E. Stern, M. W. Fanger, and C. R. Wira. 1997. Human immunodeficiency virus type 1 infection of cells and tissues from the upper and lower human female reproductive tract. *J Virol* **71**:3498–3506.

1113. Hoxie, J. A., J. D. Alpers, J. L. Rackowski, K. Huebner, B. S. Haggarty, A. J. Cedarbaum, and J. C. Reed. 1986. Alterations in T4 (CD4) protein and mRNA synthesis in cells infected with HIV. *Science* **234**:1123–1127.

1114. Hoxie, J. A., L. F. Brass, C. H. Pletcher, B. S. Haggarty, and R. H. Hahn. 1991. Cytopathic variants of an attenuated isolate of human immunodeficiency virus type 2 exhibit increased affinity for CD4. *J Virol* **65**:5096–5101.

1115. Hoxie, J. A., T. P. Fitzharris, P. R. Youngbar, D. M. Matthews, J. L. Rackowski, and S. F. Radka. 1987. Nonrandom association of cellular antigens with HTLV-III virions. *Human Immunol* **18**:39–52.

1116. Hoxie, J. A., B. S. Haggarty, J. L. Rackowski, N. Pilsbury, and J. A. Levy. 1985. Persistent noncytopathic infection of human lymphocytes with AIDS associated retrovirus (ARV). *Science* **229**:1400–1402.

1117. Hsia, K., and S. A. Spector. 1991. Human immunodeficiency virus DNA is present in a high percentage of CD4+ lymphocytes of seropositive individuals. *J Inf Dis* **164**:470–475.

1118. Hsu, D. H., R. de Waal Malefyt, D. F. Fiorentino, M. N. Dang, P. Vieira, J. DeVries, H. Spits, R. T. Mosmann, and K. W. Moore. 1990. Expression of interleukin-10 activity by Epstein-Barr virus protein BCRF1. *Science* **250**:830–832.

1119. Hsu, M.-C., U. Dhingra, J. V. Earley, M. Holly, D. Keith, C. M. Nalin, A. R. Richou, A. D. Schutt, S. Y. Tam, M. J. Potash, D. J. Volsky, and D. D. Richman. 1993. Inhibition of type 1 human immunodeficiency virus replication by a Tat antagonist to which the virus remains sensitive after prolonged exposure in vitro. *Proc Natl Acad Sci USA* **90**:6395–6399.

1120. Hsueh, F. W., C. M. Walker, D. J. Blackbourn, and J. A. Levy. 1994. Suppression of HIV replication by CD8+ cell clones derived from HIV-infected and uninfected individuals. *Cell Immunol* **159**:271–279.

1121. Hu, P. F., L. E. Hultin, P. Hultin, M. A. Hausner, K. Hirji, A. Jewett, B. Bonavida, R. Detels, and J. V. Giorgi. 1995. Natural killer cell immunodeficiency in HIV disease is manifest by profoundly decreased numbers of CD16+CD56+ cells and expansion of a population of CD16dimCD56– cells with low lytic activity. *J AIDS Hum Retrovirol* **10**:331–340.

1121a. Hu, S. L. Personal communication.

1122. Hu, S.-L., K. Abrams, G. N. Barber, P. Moran, J. M. Zarling, A. J. Langlois, L. Kuller, W. R.

Morton, and R. E. Benveniste. 1992. Protection of macaques against SIV infection by subunit vaccines of SIV envelope glycoprotein gp160. *Science* **255**:456–459.

1123. Hu, S.-L., V. Stallard, K. Abrams, G. N. Barber, L. Kuller, A. J. Langlois, W. R. Morton, and R. E. Benveniste. 1993. Protection of vaccinia-primed macaques against SIVmne infection by combination immunization with recombinant vaccinia virus and SIVmne gp160. *J Med Primatol* **22**:92–99.

1124. Hu, S. L., P. Polacino, V. Stallard, J. Klaniecki, S. Pennathur, B. M. Travis, L. Misher, H. Kornas, A. J. Langlois, W. R. Morton, and R. E. Benveniste. 1996. Recombinant subunit vaccines as an approach to study correlates of protection against primate lentivirus infection. *Immunol Let* **51**:115–119.

1125. Hu, W.-S., and H. M. Temin. 1990. Retroviral recombination and reverse transcription. *Science* **250**:1227–1233.

1126. Huang, A. S., E. L. Palma, and N. Hewlett. 1974. Pseudotype formation between enveloped RNA and DNA viruses. *Nature* **252**:743–745.

1127. Huang, Y., L. Zhang, and D. D. Ho. 1995. Characterization of nef sequences in long-term survivors of human immunodeficiency virus type 1 infection. *J Virol* **69**:93–100.

1128. Huang, Y. Q., A. Buchbinder, J. J. Li, A. Nicolaides, W. G. Zhang, and A. E. Friedman-Kien. 1992. The absence of Tat sequences in tissues of HIV-negative patients with epidemic Kaposi's sarcoma. *AIDS* **6**:1139–1142.

1129. Huang, Y. Q., J. J. Li, A. Nicolaides, and W. G. Zhang. 1992. Fibroblast growth factor 6 gene expression in AIDS-associated Kaposi's sarcoma. *Lancet* **339**:1110–1111.

1130. Huang, Y. Q., J. J. Li, and M. G. Rush. 1992. HPV-16-related DNA sequences in Kaposi's sarcoma. *Lancet* **339**:515–518.

1131. Huang, Z. B., M. J. Potash, M. Simm, M. Shahabuddin, W. Chao, H. E. Gendelman, E. Eden, and D. J. Volsky. 1993. Infection of macrophages with lymphotropic human immunodeficiency virus type 1 can be arrested after viral DNA synthesis. *J Virol* **67**:6893–6896.

1132. Hudson, C. P. 1993. Concurrent partnerships could cause AIDS epidemics. *Int J STD AIDS* **4**:249–253.

1133. Huet, T., R. Cheynier, A. Meyerhans, G. Roelants, and S. Wain-Hobson. 1990. Genetic organization of a chimpanzee lentivirus related to HIV-1. *Nature* **345**:356–359.

1134. Hufert, F. T., J. Schmitz, M. Schrieber, H. Schmitz, P. Racz, and D. D. von Laer. 1993. Human Kupffer cells infected with HIV-1 in vivo. *J AIDS* **6**:772–777.

1135. Hufert, F. T., J. van Lunzen, G. Janossy, S. Bertram, J. Schmitz, O. Haller, P. Racz, and D. von Laer. 1997. Germinal center CD4+ T cells are an important site of HIV replication *in vivo*. *AIDS* **11**:849–857.

1136. Hughes, B. P., T. F. Booth, A. S. Belyaev, D. McIlroy, J. Jowett, and P. Roy. 1993. Morphogenic capabilities of human immunodeficiency virus type 1 gag and gag-pol proteins in insect cells. *Virol* **193**:242–255.

1137. Hughes, E. S., J. E. Bell, and P. Simmonds. 1997. Investigation of the dynamics of the spread of human immunodeficiency virus to brain and other tissues by evolutionary analysis of sequences from the p17*gag* and *env* genes. *J Virol* **71**:1272–1280.

1138. Hughes, R. A., S. E. Macatonia, I. F. Rowe, A. C. S. Keat, and S. C. Knight. 1990. The detection of human immunodeficiency virus DNA in dendritic cells from the joints of patients with aseptic arthritis. *Brit J Rheum* **29**:166–170.

1139. Hugin, A. W., M. S. Vacchio, and H. C. Morse III. 1991. A virus-encoded "superantigen" in a retrovirus-induced immunodeficiency syndrome of mice. *Science* **252**:424–427.

1140. Hulskotte, E. G. J., A. M. Geretti, K. H. J. Siebelink, G. van Amerongen, M. P. Cranage, E. W. Rud, S. G. Norley, P. de Vries, and A. D. M. E. Osterhaus. 1995. Vaccine-induced virus-neutralizing antibodies and cytotoxic T cells do not protect macaques from experimental infection with simian immunodeficiency virus SIVmac32H (J5). *J Virol* **69**:6289–6296.

1141. Hunter, D. J. 1993. AIDS in sub-Saharan Africa: the epidemiology of heterosexual transmission and the prospects for prevention. *Epidemiology* **4**:63–72.

1142. Hunter, D. J., and B. N. Maggwa. 1994. Sexual behavior, sexually transmitted diseases, male circumcision and risk of HIV infection among women in Nairobi, Kenya. *AIDS* **8**:93–99.

1142a.Hurley, S. F., D. J. Jolley, and J. M. Kaldor. 1997. Effectiveness of needle-exchange programmes for prevention of HIV infection. *Lancet* **349**:1797–1800.

1143. Husch, B., M. M. Eibl, and J. W. Mannhalter. 1993. CD3, CD8 double-positive cells from HIV-1 infected chimpanzees show group-specific inhibition of HIV-1 replication. *AIDS Res Hum Retro* **9**:405–413.

1144. Hussain, L. A., C. G. Kelly, E.-M. Hecht, R. Fellowes, M. Jourdan, and T. Lehner. 1991. The expression of Fc receptors for immunoglobulin G in human rectal epithelium. *AIDS* **5**:1089–1094.

1145. Hussain, L. A., and T. Lehner. 1995. Comparative investigation of Langerhans' cells and potential receptors for HIV in oral, genitourinary and rectal epithelia. *Immunol* **85**:475–484.

1146. Hutto, C., W. P. Parks, S. Lai, M. T. Mastrucci, C. Mitchell, J. Munoz, E. Trapido, I. M. Master, and G. B. Scott. 1991. A hospital-based prospective study of perinatal infection with human immunodeficiency virus type 1. *J Peds* **118**:347–353.

1147. Hwang, S. S., T. J. Boyle, H. K. Lyerly, and B. R. Cullen. 1992. Identification of envelope V3 loop as the major determinant of CD4 neutralization sensitivity of HIV-1. *Science* **257**:535–537.

1148. Hwang, S. S., T. J. Boyle, H. K. Lyerly, and B. R. Cullen. 1991. Identification of the envelope V3 loop as the primary determinant of cell tropism in HIV-1. *Science* **253**:71–74.

1149. Hyjek, E., H. W. Lischner, T. Hyslop, J. Bartkowiak, M. Kubin, G. Trinchieri, and D. Kozbor. 1995. Cytokine patterns during progression to AIDS in children with perinatal HIV infection. *J Immunol* **155**:4060–4071.

1150. Ichimura, H., S. C. Kliks, S. Visrutaratna, C. Y. Ou, M. L. Kalish, and J. A. Levy. 1994. Biological, serological, and genetic characterization of HIV-1 subtype E isolates from Northern Thailand. *AIDS Res Hum Retro* **10**:263–269.

1151. Ichimura, H., and J. A. Levy. 1995. Polymerase substrate depletion: a novel strategy for inhibiting the replication of the human immunodeficiency virus. *Virol* **211**:554–560.

1152. Igarashi, T., Y. Ami, H. Yamamoto, R. Shibata, T. Kuwata, R. Mukai, K. Shinohara, T. Komatsu, A. Adachi, and M. Hayami. 1997. Protection of monkeys vaccinated with *vpr*- and/or *nef*-defective simian immunodeficiency virus strain mac/human immunodeficiency virus type 1 chimeric viruses: a potential candidate live-attenuated human AIDS vaccine. *J Gen Virol* **78**:985–989.

1153. Ikeuchi, K., S. Kim, R. A. Byrn, S. R. Goldring, and J. E. Groopman. 1990. Infection of non-lymphoid cells by human immunodeficiency virus type 1 or type 2. *J Virol* **64**:4226–4231.

1154. Ikonomidis, G., F. R. Frankel, D. A. Portnoy, and Y. Paterson. 1995. Listeria monocytogenes: a novel live vaccine vector, p. 317–326. *In* S. Brown, R. Chanock, H. Ginsberg, and E. Norrby (ed.), *Molecular Approaches to the Control of Infectious Diseases. Vaccines 95.* Cold Spring Harbor Laboratory Press, Cold Spring Harbor.

1155. Ilaria, G., J. L. Jacobs, B. Polsky, B. Koll, P. Baron, C. MacLow, D. Armstrong, and P. N. Schlegel. 1992. Detection of HIV-1 DNA sequences in pre-ejaculatory fluid. *Lancet* **340**:1469.

1156. Ilyinskii, P. O., M. A. Simon, S. C. Czajak, A. A. Lackner, and R. C. Desrosiers. 1997. Induction of AIDS by simian immunodeficiency virus lacking NF-κB and SP1 binding elements. *J Virol* **71**:1880–1887.

1157. Imagawa, D. T., M. H. Lee, S. M. Wolinsky, K. Sano, F. Morales, S. Kwok, J. J. Sninsky, P. G. Nishanian, J. Giorgi, J. L. Fahey, J. Dudley, B. R. Visscher, and R. Detels. 1989. Human immunodeficiency virus type 1 infection in homosexual men who remain seronegative for prolonged periods. *N Engl J Med* **320**:1458–1462.

1158. Imberti, L., A. Sottini, A. Bettinardi, M. Puoti, and D. Primi. 1991. Selective depletion in HIV infection of T cells that bear specific T cell receptor V-beta sequences. *Science* **254**:860–862.

1159. Imboden, J., A. Weiss, and J. D. Stobo. 1985. The antigen receptor on a human T cell line initiates activation by increasing cytoplasmic free calcium. *J Immunol* **134**:663–665.

1160. Imrie, A., A. Beveridge, W. Genn, J. Vizzard, and D. A. Cooper. 1997. Transmission of human immunodeficiency virus type 1 resistant to nevirapine and zidovudine. *J Inf Dis* **175**:1502–1506.

1161. **Imrie, A., A. Carr, C. Duncombe, R. Finlayson, J. Vizzard, M. Law, J. Kaldor, R. Penny, and D. A. Cooper.** 1996. Primary infection with zidovudine-resistant human immunodeficiency virus type 1 does not adversely affect outcome at 1 year. *J Inf Dis* **174**:195–198.

1162. **Indraccolo, S., M. Mion, R. Zamarchi, A. Veronesi, M. L. Veronese, M. Panozzo, C. Betterle, A. Barelli, A. Borri, A. Amadori, and L. Chieco-Bianchi.** 1993. B cell activation and human immunodeficiency virus infection. V. Phenotypic and functional alterations in CD5+ and CD5− B cell subsets. *J Clin Immunol* **13**:381–388.

1163. **Ioachim, H. L., B. Dorsett, J. Melamed, V. Adsay, and E. A. Santagada.** 1992. Cytomegalovirus, angiomatosis, and Kaposi's sarcoma: new observations of a debated relationship. *Mod Path* **5**:169–178.

1164. **Ioannidis, J. P. A., J. C. Cappelleri, J. Lau, P. R. Skolnik, B. Melville, T. C. Chalmers, and H. S. Sacks.** 1995. Early or deferred zidovudine therapy in HIV-infected patients without an AIDS-defining illness. *Ann Int Med* **122**:856–866.

1165. **Issel, C. J., D. W. Horohov, D. F. Lea, W. V. Adams, Jr., S. F. Hagius, J. M. McManus, A. C. Allison, and R. C. Montelaro.** 1992. Efficacy of inactivated whole-virus and subunit vaccines in preventing infection and disease caused by equine infectious anemia virus. *J Virol* **66**:3398–3408.

1166. **Itescu, S., J. Dalton, H. Z. Zhang, and R. Winchester.** 1993. Tissue infiltration in a CD8 lymphocytosis syndrome associated with human immunodeficiency virus-1 infection has the phenotypic appearance of an antigenically driven response. *J Clin Invest* **91**:2216–2225.

1167. **Itescu, S., U. Mathur-Wagh, M. L. Skovron, L. J. Brancato, M. Marmor, A. Zeleniuch-Jacquotte, and R. Winchester.** 1991. HLA-B35 is associated with accelerated progression to AIDS. *J AIDS* **5**:37–45.

1168. **Itescu, S., S. Rose, E. Dwyer, and R. Winchester.** 1994. Certain HLA-DR5 and -DR6 major histocompatibility complex class II alleles are associated with a CD8 lymphocytic host response to human immunodeficiency virus type 1 characterized by low lymphocyte viral strain heterogeneity and slow disease progression. *Proc Natl Acad Sci USA* **91**:11472–11476.

1169. **Itescu, S., P. F. Simonelli, R. J. Winchester, and H. S. Ginsberg.** 1994. Human immunodeficiency virus type 1 strains in the lungs of infected individuals evolve independently from those in peripheral blood and are highly conserved in the C-terminal region of the envelope V3 loop. *Proc Natl Acad Sci USA* **91**:11378–11382.

1170. **Ivanoff, L. A., J. W. Dubay, J. F. Morris, S. J. Roberts, L. Gutshall, E. J. Sternberg, E. Hunter, T. J. Matthews, and S. R. Petteway, Jr.** 1992. V3 loop region of the HIV-1 gp120 envelope protein is essential for virus infectivity. *Virol* **187**:423–432.

1171. **Iversen, A. K. N., R. W. Shafer, K. Wehrly, M. A. Winters, J. I. Mullins, B. Chesebro, and T. C. Merigan.** 1996. Multidrug-resistant human immunodeficiency virus type 1 strains resulting from combination antiretroviral therapy. *J Virol* **70**:1086–1090.

1172. **Ivey-Hoyle, M., J. S. Culp, M. A. Chaikin, B. D. Hellmig, T. J. Matthews, R. W. Sweet, and M. Rosenberg.** 1991. Envelope glycoproteins from biologically diverse isolates of immunodeficiency viruses have widely different affinities for CD4. *Proc Natl Acad Sci USA* **88**:512–516.

1173. **Iwatani, Y., S. K. Song, L. Wang, J. Planas, H. Sakai, A. Ishimoto, and M. W. Cloyd.** 1997. Human immunodeficiency virus type 1 Vpu modifies viral cytopathic effect through augmented virus release. *J Gen Virol* **78**:841–846.

1174. **Jabbar, M. A., and D. P. Nayak.** 1990. Intracellular interaction of human immunodeficiency virus type 1 (ARV-2) envelope glycoprotein gp160 with CD4 blocks the movement and maturation of CD4 to the plasma membrane. *J Virol* **64**:6297–6304.

1175. **Jacobson, D. L., J. A. McCutchan, P. L. Spechko, I. Abramson, R. S. Smith, A. Bartok, G. R. Boss, D. Durand, S. A. Bozzette, S. A. Spector, and D. D. Richman.** 1991. The evolution of lymphadenopathy and hypergammaglobulinemia are evidence for early and sustained polyclonal B lymphocyte activation during human immunodeficiency virus infection. *J Inf Dis* **163**:240–246.

1176. Jacobson, E. L., F. Pilaro, and K. A. Smith. 1996. Rational interleukin 2 therapy for HIV positive individuals: daily low doses enhance immune function without toxicity. *Proc Natl Acad Sci USA* **93**:10405–10410.

1177. Jacobson, J. M., N. Colman, N. A. Ostrow, R. W. Simson, D. Tomesch, L. Marlin, M. Rao, J. L. Mills, J. Clemens, and A. M. Prince. 1993. Passive immunotherapy in the treatment of advanced human immunodeficiency virus infection. *J Inf Dis* **168**:298–305.

1178. Jacobson, J. M., J. S. Greenspan, J. Spritzler, N. Ketter, J. L. Fahey, J. B. Jackson, L. Fox, M. Chernoff, A. W. Wu, L. A. MacPhail, G. J. Vasquez, and D. A. Wohl. 1997. Thalidomide for the treatment of oral aphthous ulcers in patients with human immunodeficiency virus infection. *N Engl J Med* **336**:1487–1493.

1179. Jacobson, M. A., R. E. Fusaro, M. Galmarini, and W. Lang. 1991. Decreased serum dehydroepiandrosterone is associated with an increased progression of human immunodeficiency virus infection in men with CD4 cell counts of 200–499. *J Inf Dis* **164**:864–868.

1180. Jacobson, M. A., M. Zegans, P. R. Pavan, J. J. O'Donnell, F. Sattler, N. Rao, S. Owens, and R. Pollard. 1997. Cytomegalovirus retinitis after initiation of highly active antiretoviral therapy. *Lancet* **439**:1443–1445.

1181. Jacquez, J. A., J. S. Koopman, C. P. Simon, and I. M. Longini, Jr. 1994. Role of primary infection in epidemics of HIV infection in gay cohorts. *J AIDS* **7**:1169–1184.

1182. Jaffe, H. W., D. J. Bregman, and R. M. Selik. 1983. Acquired immune deficiency syndrome in the United States: the first 1,000 cases. *J Inf Dis* **148**:339–345.

1183. Jameson, B. A., P. E. Rao, L. I. Kong, B. H. Hahn, G. M. Shaw, L. E. Hood, and S. B. H. Kent. 1988. Location and chemical synthesis of a binding site for HIV-1 on the CD4 protein. *Science* **240**:1335–1339.

1184. Jameson, S. C., F. R. Carbone, and M. J. Bevan. 1993. Clone-specific T cell receptor antagonists of major histocompatibility complex class I-restricted cytotoxic T cells. *J Exp Med* **177**:1541–1550.

1185. Jamieson, B. D., G. M. Aldrovandi, V. Planelles, J. B. M. Jowett, L. Gao, L. M. Bloch, I. S. Y. Chen, and J. A. Zack. 1994. Requirement of human immunodeficiency virus type 1 nef for in vivo replication and pathogenicity. *J Virol* **68**:3478–3485.

1186. Janoff, E. N., S. M. Wahl, K. Thomas, and P. D. Smith. 1995. Modulation of human immunodeficiency virus type 1 infection of human monocytes by IgA. *J Inf Dis* **172**:855–858

1186a. Janssen, R., G. Satten, S. Stramer, B. Rawal, and M. Busch. 1997. A simple strategy for identifying individuals with recent HIV infection, abstr. no. 490. *Fourth Conference on Retroviruses and Opportunistic Infections.*

1186b. Janssens, W., A. Buve, and J. N. Nkengasong. 1997. The puzzle of HIV-1 subtypes in Africa. *AIDS* **11**:705–712.

1187. Jansson, M., M. Popovic, A. Karlsson, F. Cocchi, P. Rossi, J. Albert, and H. Wigzell. 1996. Sensitivity to inhibition by β-chemokines correlates with biological phenotypes of primary HIV-1 isolates. *Proc Natl Acad Sci USA* **93**:15382–15387.

1188. Jason, J., L. A. Sleeper, S. M. Donfield, J. Murphy, I. Warrier, S. Arkin, and B. Evatt. 1995. Evidence for a shift from a type I lymphocyte pattern with HIV disease progression. *J AIDS Hum Retrovirol* **10**:471–476.

1189. Jassoy, C., R. P. Johnson, B. A. Navia, J. Worth, and B. D. Walker. 1992. Detection of a vigorous HIV-1-specific cytotoxic T lymphocyte response in cerebrospinal fluid from infected persons with AIDS dementia complex. *J Immunol* **149**:3113–3119.

1190. Jault, F. M., S. A. Spector, and D. H. Spector. 1994. The effects of cytomegalovirus on human immunodeficiency virus replication in brain-derived cells correlate with permissiveness of the cells for each virus. *J Virol* **68**:959–973.

1191. Javaherian, K., A. J. Langlois, G. J. LaRosa, A. T. Profy, D. P. Bolognesi, W. C. Herlihy, S. D. Putney, and T. J. Matthews. 1990. Broadly neutralizing antibodies elicted by the hypervariable neutralizing determinant of HIV-1. *Science* **250**:1590–1593.

1192. Javaherian, K., A. J. Langlois, C. McDanal, K. L. Ross, L. I. Eckler, C. L. Jellis, A. T. Profy, J. R. Rusche, D. P. Bolognesi, S. D. Putney, and T. J. Matthews. 1989. Principal neutralizing domain of the human immunodeficiency virus type 1 envelope protein. *Proc Natl Acad Sci USA* **86**:6768–6772.

1193. Jeffrey, A. A., D. Israel-Biet, J.-M. Andrieu, P. Even, and A. Venet. 1991. HIV isolation from pulmonary cells derived from bronchoalveolar lavage. *Clin Exp Immunol* **84**:488–492.

1194. Jehuda-Cohen, T., J. Powell, K. W. Sell, F. Villinger, E. Lockwood, H. M. McClure, and A. Ahmed-Ansari. 1991. Transmission of retrovirus infection by transfusion of seronegative blood in nonhuman primates. *J Inf Dis* **163**:1223–1228.

1195. Jehuda-Cohen, T., B. A. Slade, J. D. Powell, F. Villinger, B. De, T. M. Folks, H. M. McClure, K. W. Sell, and A. Ahmed-Ansari. 1990. Polyclonal B-cell activation reveals antibodies against human immunodeficiency virus type 1 (HIV-1) in HIV-1-seronegative individuals. *Proc Natl Acad Sci USA* **87**:3972–3976.

1196. Jelinek, D. F., and P. E. Lipsky. 1987. Enhancement of human B cell proliferation and differentiation by tumor necrosis factor-alpha and interleukin 1. *J Immunol* **139**:2970–2976.

1197. Jelinek, D. F., J. B. Splawski, and P. E. Lipsky. 1986. The roles of interleukin-2 and interferon-gamma in human B cell activation, growth and differentiation. *Eur J Immunol* **16**:925.

1198. Jelonek, M. T., J. L. Maskrey, K. S. Steimer, B. J. Potts, K. W. Higgins, and M. A. Keller. 1995. Inhibition of the offspring anti-recombinant gp120 antibody response to a human immunodeficiency virus vaccine by maternal immunization in a murine model. *J Inf Dis* **172**:539–542.

1199. Jeng, C. R., R. V. English, T. Childers, M. B. Tompkins, and W. A. F. Tompkins. 1996. Evidence for CD8+ antiviral activity in cats infected with feline immunodeficiency virus. *J Virol* **70**:2474–2480.

1200. Jewett, A., and B. Bonavida. 1990. Peripheral blood monocytes derived from HIV+ individuals mediate antibody-dependent cellular cytotoxicity (ADCC). *Clin Immunol Immunopathol* **54**:192–199.

1201. Jewett, A., M. Cavalcanti, J. Giorgi, and B. Bonavida. 1997. Concomitant killing *in vitro* of both gp120-coated CD4+ peripheral T lymphocytes and natural killer cells in the antibody-dependent cellular cytotoxicity (ADCC) system. *J Immunol* **158**:5492–5500.

1201a. Jiang, J.-D., F.-N. Chu, P. H. Naylor, J. E. Kirkley, J. Mandeli, J. L. Wallace, P. S. Sarin, A. L. Goldstein, J. F. Holland, and J. G. Bekesi. 1992. Specific antibody responses to synthetic peptides of HIV-1 p17 correlate with different stages of HIV-1 infection. *J AIDS* **5**:382–390.

1202. Jiang, S., K. Lin, and A. R. Neurath. 1991. Enhancement of human immunodeficiency virus type 1 infection by antisera to peptides from the envelope glycoproteins gp120/gp41. *J Exp Med* **174**:1557–1563.

1203. Jiang, S., and A. R. Neurath. 1992. Potential risks of eliciting antibodies enhancing HIV-1 infection of monocytic cells by vaccination with V3 loops of unmatched HIV-1 isolates. *AIDS* **6**:331–342.

1203a. Joag, S. V., I. Adany, Z. Li, L. Foresman, D. M. Pinson, C. Wang, E. B. Stephens, R. Raghavan, and O. Narayan. 1997. Animal model of mucosally transmitted human immunodeficiency virus type 1 disease: intravaginal and oral deposition of simian/human immunodeficiency virus in macaques results in systemic infection, elimination of CD4+ T cells, and AIDS. *J Virol* **71**:4016–4023.

1204. Joag, S. V., Z. Li, L. Foresman, E. B. Stephens, L.-J. Zhao, I. Adany, D. M. Pinson, H. M. McClure, and O. Narayan. 1996. Chimeric simian/human immunodeficiency virus that causes progressive loss of CD4+ T cells and AIDS in pig-tailed macaques. *J Virol* **70**:3189–3197.

1205. Joag, S. V., E. B. Stephens, D. Galbreath, G. W. Zhu, Z. Li, L. Foresman, L. J. Zhao, D. M. Pinson, and O. Narayan. 1995. Simian immunodeficiency virus SIV$_{mac}$ chimeric virus whose *env* gene was derived from SIV-encephalitic brain is macrophage-tropic but not neurovirulent. *J Virol* **69**:1367–1369.

1206. John, G. C., R. W. Nduati, D. Mbori-Ngacha, J. Overbaugh, M. Welch, B. A. Richardson, J. Ndinya-Achola, J. Bwayo, J. Krieger, F. Onyango, and J. K. Kreiss. 1997. Genital shedding of human immunodeficiency virus type 1 DNA during pregnancy: association with immunosuppression, abnormal cervical or vaginal discharge, and severe vitamin A deficiency. *J Inf Dis* **175**:57–62.

1206a.Johnson, R. P., R. L. Glickman, J. Q. Yang, A. Kaur, J. T. Dion, M. J. Mulligan, and R. C. Desrosiers. 1997. Induction of vigorous cytotoxic T-lymphocyte responses by live attenuated simian immunodeficiency virus. *J Virol* 71:7711–7718.

1207. Johnson, P. R., D. C. Montefiori, S. Goldstein, T. E. Hamm, Y. Zhou, S. Kitov, N. L. Haigwood, L. Misher, W. T. London, J. L. Gerin, A. Allison, R. H. Purcell, R. M. Chanock, and V. M. Hirsch. 1992. Inactivated whole-virus vaccine derived from a proviral DNA clone of simian immunodeficiency virus induces high levels of neutralizing antibodies and confers protection against heterologous challenge. *Proc Natl Acad Sci USA* 89:2175–2179.

1208. Johnston, M. I., and D. F. Hoth. 1993. Present status and future prospects for HIV therapies. *Science* 260:1286–1293.

1209. Joling, P., L. J. Bakker, J. A. G. Van Strijp, T. Meerloo, L. deGraaf, M. E. M. Dekker, J. Goudsmit, J. Verhoef, and H. J. Schuurman. 1993. Binding of human immunodeficiency virus type-1 to follicular dendritic cells *in vitro* is complement dependent. *J Immunol* 150:1065–1073.

1210. Joly, P., J. M. Guillon, C. Mayaud, F. Plata, I. Theodorou, P. Denis, P. Debre, and B. Autran. 1989. Cell mediated suppression of HIV-specific cytotoxic T lymphocytes. *J Immunol* 143:2193–2201.

1211. Jonassen, T. O., K. Stene-Johansen, E. S. Berg, O. Hungnes, C. F. Lindboe, S. S. Froland, and B. Grinde. 1997. Sequence analysis of HIV-1 group O from Norwegian patients infected in the 1960s. *Virol* 231:43–47.

1212. Jones, K. A., J. T. Kadonaga, P. A. Luciw, and R. Tjian. 1986. Activation of the AIDS retrovirus promoter by the cellular transcription factor, Sp1. *Science* 232:755–759.

1213. Jordan, C. A., B. A. Watkins, C. Kufta, and M. Dubois-Dalcq. 1991. Infection of brain microglial cells by human immunodeficiency virus type 1 is CD4 dependent. *J Virol* 65:736–742.

1214. Jovaisas, E., M. A. Koch, A. Schafer, M. Stauber, and D. Lowenthal. 1985. LAV/HTLV-III in 20-week fetus. *Lancet* ii:1129.

1215. Jurriaans, S., J. T. Dekker, and A. de Ronde. 1992. HIV-1 viral DNA load in peripheral blood mononuclear cells from seroconverters and long-term infected individuals. *AIDS* 6:635–641.

1216. Jurriaans, S., B. Van Gemen, G. J. Weverling, D. Van Strijp, P. Nara, R. Coutinho, M. Koot, H. Schuitemaker, and J. Goudsmit. 1994. The natural history of HIV-1 infection: virus load and virus phenotype independent determinants of clinical course? *Virol* 204:223–233.

1217. Juszczak, R. J., H. Turchin, A. Truneh, J. Culp, and S. Kassis. 1991. Effect of human immunodeficiency virus gp120 glycoprotein on the association of the protein tyrosine kinase p56lck with CD4 in human T lymphocytes. *J Biol Chem* 266:11176–11183.

1218. Kahn, J. O., F. Sinangil, J. Baenziger, N. Murcar, D. Wynne, R. L. Coleman, K. S. Steimer, C. L. Dekker, and D. Chernoff. 1994. Clinical and immunologic responses to human immunodeficiency virus (HIV) type 1_{SF2} gp120 subunit vaccine combined with MF59 adjuvant with or without muramyl tripeptide dipalmitoyl phosphatidylethanolamine in non-HIV-infected human volunteers. *J Inf Dis* 170:1288–1291.

1219. Kahn, J. O., S. W. Lagakos, D. D. Richman, A. Cross, C. Pettinelli, S. Liou, M. Brown, P. A. Volberding, C. S. Crumpacker, G. Beall, H. S. Sacks, T. C. Merigan, M. Beltangady, L. Smaldone, and R. Dolin. 1992. A controlled trial comparing continued zidovudine with didanosine in human immunodeficiency virus infection. *N Engl J Med* 327:583–587.

1220. Kahn, J. O., K. S. Steimer, J. Baenziger, A. M. Duliege, M. Feinberg, T. Elbeik, M. Chesney, N. Murcar, D. Chernoff, and F. Sinangil. 1995. Clinical, immunologic, and virologic observations related to human immunodeficiency virus (HIV) type 1 infection in a volunteer in an HIV-1 vaccine clinical trial. *J Inf Dis* 171:1343–1347.

1221. Kaiser, P. K., J. T. Offermann, and S. A. Lipton. 1990. Neuronal injury due to HIV-1 envelope protein is blocked by anti-gp120 antibodies but not by anti-CD4 antibodies. *Neurol* 40:1757–1761.

1222. Kaldor, J. M., B. Tindall, P. Williamson, J. Elford, and D. A. Cooper. 1993. Factors associated with Kaposi's sarcoma in a cohort of homosexual and bisexual men. *J AIDS* 6:1145–1149.

1223. Kalish, L. A., J. Pitt, J. Lew, S. Landesman, C. Diaz, R. Hershow, F. B. Hollinger, M. Pagano, B. Smeriglio, and J. Moye. 1997. Defining the time of fetal or perinatal acquisition of human immunodeficiency virus type 1 infection on the basis of age at first positive culture. *J Inf Dis* **175**:712–715.

1224. Kalish, M., K. Potts, C. Bandea, G. Orloff, C. C. Luo, N. de la Torre, G. Schochetman, and C. Y. Ou. 1991. Genetic diversity in the principal neutralizing domain (V3 region) of HIV-1 strains from nine countries. *In International Conference on Advances in AIDS Vaccine Development, Fourth Annual Meeting of the NCVDG.*

1225. Kalter, D. C., H. E. Gendelman, and M. S. Meltzer. 1990. Infection of human epidermal Langerhans' cells by HIV (reply). *AIDS* **4**:266–268.

1226. Kalter, D. C., H. E. Gendelman, and M. S. Meltzer. 1991. Inhibition of human immunodeficiency virus infection in monocytes by monoclonal antibodies against leukocyte adhesion molecules. *Immunol Let* **30**:219–228.

1227. Kamel-Reid, S., and J. E. Dick. 1988. Engraftment of immune-deficient mice with human hematopoietic stem cells. *Science* **242**:1706–1709.

1228. Kameoka, M., T. Kimura, Y.-H. Zheng, S. Suzuki, K. Fujinaga, R. B. Luftig, and K. Ikuta. 1997. Protease-defective, gp120-containing human immunodeficiency virus type 1 particles induce apoptosis more efficiently than does wild-type virus or recombinant gp120 protein in healthy donor-derived peripheral blood T cells. *J Clin Micro* **35**:41–47.

1229. Kamine, J., B. Elangovan, T. Subramanian, D. Coleman, and G. Chinnadurai. 1996. Identification of a cellular protein that specifically interacts with the essential cysteine region of the HIV-1 Tat transactivator. *Virol* **216**:357–366.

1230. Kaminsky, L. S., T. McHugh, D. Stites, P. Volberding, G. Henle, W. Henle, and J. A. Levy. 1985. High prevalence of antibodies to AIDS-associated retroviruses (ARV) in acquired immune deficiency syndrome and related conditions and not in other disease states. *Proc Natl Acad Sci USA* **82**:5535–5539.

1231. Kampinga, G. A., A. Simonon, P. Van de Perre, E. Karita, P. Msellati, and J. Goudsmit. 1997. Primary infections with HIV-1 of women and their offspring in Rwanda: findings of heterogeneity at seroconversion, coinfection, and recombinants of HIV-1 subtypes A and C. *Virol* **227**:63–76.

1232. Kaneshima, H., L. Su, M. L. Bonyhadi, R. I. Connor, D. D. Ho, and J. M. McCune. 1994. Rapid-high, syncytium-inducing isolates of human immunodeficiency virus type 1 induce cytopathicity in the human thymus of the SCID-hu mouse. *J Virol* **68**:8188–8192.

1233. Kang, C.-Y., K. Hariharan, P. L. Nara, J. Sodroski, and J. P. Moore. 1994. Immunization with a soluble CD4-gp120 complex preferentially induces neutralizing anti-human immunodeficiency virus type 1 antibodies directed to conformation-dependent epitopes of gp120. *J Virol* **68**:5854–5862.

1234. Kang, C.-Y., K. Hariharan, M. R. Posner, and P. Nara. 1993. Identification of a new neutralizing epitope conformationally affected by the attachment of CD4 to gp120. *J Immunol* **151**:449–457.

1235. Kang, C.-Y., P. Nara, S. Chamat, V. Caralli, T. Ryskamp, N. Haigwood, R. Newman, and H. Kohler. 1991. Evidence for non-V3-specific neutralizing antibodies that interfere with gp120/CD4 binding in human immunodeficiency virus-1-infected humans. *Proc Natl Acad Sci USA* **88**:6171–6175.

1236. Kanitakis, J., C. Marchand, H. Su, J. Thivolet, G. Zambruno, D. Schmitt, and L. Gazzolo. 1989. Immunohistochemical study of normal skin of HIV-1-infected patients shows no evidence of infection of epidermal Langerhans cells by HIV. *AIDS Res Hum Retro* **5**:293–302.

1237. Kanki, P., S. M'Boup, and R. Marlink. 1992. Prevalence and risk determinants of human immunodeficiency virus type 2 (HIV-2) and human immunodeficiency virus type 1 (HIV-1) in West African female prostitutes. *Am J Epidemiol* **136**:895–907.

1238. Kannagi, M., L. V. Chalifoux, C. I. Lord, and N. L. Letvin. 1988. Suppression of simian immunodeficiency virus replication *in vitro* by CD8+ lymphocytes. *J Immunol* **140**:2237–2242.

1239. Kannagi, M., T. Masuda, T. Hattori, T. Kanoh, K. Nasu, N. Yamamoto, and S. Harada.

1990. Interference with human immunodeficiency virus (HIV) replication by CD8+ T cells in peripheral blood leukocytes of asymptomatic HIV carriers *in vitro. J Virol* **64**:3399–3406.

1240. **Kaposi, M.** 1872. Idiopathisches multiples Pigment Sarkom der Haut. *Arch Dermatol Syphillis* **4**:265–273.

1241. **Karin, M.** 1992. Signal transduction from cell surface to nucleus in development and disease. *FASEB J* **6**:2581–2590.

1242. **Karlsson, A., K. Parsmyr, E. Sandstrom, E. M. Fenyo, and J. Albert.** 1994. MT-2 cell tropism as prognostic marker for disease progression in human immunodeficiency virus type 1 infection. *J Clin Micro* **32**:364–370.

1243. **Karlsson, G. B., F. Gao, J. Robinson, B. Hahn, and J. Sodroski.** 1996. Increased envelope spike density and stability are not required for the neutralization resistance of primary human immunodeficiency viruses. *J Virol* **70**:6136–6142.

1244. **Karlsson, G. B., M. Halloran, J. Li, I. W. Park, R. Gomila, K. A. Reimann, M. K. Axthelm, S. A. Iliff, N. A. Letvin, and J. Sodroski.** 1997. Characterization of molecularly cloned simian-human immunodeficiency viruses causing rapid CD4+ lymphocyte depletion in rhesus monkeys. *J Virol* **71**:4218–4225.

1245. **Karpas, A., I. K. Hewlett, F. Hill, J. Gray, N. Byron, D. Gilgen, V. Bally, J. K. Oates, B. Gazzard, and J. E. Epstein.** 1990. Polymerase chain reaction evidence of human immunodeficiency virus 1 neutralization by passive immunization in patients with AIDS and AIDS-related complex. *Proc Natl Acad Sci USA* **87**:7613–7617.

1246. **Karpatkin, S., M. A. Nardi, and Y. H. Kouri.** 1992. Internal-image anti-idiotype HIV-1 gp120 antibody in human immunodeficiency virus 1 (HIV-1)-seropositive individuals with thrombocytopenia. *Proc Natl Acad Sci USA* **89**:1487–1491.

1247. **Karpus, W. J., N. W. Lukacs, K. J. Kennedy, W. S. Smith, S. D. Hurst, and T. A. Barrett.** 1997. Differential CC chemokine-induced enhancement of T helper cell cytokine production. *J Immunol* **158**:4129–4136.

1248. **Karray, S., and M. Zouali.** 1997. Identification of the B cell superantigen-binding site of HIV-1 gp120. *Proc Natl Acad Sci USA* **94**:1356–1360.

1249. **Karzon, D. T., D. P. Bolognesi, and W. C. Koff.** 1992. Development of a vaccine for the prevention of AIDS, a critical appraisal. *Vaccine* **10**:1039–1052.

1250. **Kaslow, R. A., W. C. Blackwelder, D. G. Ostrow, D. Yerg, J. Palenicek, A. H. Coulson, and R. O. Valdiserri.** 1989. No evidence for a role of alcohol or other psychoactive drugs in acceleratng immunodeficiency in HIV-1-positive individuals. *J Am Med Assoc* **261**:3424–3429.

1251. **Kaslow, R. A., M. Carrington, R. Apple, L. Park, A. Munoz, A. J. Saah, J. J. Goedert, C. Winkler, S. J. O'Brien, C. Rinaldo, R. Detels, W. Blattner, J. Phair, H. Erlich, and D. L. Mann.** 1996. Influence of combinations of human major histocompatibility complex genes on the course of HIV-1 infection. *Nature Med* **2**:405–411.

1251a. **Kaslow, R. A., R. Duquesnoy, M. VanRaden, L. Kingsley, M. Marrari, H. Friedman, S. Su, A. J. Saah, R. Detels, J. Phair, and C. Rinaldo.** 1990. A1, Cw7, B8, DR3 antigen combination associated with rapid decline of T-helper lymphocytes in HIV-1 infection. *Lancet* **335**:927–930.

1252. **Kato, H., M. Horikoshi, and R. G. Roeder.** 1991. Repression of HIV-1 transcription by a cellular protein. *Science* **251**:1476–1479.

1253. **Katz, M. H., N. A. Hessol, S. P. Buchbinder, A. Hirozawa, P. O'Malley, and S. D. Holmberg.** 1994. Temporal trends of opportunistic infections and malignancies in homosexual men with AIDS. *J Inf Dis* **170**:198–202.

1254. **Katzenstein, T. L., C. Pedersen, C. Nielsen, J. D. Lundgren, P. H. Jakobsen, and J. Gerstoft.** 1996. Longitudinal serum HIV RNA quantification: correlation to viral phenotype at seroconversion and clinical outcome. *AIDS* **10**:167–173.

1255. **Kawashima, H., S. Bandyopadhyay, R. Rutstein, and S. A. Plotkin.** 1991. Excretion of human immunodeficiency type 1 in the throat but not in urine by infected children. *J Peds* **118**:80–82.

1256. **Kazazi, F., J. M. Mathijs, P. Foley, and A. L. Cunningham.** 1989. Variations in CD4 expression by human monocytes and macrophages and their relationship to infection with the human immunodeficiency virus. *J Gen Virol* **70**:2661–2672.

1257. Kazi, S., P. R. Cohen, F. Williams, R. Schempp, and J. D. Reveille. 1996. The diffuse infiltrative lymphocytosis syndrome: clinical and immunogenetic features in 35 patients. *AIDS* **10**:385–391.

1258. Keay, S., C. O. Tacket, J. R. Murphy, and B. S. Handwerger. 1992. Anti-CD4 anti-idiotype antibodies in volunteers immunized with rgp160 of HIV-1 or infected with HIV-1. *AIDS Res Hum Retro* **8**:1091–1098.

1259. Kedes, D. H., E. Operskalski, M. Busch, R. Kohn, J. Flood, and D. Ganem. 1996. The seroepidemiology of human herpesvirus 8 (Kaposi's sarcoma-associated herpesvirus): distribution of infection in KS risk groups and evidence for sexual transmission. *Nature Med* **2**:918–924.

1259a. Keet, I. M. P., M. Janssen, P. J. Veugelers, F. Miedema, M. R. Klein, J. Goudsmit, R. A. Coutinho, and F. de Wolf. 1997. Longitudinal analysis of CD4 T cell counts, T cell reactivity, and human immunodeficency virus type 1 RNA levels in persons remaining AIDS-free despite CD4 cell counts <200 for >5 years. *J Inf Dis* **176**:665–671.

1260. Keet, I. P. M., P. Krijnen, M. Koot, J. M. A. Lange, F. Miedema, J. Goudsmit, and R. A. Coutinho. 1993. Predictors of rapid progression to AIDS in HIV-1 seroconverters. *AIDS* **7**:51–57.

1261. Kehrl, J. H., M. Alvarez-Mon, G. A. Delsing, and A. S. Fauci. 1987. Lymphotoxin is an important T cell-derived growth factor for human B cells. *Science* **242**:1144–1146.

1262. Kelker, H. C., M. Seidlin, M. Vogler, and F. T. Valentine. 1992. Lymphocytes from some long-term seronegative heterosexual partners of HIV-infected individuals proliferate in response to HIV antigens. *AIDS Res Hum Retro* **8**:1355–1359.

1263. Kellam, P., C. A. B. Bouchers, and B. A. Larder. 1992. Fifth mutation in human immunodeficiency virus type 1 reverse transcriptase contributes to the development of high-level resistance to zidovudine. *Proc Natl Acad Sci USA* **89**:1934–1938.

1264. Kelleher, A. D., L. Al-Harthi, and A. L. Landay. 1997. Immunological effects of antiretroviral and immune therapies of HIV. *AIDS 1997* **11**(Suppl A):S149–S155.

1265. Kelleher, A. D., A. Carr, J. Zaunders, and D. A. Cooper. 1996. Alterations in the immune response of human immunodeficiency virus (HIV)-infected subjects treated with an HIV-specific protease inhibitor, ritonavir. *J Inf Dis* **173**:321–329.

1266. Keller, A., E. D. Garrett, and B. R. Cullen. 1992. The Bel-1 protein of human foamy virus activates human immunodeficiency virus type 1 gene expression via a novel DNA target site. *J Virol* **66**:3946–3949.

1267. Keller, R., K. Peden, S. Paulous, L. Montagnier, and A. Cordonnier. 1993. Amino acid changes in the fourth conserved region of human immunodeficiency virus type 2 strain HIV-2ROD envelope glycoprotein modulate fusion. *J Virol* **67**:6253–6258.

1268. Kenney, S., J. Kamine, D. Markovitz, R. Fenrick, and J. Pagano. 1988. An Epstein-Barr virus immediate-early gene product trans-activates gene expression from the human immunodeficiency virus long terminal repeat. *Proc Natl Acad Sci USA* **85**:1652–1656.

1269. Kensil, C. R., U. Patel, M. Lennick, and D. Marciani. 1991. Separation and characterization of saponins with adjuvant activity from Quillaja saponaria molina cortex. *J Immunol* **146**:431–437.

1270. Kent, K. A., P. Kitchin, K. H. G. Mills, M. Page, F. Taffs, T. Corcoran, P. Silvera, B. Flanagan, C. Powell, J. Rose, C. Ling, A. M. Aubertin, and E. J. Stott. 1994. Passive immunization of cynomolgus macaques with immune sera or a pool of neutralizing monoclonal antibodies failed to protect against challenge with SIVmac251. *AIDS Res Hum Retro* **10**:189–194.

1271. Kent, S. J., P. D. Greenberg, M. C. Hoffman, R. E. Akridge, and M. J. McElrath. 1997. Antagonism of vaccine-induced HIV-1-specific CD4+ T cells by primary HIV-1 infection. *J Immunol* **158**:807–815.

1272. Kent, S. J., S.-L. Hu, L. Corey, W. R. Morton, and P. D. Greenberg. 1996. Detection of simian immunodeficiency virus (SIV)-specific CD8+ T cells in macaques protected from SIV challenge by prior SIV subunit vaccination. *J Virol* **70**:4941–4947.

1273. Kerkau, T., R. Schmitt-Landgraf, A. Schimpl, and E. Wecker. 1989. Downregulation of HLA class I antigens in HIV-1-infected cells. *AIDS Res Hum Retro* 5:613–620.

1274. Kerr, J. F. R., and B. V. Harmon. 1991. Definition and incidence of apoptosis: an historical perspective, p. 5–30. In L. D. Tomei and F. O. Cope (ed.), *Apoptosis: The Molecular Basis of Cell Death*, vol. 3. Cold Spring Harbor Laboratory, Cold Spring Harbor.

1275. Kerr, J. F. R., A. H. Wyllie, and A. R. Currie. 1972. Apoptosis: a basic biological phenomenon with wide-ranging implications in tissue kinetics. *Brit J Cancer* 26:239–257.

1276. Kersten, M. J., M. R. Klein, A. M. Holwerda, F. Miedema, and M. H. J. van Oers. 1997. Epstein-Barr virus-specific cytotoxic T cell responses in HIV-1 infection. *J Clin Invest* 99:1525–1533.

1277. Keshet, E., and H. M. Temin. 1979. Cell killing by spleen necrosis virus is correlated with a transient accumulation of spleen necrosis virus DNA. *J Virol* 31:376–388.

1278. Kestens, L., M. Melbye, R. J. Biggar, W. J. Stevens, P. Piot, A. De Muynck, H. Taelman, M. De Feyter, L. Paluku, and P. L. Gigase. 1985. Endemic African Kaposi's sarcoma is not associated with immunodeficiency. *Int J Cancer* 36:49–54.

1279. Kestens, L., J. Vingerhoets, M. Peeters, G. Vanham, C. Vereecken, G. Penne, H. Niphuis, P. van Eerd, G. van der Groen, P. Gigase, and J. Heeney. 1995. Phenotypic and functional parameters of cellular immunity in a chimpanzee with a naturally acquired simian immunodeficiency virus infection. *J Inf Dis* 172:957–963.

1280. Kestler, H., T. Kodama, D. Ringler, M. Marthas, N. Pedersen, A. Lackner, D. Regier, P. Sehgal, M. Daniel, N. King, and R. Desrosiers. 1990. Induction of AIDS in rhesus monkeys by molecularly cloned simian immunodeficiency virus. *Science* 248:1109–1112.

1281. Kestler, H. W., III, D. J. Ringler, K. Mori, D. L. Panicali, P. K. Sehgal, M. D. Daniel, and R. C. Desrosiers. 1991. Importance of the *nef* gene for maintenance of high virus loads and for development of AIDS. *Cell* 65:651–662.

1282. Ketzler, S., S. Weis, H. Haug, and H. Budka. 1990. Loss of neurons in the frontal cortex in AIDS brains. *Acta Neuropathol* 80:92–94.

1283. Keys, B., J. Karis, B. Fadeel, A. Valentin, G. Norkrans, L. Hagberg, and F. Chiodi. 1993. V3 sequences of paired HIV-1 isolates from blood and cerebrospinal fluid cluster according to host and show variation related to the clinical stage of disease. *Virol* 196:475–483.

1284. Khabbaz, R. F., W. Heneine, J. R. George, B. Parekh, T. Rowe, T. Woods, W. M. Switzer, H. M. McClure, M. Murphey-Corb, and T. M. Folks. 1994. Infection of a laboratory worker with simian immunodeficiency virus. *N Engl J Med* 330:172–177.

1285. Khansari, D. N., A. J. Murgo, and R. E. Faith. 1990. Effects of stress on the immune system. *Immunol Today* 11:170–175.

1286. Kido, H., A. Fukutomi, and N. Katunuma. 1990. A novel membrane-bound serine esterase in human T4+ lymphocytes immunologically reactive with antibody inhibiting syncytia induced by HIV-1. Purification and characterization. *J Biol Chem* 265:21979–21985.

1287. Kido, H., A. Fukutomi, and N. Katunuma. 1991. Tryptase TL_2 in the membrane of human T4+ lymphocytes is a novel binding protein of the V3 domain of HIV-1 envelope glycoprotein gp120. *FEBS Letters* 286:233–236.

1288. Kikukawa, R., Y. Koyanagi, S. Harada, N. Kobayashi, M. Hatanaka, and N. Yamamoto. 1986. Differential susceptibility to the acquired immunodeficiency syndrome retrovirus in cloned cells of human leukemic T cell line Molt-4. *J Virol* 57:1159–1162.

1289. Kim, J. H., J. D. Mosca, M. T. Vahey, R. J. McLinden, D. S. Burke, and R. R. Redfield. 1993. Consequences of human immunodeficiency virus type 1 superinfection of chronically infected cells. *AIDS Res Hum Retro* 9:875–882.

1290. Kim, S., R. Byrn, J. Groopman, and D. Baltimore. 1989. Temporal aspects of DNA and RNA synthesis during human immunodeficiency virus infection: evidence for differential gene expression. *J Virol* 63:3708–3713.

1291. Kim, S., K. Ikeuchi, R. Byrn, J. Groopman, and D. Baltimore. 1989. Lack of a negative influence on viral growth by the *nef* gene of human immunodeficiency virus type 1. *Proc Natl Acad Sci USA* 86:9544–9548.

1292. Kim, S., K. Ikeuchi, J. Groopman, and D. Baltimore. 1990. Factors affecting cellular tropism of human immunodeficiency virus. *J Virol* 64:5600–5604.

1293. Kimmel, P. L., T. M. Phillips, A. Ferreira-Centeno, T. Farkas-Szallasi, A. A. Abraham, and C. T. Garrett. 1992. Idiotypic IgA nephropathy in patients with human immunodeficiency virus infection. *N Engl J Med* 327:702–706.

1294. Kimpton, J., and M. Emerman. 1992. Detection of replication-competent and pseudotyped human immunodeficiency virus with a sensitive cell line on the basis of activation of an integrated beta-galactosidase gene. *J Virol* 66:2232–2239.

1295. Kinlen, L. J. 1982. Immunosuppressive therapy and cancer. *Cancer Survey* 1:567–583.

1296. Kinloch-De Loes, S., B. J. Hirschel, B. Hoen, D. A. Cooper, B. Tindall, A. Carr, J.-H. Saurat, N. Clumeck, A. Lazzarin, L. Mathiesen, F. Raffi, F. Antunes, J. von Overbeck, R. Luthy, M. Glauser, D. Hawkins, C. Baumberger, S. Yerly, T. V. Perneger, and L. Perrin. 1995. A controlled trial of zidovudine in primary human immunodeficiency virus infection. *N Engl J Med* 333:408–413.

1297. Kinter, A. L., S. M. Bende, E. C. Hardy, R. Jackson, and A. S. Fauci. 1995. Interleukin 2 induces CD8+ T cell-mediated suppression of human immunodeficiency virus replication in CD4+ T cells and this effect overrides its ability to stimulate virus expression. *Proc Natl Acad Sci USA* 92:10985–10989.

1298. Kinter, A. L., M. Ostrowski, D. Goletti, A. Oliva, D. Weissman, K. Gantt, E. Hardy, R. Jackson, L. Ehler, and A. S. Fauci. 1996. HIV replication in CD4+ T cells of HIV-infected individuals is regulated by a balance between the viral suppressive effects of endogenous β-chemokines and the viral inductive effects of other inductive cytokines. *Proc Natl Acad Sci USA* 93:14076–14081.

1299. Kinter, A. L., G. Poli, W. Maury, T. M. Folks, and A. S. Fauci. 1990. Direct and cytokine-mediated activation of protein kinase C induces human immunodeficiency virus expression in chronically infected promonocytic cells. *J Virol* 64:4306–4312.

1300. Kion, T. A., and G. W. Hoffmann. 1991. Anti-HIV and anti-anti-MHC antibodies in alloimmune and autoimmune mice. *Science* 253:1138–1140.

1300a. Kiprov, D. Personal communication.

1301. Kiprov, D., W. Pfaeffl, G. Parry, R. Lippert, W. Lang, and R. Miller. 1988. Antibody-mediated peripheral neuropathies associated with ARC and AIDS: successful treatment with plasmapheresis. *J Clin Apheresis* 4:3–7.

1302. Kiprov, D. D., B. J. Kwiatkowska, and R. G. Miller. 1990. Therapeutic apheresis in human immunodeficiency virus-related syndromes. *Curr Studies Hem Blood Trans* 57:184–197.

1303. Kirchhoff, F., T. C. Greenough, D. B. Brettler, J. L. Sullivan, and R. C. Desrosiers. 1995. Brief report: absence of intact nef sequences in a long-term survivor with nonprogressive HIV-1 infection. *N Engl J Med* 332:228–232.

1304. Kirchhoff, F., T. C. Greenough, M. Hamacher, J. L. Sullivan, and R. C. Desrosiers. 1997. Activity of human immunodeficiency virus type 1 promoter/TAR regions and *tat*1 genes derived from individuals with different rates of disease progression. *Virol* 232:319–331.

1305. Kishi, M., K. Tokunaga, Y.-H. Zheng, M. K. Bahmani, M. Kakinuma, M. Nonoyama, P. K. Lai, and K. Ikuta. 1995. Superinfection of a defective human immunodeficiency virus type 1 provirus-carrying T cell clone with *vif* or *vpu* mutants gives cytopathic virus particles by homologous recombination. *AIDS Res Hum Retro* 11:45–53.

1306. Kiviat, N. B., C. W. Critchlow, K. K. Holmes, J. Kuypers, J. Sayer, C. Dunphy, C. Surawicz, P. Kirby, R. Wood, and J. R. Daling. 1992. Association of anal dysplasia and human papillomavirus with immunosuppression and HIV infection among homosexual men. *AIDS* 7:43–49.

1307. Klaassen, R. J. L., R. Goldschmeding, K. M. Dolman, A. B. J. Vlekke, H. M. Weigel, J. K. M. Eeftinck Schattenkerk, J. W. Mulder, M. L. Westedt, and A. E. G. K. von dem Borne. 1992. Anti-neutrophil cytoplasmic autoantibodies in patients with symptomatic HIV infection. *Clin Exp Immunol* 87:24–30.

1308. Klaassen, R. J. L., J. W. Mulder, A. B. J. Vlekke, J. K. M. Eeftinck Schattenkerk, H. M.

Weigel, J. M. A. Lange, and A. E. G. K. von dem Borne. 1990. Autoantibodies against peripheral blood cells appear early in HIV infection and their prevalence increases with disease progression. *Clin Exp Immunol* **81**:11–17.

1309. Klasse, P. J., J. A. McKeating, M. Schutten, M. S. Reitz, Jr., and M. Robert-Guroff. 1993. An immune-selected point mutation in the transmembrane protein of human immunodeficiency virus type 1 (HXB2-Env:Ala 582 (→Thr) decreases viral neutralization by monoclonal antibodies to the CD4-binding site. *Virol* **196**:332–337.

1310. Klatzmann, D., F. Barre-Sinoussi, M. T. Nugeyre, C. Dauquet, E. Vilmer, C. Griscelli, F. Brun-Vezinet, C. Rouzioux, J. C. Gluckman, and J. C. Chermann. 1984. Selective tropism of lymphadenopathy-associated virus (LAV) for helper-inducer T-lymphocytes. *Science* **225**:59–62.

1311. Klatzmann, D., E. Champagne, S. Chamaret, J. Gurest, D. Guetard, T. Hercend, J. C. Gluckman, and L. Montagnier. 1984. T-lymphocyte T4 molecule behaves as receptor for human retrovirus LAV. *Nature* **312**:767–778.

1312. Klebanoff, S. J., and R. W. Coombs. 1992. Viricidal effect of polymorphonuclear leukocytes on human immunodeficiency virus-1. *J Clin Invest* **89**:2014–2017.

1313. Kleburtz, K. D., D. W. Giang, R. B. Schiffer, and N. Vakil. 1991. Abnormal vitamin B12 metabolism in human immunodeficiency virus infection: association with neurological dysfunction. *Arch Neurol* **48**:312–314.

1314. Kleim, J.-P., A. Ackermann, H. H. Brackmann, M. Gahr, and K. E. Schneweis. 1991. Epidemiologically closely related viruses from hemophilia B patients display high homology in two hypervariable regions of the HIV-1 *env* gene. *AIDS Res Hum Retro* **7**:417–421.

1315. Klein, G. 1981. The role of gene dosage and genetic transpositions in carcinogenesis. *Nature* **294**:313–318.

1316. Klein, M. R., I. P. M. Keet, J. D'Amaro, R. J. Bende, A. Hekman, B. Mesman, M. Koot, L. P. de Waal, R. A. Coutinho, and F. Miedema. 1994. Associations between HLA frequencies and pathogenic features of human immunodefiency virus type 1 infection in seroconverters from the Amsterdam cohort of homosexual men. *J Inf Dis* **169**:1244–1249.

1317. Klein, M. R., C. A. van Baalen, A. M. Holwerda, S. R. Kerkhof Garde, R. J. Bende, I. P. M. Keet, J. K. Eeftinck-Schattenkerk, A. D. M. E. Osterhaus, H. Schuitemaker, and F. Miedema. 1995. Kinetics of Gag-specific cytotoxic T lymphocyte responses during the clinical course of HIV-1 infection: a longitudinal analysis of rapid progressors and long-term asymptomatics. *J Exp Med* **181**:1365–1372.

1317a. Klein, S. A., J. M. Dobmeyer, T. S. Dobmeyer, M. Pape, O. G. Ottmann, E. B. Helm, D. Hoelzer, and R. Rossol. 1997. Demonstration of the Th1 to TH2 cytokine shift during the course of HIV-1 infection using cytoplasmic cytokine detection on single cell level by flow cytometry. *AIDS* **11**:1111–1118.

1318. Klenerman, P., R. Phillips, and A. McMichael. 1996. Cytotoxic T cell antagonism in HIV. *Sem Virol* **7**:31–39.

1319. Klenerman, P., R. E. Phillips, C. R. Rinaldo, L. M. Wahl, G. Ogg, R. M. May, A. J. McMichael, and M. A. Nowak. 1996. Cytotoxic T lymphocytes and viral turnover in HIV type 1 infection. *Proc Natl Acad Sci USA* **93**:15323–15328.

1319a. Kliks, S., and J. A. Levy. Unpublished observations.

1319b. Kliks, S., C. P. Locher, and J. A. Levy. Unpublished observations.

1320. Kliks, S. C., A. Nisalak, W. E. Brandt, L. Wahl, and D. S. Burke. 1989. Antibody-dependent enhancement of dengue virus growth in human monocytes as a risk factor for dengue hemorrhagic fever. *Am J Trop Med Hyg* **40**:444–451.

1321. Kliks, S. C., T. Shioda, N. L. Haigwood, and J. A. Levy. 1993. V3 variability can influence the ability of an antibody to neutralize or enhance infection by diverse strains of human immunodeficiency virus type 1. *Proc Natl Acad Sci USA* **90**:11518–11522.

1322. Kliks, S. C., D. W. Wara, D. V. Landers, and J. A. Levy. 1994. Features of HIV-1 that could influence maternal-child transmission. *J Am Med Assoc* **272**:467–474.

1323. Klimas, N., R. Patarca, J. Walling, R. Garcia, V. Mayer, D. Moody, T. Okarma, and M. A.

Fletcher. 1994. Clinical and immunological changes in AIDS patients following adoptive therapy with activated autologous CD8 T cells and interleukin-2 infusion. *AIDS* 8:1073–1081.

1324. Klimas, N. G., J. B. Page, R. Patarca, D. Chitwood, R. Morgan, and M. A. Fletcher. 1993. Effects of retroviral infections on immune function in African-American intravenous drug users. *AIDS* 7:331–335.

1325. Kloster, B. E., R. H. Tomar, and T. J. Spira. 1984. Lymphocytotoxic antibodies in the acquired immune deficiency syndrome (AIDS). *Clin Immunol Immunopathol* 30:330–335.

1326. Knight, S. C. 1996. Bone-marrow-derived dendritic cells and the pathogenesis of AIDS. *AIDS* 10:807–817.

1327. Knight, S. C., and S. Patterson. 1997. Bone marrow-derived dendritic cells, infection with human immunodeficiency virus, and immunopathology. *Annu Rev Immunol* 15:593–615.

1328. Kobayashi, J., A. Takeda, S. Green, C. U. Tuazon, and F. A. Ennis. 1993. Direct detection of infectious human immunodeficiency virus type 1 (HIV-1) immune complexes in the sera of HIV-1-infected persons. *J Inf Dis* 168:729–732.

1329. Kodama, T., K. Mori, T. Kawahara, D. J. Ringler, and R. C. Desrosiers. 1993. Analysis of simian immunodeficiency virus sequence variation in tissues of rhesus macaques with simian AIDS. *J Virol* 67:6522–6534.

1330. Koenig, S., A. J. Conley, Y. A. Brewah, G. M. Jones, S. Leath, L. J. Boots, V. Davey, G. Pantaleo, J. F. Demarest, C. Carter, C. Wannebo, J. R. Yannelli, S. A. Rosenberg, and H. C. Lane. 1995. Transfer of HIV-1-specific cytotoxic T lymphocytes to an AIDS patient leads to selection for mutant HIV variants and subsequent disease progression. *Nature Med* 1:330–336.

1331. Koenig, S., H. E. Gendelman, J. M. Orenstein, M. C. Dal Canto, G. H. Pezeshkpour, M. Yungbluth, F. Janotta, A. Aksamit, M. A. Martin, and A. S. Fauci. 1986. Detection of AIDS virus in macrophages in brain tissue from AIDS patients with encephalopathy. *Science* 233:1089–1093.

1332. Koerper, M. A. 1989. AIDS and hemophilia, p. 79–95. *In* J. A. Levy (ed.), *AIDS: Pathogenesis and Treatment.* Marcel Dekker, Inc., New York.

1333. Koga, Y., M. Sasaki, H. Yoshida, M. Oh-Tsu, G. Kimura, and K. Nomoto. 1991. Disturbance of nuclear transport of proteins in CD4+ cells expressing gp160 of human immunodeficiency virus. *J Virol* 65:5609–5612.

1334. Koga, Y., M. Sasaki, H. Yoshida, H. Wigzell, G. Kimura, and K. Nomoto. 1990. Cytopathic effect determined by the amount of CD4 molecules in human cell lines expressing envelope glycoprotein of HIV. *J Immunol* 144:94–102.

1335. Kohler, H., J. Goudsmit, and P. Nara. 1992. Clonal dominance: cause for a limited and failing immune response to HIV-1 infection and vaccination. *J AIDS* 5:1158–1168.

1336. Kohler, H., S. Muller, and P. L. Nara. 1994. Deceptive imprinting in the immune response against HIV-1. *Immunol Today* 15:475–478.

1337. Kohlstaedt, L. A., J. Wang, J. M. Friedman, P. A. Rice, and T. A. Steitz. 1992. Crystal structure at 3.5 angstrom resolution of HIV-1 reverse transcriptase complexed with an inhibitor. *Science* 256:1783–1790.

1338. Koito, A., G. Harrowe, J. A. Levy, and C. Cheng-Mayer. 1994. Functional role of the V1/V2 region of human immunodeficiency virus type 1 envelope glycoprotein gp120 in infection of primary macrophages and sCD4 neutralization. *J Virol* 68:2253–2259.

1339. Koito, A., T. Hattori, T. Murakami, S. Matsushita, Y. Maeda, T. Yamamoto, and K. Takatsuki. 1989. A neutralizing epitope of human immunodeficiency virus type 1 has homologous amino acid sequences with the active site of inter-alpha-trypsin inhibitor. *Int Immunol* 1:613–618.

1340. Koito, A., L. Stamatatos, and C. Cheng-Mayer. 1995. Small amino acid sequence changes within the V2 domain can affect the function of a T-cell line-tropic human immunodeficiency virus type 1 envelope gp120. *Virol* 206:878–884.

1341. Kolesnitchenko, V., L. M. Wahl, H. Tian, I. Sunila, Y. Tani, D.-P. Hartmann, J. Cossman,

M. Raffeld, J. Orenstein, L. E. Samelson, and D. I. Cohen. 1995. Human immunodeficiency virus 1 envelope-initiated G2-phase programmed cell death. *Proc Natl Acad Sci USA* **92**:11889–11893.

1342. Kollmann, T. R., M. Pettoello-Mantovani, N. F. Katopodis, M. Hachamovitch, A. Rubinstein, A. Kim, and H. Goldstein. 1996. Inhibition of acute *in vivo* human immunodeficiency virus infection by human interleukin 10 treatment of SCID mice implanted with human fetal thymus and liver. *Proc Natl Acad Sci USA* **93**:3126–3131.

1343. Kolson, D. L., J. Buchhalter, R. Collman, B. Hellmig, C. F. Farrell, C. Debouck, and F. Gonzalez-Scarano. 1993. HIV-1 Tat alters normal ogranization of neurons and astrocytes in primary rodent brain cell cultures: RGD sequence dependence. *AIDS Res Hum Retro* **9**:677–685.

1344. Komanduri, K. V., J. A. Luce, M. S. McGrath, B. G. Herndier, and V. L. Ng. 1996. The natural history and molecular heterogeneity of HIV-associated primary malignant lymphomatous effusions. *J AIDS Hum Retrovirol* **13**:215–226.

1345. Kong, L. I., S.-W. Lee, J. C. Kappes, J. S. Parkin, D. Decker, J. A. Hoxie, B. H. Hahn, and G. M. Shaw. 1988. West African HIV-2-related human retrovirus with attenuated cytopathicity. *Science* **240**:1525–1529.

1346. Koot, M., I. P. M. Keet, A. H. V. Vos, R. E. Y. de Goede, J. T. L. Roos, R. A. Coutinho, F. Miedema, P. T. A. Schellekens, and M. Tersmette. 1993. Prognostic value of HIV-1 syncytium-inducing phenotype for rate of CD4+ cell depletion and progression to AIDS. *Ann Int Med* **118**:681–688.

1347. Koot, M., A. H. V. Vos, R. P. M. Keet, R. E. Y. de Goede, M. W. Dercksen, F. G. Terpstra, R. A. Coutinho, F. Miedema, and M. Tersmette. 1992. HIV-1 biological phenotype in long-term infected individuals evaluated with an MT-2 cocultivation assay. *AIDS* **6**:49–54.

1348. Kootstra, N. A., A. B. van't Wout, H. G. Huisman, F. Miedema, and H. Schuitemaker. 1994. Interference of interleukin-10 with human immunodeficiency virus type 1 replication in primary monocyte-derived macrophages. *J Virol* **68**:6967–6975.

1349. Kopf, M., G. Le Gros, M. Bachmann, M. C. Lamers, H. Bluethmann, and G. Köhler. 1993. Disruption of murine IL-4 gene blocks Th2 cytokine responses. *Science* **362**:245–247.

1350. Korber, B. T. M., K. J. Kuntsman, B. K. Patterson, M. Furtado, M. M. McEvilly, R. Levy, and S. M. Wolinsky. 1994. Genetic differences between blood-and brain-derived viral sequences from human immunodeficiency virus type 1-infected patients: evidence of conserved elements in the V3 region of the envelope protein of brain-derived sequences. *J Virol* **68**:7467–7481.

1351. Korber, B. T. M., K. MacInnes, R. F. Smith, and G. Myers. 1994. Mutational trends in V3 loop protein sequences observed in different genetic lineages of human immunodeficiency virus type 1. *J Virol* **68**:6730–6744.

1352. Korneyeva, M., P. Stalhandske, and B. Asjo. 1993. Jurkat-Tat but not other Tat-expressing cell lines support replication of slow/low type HIV. *J AIDS* **6**:231–236.

1353. Kornfeld, H., W. W. Cruikshank, S. W. Pyle, J. S. Berman, and D. M. Center. 1988. Lymphocyte activation by HIV-1 envelope glycoprotein. *Nature* **335**:445–448.

1354. Kostrikis, L. G., E. Bagdades, Y. Cao, L. Zhang, D. Dimitriou, and D. D. Ho. 1995. Genetic analysis of human immunodeficiency virus type 1 strains from patients in Cyprus: identification of a new subtype designated subtype I. *J Virol* **69**:6122–6130.

1355. Kotler, D. P., H. P. Gaetz, M. Lange, E. B. Klein, and P. R. Holt. 1984. Enteropathy associated with the acquired immunodeficiency syndrome. *Ann Int Med* **101**:421–428.

1356. Kotler, D. P., S. Reka, A. Borcich, and W. J. Cronin. 1991. Detection, localization, and quantitation of HIV-associated antigens in intestinal biopsies from patients with AIDS. *Am J Path* **139**:823–830.

1357. Koup, R. A., J. T. Safrit, Y. Cao, C. A. Andrews, G. McLeod, W. Borkowsky, C. Farthing, and D. D. Ho. 1994. Temporal association of cellular immune responses with the initial control of viremia in primary human immunodeficiency virus type 1 syndrome. *J Virol* **68**:4650–4655.

1358. Koup, R. A., J. L. Sullivan, P. H. Levine, D. Brettler, A. Mahr, G. Mazzara, S. McKenzie, and

D. Panicali. 1989. Detection of major histocompatibility complex class I-restricted, HIV-specific cytotoxic T lymphocytes in the blood of infected hemophiliacs. *Blood* 73:1909–1914.

1359. Koup, R. A., J. L. Sullivan, P. H. Levine, F. Brewster, A. Mahr, G. Mazzara, S. McKenzie, and D. Panicali. 1989. Antigenic specificity of antibody-dependent cell-mediated cytotoxicity directed against human immunodeficiency virus in antibody-positive sera. *J Virol* 63:584–590.

1360. Kourtis, A. P., C. Ibegbu, A. J. Nahmias, F. K. Lee, W. S. Clark, M. K. Sawyer, and S. Nesheim. 1996. Early progression of disease in HIV-infected infants with thymus dysfunction. *N Engl J Med* 335:1431–1436.

1361. Kovacs, J. A., M. Baseler, R. J. Dewar, S. Vogel, R. T. Davey, Jr., J. Falloon, M. A. Polis, R. E. Walker, R. Stevens, N. P. Salzman, J. A. Metcalf, H. Masur, and H. C. Lane. 1995. Increases in CD4 T lymphocytes with intermittent courses of interleukin-2 in patients with human immunodeficiency virus infection. *N Engl J Med* 332:567–575.

1362. Kovacs, J. A., M. B. Vasudevachari, M. Easter, R. T. Davey, Jr., J. Falloon, M. A. Polis, J. A. Metcalf, N. Salzman, M. Baseler, G. E. Smith, F. Volvovitz, H. Masur, and H. C. Lane. 1993. Induction of humoral and cell-mediated anti-human immunodefiency virus (HIV) responses in HIV seronegative volunteers by immunization with recombinant gp160. *J Clin Invest* 92:919–928.

1363. Kovacs, J. A., S. Vogel, J. M. Albert, J. Falloon, R. T. Davey, Jr., R. E. Walker, M. A. Polis, K. Spooner, J. A. Metcalf, M. Baseler, G. Fyfe, and H. C. Lane. 1996. Controlled trial of interleukin-2 infusions in patients infected with the human immunodeficiency virus. *N Engl J Med* 335:1350–1356.

1364. Koval, V., C. Clark, M. Vaishnav, S. A. Spector, and D. H. Spector. 1991. Human cytomegalovirus inhibits human immunodeficiency virus replication in cells productively infected by both viruses. *J Virol* 65:6969–6978.

1365. Kowalski, M., L. Bergeron, T. Dorfman, W. Haseltine, and J. Sodroski. 1991. Attenuation of human immunodeficiency virus type 1 cytopathic effect by a mutation affecting the transmembrane envelope glycoprotein. *J Virol* 65:281–291.

1366. Kowalski, M., J. Potz, L. Basiripour, T. Dorfman, W. C. Goh, E. Terwilliger, A. Dayton, C. Rosen, W. Haseltine, and J. Sodroski. 1987. Functional regions of the envelope glycoprotein of human immunodeficiency virus type 1. *Science* 237:1351–1355.

1367. Koyanagi, Y., S. Miles, R. T. Mitsuyasu, J. E. Merrill, H. V. Vinters, and I. S. Y. Chen. 1987. Dual infection of the central nervous system by AIDS viruses with distinct cellular tropisms. *Science* 236:819–822.

1368. Koyanagi, Y., W. A. O'Brien, J. Q. Zhao, D. W. Golde, J. C. Gasson, and I. S. Y. Cheng. 1988. Cytokines alter production of HIV-1 from primary mononuclear phagocytes. *Science* 241:1673–1675.

1369. Kozak, S. L., E. J. Platt, N. Madani, F. E. Ferro, K. Peden, and D. Kabat. 1997. CD4, CXCR-4, amd CCR-5 dependencies for infections by primary patient and laboratory-adapted isolates of human immunodeficiency virus type 1. *J Virol* 71:873–882.

1370. Kozal, M. J., R. W. Shafer, M. A. Winters, D. A. Katzenstein, and T. C. Merigan. 1993. A mutation in human immunodeficiency virus reverse transcriptase and decline in CD4 lymphocyte numbers in long-term zidovudine recipients. *J Inf Dis* 167:526–532.

1371. Kozlowski, P. A., K. P. Black, and S. Jackson. 1995. High prevalence of serum IgA HIV-1 infection-enhancing antibodies in HIV-infected persons. *J Immunol* 154:6163–6173.

1372. Kreiss, J., E. Ngugi, K. Holmes, J. Ndinya-Achola, P. Waiyaki, P. L. Roberts, I. Ruminjo, R. Sajabi, J. Kimata, T. R. Fleming, A. Anzala, D. Holton, and F. Plummer. 1992. Efficacy of nonoxynol 9 contraceptive sponge use in preventing heterosexual acquisition of HIV in Nairobi prostitutes. *J Am Med Assoc* 268:477–482.

1373. Kreiss, J. K., R. Coombs, F. Plummer, K. K. Holmes, B. Nikora, W. Cameron, E. Ngugu, J. O. N. Achola, and L. Corey. 1989. Isolation of human immunodeficiency virus from genital ulcers in Nairobi prostitutes. *J Inf Dis* 160:380–384.

1374. Kreiss, J. K., and S. G. Hopkins. 1993. The association between circumcision status and human immunodeficiency virus infection among homosexual men. *J Inf Dis* 168:1404–1408.

1375. Krieger, J. N., R. W. Coombs, A. C. Collier, S. O. Ross, K. Chaloupka, D. K. Cummings, V. L. Murphy, and L. Corey. 1991. Recovery of human immunodeficiency virus type 1 from semen: minimal impact of stage of infection and current antiviral chemotherapy. *J Inf Dis* **163**:386–388.

1376. Krieger, J. N., R. W. Coombs, A. C. Collier, S. O. Ross, C. Speck, and L. Corey. 1995. Seminal shedding of human immunodeficiency virus type 1 and human cytomegalovirus: evidence for different immunologic controls. *J Inf Dis* **171**:1018–1022.

1377. Krivine, A., G. Firtion, L. Cao, C. Francoual, R. Henrion, and P. Lebon. 1992. HIV replication during the first weeks of life. *Lancet* **339**:1187–1189.

1377a. Krivine, A., S. Le Bourdelles, G. Firtion, and P. Lebon. 1997. Viral kinetics in HIV-1 perinatal infection. *Lancet* **350**:493.

1377b. Kroner, B. L., P. S. Rosenberg, L. M. Aledort, W. G. Alvord, and J. J. Goedert. 1994. HIV-1 infection incidence among persons with hemophilia in the United States and Western Europe, 1978–1990. *J AIDS* **7**:279–286.

1378. Krown, S. E. 1988. AIDS-associated Kaposi's sarcoma: pathogenesis, clinical course and treatment. *AIDS* **2**:71–80.

1378a. Kubo, M., T. Ohashi, M. Fujii, S. Oka, A. Iwamoto, S. Harada, and M. Kannagi. 1997. Abrogation of in vitro suppression of human immunodeficiency virus type 1 (HIV-1) replication mediated by CD8+ T lymphocytes of asymptomatic HIV-1 carriers by staphyloccal enterotoxin B and phorbol esters through induction of tumor necrosis factor alpha. *J Virol* **71**:7560–7566.

1379. Kuhn, L., E. J. Abrams, P. B. Matheson, P. A. Thomas, G. Lambert, M. Bamji, B. Greenberg, R. W. Steketee, and D. M. Thea. 1997. Timing of maternal-infant HIV transmission: associations between intrapartum factors and early polymerase chain reaction results. *AIDS* **11**:429–435.

1380. Kuhn, L., R. Bobat, A. Coutsoudis, D. Moodley, H. M. Coovadia, W.-Y. Tsai, and Z. A. Stein. 1996. Cesarean deliveries and maternal-infant HIV transmission: results from a prospective study in South Africa. *J AIDS Hum Retrovirol* **11**:478–483.

1381. Kuhnel, H., H. von Briesen, U. Dietrich, M. Adamski, D. Mix, L. Biesert, R. Kreutz, A. Immelmann, K. Henco, C. Meichsner, R. Adreesen, H. Gelderblom, and H. Rubsamen-Waigmann. 1989. Molecular cloning of two West African human immunodeficiency virus type 2 isolates that replicate well in macrophages: a Gambian isolate, from a patient with neurologic acquired immunodeficiency syndrome, and a highly divergent Ghanian isolate. *Proc Natl Acad Sci USA* **86**:2383–2387.

1382. Kuiken, C. A., J.-J. deJong, E. Baan, W. Keulen, M. Tersmette, and J. Goudsmit. 1992. Evolution of the V3 envelope domain in proviral sequences and isolates of human immunodeficiency virus type 1 during transition of the viral biological phenotype. *J Virol* **66**:4622–4627.

1383. Kuiken, C. L., G. Zwart, E. Baan, R. A. Coutinho, A. R. van den Hoek, and J. Goudsmit. 1993. Increasing antigenic and genetic diversity of the V3 variable domain of the human immunodeficiency virus envelope protein in the course of the AIDS epidemic. *Proc Natl Acad Sci USA* **90**:9061–9065.

1384. Kumar, M., L. Resnick, D. Loewenstein, J. Berger, and C. Eisdorfer. 1989. Brain reactive antibodies and the AIDS dementia complex. *J AIDS* **2**:469–471.

1385. Kumar, P., H. X. Hui, J. C. Kappes, B. S. Haggarty, J. A. Hoxie, S. K. Arya, G. M. Shaw, and B. H. Hahn. 1990. Molecular characterization of an attenuated human immunodeficiency virus type 2 isolate. *J Virol* **64**:890–901.

1386. Kunanusont, C., H. M. Foy, J. K. Kreiss, S. Rerks-Ngarm, P. Phanuphak, S. Raktham, C.-P. Pau, and N. L. Young. 1995. HIV-1 subtypes and male-to-female transmission in Thailand. *Lancet* **345**:1078–1083.

1387. Kundu, S. K., D. Katzenstein, L. E. Moses, and T. C. Merigan. 1992. Enhancement of human immunodeficiency virus HIV-specific CD4+ and CD8+ cytotoxic T-lymphocyte activities in HIV-infected asymptomatic patients given recombinant gp160 vaccine. *Proc Natl Acad Sci USA* **89**:11204–11208.

1388. **Kundu, S. K., and T. C. Merigan.** 1992. Equivalent recognition of HIV proteins, *env, gag* and *RT* by CD4+ and CD8+ cytotoxic T lymphocytes. *AIDS* **6**:643–649.

1389. **Kunsch, C., H. T. Hartle, and B. Wigdahl.** 1989. Infection of human fetal dorsal root ganglion glial cells with human immunodeficiency virus type 1 involves an entry mechanism independent of the CD4 T4A epitope. *J Virol* **63**:5054–5061.

1390. **Kunzi, M. S., H. Farzadegan, J. B. Margolick, D. Vlahov, and P. M. Pitha.** 1995. Identification of human immunodeficiency virus primary isolates resistant to interferon-α and correlation of prevalence to disease progression. *J Inf Dis* **171**:822–828.

1391. **Kunzi, M. S., and J. E. Groopman.** 1993. Identification of a novel human immunodeficiency virus strain cytopathic to megakaryocytic cells. *Blood* **81**:3336–3342.

1392. **Kusumi, K., B. Conway, S. Cunningham, A. Berson, C. Evans, A. K. N. Iversen, D. Colvin, M. V. Gallo, S. Coutre, E. G. Shpaer, D. V. Faulkner, A. DeRonde, S. Volkman, C. Williams, M. S. Hirsch, and J. I. Mullins.** 1992. Human immunodeficiency virus type 1 envelope gene structure and diversity *in vivo* and after cocultivation *in vitro*. *J Virol* **66**:875–885.

1392a.**Kuwata, T., Y. Miyazaki, T. Igarashi, J. Takehisa, and M. Hayami.** 1997. The rapid spread of recombinants during a natural in vitro infection with two human immunodeficiency virus type 1 strains. *J Virol* **71**:7088–7091.

1393. **Kwak, L. W., M. Wilson, L. M. Weiss, S. J. Horning, R. A. Warnke, and R. F. Dorfman.** 1991. Clinical significance of morphologic subdivision in diffuse large cell lymphoma. *Cancer* **68**:1988–1993.

1394. **Kwok, S., D. H. Mack, K. B. Mullis, B. Poiesz, G. Ehrlich, D. Blair, A. Friedman-Kien, and J. J. Sninsky.** 1987. Identification of human immunodeficiency virus sequences by using *in vitro* enzymatic amplification and oligomer cleavage detection. *J Virol* **61**:1690–1694.

1395. **Lackritz, E. M., G. A. Satten, J. Aberle-Grasse, R. Y. Dodd, V. P. Raimondi, R. S. Janssen, W. F. Lewis, E. P. Notari IV, and L. R. Petersen.** 1995. Estimated risk of transmission of the human immunodeficiency virus by screened blood in the United States. *N Engl J Med* **333**:1721–1725.

1396. **Lafeuillade, A., C. Poggi, G. Hittinger, L. Chollet, and N. Profizi.** Early events in lymph nodes during primary HIV-1 infection. *AIDS*, in press.

1397. **Lafeuillade, A., C. Poggi, N. Profizi, C. Tamalet, and O. Costes.** 1996. Human immunodeficiency virus type 1 kinetics in lymph nodes compared with plasma. *J Inf Dis* **174**:404–407.

1398. **Lafeuillade, A., C. Poggi, and C. Tamalet.** 1996. GM-CSF increases HIV-1 load. *Lancet* **347**:1123–1124.

1399. **Lafeuillade, A., C. Poggi, C. Tamalet, N. Profizi, C. Tourres, and O. Costes.** 1997. Effects of a combination of zidovudine, didanosine, and lamivudine on primary human immunodeficiency virus type 1 infection. *J Inf Dis* **175**:1051–1055.

1400. **Lafon, M., M. Lafage, A. Martinez-Arends, R. Ramirez, F. Vuillier, D. Charron, V. Lotteau, and D. Scott-Algara.** 1992. Evidence for a viral superantigen in humans. *Nature* **358**:507–510.

1401. **Lafon, M.-E., A.-M. Steffan, C. Royer, D. Jaeck, A. Beretz, A. Kirn, and J.-L. Gendrault.** 1994. HIV-1 infection induces functional alterations in human liver endothelial cells in primary culture. *AIDS* **8**:747–752.

1402. **Lafon, M.-E., A. M. Steffan, J. L. Gendrault, C. Klein-Soyer, L. Gloeckler-Tondre, C. Royer, and A. Kirn.** 1992. Interaction of human immunodeficiency virus with human macrovascular endothelial cells *in vitro*. *AIDS Res Hum Retro* **8**:1567–1570.

1403. **Lafrenie, R. M., L. M. Wahl, J. S. Epstein, I. K. Hewlett, K. M. Yamada, and S. Dhawan.** 1996. HIV-1-Tat modulates the function of monocytes and alters their interactions with microvessel endothelial cells. *J Immunol* **156**:1638–1645.

1404. **Laga, M., A. Manoka, M. Kivuvu, B. Malele, M. Tuliza, N. Nzila, J. Goeman, F. Behets, V. Batter, M. Alary, W. L. Heyward, R. W. Ryder, and P. Piot.** 1993. Non-ulcerative sexually transmitted diseases as risk factors for HIV-1 transmission in women: results from a cohort study. *AIDS* **7**:95–102.

1405. **Lahdevirta, J., C. P. J. Maury, A. M. Teppo, and H. Repo.** 1988. Elevated levels of circulating cachectin/tumor necrosis factor in patients with acquired immunodeficiency syndrome. *Am J Med* **85**:289–291.

1406. Lallemant, M., A. Baillou, S. Lallemant-Le Coeur, S. Nzingoula, M. Mampaka, P. M. Pele, F. Barin, and M. Essex. 1994. Maternal antibody response at delivery and perinatal transmission of human immunodeficiency virus type 1 in African women. *Lancet* **343**:1001–1005.

1407. Lamarre, D., A. Ashkenazi, S. Fleury, D. H. Smith, R.-P. Sekaly, and D. J. Capon. 1989. The MHC-binding and gp120-binding functions of CD4 are separable. *Science* **245**:743–746.

1408. Lamb, R. A., and L. H. Pinto. 1997. Do Vpu and Vpr of human immunodeficiency virus type 1 and NB of influenza B virus have ion channel activities in the viral life cycles? *Virol* **229**:1–11.

1409. Lamers, S. L., J. W. Sleasman, J. X. She, K. A. Barrie, S. M. Pomeroy, D. J. Barrett, and M. M. Goodenow. 1993. Independent variation and positive selection in env V1 and V2 domains within maternal-infant strains of human immunodeficiency virus type 1 in vivo. *J Virol* **67**:3951–3960.

1410. Lamers, S. L., J. W. Sleasman, J. X. She, K. A. Barrie, S. M. Pomeroy, D. J. Barrett, and M. M. Goodenow. 1994. Persistence of multiple maternal genotypes of human immunodeficiency virus type 1 in infants by vertical transmission. *J Clin Invest* **93**:380–390.

1411. Lamhamedi-Cherradi, S., B. Culmann-Penciolelli, B. Guy, T. D. Ly, C. Goujard, J.-G. Guillet, and E. Gomard. 1995. Different patterns of HIV-1-specific cytotoxic T-lymphocyte activity after primary infection. *AIDS* **9**:421–426.

1412. Landau, N. R., K. A. Page, and D. R. Littman. 1991. Pseudotyping with human T-cell leukemia virus type I broadens the human immunodeficiency virus host range. *J Virol* **65**:162–169.

1413. Landay, A., H. A. Kessler, C. A. Benson, J. C. Pottage, Jr., R. Murphy, P. Urbanski, S. Kucik, and J. Phair. 1990. Isolation of HIV-1 from monocytes of individuals negative by conventional culture. *J Inf Dis* **161**:706–710.

1414. Landay, A., B. Ohlsson-Wilhelm, and J. V. Giorgi. 1990. Application of flow cytometry to the study of HIV infection. *AIDS* **4**:479–497.

1415. Landay, A. L., M. Clerici, F. Hashemi, H. Kessler, J. A. Berzofsky, and G. M. Shearer. 1996. *In vitro* restoration of T cell immune function in human immunodeficiency virus-positive persons: effects of interleukin (IL)-12 and anti-IL-10. *J Inf Dis* **173**:1085–1091.

1416. Landay, A. L., C. Mackewicz, and J. A. Levy. 1993. An activated CD8 + T cell phenotype correlates with anti-HIV activity and asymptomatic clinical status. *Clin Immunol Immunopathol* **69**:106–116.

1417. Landay, A. L., S. Z. Schade, D. M. Takefman, M. C. Kuhns, A. L. McNamara, R. L. Rosen, H. A. Kessler, and G. T. Spear. 1993. Detection of HIV-1 provirus in bronchoalveolar lavage cells by polymerase chain reaction. *J AIDS* **6**:171–175.

1418. Landesman, S., B. Weiblen, H. Mendez, A. Willoughby, J. J. Goedert, A. Rubinstein, H. Minkoff, G. Moroso, and R. Hoff. 1991. Clinical utility of HIV-IgA immunoblot assay in the early diagnosis of perinatal HIV infection. *J Am Med Assoc* **266**:3443–3446.

1419. Landesman, S. H., L. A. Kalish, D. N. Burns, H. Minkoff, H. E. Fox, C. Zorrilla, P. Garcia, M. G. Fowler, L. Mofenson, and R. Tuomala. 1996. Obstetrical factors and the transmission of human immunodeficiency virus type 1 from mother to child. *N Engl J Med* **334**:1617–1623.

1420. Lane, H. C., J. M. Depper, W. C. Greene, G. Whalen, T. A. Walkmann, and A. S. Fauci. 1985. Qualitative analysis of immune function in patients with the acquired immunodeficiency syndrome. *N Engl J Med* **313**:79–84.

1421. Lane, H. C., H. Masur, L. C. Edgar, G. Whalen, A. H. Rook, and A. S. Fauci. 1983. Abnormalities of B-cell activation and immunoregulation in patients with the acquired immunodeficiency syndrome. *N Engl J Med* **309**:453–458.

1422. Lang, W., H. Perkins, R. E. Anderson, R. Royce, N. Jewell, and W. Winkelstein, Jr. 1989. Patterns of T lymphocyte changes with human immunodeficiency virus infection: from seroconversion to the development of AIDS. *J AIDS* **2**:63–69.

1423. **Lange, J. M. A.** 1997. Current problems and the future of antiretroviral drug trials. *Science* **276**:548–550.

1423a.**Lange, J. M. A., F. de Wolf, W. J. A. Krone, S. A. Danner, R. A. Coutinho, and J. Goudsmit.** 1987. Decline of antibody reactivity to outer viral core protein p17 is an earlier serological marker of disease progression in human immunodeficiency virus infection than anti-p24 decline. *AIDS* **1**:155–159.

1424. **Lange, J. M. A., D. A. Paul, H. G. Huisman, F. de Wolf, H. van den Berg, R. A. Coutinho, S. A. Danner, J. van der Noordaa, and J. Goudsmit.** 1986. Persistent HIV antigenaemia and decline of HIV core antibodies associated with transition to AIDS. *Brit Med J* **293**:1459–1462.

1425. **Langhoff, E., E. F. Terwilliger, H. J. Bos, K. H. Kalland, M. C. Poznansky, O. M. L. Bacon, and W. A. Haseltine.** 1991. Replication of human immunodeficiency virus type 1 in primary dendritic cell cultures. *Proc Natl Acad Sci USA* **88**:7998–8002.

1426. **Langlade-Demoyen, P., N. Ngo-Giang-Huong, F. Ferchal, and E. Oksenhendler.** 1994. Human immunodeficiency virus (HIV) *nef*-specific cytotoxic T lymphocytes in noninfected heterosexual contacts of HIV-infected patients. *J Clin Invest* **93**:1293–1297.

1427. **Langlois, A. J., K. J. Weinhold, T. J. Matthews, M. L. Greenberg, and D. P. Bolognesi.** 1992. The ability of certain SIV vaccines to provoke reactions against normal cells. *Science* **255**:292–293.

1428. **Lanzavecchia, A., E. Roosnek, T. Gregory, P. Berman, and S. Abrignani.** 1988. T cells can present antigens such as HIV gp120 targeted to their own surface molecules. *Nature* **334**:530–532.

1429. **Lapham, C. K., J. Ouyang, B. Chandrasekhar, N. Y. Nguyen, D. S. Dimitrov, and H. Golding.** 1996. Evidence for cell-surface association between fusin and the CD4-gp120 complex in human cell lines. *Science* **274**:602–605.

1430. **Larder, B. A., P. Kellam, and S. D. Kemp.** 1993. Convergent combination therapy can select viable multidrug-resistant HIV-1 in vitro. *Nature* **365**:451–453.

1431. **Larder, B. A., and S. D. Kemp.** 1989. Multiple mutations in HIV-1 reverse transcriptase confer high-level resistance to zidovudine (AZT). *Science* **246**:1155–1158.

1432. **Larder, B. A., S. D. Kemp, and P. R. Harrigan.** 1995. Potential mechanism for sustained antiretroviral efficacy of AZT-3TC combination therapy. *Science* **269**:696–699.

1433. **LaRosa, G. J., J. P. Davide, K. Weinhold, J. A. Waterbury, A. T. Profy, J. A. Lewis, A. J. Langlois, G. R. Dreesman, R. N. Boswell, P. Shadduck, L. H. Holley, M. Karplus, D. P. Bolognesi, T. J. Matthews, E. A. Emini, and S. D. Putney.** 1990. Conserved sequence and structural elements in the HIV-1 principal neutralizing determinant. *Science* **249**:932–935.

1434. **Lasky, L. A., G. Nakamura, D. H. Smith, C. Fennie, C. Shimasaki, E. Patzer, P. Berman, T. Gregory, and D. J. Capon.** 1987. Delineation of a region of the human immunodeficiency virus type 1 gp120 glycoprotein critical for interaction with the CD4 receptor. *Cell* **50**:975–985.

1435. **Lassman, H., M. Schmied, K. Vass, and W. F. Hickey.** 1993. Bone marrow derived elements and resident microglia in brain inflammation. *Glia* **7**:19–24.

1436. **Lassoued, K., J. P. Clauvel, S. Fegueux, S. Matheron, I. Gorin, and E. Oksenhandler.** 1991. AIDS-associated Kaposi's sarcoma in female patients. *AIDS* **5**:877–880.

1437. **Lathey, J. L., R. D. Pratt, and S. A. Spector.** 1997. Appearance of autologous neutralizing antibody correlates with reduction in virus load and phenotype switch during primary infection with human immunodeficiency virus type 1. *J Inf Dis* **175**:231–232.

1438. **Lauener, R. P., S. Huttner, M. Buisson, J. P. Hossle, M. Albisetti, J.-M. Seigneurin, R. A. Seger, and D. Nadal.** 1995. T-cell death by apoptosis in vertically human immunodeficiency virus-infected children coincides with expansion of CD8+/interleukin-2 receptor− /HLA-DR+ T cells: sign of a possible role for herpes viruses as cofactors? *Blood* **86**:1400–1407.

1439. **Laughlin, M. A., S. Zeichner, D. Kolson, J. C. Alwine, T. Seshamma, R. J. Pomerantz, and F. Gonzalez-Scarano.** 1993. Sodium butyrate treatment of cells latently infected with HIV-1 results in the expression of unspliced viral RNA. *Virol* **196**:496–505.

1440. **Laurence, J.** 1990. Molecular interactions among herpesviruses and human immunodeficiency viruses. *J Inf Dis* **162**:338–346.

1441. Laurence, J. 1990. Novel vaccination and antireceptor strategies against HIV. *AIDS Res Hum Retro* **6**:175–181.

1442. Laurence, J., and S. M. Astrin. 1991. Human immunodeficiency virus induction of malignant transformation in human B lymphocytes. *Proc Natl Acad Sci USA* **88**:7635–7639.

1443. Laurence, J., A. B. Gottlieb, and H. G. Kunkel. 1983. Soluble suppressor factors in patients with acquired immune deficiency syndrome and its prodrome. *J Clin Invest* **72**:2072–2081.

1444. Laurence, J., A. S. Hodtsev, and D. N. Posnett. 1992. Superantigen implicated in dependence of HIV-1 replication in T cells on TCR V beta expression. *Nature* **358**:255–259.

1445. Laurence, J., D. Mitra, M. Steiner, D. H. Lynch, F. P. Siegal, and L. Staiano-Coico. 1996. Apoptotic depletion of CD4+ T cells in idiopathic CD4+ T lymphocytopenia. *J Clin Invest* **97**:672–680.

1446. Laurence, J., A. Saunders, E. Early, and J. E. Salmon. 1990. Human immunodeficiency virus infection of monocytes: relationship to Fc-gamma receptors and antibody-dependent viral enhancement. *Immunol* **70**:338–343.

1447. Laurence, J., M. B. Sellers, and S. Sikder. 1989. Effect of glucocorticoids on chronic human immunodeficiency virus (HIV) infection and HIV promoter-mediated transcription. *Blood* **74**:291–297.

1448. Laurent, A. G., A. G. Hovanessian, Y. Riviere, B. Krust, A. Regnault, L. Montagnier, A. Finddeli, M. P. Kieny, and B. Guy. 1990. Production of a non-functional *nef* protein in human immunodeficiency virus type 1-infected CEM cells. *J Gen Virol* **71**:2273–2281.

1449. Laurent-Crawford, A. G., B. Krust, S. Muller, Y. Riviere, M.-A. Rey-Cuille, J.-M. Bechet, L. Montagnier, and A. G. Hovanessian. 1991. The cytopathic effect of HIV is associated with apoptosis. *Virol* **185**:829–839.

1450. Laurent-Crawford, A. G., B. Krust, Y. Riviere, C. Desgranges, S. Muller, M. P. Kieny, C. Dauguet, and A. G. Hovanessian. 1993. Membrane expression of HIV envelope glycoproteins triggers apoptosis in CD4 cells. *AIDS Res Hum Retro* **9**:761–773.

1451. Layne, S. P., M. J. Merges, M. Dembo, J. L. Spouge, S. R. Conley, J. P. Moore, J. L. Raina, H. Renz, H. R. Gelderblom, and P. L. Nara. 1992. Factors underlying spontaneous inactivation and susceptibility to neutralization of human immunodeficiency virus. *Virol* **189**:695–714.

1452. Layne, S. P., M. J. Merges, J. L. Spouge, M. Dembo, and P. L. Nara. 1991. Blocking of human immunodeficiency virus infection depends on cell density and viral stock age. *J Virol* **65**:3293–3300.

1453. Layton, G. T., S. J. Harris, A. J. H. Gearing, M. Hill-Perkins, J. S. Cole, J. C. Griffiths, N. R. Burns, A. J. Kingsman, and S. E. Adams. 1993. Induction of HIV-specific cytotoxic T lymphocytes in vivo with hybrid HIV-1 V3: Ty-virus-like particles. *J Immunol* **151**:1097–1107.

1454. Le Grand, R., M. Nadal, A. Cheret, P. Roques, B. Vaslin, F. Matheux, F. Theodoro, G. Gras, L. Gauthier, A. M. Aubertin, and D. Dormont. 1995. Infection of macaques after vaginal exposure to a primary isolate of SIVmac251. *AIDS* **9**:308–309.

1455. Leal, M., Y. Torres, F. J. Medrano, E. J. Calderon, C. Rey, and E. Lissen. 1994. Does early zidovudine treatment prevent the emergence of syncytium-inducing human immunodeficiency virus? *J Inf Dis* **170**:1041–1042.

1456. Lebbé, C., C. Pellet, R. Tatoud, F. Agbalika, P. Dosquet, G. P. Desgrez, P. Morel, and F. Calvo. 1997. Absence of human herpesvirus 8 sequences in prostate specimens. *AIDS* **11**:270.

1457. Lecatsas, G., S. Houff, A. Macher, E. Gelman, R. Steis, C. Reichert, H. Masur, and J. L. Sever. 1985. Retrovirus-like particles in salivary glands, prostate and testes of AIDS patients. *Proc Soc Exp Biol Med* **178**:653–655.

1458. Lech, W. J., G. Wang, Y. L. Yang, Y. Chee, K. Dorman, D. McCrae, L. C. Lazzeroni, J. W. Erickson, J. S. Sinsheimer, and A. H. Kaplan. 1996. In vivo sequence diversity of the protease of human immunodeficiency virus type 1: presence of protease inhibitor-resistant variants in untreated subjects. *J Virol* **70**:2038–2043.

1459. Lederman, M. M., S. F. Purvis, E. I. Walter, J. T. Carey, and M. E. Medof. 1989. Heightened complement sensitivity of acquired immunodeficiency syndrome lymphocytes related to diminished expression of decay-accelerating factor. *Proc Natl Acad Sci USA* **86**:4205–4209.

1460. **Lee, M. R., D. D. Ho, and M. E. Gurney.** 1987. Functional interaction and partial homology between human immunodeficiency virus and neuroleukin. *Science* **237**:1047–1051.

1461. **Lee, T. H., H. W. Sheppard, M. Reis, D. Dondero, D. Osmond, and M. P. Busch.** 1994. Circulating HIV-1-infected cell burden from seroconversion to AIDS: importance of postseroconversion viral load on disease course. *J AIDS* **7**:381–388.

1462. **Lee, W.-R., W.-J. Syu, B. Du, M. Matsuda, S. Tan, A. Wolf, M. Essex, and T.-H. Lee.** 1992. Nonrandom distribution of gp120 N-linked glycosylation sites important for infectivity of human immunodeficiency virus type 1. *Proc Natl Acad Sci USA* **89**:2213–2217.

1463. **Legrain, P., B. Goud, and G. Buttin.** 1986. Increase of retroviral infection *in vitro* by the binding of antiretrovirus antibodies. *J Virol* **60**:1141–1144.

1463a. **LeGuern, M., and J. A. Levy.** Unpublished observations.

1464. **LeGuern, M., and J. A. Levy.** 1992. HIV-1 can superinfect HIV-2-infected cells: pseudotype virions produced with expanded cellular host range. *Proc Natl Acad Sci USA* **89**:363–367.

1465. **LeGuern, M., T. Shioda, J. A. Levy, and C. Cheng-Mayer.** 1993. Single amino acid change in Tat determines the different rates of replication of two sequential HIV-1 isolates. *Virol* **195**:441–447.

1466. **Lehner, T., L. A. Bergmeier, C. Panagiotidi, L. Tao, R. Brookes, L. S. Klavinskis, P. Walker, J. Walker, R. G. Ward, L. Hussain, A. J. H. Gearing, and S. E. Adams.** 1992. Induction of mucosal and systemic immunity to a recombinant simian immunodeficiency viral protein. *Science* **258**:1365–1369.

1467. **Lehner, T., L. A. Bergmeier, L. Tao, C. Panagiotidi, L. S. Klavinskis, L. Hussain, R. G. Ward, N. Meyers, S. E. Adams, A. J. H. Gearing, and R. Brookes.** 1994. Targeted lymph node immunization with simian immunodeficiency virus p27 antigen to elicit genital, rectal, and urinary immune responses in nonhuman primates. *J Immunol* **153**:1858–1868.

1468. **Lehner, T., R. Brookes, C. Panagiotodi, L. Tao, L. S. Klavinskis, J. Walker, P. Walker, R. Ward, L. Hussain, A. J. H. Gearing, S. E. Adams, and L. A. Bergmeier.** 1993. T- and B-cell functions and epitope expression in nonhuman primates immunized with simian immunodeficiency virus antigen by the rectal route. *Proc Natl Acad Sci USA* **90**:8638–8642.

1469. **Lehner, T., Y. Wang, M. Cranage, L. A. Bergmeier, E. Mitchell, L. Tao, G. Hall, M. Dennis, N. Cook, R. Brookes, L. Klavinskis, I. Jones, C. Doyle, and R. Ward.** 1996. Protective mucosal immunity elicited by targeted iliac lymph node immunization with a subunit SIV envelope and core vaccine in macaques. *Nature Med* **2**:767–775.

1470. **Leiderman, I. Z., M. L. Greenberg, B. R. Adelsberg, and F. P. Siegal.** 1987. A glycoprotein inhibitor of in vitro granulopoiesis associated with AIDS. *Blood* **70**:1267–1272.

1471. **Leigh Brown, A. J., and E. C. Holmes.** 1994. Evolutionary biology of human immunodeficiency virus. *Annu Rev Ecol Syst* **25**:127–165.

1472. **Leis, J., D. Baltimore, J. M. Bishop, J. Coffin, E. Fleissner, S. P. Goff, S. Oroszlan, H. Robinson, A. M. Skalka, H. M. Temin, and V. Vogt.** 1988. Standardized and simplified nomenclature for proteins common to all retroviruses. *J Virol* **62**:1808–1809.

1473. **Leith, J. G., K. F. T. Copeland, P. J. McKay, C. D. Richards, and K. L. Rosenthal.** 1997. CD8+ T-cell-mediated suppression of HIV-1 long terminal repeat-driven gene expression is not modulated by the CC chemokines RANTES, macrophage inflammatory protein (MIP)-1α and MIP-1β. *AIDS* **11**:575–580.

1474. **Lekutis, C., J. W. Shiver, M. A. Liu, and N. L. Letvin.** 1997. HIV-1 env DNA vaccine administered to rhesus monkeys elicits MHC class II-restricted CD4+ T helper cells that secrete IFN-γ and TNF-α. *J Immunol* **158**:4471–4477.

1475. **Lemaitre, M., D. Guetard, Y. Henin, L. Montagnier, and A. Zerial.** 1990. Protective activity of tetracycline analogs against the cytopathic effect of the human immunodeficiency viruses in CEM cells. *Res Virol* **141**:5–16.

1476. **Lenberg, M. E., and N. R. Landau.** 1993. Vpu-induced degradation of CD4: requirement for specific amino acid residues in the cytoplasmic domain of CD4. *J Virol* **67**:7238–7245.

1477. **Lenderking, W. R., R. D. Gelber, D. J. Cotton, B. F. Cole, A. Goldhirsch, P. A. Volberding, and M. A. Testa.** 1994. Evaluation of the quality of life associated with zidovudine treatment in asymptomatic human immunodeficiency virus infection. *N Engl J Med* **330:**738–743.

1478. **Lennette, E. T., D. J. Blackbourn, and J. A. Levy.** 1996. Antibodies to human herpesvirus type 8 in the general population and in Kaposi's sarcoma patients. *Lancet* **348:**858–861.

1479. **Leonard, C. K., M. W. Spellman, L. Riddle, R. J. Harris, J. N. Thomas, and T. J. Gregory.** 1990. Assignment of intrachain disulfide bonds and characterization of potential glycosylation sites of the type 1 recombinant human immunodeficiency virus envelope glycoprotein (gp120) expressed in Chinese hamster ovary cells. *J Biol Chem* **265:**10373–10382.

1480. **Leonard, G., A. Chaput, V. Courgnaud, A. Sangare, F. Denis, and C. Brechot.** 1993. Characterization of dual HIV-1 and HIV-2 serological profiles by polymerase chain reaction. *AIDS* **7:**1185–1189.

1481. **Letvin, N. L., J. Li, M. Halloran, M. P. Cranage, E. W. Rud, and J. Sodroski.** 1995. Prior infection with a nonpathogenic chimeric simian-human immunodeficiency virus does not efficiently protect macaques against challenge with simian immunodefiency virus. *J Virol* **69:**4569–4571.

1481a.**Letvin, N. L., D. C. Montefiori, Y. Yasutomi, H. C. Perry, M. E. Davies, C. Lekutis, M. Alroy, D. C. Freed, C. I. Lord, L. K. Handt, M. A. Liu, and J. W. Shiver.** 1997. Potent, protective anti-HIV immune responses generated by bimodal HIV Env DNA+ protein vaccination. *Proc Natl Acad Sci USA* **94:**9378–9383.

1482. **Levacher, M., F. Hulstaert, S. Tallet, S. Ullery, J. J. Pocidalo, and B. A. Bach.** 1992. The significance of activation markers on CD8 lymphocytes in human immunodeficiency syndrome: staging and prognostic value. *Clin Exp Immunol* **90:**376–382.

1483. **Levi, G., M. Patrizio, A. Bernardo, T. C. Petrucci, and C. Agresti.** 1993. Human immunodeficiency virus coat protein gp120 inhibits the beta-adrenergic regulation of astroglial and microglial functions. *Proc Natl Acad Sci USA* **90:**1541–1545.

1484. **Levine, A. M.** 1992. Acquired immunodeficiency syndrome-related lymphoma. *Blood* **80:**8–20.

1485. **Levine, A. M., S. Groshen, J. Allen, K. M. Munson, D. J. Carlo, A. E. Daigle, F. Ferre, F. C. Jensen, S. P. Richieri, R. J. Trauger, J. W. Parker, P. L. Salk, and J. Salk.** 1996. Initial studies on active immunization of HIV-infected subjects using a gp120-depleted HIV-1 immunogen: long-term follow-up. *J AIDS Hum Retrovirol* **11:**351–364.

1486. **Levine, B. L., J. D. Mosca, J. L. Riley, R. G. Carroll, M. T. Vahey, L. L. Jagodzinski, K. F. Wagner, D. L. Mayers, D. S. Burke, O. S. Weislow, D. C. St. Louis, and C. H. June.** 1996. Antiviral effect and *ex vivo* CD4+ T cell proliferation in HIV-positive patients as a result of CD28 costimulation. *Science* **272:**1939–1943.

1487. **Levy, D. N., L. S. Fernandes, W. V. Williams, and D. B. Weiner.** 1993. Induction of cell differentiation of human immunodeficiency virus 1 vpr. *Cell* **72:**541–550.

1488. **Levy, D. N., Y. Refaeli, and D. B. Weiner.** 1995. Extracellular Vpr protein increases cellular permissiveness to human immunodeficiency virus replication and reactivates virus from latency. *J Virol* **69:**1243–1252.

1489. **Levy, J. A.** 1988. Can an AIDS vaccine be developed? *Trans Med Rev* **2:**265–271.

1490. **Levy, J. A.** 1990. Changing concepts in HIV infection: challenges for the 1990's. *AIDS* **4:**1051–1058.

1491. **Levy, J. A.** 1993. HIV pathogenesis and long-term survival. *AIDS* **7:**1401–1410.

1492. **Levy, J. A.** 1995. HIV research: a need to focus on the right target. *Lancet* **345:**1619–1621.

1493. **Levy, J. A.** 1989. The human immunodeficiency viruses (HIV): detection and pathogenesis, p. 159–229. *In* J. A. Levy (ed.), *AIDS: Pathogenesis and Treatment*. Marcel Dekker, Inc., New York.

1494. **Levy, J. A.** 1989. Human immunodeficiency viruses and the pathogenesis of AIDS. *J Am Med Assoc* **261:**2997–3006.

1495. **Levy, J. A.** 1996. Infection by human immunodeficiency virus—CD4 is not enough. *N Engl J Med* **335:**1528–1530.

1496. Levy, J. A. 1986. The multifaceted retrovirus. *Cancer Res* **46**:5457–5468.

1497. Levy, J. A. 1988. The mysteries of HIV: challenges for therapy and prevention. *Nature* **333**:519–522.

1498. Levy, J. A. 1995. A new human herpesvirus: KSHV or HHV8? *Lancet* **346**:786.

1499. Levy, J. A. 1996. Surrogate markers in AIDS research. Is there truth in numbers? *J Am Med Assoc* **276**:161–162.

1500. Levy, J. A. 1997. Three new human herpesviruses (HHV6, 7, and 8). *Lancet* **349**:558–563.

1501. Levy, J. A. 1988. The transmission of AIDS: the case of the infected cell. *J Am Med Assoc* **259**:3037–3038.

1502. Levy, J. A. 1993. The transmission of HIV and factors influencing progression to disease. *Am J Med* **95**:86–100.

1503. Levy, J. A. 1977. Type C RNA viruses and autoimmune disease, p. 403–453. *In* N. Talal (ed.), *Autoimmunity: Genetic, Immunologic, Virology and Clinical Aspects.* Academic Press, New York.

1504. Levy, J. A. 1996. The value of primate models for studying human immunodeficiency virus pathogenesis. *J Med Primatol* **25**:163–174.

1505. Levy, J. A. 1978. Xenotropic type C viruses. *Curr Top Micro Immunol* **79**:111–213.

1505a. Levy, J. A. Unpublished observations.

1506. Levy, J. A., C. Cheng-Mayer, D. Dina, and P. A. Luciw. 1986. AIDS retrovirus (ARV-2) clone replicates in transfected human and animal fibroblasts. *Science* **232**:998–1001.

1507. Levy, J. A., L. Evans, C. Cheng-Mayer, L.-Z. Pan, A. Lane, C. Staben, D. Dina, C. Wiley, and J. Nelson. 1987. The biologic and molecular properties of the AIDS-associated retrovirus that affect antiviral therapy. *Ann Inst Pasteur* **138**:101–111.

1508. Levy, J. A., and A. H. Fieldsteel. 1982. Freeze-drying is an effective method for preserving infectious type C retroviruses. *J Virol Meth* **5**:165–171.

1508a. Levy, J. A., and R. Glogau. Unpublished observations.

1509. Levy, J. A., and D. Greenspan. 1988. HIV in saliva. *Lancet* **ii**:1248.

1510. Levy, J. A., A. D. Hoffman, S. M. Kramer, J. A. Landis, J. M. Shimabukuro, and L. S. Oshiro. 1984. Isolation of lymphocytopathic retroviruses from San Francisco patients with AIDS. *Science* **225**:840–842.

1511. Levy, J. A., H. Hollander, J. Shimabukuro, J. Mills, and L. Kaminsky. 1985. Isolation of AIDS-associated retroviruses from cerebrospinal fluid and brain of patients with neurological symptoms. *Lancet* **ii**:586–588.

1511a. Levy, J. A., F. Hsueh, D. J. Blackbourn, D. Wara, and P. S. Weintrub. CD8+ cell noncytotoxic antiviral activity in HIV-infected and uninfected children. *J Inf Dis* in press.

1512. Levy, J. A., L. S. Kaminsky, W. J. W. Morrow, K. Steimer, P. Luciw, D. Dina, J. Hoxie, and L. Oshiro. 1985. Infection by the retrovirus associated with the acquired immunodeficiency syndrome. *Ann Int Med* **103**:694–699.

1513. Levy, J. A., A. Landay, and E. T. Lennette. 1990. HHV-6 inhibits HIV-1 replication in cell culture. *J Clin Micro* **28**:2362–2364.

1514. Levy, J. A., C. Mackewicz, and C. Cheng-Mayer. 1991. Natural antiviral responses in HIV infection, vol. 1, p. 58. *In Seventh International Conference on AIDS, Florence, Italy.*

1515. Levy, J. A., C. E. Mackewicz, and E. Barker. 1996. Controlling HIV pathogenesis: the role of noncytotoxic anti-HIV activity of CD8+ cells. *Immunol Today* **17**:217–224.

1516. Levy, J. A., W. Margaretten, and J. Nelson. 1989. Detection of HIV in enterochromaffin cells in the rectal mucosa of an AIDS patient. *Am J Gastro* **84**:787–789.

1517. Levy, J. A., G. Mitra, and M. M. Mozen. 1984. Recovery and inactivation of infectious retroviruses added to factor VIII concentrates. *Lancet* **ii**:722–723.

1518. Levy, J. A., G. A. Mitra, M. F. Wong, and M. M. Mozen. 1985. Inactivation by wet and dry heat procedures of AIDS-associated retrovirus (ARV) during factor VIII purification from plasma. *Lancet* **i**:1456–1457.

1518a.Levy, J. A., and R. Orque. Unpublished observations.

1519. Levy, J. A., B. Ramachandran, E. Barker, J. Guthrie, and T. Elbeik. 1996. Plasma viral load, CD4+ cell counts, and HIV-1 production by cells. *Science* 271:670–671.

1520. Levy, J. A., and A. Sato. Unpublished observations.

1521. Levy, J. A., J. Shimabukuro, T. McHugh, C. Casavant, D. Stites, and L. Oshiro. 1985. AIDS-associated retroviruses (ARV) can productively infect other cells besides human T helper cells. *Virol* 147:441–448.

1522. Levy, J. A., and J. Ziegler. 1983. Acquired immune deficiency syndrome (AIDS) is an opportunistic infection and Kaposi's sarcoma results from secondary immune stimulation. *Lancet* ii:78–81.

1523. Levy, Y., and J. C. Brouet. 1994. Interleukin-10 prevents spontaneous death of germinal center B cells by induction of the bcl-1 protein. *J Clin Invest* 93:424–428.

1524. Lewin, S. R., P. Lambert, N. J. Deacon, J. Mills, and S. M. Crowe. 1997. Constitutive expression of p50 homodimer in freshly isolated human monocytes decreases with in vitro and in vivo differentiation: a possible mechanism influencing human immunodeficiency virus replication in monocytes and mature macrophages. *J Virol* 71:2114–2119.

1525. Lewis, D. E., D. S. N. Tang, A. Adu-Oppong, W. Schober, and J. R. Rodgers. 1994. Anergy and apoptosis in CD8+ T cells from HIV-infected persons. *J Immunol* 153:412–420.

1525a.Lewis, M. G., F. Novembre, R. Desrosiers, Y. Lu, D. Montefiori, J. Yalley-Ogunro, J. Greenhouse, T. Brennan, and G. Eddy. 1997. Attenuated SIV vaccines: degree of protection from homologous and heterologous challenge, p. 88. Presented at the Ninth Annual Meeting of the National Cooperative Vaccine Development Groups for AIDS, Bethesda, Md.

1525b.Lewis, M. G. Personal communication.

1526. Lewis, P., M. Hensel, and M. Emerman. 1992. Human immunodeficiency virus infection of cells arrested in the cell cycle. *EMBO J* 11:3053–3058.

1527. Lewis, P. F., and M. Emerman. 1994. Passage through mitosis is required for oncoretroviruses but not for the human immunodeficiency virus. *J Virol* 68:510–516.

1528. Lewis, S. H., C. Reynolds-Kohler, H. E. Fox, and J. A. Nelson. 1990. HIV-1 in trophoblastic and villous Hofbauer cells, and haematological precursors in eight-week fetuses. *Lancet* 335:565–568.

1529. Li, C. J., D. J. Friedman, C. Wang, V. Metelev, and A. B. Pardee. 1995. Induction of apoptosis in uninfected lymphocytes by HIV-1 Tat protein. *Science* 268:429–431.

1530. Li, C. J., L. J. Zhang, B. J. Dezube, C. S. Crumpacker, and A. B. Pardee. 1993. Three inhibitors of type 1 human immunodeficiency virus long terminal repeat-directed gene expression and virus replication. *Proc Natl Acad Sci USA* 90:1839–1842.

1531. Li, G., M. Simm, M. J. Potash, and D. J. Volsky. 1993. Human immunodeficiency virus type 1 DNA synthesis, integration, and efficient viral replication in growth-arrested T cells. *J Virol* 67:3969–3977.

1532. Li, J. J., A. E. Friedman-Kien, Y.-Q. Huang, M. Mirabile, and Y. Z. Cao. 1990. HIV-1 DNA proviral sequences in fresh urine pellets from HIV-1 seropositive persons. *Lancet* 335:1590–1591.

1533. Li, J. J., Y. Q. Huang, C. J. Cockerell, and A. E. Friedman-Kien. 1996. Localization of human herpes-like virus type 8 in vascular endothelial cells and perivascular spindle-shaped cells of Kaposi's sarcoma lesions by *in situ* hybridization. *Am J Path* 148:1741–1748.

1534. Li, P., L. J. Kuiper, A. J. Stephenson, and C. J. Burrell. 1992. *De novo* reverse transcription is a crucial event in cell-to-cell transmission of human immunodeficiency virus. *J Gen Virol* 73:955–959.

1534a.Li, Q., K. Gebhard, T. Schacker, K. Henry, and A. T. Haase. 1997. The relationship between tumor necrosis factor and human immunodeficiency virus gene expression in lymphoid tissue. *J Virol* 71:7080–7082.

1535. Li, S., V. Polonis, H. Isobe, H. Zaghouani, R. Guinea, T. Moran, C. Bona, and P. Palese. 1993. Chimeric influenza virus induces neutralizing antibodies and cytotoxic T cells against human immunodeficiency virus type 1. *J Virol* 67:6659–6666.

1536. Li, X. D., B. Moore, and M. W. Cloyd. 1996. Gradual shutdown of virus production resulting in latency is the norm during the chronic phase of human immunodeficiency virus replication and differential rates and mechanisms of shutdown are determined by viral sequences. *Virol* **225**:196–212.

1537. Li, Y., J. C. Kappes, J. A. Conway, R. W. Price, G. M. Shaw, and B. H. Hahn. 1991. Molecular characterization of human immunodeficiency virus type 1 cloned directly from uncultured human brain tissue: identification of replication-competent and -defective viral genomes. *J Virol* **65**:3973–3985.

1537a. Liao, F., G. Alkhatib, K. W. Peden, O. Sharma, E. A. Berger, and J. M. Farber. 1997. STRL33, a novel chemokine receptor-like protein, functions as a fusion cofactor for both macrophage-tropic and T cell line-tropic HIV-1. *J Exp Med* **185**:2015–2023.

1538. Lieberman, A. P., P. M. Pitha, H. S. Shin, and M. L. Shin. 1989. Production of tumor necrosis factor and other cytokines by astrocytes stimulated with lipopolysaccharide of a neurotropic virus. *Proc Natl Acad Sci USA* **86**:6348–6352.

1538a. Lieberman, J., P. R. Skolnik, G. R. Parkerson, III, J. A. Fabry, B. Landry, J. Bethel, and J. Kagan. 1997. Safety of autologous, *ex vivo*-expanded human immunodeficiency virus (HIV)-specific cytotoxic T-lymphocyte infusion in HIV-infected patients. *Blood* **90**:2196–2206.

1539. Lifson, A. R., S. P. Buchbinder, H. W. Sheppard, A. C. Mawle, J. C. Wilber, M. Stanley, C. E. Hart, N. A. Hessol, and S. D. Holmberg. 1991. Long-term human immunodeficiency virus infection in asymptomatic homosexual and bisexual men with normal CD4+ lymphocyte counts: immunologic and virologic characteristics. *J Inf Dis* **163**:959–965.

1540. Lifson, A. R., W. W. Darrow, and N. A. Hessol. 1990. Kaposi's sarcoma in a cohort of homosexual and bisexual men. *Am J Epidemiol* **131**:221–231.

1541. Lifson, A. R., N. A. Hessol, S. P. Buchbinder, P. M. O'Malley, L. Barnhart, M. Segal, M. H. Katz, and S. D. Holmberg. 1992. Serum beta$_2$-microglobulin and prediction of progression to AIDS in HIV infection. *Lancet* **339**:1436–1440.

1542. Lifson, A. R., P. M. O'Malley, N. A. Hessol, S. P. Buchbinder, L. Cannon, and G. W. Rutherford. 1990. HIV seroconversion in two homosexual men after receptive oral intercourse with ejaculation: implications for counseling concerning safe sexual practices. *Am J Pub Health* **80**:1509–1511.

1543. Lifson, A. R., M. Stanley, J. Pane, P. M. O'Malley, J. C. Wilber, A. Stanley, B. Jeffery, G. W. Rutherford, and P. R. Sohmer. 1990. Detection of human immunodeficiency virus DNA using the polymerase chain reaction in a well-characterized group of homosexual and bisexual men. *J Inf Dis* **161**:436–439.

1544. Lifson, J., S. Coutre, E. Huang, and E. Engleman. 1986. Role of envelope glycoprotein carbohydrate in human immunodeficiency virus (HIV) infectivity and virus-induced cell fusion. *J Exp Med* **164**:2101–2106.

1545. Lifson, J. D., M. B. Feinberg, G. R. Reyes, L. Rabin, B. Banapour, S. Chakrabarti, B. Moss, F. Wong-Staal, K. S. Steimer, and E. G. Engleman. 1986. Induction of CD4-dependent cell fusion by the HTLV-III/LAV envelope glycoprotein. *Nature* **323**:725–728.

1546. Lifson, J. D., K. M. Hwang, P. L. Nara, B. Fraser, M. Padgett, N. M. Dunlop, and L. E. Eiden. 1988. Synthetic CD4 peptide derivatives that inhibit HIV infection and cytopathicity. *Science* **241**:712–716.

1547. Lifson, J. D., D. M. Rausch, V. S. Kalyanaraman, K. M. Hwang, and L. E. Eiden. 1991. Synthetic peptides allow discrimination of structural features of CD4 (81–92) important for HIV-1 infection versus HIV-1-induced syncytium formation. *AIDS Res Hum Retro* **7**:449–455.

1548. Lifson, J. D., G. R. Reyes, M. S. McGrath, B. S. Stein, and E. G. Engleman. 1986. AIDS retrovirus induced cytopathology: giant cell formation and involvement of CD4 antigen. *Science* **232**:1123–1127.

1549. Liles, W. C., and W. C. Van Voorhis. 1995. Nomenclature and biologic significance of cytokines involved in inflammation and the host immune response. *J Inf Dis* **172**:1573–1580.

1550. Lim, S. G., A. Condez, C. A. Lee, M. A. Johnson, C. Elia, and L. W. Poulter. 1993. Loss of mucosal CD4 lymphocytes is an early feature of HIV infection. *Clin Exp Immunol* **92**:448–454.

1551. Lim, S. G., A. Condez, and L. W. Poulter. 1993. Mucosal macrophage subsets of the gut in HIV: decrease in antigen-presenting cell phenotype. *Clin Exp Immunol* 92:442–447.

1552. Lin, J. C., S. C. Lin, E. C. Mar, P. E. Pellett, F. R. Stamey, J. A. Stewart, and T. J. Spira. 1995. Is Kaposi's sarcoma-associated herpesvirus detectable in semen of HIV-infected homosexual men? *Lancet* 346:1601–1602.

1553. Lindboe, C. F., S. S. Froland, K. W. Wefring, P. J. Linnestad, T. Bohmer, A. Foerster, and A. C. Loken. 1986. Autopsy findings in three family members with a presumably acquired immunodeficiency syndrome of unknown etiology. *Acta Pathol Microbiol Immunol Scand* 94:117–123.

1554. Lindenmann, J. 1974. Viruses as immunological adjuvants in cancer. *Biochim Biophys Acta* 355:49–75.

1555. Linette, G. P., R. J. Hartzmann, J. A. Ledbetter, and C. H. June. 1988. HIV-1-infected T cells show a selective signaling defect after perturbation of CD3/antigen receptor. *Science* 241:573–576.

1556. Ling, E. A., and W.-C. Wong. 1993. The origin and nature of ramified and amoeboid microglia: a historical review and current concepts. *Glia* 7:9–18.

1557. Linhart, H., B. R. Gundlach, S. Sopper, U. Dittmer, K. Matz-Rensing, E.-M. Kuhn, J. Muller, G. Hunsmann, C. Stahl-Henning, and K. Uberla. 1997. Live attenuated SIV vaccines are not effective in a postexposure vaccination model. *AIDS Res Hum Retro* 13:593–599.

1558. Linsley, P. S., and J. A. Ledbetter. 1993. The role of the CD28 receptor during T cell responses to antigen. *Annu Rev Immunol* 11:191–212.

1559. Linsley, P. S., J. L. Greene, P. Tan, J. Bradshaw, J. A. Ledbetter, C. Anasetti, and N. K. Damle. 1992. Coexpression and functional cooperation of CTLA-4 and CD28 on activated T lymphocytes. *J Exp Med* 176:1595–1604.

1560. Linsley, P. S., J. A. Ledbetter, E. Kinney-Thomas, and S.-L. Hu. 1988. Effects of anti-gp120 monoclonal antibodies on CD4 receptor binding by the *env* protein of human immunodeficiency virus type 1. *J Virol* 62:3695–3702.

1561. Lioy, J., W.-Z. Ho, J. R. Cutilli, R. A. Polin, and S. D. Douglas. 1993. Thiol suppression of human immunodeficiency virus type 1 replication in primary cord blood monocyte-derived macrophages in vitro. *J Clin Invest* 91:495–498.

1562. Lipshultz, S. E., C. H. Fox, A. R. Perez-Atayde, S. P. Sanders, S. D. Colan, K. McIntosh, and H. S. Winter. 1990. Identification of human immunodeficiency virus-1 RNA and DNA in the heart of a child with cardiovascular abnormalities and congenital acquired immune deficiency syndrome. *Am J Cardiol* 66:246–250.

1563. Lipton, S. A. 1991. Calcium channel antagonists and human immunodeficiency virus coat protein-mediated neuronal injury. *Ann Neurol* 30:110–114.

1564. Lipton, S. A., N. J. Sucher, P. K. Kaiser, and E. B. Dreyer. 1991. Synergistic effects of HIV coat protein and NMDA receptor-mediated neurotoxicity. *Neuron* 7:111–118.

1565. Lisignoli, G., M. C. Monaco, A. Degrassi, S. Toneguzzi, E. Ricchi, P. Costigliola, and A. Facchini. 1993. In vitro immunotoxicity of +/− 2'-deoxy-3'-thiacytidine, a new anti-HIV agent. *Clin Exp Immunol* 92:455–459.

1566. Little, D., J. W. Said, and R. J. Siegel. 1986. Endothelial cell markers in vascular neoplasms: an immunohistochemical study comparing factor VIII-related antigen, blood group specific antignes, 6-Keto-PGF1 alpha, and *Ulex europaeus* 1. *J Pathol* 149:89–95.

1567. Liu, H., X. Wu, M. Newman, G. M. Shaw, B. H. Hahn, and J. C. Kappes. 1995. The vif protein of human and simian immunodeficiency viruses is packaged into virions and associates with viral core structures. *J Virol* 69:7630–7638.

1568. Liu, R., W. A. Paxton, S. Choe, D. Ceradini, S. R. Martin, R. Horuk, M. E. MacDonald, H. Stuhlmann, R. A. Koup, and N. R. Landau. 1996. Homozygous defect in HIV-1 coreceptor accounts for resistance for some multiply-exposed individuals to HIV-1 infection. *Cell* 86:367–377.

1569. Liu, Z.-Q., C. Wood, J. A. Levy, and C. Cheng-Mayer. 1990. The viral envelope gene is involved in the macrophage tropism of an HIV-1 strain isolated from the brain. *J Virol* **64**:6143–6153.

1570. Liuzzi, G., P. Bagnarelli, A. Chirianni, M. Clementi, S. Nappa, P. Juillio Cataldo, A. Valenza, and M. Piazza. 1995. Quantitation of HIV-1 genome copy number in semen and saliva. *AIDS* **9**:651–653.

1571. Livingstone, W. J., M. Moore, D. Innes, J. E. Bell, and P. Simmonds. 1996. Frequent infection of peripheral blood CD8-positive T-lymphocytes with HIV-1. *Lancet* **348**:649–654.

1572. Ljunggren, K., G. Biberfeld, M. Jondal, and E.-M. Fenyo. 1989. Antibody-dependent cellular cytotoxicity detects type- and strain-specific antigens among human immunodeficiency virus types 1 and 2 and simian immunodeficiency virus SIV$_{mac}$ isolates. *J Virol* **63**:3376–3381.

1573. Ljunggren, K., P. A. Broliden, L. Morfeldt-Manson, M. Jondal, and B. Wahren. 1988. IgG subclass response to HIV in relation to antibody-dependent cellular cytotoxicity at different clinical stages. *Clin Exp Immunol* **73**:343–347.

1574. Lloyd, T. E., L. Yang, D. N. Tang, T. Bennett, W. Schober, and D. E. Lewis. 1997. Regulation of CD28 costimulation in human CD8+ T cells. *J Immunol* **158**:1551–1558.

1575. Lo, S.-C. 1986. Isolation and identification of a novel virus from patients with AIDS. *Am J Trop Med Hyg* **35**:675–676.

1576. Lo, S.-C., R. Y.-H. Wang, P. B. Newton III, N.-Y. Yang, M. A. Sonoda, and J. W.-K. Shih. 1989. Fatal infection of silvered leaf monkeys with a virus-like infectious agent (VLIA) derived from a patient with AIDS. *Am J Trop Med Hyg* **40**:399–409.

1577. Locher, C. P., D. J. Blackbourn, S. W. Barnett, K. K. Murthy, E. K. Cobb, S. Rouse, G. Greco, G. Reyes-Teran, K. M. Brasky, K. D. Carey, and J. A. Levy. 1997. Superinfection with HIV-2 can reactivate virus production in baboons but is contained by a CD8+ T-cell antiviral response. *J Inf Dis* **176**:948–959.

1577a. Locher, C., D. Blackbourn, and J. A. Levy. Unpublished observations.

1577b. Locher, C. P., S. Kliks, and J. A. Levy. Unpublished observations.

1578. Lohman, B. L., M. B. McChesney, C. J. Miller, E. McGowan, S. M. Joye, K. K. A. Van Rompay, E. Reay, L. Antipa, N. C. Pedersen, and M. L. Marthas. 1994. A partially attenuated simian immunodeficiency virus induces host immunity that correlates with resistance to pathogenic virus challenge. *J Virol* **68**:7021–7029.

1579. Lohman, B. L., M. B. McChesney, C. J. Miller, M. Otsyula, C. J. Berardi, and M. L. Marthas. 1994. Mucosal immunization with a live, virulence-attenuated simian immunodeficiency virus (SIV) vaccine elicits antiviral cytotoxic T lymphocytes and antibodies in rhesus macaques. *J Med Primatol* **23**:95–101.

1580. Lohman, B. L., C. J. Miller, and M. B. McChesney. 1995. Antiviral cytotoxic T lymphocytes in vaginal mucosa of simian immunodeficiency virus-infected rhesus macaques. *J Immunol* **155**:5855–5860.

1581. Lohse, A. W., F. Mor, N. Karin, and I. R. Cohen. 1989. Control of experimental autoimmune encephalomyelitis by T cells responding to activated T cells. *Science* **244**:820–822.

1582. Lokensgard, J. R., G. Gekkar, L. C. Ehrlich, S. Hu, C. C. Chao, and P. K. Peterson. 1997. Proinflammatory cytokines inhibit HIV-1$_{SF162}$ expression in acutely infected human brain cell cultures. *J Immunol* **158**:2449–2455.

1583. Lombardi, V., R. Placido, G. Scarlatti, M. L. Romiti, M. Mattei, F. Mariani, F. Poccia, P. Rossi, and V. Colizzi. 1993. Epitope specificity, antibody-dependent cellular cytotoxicity, and neutralizing activity of antibodies to human immunodeficiency virus type 1 in autoimmune MRL/lpr mice. *J Inf Dis* **167**:1267–1273.

1584. Looney, D. J., A. G. Fisher, S. D. Putney, J. R. Rusche, R. R. Redfield, D. S. Burke, R. C. Gallo, and F. Wong-Staal. 1988. Type-restricted neutralization of molecular clones of human immunodeficiency virus. *Science* **241**:357–359.

1585. Lori, F., F. Veronese, A. L. de Vico, P. Lusso, M. S. Reitz, Jr., and R. C. Gallo. 1992. Viral DNA carried by human immunodeficiency virus type 1 virions. *J Virol* **66**:5067–5074.

1585a. Louie, B., et al. Personal communication.

1586. Louwagie, J., W. Janssens, J. Mascola, L. Heyndrickx, P. Hegerich, G. van der Groen, F. E. McCutchan, and D. S. Burke. 1995. Genetic diversity of the envelope glycoprotein from human immunodeficiency virus type 1 isolates of African origin. *J Virol* **69**:263–271.

1587. Louwagie, J., F. E. McCutchan, M. Peeters, T. P. Brennan, E. Sanders-Buell, G. A. Eddy, G. van der Groen, K. Fransen, G.-M. Gershy-Damet, R. Deleys, and D. S. Burke. 1993. Phylogenetic analysis of gag genes from 70 international HIV-1 isolates provides evidence for multiple genotypes. *AIDS* **7**:769–780.

1588. Loveday, C., S. Kaye, M. Tenant-Flowers, M. Semple, U. Ayliffe, I. V. D. Weller, and R. S. Tedder. 1995. HIV-1 RNA serum-load and resistant viral genotypes during early zidovudine therapy. *Lancet* **345**:820–824.

1589. Lu, S., J. Arthos, D. C. Montefiori, Y. Yasutomi, K. Manson, F. Mustafa, E. Johnson, J. C. Santoro, J. Wissink, J. I. Mullins, J. R. Haynes, N. L. Letvin, M. Wyand, and H. L. Robinson. 1996. Simian immunodeficiency virus DNA vaccine trial in macaques. *J Virol* **70**:3978–3991.

1590. Lu, W., J. W. Shih, J. M. Tourani, D. Eme, H. J. Alter, and J. M. Andrieu. 1993. Lack of isolate-specific neutralizing activity is correlated with an increased viral burden in rapidly progressing HIV-1-infected patients. *AIDS* **7**:S91-S99.

1591. Lu, Y., P. Brosio, M. Lafaile, J. Li, R. G. Collman, J. Sodroski, and C. J. Miller. 1996. Vaginal transmission of chimeric simian/human immunodeficiency virsuses in rhesus macaques. *J Virol* **70**:3045–3050.

1592. Lu, Y., M. S. Salvato, C. D. Pauza, J. Li, J. Sodroski, K. Manson, M. Wyand, N. Letvin, S. Jenkins, N. Touzjian, C. Chutkowski, N. Kushner, M. LeFaile, L. G. Payne, and B. Roberts. 1996. Utility of SHIV for testing HIV-1 vaccine candidates in macaques. *J AIDS Hum Retrovirol* **12**:99–106.

1593. Lu, Y. L., P. Spearman, and L. Ratner. 1993. Human immunodeficiency virus type 1 viral protein R localization in infected cells and virions. *J Virol* **67**:6542–6550.

1594. Lu, Y. Y., Y. Koga, K. Tanaka, M. Sasaki, G. Kimura, and K. Nomoto. 1994. Apoptosis induced in CD4+ cells expressing gp160 of human immunodeficiency virus type 1. *J Virol* **68**:390–399.

1595. Lu, Z., J. F. Berson, Y. Chen, J. D. Turner, T. Zhang, M. Sharron, M. H. Jenks, Z. Wang, J. Kim, J. Rucker, J. A. Hoxie, S. C. Peiper, and R. W. Doms. 1997. Evolution of HIV-1 coreceptor usage through interactions with distinct CCR5 and CXCR4 domains. *Proc Natl Acad Sci USA* **94**:6426–6431.

1595a. Luban, J. 1996. Absconding with the chaperone: essential cyclophilin-gag interaction in HIV-1 virions. *Cell* **87**:1157–1159.

1596. Luban, J., K. L. Bossolt, E. K. Franke, G. V. Kalpana, and S. P. Goff. 1993. Human immunodeficiency virus type 1 Gag protein binds to cyclophilins A and B. *Cell* **73**:1067–1078.

1596a. Lubeck, M. D., R. Natuk, M. Myagkikh, N. Kalyan, K. Aldrich, F. Sinangil, S. Alipanah, S. C. Murthy, P. K. Chanda, S. M. Nigida, Jr., P. D. Markham, S. Zolla-Pazner, K. Steimer, M. Wade, M. S. Reitz, Jr., L. O. Arthur, S. Mizutani, A. Davis, P. P. Hung, R. C. Gallo, J. Eichberg, and M. Robert-Guroff. 1997. Long-term protection of chimpanzees against high-dose HIV-1 challenge induced by immunization. *Nat Med* **3**:651–658.

1597. Lucey, D. R., M. Clerici, and G. M. Shearer. 1996. Type 1 and type 2 cytokine dysregulation in human infectious, neoplastic, and inflammatory diseases. *Clin Microbiol Rev* **9**:532–562.

1597a. Luciw, P. A. Personal communication.

1598. Luciw, P. A., C. Cheng-Mayer, and J. A. Levy. 1987. Mutational anlaysis of the human immunodeficiency virus (HIV): the orf-B region down-regulates virus replication. *Proc Natl Acad Sci USA* **84**:1434–1438.

1599. Luciw, P. A., S. J. Potter, K. Steimer, D. Dina, and J. A. Levy. 1984. Molecular cloning of AIDS-associated retrovirus. *Nature* **312**:760–763.

1600. Luciw, P. A., E. Pratt-Lowe, K. E. S. Shaw, J. A. Levy, and C. Cheng-Mayer. 1995. Persistent infection of rhesus macques with T-cell-line-tropic and macrophage-tropic clones of simian/human immunodeficiency viruses (SHIV). *Proc Natl Acad Sci USA* **92**:7490–7494.

1601. Ludvigsen, A., T. Werner, W. Gimbel, V. Erfle, and R. Brack-Werner. 1996. Down-modulation of HIV-1 LTR activity by an extra-LTR *nef* gene fragment. *Virol* **216**:245–251.

1602. Luizzi, G. M., C. M. Mastroinni, V. Vullo, E. Jirillo, S. Delia, and P. Riccio. 1992. Cerebrospinal fluid myelin basic protein as predictive marker of demyelination in AIDS dementia complex. *J Neuroimmunol* **36**:251–254.

1603. Lukashov, V. V., and J. Goudsmit. 1995. Increasing genotypic and phenotypic selection from the original genomic RNA populations of HIV-1 strains LAI and MN (NM) by peripheral blood mononuclear cell culture, B-cell-line propagation and T-cell-line adaptation. *AIDS* **9**:1307–1311.

1604. Lukashov, V. V., C. L. Kuiken, and J. Goudsmit. 1995. Intrahost human immunodeficiency virus type 1 evolution is related to length of the immunocompetent period. *J Virol* **69**:6911–6916.

1605. Luke, W., C. Coulibaly, U. Dittmer, G. Voss, R. Oesterle, B. Makoschey, U. Sauermann, E. Jurkiewicz, C. Stahl-Henning, H. Petry, and G. Hunsmann. 1996. Simian immunodeficiency virus (SIV) gp130 oligomers protect rhesus macaques (Macaca mulatta) against the infection with SIVmac32H grown on T-cells or derived *ex vivo. Virol* **216**:444–450.

1606. Lunardi-Iskandar, Y., J. L. Bryant, R. A. Zeman, V. H. Lam, F. Samaniego, J. M. Besnier, P. Hermans, A. R. Thierry, P. Gill, and R. C. Gallo. 1995. Tumorigenesis and metastasis of neoplastic Kaposi's sarcoma cell line in immunodeficient mice blocked by a human pregnancy hormone. *Nature* **375**:64–68.

1607. Luo, L., Y. Li, P. M. Cannon, S. Kim, and C. Yong Kang. 1992. Chimeric gag-V3 virus-like particles of human immunodeficiency virus induce virus-neutralizing antibodies. *Proc Natl Acad Sci USA* **89**:10527–10531.

1608. Luria, S., I. Chambers, and P. Berg. 1991. Expression of the type 1 human immunodeficiency virus *nef* protein in T cells prevents antigen receptor-mediated induction of interleukin 2 mRNA. *Proc Natl Acad Sci USA* **88**:5326–5330.

1609. Lusso, P., A. DeMaria, M. Malnati, and F. Lori. 1991. Induction of CD4 and susceptibility to HIV-1 infection in human CD8+ T lymphocytes by human herpesvirus-6. *Nature* **349**:533–535.

1610. Lusso, P., B. Ensoli, P. D. Markham, D. V. Ablashi, S. Z. Salahuddin, E. Tschachler, F. Wong-Staal, and R. C. Gallo. 1989. Productive dual infection of human CD4+ T lymphocytes by HIV-1 and HHV-6. *Nature* **337**:370–373.

1611. Lusso, P., M. S. Malnati, A. Garzino-Demo, R. W. Crowley, E. O. Long, and R. C. Gallo. 1993. Infection of natural killer cells by human herpesvirus 6. *Nature* **362**:458–462.

1612. Lusso, P., P. Secchiero, R. W. Crowley, A. Garzino-Demo, Z. N. Berneman, and R. C. Gallo. 1994. CD4 is a critical component of the receptor for human herpesvirus 7: interference with human immunodeficiency virus. *Proc Natl Acad Sci USA* **91**:3872–3876.

1613. Lusso, P., F. D. M. Veronese, B. Ensoli, G. Franchini, C. Jemma, S. E. de Rocco, V. S. Kalyanaraman, and R. C. Gallo. 1990. Expanded HIV-1 cellular tropism by phenotypic mixing with murine endogenous retroviruses. *Science* **247**:848–852.

1614. Lyketsos, C. G., D. R. Hoover, M. Guccione, W. Senterfitt, M. A. Dew, J. Wesch, M. J. VanRaden, G. J. Treisman, and H. Morgenstern. 1993. Depressive symptoms as predictors of medical outcomes in HIV infection. *J Am Med Assoc* **270**:2563–2567.

1615. Lyman, W. D., R. Soeiro, and A. Rubinstein. 1993. Viral culture of HIV in neonates. *N Engl J Med* **328**:814–815.

1616. Lynn, W. S., A. Tweedale, and M. W. Cloyd. 1988. Human immunodeficiency virus (HIV-1) cytotoxicity: perturbation of the cell membrane and depression of phospholipid synthesis. *Virol* **163**:43–51.

1617. Lyter, D. W., J. Bryant, R. Thackeray, C. R. Rinaldo, and L. A. Kingsley. 1995. Incidence of human immunodeficiency virus-related and nonrelated malignancies in a large cohort of homosexual men. *J Clin Oncol* **13**:2540–2546.

1618. Ma, M., J. D. Geiger, and A. Nath. 1994. Characterization of a novel binding site for the human immunodeficiency virus type 1 envelope protein gp120 on human fetal astrocytes. *J Virol* **68**:6824–6828.

1619. Macatonia, S. E., M. Compels, A. J. Pinching, S. Patterson, and S. C. Knight. 1992. Antigen presentation by macrophages but not by dendritic cells in human immunodeficiency virus (HIV) infection. *Immunol* **75**:576–581.

1620. Macatonia, S. E., N. A. Hosken, M. Litton, P. Vieira, C.-S. Hsieh, J. A. Culpepper, M. Wysocka, G. Trinchieri, K. M. Murphy, and A. O'Garra. 1995. Dendritic cells produce IL-12 and direct the development of Th1 cells from naive CD4+ T cells. *J Immunol* **154**:5071–5079.

1621. Macatonia, S. E., R. Lau, S. Patterson, J. Pinching, and S. C. Knight. 1990. Dendritic cell infection, depletion and dysfunction in HIV-infected individuals. *Immunol* **71**:38–45.

1622. Macatonia, S. E., S. Patterson, and S. C. Knight. 1991. Primary proliferative and cytotoxic T-cell responses to HIV induced *in vitro* by human dendritic cells. *Immunol* **74**:399–406.

1623. Macatonia, S. E., S. Patterson, and S. C. Knight. 1989. Suppression of immune responses by dendritic cells infected with HIV. *Immunol* **67**:285–289.

1624. Macatonia, S. E., P. M. Taylor, S. C. Knight, and B. A. Askonas. 1989. Primary stimulation by dendritic cells induces antiviral proliferative and cytotoxic T cell responses in vitro. *J Exp Med* **169**:1255–1264.

1625. Macchia, D., C. Simonelli, P. Parronchi, M. P. Piccinni, P. Biswas, M. Mazzetti, A. Ravina, E. Maggi, and S. Romagnani. 1991. In vitro infection with HIV of antigen-specific T cell clones derived from HIV-seronegative individuals. Effects on cytokine production and helper function. *Ric Clin Lab* **21**:85–90.

1626. MacDonald, T. T., and J. Spencer. 1992. Cell-mediated immune injury in the intestine. *Gastroenterol Clin North Am* **21**:367–386.

1627. Maciejewski, J. P., F. F. Weichold, and N. S. Young. 1994. HIV-1 suppression of hematopoiesis in vitro mediated by envelope glycoprotein and TNF-alpha. *J Immunol* **153**:4303–4310.

1628. Mackall, C. L., T. A. Fleisher, M. R. Brown, M. P. Andrich, C. C. Chen, I. M. Feuerstein, M. E. Horowitz, I. T. Magrath, A. T. Shad, S. M. Steinberg, L. H. Wexler, and R. E. Gress. 1995. Age, thymopoiesis, and CD4+ T-lymphocyte regeneration after intensive chemotherapy. *N Engl J Med* **332**:143–149.

1629. Mackewicz, C., and J. A. Levy. 1992. CD8+ cell anti-HIV activity: nonlytic suppression of virus replication. *AIDS Res Hum Retro* **8**:1039–1050.

1630. Mackewicz, C. E., E. Barker, G. Greco, G. Reyes-Teran, and J. A. Levy. 1997. Do β-chemokines have clinical relevance in HIV infection? *J Clin Invest,* **100**:921–930.

1631. Mackewicz, C. E., E. Barker, and J. A. Levy. 1996. Role of β-chemokines in suppressing HIV replication. *Science* **274**:1393–1395.

1632. Mackewicz, C. E., D. J. Blackbourn, and J. A. Levy. 1995. CD8+ cells suppress HIV replication by inhibiting viral transcription. *Proc Natl Acad Sci USA* **92**:2308–2312.

1633. Mackewicz, C. E., A. Landay, H. Hollander, and J. A. Levy. 1994. Effect of zidovudine therapy on CD8+ T cell anti-HIV activity. *Clin Immunol Immunopathol* **73**:80–87.

1633a. Mackewicz, C. E., and J. A. Levy. Unpublished observations.

1634. Mackewicz, C. E., J. A. Levy, W. W. Cruikshank, H. Kornfeld, and D. M. Center. 1996. Role of IL-16 in HIV replication. *Nature* **383**:488–489.

1635. Mackewicz, C. E., H. Ortega, and J. A. Levy. 1994. Effect of cytokines on HIV replication in CD4+ lymphocytes: lack of identity with the CD8+ cell antiviral factor. *Cell Immunol* **153**:329–343.

1636. Mackewicz, C. E., H. W. Ortega, and J. A. Levy. 1991. CD8+ cell anti-HIV activity correlates with the clinical state of the infected individual. *J Clin Invest* **87**:1462–1466.

1636a. Mackewicz, C. E., B. Patterson, and J. A. Levy. Unpublished observations.

1637. Mackewicz, C. E., L. C. Yang, J. D. Lifson, and J. A. Levy. 1994. Non-cytolytic CD8 T-cell anti-HIV responses in primary infection. *Lancet* **344**:1671–1673.

1638. Maclean, C., P. J. Flegg, and D. C. Kilpatrick. 1990. Anti-cardiolipin antibodies and HIV infection. *Clin Exp Immunol* **81**:263–266.

1639. MacMahon, E. M. E., J. D. Glass, S. D. Hayward, R. B. Mann, P. S. Becker, P. Charache, J. C. McArthur, and R. F. Ambinder. 1991. Epstein-Barr virus in AIDS-related primary central nervous system lymphoma. *Lancet* **338**:969–973.

1640. Maddon, P. J., A. G. Dalgleish, J. S. McDougal, P. R. Clapham, R. A. Weiss, and R. Axel. 1986. The T4 gene encodes the AIDS virus receptor and is expressed in the immune system and the brain. *Cell* 47:333–348.

1641. Maeda, Y., S. Matsushita, T. Hattori, T. Murakami, and K. Takatsuki. 1992. Changes in the reactivity and neutralizing activity of a type-specific neutralizing monoclonal antibody induced by interaction of soluble CD4 with gp120. *AIDS Res Hum Retro* 8:2049–2054.

1642. Maggi, E., M. G. Giudizi, R. Biagiotti, F. Annunziato, R. Manetti, M.-P. Piccinni, P. Parronchi, S. Sampognaro, L. Giannarini, G. Zuccati, and S. Romagnani. 1994. Th2-like CD8+ T cells showing B cell helper function and reduced cytolytic activity in human immunodeficiency virus type 1 infection. *J Exp Med* 180:489–495.

1643. Maggi, E., D. Macchia, P. Parronchi, M. Mazzatti, A. Ravina, D. Milo, and S. Romagnani. 1987. Reduced production of interleukin 2 and interferon-gamma and enhanced helper activity for IgG synthesis by cloned CD4+ T cells from patients with AIDS. *Eur J Immunol* 17:1685–1690.

1644. Maggi, E., M. Mazzetti, A. Ravina, F. Annunziato, M. de Carli, M. P. Piccinni, R. Manetti, M. Carbonari, A. M. Pesce, G. del Prete, and S. Romagnani. 1994. Ability of HIV to promote a Th1 to Th0 shift and to replicate preferentially in Th2 and Th0 cells. *Science* 265:244–248.

1645. Magnuson, D. S. K., B. E. Knudsen, J. D. Geiger, R. M. Brownstone, and A. Nath. 1995. Human immunodeficiency virus type 1 Tat activates non-N-methyl-D-aspartate excitatory amino acid receptors and causes neurotoxicity. *Ann Neurol* 37:373–380.

1646. Magrath, I. 1990. The pathogenesis of Burkitt's lymphoma. *Adv Cancer Res* 55:133–270.

1647. Mahoney, S. E., M. Duvic, and B. J. Nickoloff. 1991. Human immunodeficiency virus (HIV) transcripts identified in HIV-related psoriasis and Kaposi's sarcoma lesions. *J Clin Invest* 88:174–185.

1648. Maiman, M., R. G. Fruchter, M. Clark, C. D. Arrastia, R. Matthews, and E. J. Gates. 1997. Cervical cancer as an AIDS-defining illness. *Obstet Gynecol* 89:76–80.

1649. Maiman, M., R. G. Fruchter, L. Guy, S. Cuthill, P. Levine, and E. Serur. 1993. Human immunodeficiency virus infection and invasive cervical carcinoma. *Cancer* 71:402–406.

1650. Maitra, R. K., N. Ahmad, S. M. Holland, and S. Venkatesan. 1991. Human immunodeficiency virus type 1 (HIV-1) provirus expression and LTR transcription are repressed in *nef*-expressing cell lines. *Virol* 182:522–533.

1651. Malamud, D., C. Davis, P. Berthold, E. Roth, and H. Friedman. 1993. Human submandibular saliva aggregates HIV. *AIDS Res Hum Retro* 9:633–637.

1652. Maldarelli, F., H. Sato, E. Berthold, J. Orenstein, and M. A. Martin. 1995. Rapid induction of apoptosis by cell-to-cell transmission of human immunodeficiency virus type 1. *J Virol* 69:6457–6465.

1653. Malley, S. D., J. M. Grange, F. Hamedi-Sangsari, and J. R. Vila. 1994. Synergistic anti-human immunodeficiency virus type 1 effect of hydroxamate compounds with 2′,3′-dideoxyinosine in infected resting human lymphocytes. *Proc Natl Acad Sci USA* 91:11017–11021.

1654. Manetti, R., P. Parronchi, M. G. Giudizi, M.-P. Piccinni, E. Maggi, G. Trinchieri, and S. Romagnani. 1993. Natural killer cell stimulatory factor (interleukin 12 [IL-12]) induces T helper type 1 (Th1)-specific immune responses and inhibits the development of IL-4-producing Th cells. *J Exp Med* 177:1199–1204.

1655. Mangan, D. F., B. Robertson, and S. M. Wahl. 1992. IL-4 enhances programmed cell death (apoptosis) in stimulated human monocytes. *J Immunol* 148:1812–1816.

1656. Mangkornkanok-Mark, M., A. S. Mark, and J. Dong. 1984. Immunoperoxidase evaluation of lymph nodes from acquired immune deficiency patients. *Clin Exp Immunol* 55:581–586.

1656a. Mankowski, J. L., M. T. Flaherty, J. P. Spelman, D. A. Hauer, P. J. Didier, A. M. Amedee, M. Murphey-Corb, L. M. Kirstein, A. Munoz, J. E. Clements, and M. C. Zink. 1997. Pathogenesis of simian immunodeficiency virus encephalitis: viral determinants of neurovirulence. *J Virol* 71:6055–6060.

1657. Mankowski, J. L., J. P. Spelman, H. G. Ressetar, J. D. Strandberg, J. Laterra, D. L. Carter, J.

E. Clements, and M. C. Zink. 1994. Neurovirulent simian immunodeficiency virus replicates productively in endothelial cells of the central nervous system in vivo and in vitro. *J Virol* **68**:8202–8208.

1658. Mann, D. L., F. Lasane, M. Popovic, L. O. Arthur, W. G. Robey, W. A. Blattner, and M. J. Newman. 1987. HTLV-III large envelope protein (gp120) suppresses PHA-induced lymphocyte blastogenesis. *J Immunol* **138**:2640–2644.

1659. Mann, D. L., C. Murray, R. Yarchoan, W. A. Blattner, and J. J. Goedert. 1988. HLA antigen frequencies in HIV-1 seropositive disease-free individuals and patients with AIDS. *J AIDS* **1**:13–17.

1660. Mann, J., and D. Tarantola. 1996. *AIDS in the World II.* Oxford University Press, New York.

1661. Mannino, R. J., and S. Gould-Fogerite. 1995. Lipid matrix-based vaccines for systemic and mucosal immunization, p. 363–379. *In* M. T. Powell and M. J. Newman (ed.), *Vaccine Design: The Subunit Approach.* Plenum Press, New York.

1662. Mano, H., and J.-C. Chermann. 1991. Fetal human immunodeficiency virus type 1 infection of different organs in the second trimester. *AIDS Res Hum Retro* **7**:83–88.

1663. Marandin, A., A. Katz, E. Oksenhendler, M. Tulliez, F. Picard, W. Vainchenker, and F. Louache. 1996. Loss of primitive hematopoietic progenitors in patients with human immunodeficiency virus infection. *Blood* **88**:4568–4578.

1664. Marasco, W. A., W. A. Haseltine, and S. Chen. 1993. Design, intracellular expression, and activity of a human anti-human immunodeficiency virus type 1 gp120 single-chain antibody. *Proc Natl Acad Sci USA* **90**:7889–7893.

1665. Marcon, L., and J. Sodroski. 1994. gp120-independent fusion mediated by the human immunodeficiency virus type 1 gp41 envelope glycoprotein: a reassessment. *J Virol* **68**:1977–1982.

1666. Margolick, J. B., A. Munoz, A. D. Donnenberg, L. P. Park, N. Galai, J. V. Giorgi, M. R. G. O'Gorman, and J. Ferbas. 1995. Failure of T-cell homeostasis preceding AIDS in HIV-1 infection. *Nature Med* **1**:674–680.

1667. Margolick, J. B., D. J. Volkman, T. M. Folks, and A. S. Fauci. 1987. Amplification of HTLV-III/LAV infection by antigen-induced activation of T cells and direct suppression by virus of lymphocyte blastogenic responses. *J Immunol* **138**:1719–1723.

1668. Margolis, D. M., M. Somasundaran, and M. R. Green. 1994. Human transcription factor YY1 represses human immunodeficiency virus type 1 transcription and virion production. *J Virol* **68**:905–910.

1669. Mariani, R., and J. Skowronski. 1993. CD4 down-regulation by nef alleles isolated from human immunodeficiency virus type 1-infected individuals. *Proc Natl Acad Sci USA* **90**:5549–5553.

1670. Mariotti, M., J.-J. Lefrere, B. Noel, F. Ferrer-Le-Coeur, D. Vittecoq, R. Girot, C. Bosser, A.-M. Courouce, C. Salmon, and P. Rouger. 1990. DNA amplification of HIV-1 in seropositive individuals and in seronegative at-risk individuals. *AIDS* **4**:633–637.

1671. Markert, M. L., D. D. Kostyu, F. E. Ward, T. M. McLaughlin, T. J. Watson, R. H. Buckley, S. E. Schiff, R. M. Ungerleider, J. W. Gaynor, K. T. Oldham, S. M. Mahaffey, M. Ballow, D. A. Driscoll, L. P. Hale, and B. F. Haynes. 1997. Successful formation of a chimeric human thymus allograft following transplantation of cultured postnatal human thymus. *J Immunol* **158**:998–1005.

1672. Markham, R. B., J. Coberly, A. J. Ruff, D. Hoover, J. Gomez, E. Holt, J. Desormeaux, R. Boulos, T. C. Quinn, and N. A. Halsey. 1994. Maternal IgG1 and IgA antibody to V3 loop consensus sequence and maternal-infant HIV-1 transmission. *Lancet* **343**:390–391.

1672a. Markowitz, M. 1997. *Combination Therapy for HIV Infection.* International Association of Physicians in AIDS Care, Chicago.

1673. Markwell, M. A. K., L. Svennerholm, and J. C. Paulson. 1981. Specific gangliosides function as host cell receptors for Sendai virus. *Proc Natl Acad Sci USA* **78**:5406–5410.

1674. Marlink, R. 1996. Lessons from the second AIDS virus, HIV-2. *AIDS* **10**:689–699.

1675. Marmor, M., A. E. Friedman-Kien, and S. Zolla-Pazner. 1984. Kaposi's sarcoma in homosexual men. *Ann Int Med* **100**:809–815.

1676. Marriott, D. J. E., and M. McMurchie. 1997. HIV and advanced immune deficiency. *Managing HIV* **164**:15–16.

1677. Marsh, J. W., B. Herndier, A. Tsuzuki, V. L. Ng, B. Shiramizu, N. Abbey, and M. S. McGrath. 1995. Cytokine expression in large cell lymphoma associated with acquired immunodeficiency syndrome. *J Interferon Cytokine Res* **15**:261–268.

1678. Marschang, P., U. Kruger, C. Ochsenbauer, L. Gurtler, A. Hittmair, V. Bosch, J. R. Patsch, and M. P. Dierich. 1997. Complement activation by HIV-1-infected cells: the role of transmembrane glycoprotein gp41. *J AIDS Hum Retrovirol* **14**:102–109.

1679. Marthas, M. L., S. Sutjipto, J. Higgins, B. Lohman, J. Torten, P. A. Luciw, P. A. Marx, and N. C. Pedersen. 1990. Immunization with a live, attenuated simian immunodeficiency virus (SIV) prevents early disease but not infection in rhesus macaques challenged with pathogenic SIV. *J Virol* **64**:3694–3700.

1679a. Marthas, M. L., K. K. A. Van Rompay, M. Otsyula, C. J. Miller, D. R. Canfield, N. C. Pedersen, and M. B. McChesney. 1995. Viral factors determine progression to AIDS in simian immunodeficiency virus-infected newborn rhesus macaques. *J Virol* **69**:4198–4205.

1680. Martin, N. L., J. A. Levy, H. S. Legg, P. S. Weintrub, M. J. Cowan, and D. W. Wara. 1991. Detection of infection with human immunodeficiency virus (HIV) type 1 in infants by an anti-immunoglobulin A assay using recombinant proteins. *J Peds* **118**:354–358.

1681. Martin, S. J., P. M. Matear, and A. Vyakarnam. 1994. HIV-1 infection of human CD4+ T cells in vitro. *J Immunol* **152**:330–342.

1682. Martinez, O. M., R. S. Gibbons, M. R. Garavoy, and F. R. Aronson. 1990. IL-4 inhibits IL-2 receptor expression and Il-2 dependent proliferation of human T-cells. *J Immunol* **144**:2211–2215.

1683. Martins, L. P., N. Chenciner, B. Asjo, A. Meyerhans, and S. Wain-Hobson. 1991. Independent fluctuation of human immunodeficiency virus type 1 *rev* and gp41 quasispecies in vivo. *J Virol* **65**:4502–4507.

1684. Marx, P. A., R. W. Compans, A. Gettie, J. K. Staas, R. M. Gilley, M. J. Mulligan, G. V. Yamshchikov, D. Chen, and J. H. Eldridge. 1993. Protection against vaginal SIV transmission with microencapsulated vaccine. *Science* **260**:1323–1327.

1685. Marx, P. A., Y. Li, N. W. Lerche, S. Sutjipto, A. Gettie, J. A. Yee, B. H. Brotman, A. M. Prince, A. Hanson, R. G. Webster, and R. C. Desrosiers. 1991. Isolation of a simian immunodeficiency virus related to human immunodeficiency virus type 2 from a West African pet sooty mangabey. *J Virol* **65**:4480–4485.

1686. Marx, P. A., A. I. Spira, A. Gettie, P. J. Dailey, R. S. Veazey, A. A. Lackner, C. J. Mahoney, C. J. Miller, L. E. Claypool, D. D. Ho, and N. J. Alexander. 1996. Progesterone implants enhance SIV vaginal transmission and early virus load. *Nature Med* **2**:1084–1089.

1687. Mascola, J. R., M. K. Louder, S. R. Surman, T. C. Vancott, X. F. Yu, J. Bradac, K. R. Porter, K. E. Nelson, M. Girard, J. G. McNeil, F. E. McCutchan, D. L. Birx, and D. S. Burke. 1996. Human immunodeficiency virus type 1 neutralizing antibody serotyping using serum pools and an infectivity reduction assay. *AIDS Res Hum Retro* **12**:1319–1328.

1688. Mascola, J. R., J. Louwagie, F. E. McCutchen, C. L. Fischer, P. A. Hegerich, K. F. Wagner, A. K. Fowler, J. G. McNeil, and D. S. Burke. 1994. Two antigenically distinct subtypes of human immunodeficiency virus type 1: viral genotype predicts neutralization serotype. *J Inf Dis* **169**:48–54.

1689. Mascola, J. R., B. J. Mathieson, P. M. Zack, M. C. Walker, S. B. Halstead, and D. S. Burke. 1993. Summary report: workshop on the potential risks of antibody-dependent enhancement in human HIV vaccine trials. *AIDS Res Hum Retro* **9**:1175–1184.

1690. Mascola, J. R., S. W. Snyder, O. W. Weislow, S. M. Belay, R. B. Belshe, D. H. Schwartz, M. L. Clements, R. Dolin, B. S. Graham, G. J. Gorse, M. C. Keefer, M. J. McElrath, M. C. Walker, K. F. Wagner, J. G. McNeil, F. E. McCutchan, and D. S. Burke. 1996. Immunization with envelope subunit vaccine products elicits neutralizing antibodies against laboratory-adapted but not primary isolates of human immunodeficiency virus type 1. *J Inf Dis* **173**:340–348.

1691. Masood, R., Y. Zhang, M. W. Bond, D. T. Scadden, T. Moudgil, R. E. Law, M. H. Kaplan,

B. Jung, B. M. Espina, and Y. Lunardi-Iskandar. 1995. Interleukin-10 is an autocrine growth factor for acquired immunodeficiency syndrome-related B-cell lymphoma. *Blood* **85**:3423–3430.

1692. **Massiah, M. A., M. R. Starich, C. Paschall, M. F. Summers, A. M. Christensen, and W. I. Sundquist.** 1994. Three-dimensional structure of the human immunodeficiency virus type 1 matrix protein. *J Mol Biol* **244**:198–223.

1693. **Master, S., J. Taylor, S. Kyalwazi, and J. L. Ziegler.** 1970. Immunological studies in Kaposi's sarcoma in Uganda. *Brit Med J* **1**:600–602.

1694. **Masuda, M., P. M. Hoffman, and S. K. Ruscetti.** 1993. Viral determinants that control the neuropathogenicity of PVC-211 murine leukemia virus in vivo determine brain capillary endothelial cell tropism of the virus in vitro. *J Virol* **67**:4580–4587.

1695. **Masur, H., M. A. Michelis, and J. B. Greene.** 1981. An outbreak of community-acquired *Pneumocystis carinii* pneumonia. *N Engl J Med* **305**:1431–1438.

1696. **Mathijs, J. M., M. C. Hing, J. Grierson, D. E. Dwyer, C. Goldschmidt, D. A. Cooper, and A. L. Cunningham.** 1988. HIV infection of rectal mucosa. *Lancet* **i**:1111.

1697. **Matsuyama, T., N. Kobayashi, and N. Yamamoto.** 1991. Cytokines and HIV infection: is AIDS a tumor necrosis factor disease? *AIDS* **5**:1405–1417.

1698. **Matteucci, D., M. Pistello, P. Mazzetti, S. Giannecchini, D. Del Mauro, L. Zaccaro, P. Bandecchi, F. Tozzini, and M. Bendinelli.** 1996. Vaccination protects against in-vivo-grown feline immunodeficiency virus even in the absence of detectable neutralizing antibodies. *J Virol* **70**:617–622.

1699. **Matthews, T. J., A. J. Langlois, W. G. Robey, N. T. Chang, R. C. Gallo, P. J. Fischinger, and D. P. Bolognesi.** 1986. Restricted neutralization of divergent human T-lymphotropic virus type III isolates by antibodies to the major envelope glycoprotein. *Proc Natl Acad Sci USA* **83**:9709–9713.

1700. **Matthews, T. J., K. J. Weinhold, H. K. Lyerly, A. J. Langlois, H. Wigzell, and D. P. Bolognesi.** 1987. Interaction between the human T-cell lymphotropic virus type IIIB envelope glycoprotein gp120 and the surface antigen CD4: role of carbohydrate in binding and cell fusion. *Proc Natl Acad Sci USA* **84**:5424–5428.

1701. **Maury, W., B. J. Potts, and A. B. Rabson.** 1989. HIV-1 infection of first-trimester and term human placental tissue: a possible mode of maternal-fetal transmission. *J Inf Dis* **160**:583–588.

1702. **Mayaux, M.-J., M. Burgard, J.-P. Teglas, J. Cottalorda, A. Krivine, F. Simon, J. Puel, C. Tamalet, D. Dormont, B. Masquelier, A. Doussin, C. Rouzioux, and S. Blanche.** 1996. Neonatal characteristics in rapidly progressive perinatally acquired HIV-1 disease. *J Am Med Assoc* **275**:606–610.

1703. **Mayer, K. H., and D. J. Anderson.** 1995. Heterosexual HIV transmission. *Infect Agents Dis* **4**:273–284.

1703a. **Mazzoli, S., D. Trabattoni, S. Lo Caputo, S. Piconi, C. Ble, F. Meacci, S. Ruzzante, A. Salvi, F. Semplici, R. Longhi, M. L. Fusi, N. Tofani, M. Biasin, M. L. Villa, F. Mazzotta, and M. Clerici.** HIV-specific mucosal and cellular immunity in HIV-seronegative partners of HIV-seropositive individuals. *Nature Med*, in press.

1704. **McCarthy, M.** 1997. Keep guard up against HIV-1-related lung infections, say experts. *Lancet* **349**:1607.

1705. **McClain, K. L., C. T. Leach, H. B. Jenson, V. V. Joshi, B. H. Pollock, R. T. Parmley, F. J. DiCarlo, E. G. Chadwick, and S. B. Murphy.** 1995. Association of Epstein-Barr virus with leiomyosarcomas in young people with AIDS. *N Engl J Med* **332**:12–18.

1706. **McCloskey, T. W., M. Ott, E. Tribble, S. A. Khan, S. Teichberg, M. O. Paul, S. Pahwa, E. Verdin, and N. Chirmule.** 1997. Dual role of HIV Tat in regulation of apoptosis in T cells. *J Immunol* **158**:1014–1019.

1707. **McClure, H. M., D. C. Anderson, P. N. Fultz, A. A. Ansari, T. Jehuda-Cohen, F. Villinger, S. A. Klumpp, W. Switzer, E. Lockwood, A. Brodie, and H. Keyserling.** 1991. Maternal transmission of SIV$_{smm}$ in rhesus macaques. *J Med Primatol* **20**:182–187.

1708. McClure, M. O., P. J. Goulder, G. Ogg, A. J. McMichael, and J. N. Weber. 1996. HIV clearance in infants. *Lancet* 347:1122.

1709. McClure, M. O., M. Marsh, and R. A. Weiss. 1988. Human immunodeficiency virus infection of CD4-bearing cells occurs by a pH-independent mechanism. *EMBO Journal* 7:513–518.

1710. McClure, M. O., J. P. Moore, D. F. Blanc, P. Scotting, G. M. W. Cook, R. J. Keynes, J. N. Weber, D. Davies, and R. A. Weiss. 1992. Investigations into the mechanism by which sulfated polysaccharides inhibit HIV infection *in vitro*. *AIDS Res Hum Retro* 8:19–26.

1711. McCune, J. M. 1995. Viral latency in HIV disease. *Cell* 82:183–188.

1711a. McCune, J. M. Thymic function in HIV-1 disease. *Sem Immunol* 9:in press.

1712. McCune, J. M., L. B. Rabin, M. B. Feinberg, M. Lieberman, J. C. Kosek, G. R. Reyes, and I. L. Weissman. 1988. Endoproteolytic cleavage of gp160 is required for the activation of human immunodeficiency virus. *Cell* 53:55–67.

1713. McCusker, J., A. M. Stoddard, K. H. Mayer, D. N. Cowan, and J. E. Groopman. 1988. Behavioral risk factors for HIV infection among homosexual men at a Boston community health center. *Am J Pub Health* 78:68–71.

1714. McCutchan, F. E., P. A. Hegerich, T. P. Brennan, P. Phanuphak, P. Singharaj, A. Jugsudee, P. W. Berman, A. M. Gray, A. K. Fowler, and D. S. Burke. 1992. Genetic variants of HIV-1 in Thailand. *AIDS Res Hum Retro* 8:1887–1895.

1715. McCutchan, F. E., E. Sanders-Buell, C. W. Oster, R. R. Redfield, S. K. Hira, P. L. Perine, B. L. P. Ungar, and D. S. Burke. 1991. Genetic comparison of human immunodeficiency virus (HIV-1) isolates by polymerase chain reaction. *J AIDS* 4:1241–1250.

1716. McDonald, R. A., D. L. Mayers, R. C. Y. Chung, K. F. Wagner, S. Ratto-Kim, D. L. Birx, and N. L. Michael. 1997. Evolution of human immunodeficiency virus type 1 *env* sequence variation in patients with diverse rates of disease progression and T-cell function. *J Virol* 71:1871–1879.

1717. McDougal, J. S., M. S. Kennedy, J. K. A. Nicholson, T. J. Spira, H. W. Jaffe, J. E. Kaplan, D. B. Fishbein, P. O'Malley, C. H. Aloisio, C. M. Black, M. Hubbard, and C. B. Reimer. 1987. Antibody response to human immunodeficiency virus in homosexual men. *J Clin Invest* 80:316–324.

1718. McDougal, J. S., M. S. Kennedy, S. L. Orloff, J. K. A. Nicholson, and T. J. Spira. 1996. Mechanisms of human immunodeficiency virus type 1 (HIV-1) neutralization: irreversible inactivation of infectivity by anti-HIV-1 antibody. *J Virol* 70:5236–5245.

1719. McDougal, J. S., M. S. Kennedy, J. M. Sligh, S. P. Cort, A. Mawle, and J. K. A. Nicholson. 1986. Binding of HTLV-III/LAV to T4+ T cells by a complex of the 110K viral protein and the T4 molecule. *Science* 231:382–385.

1720. McDougal, J. S., L. S. Martin, S. P. Cort, M. Mozen, C. M. Heldebrant, and B. L. Evatt. 1985. Thermal inactivation of the acquired immunodeficiency syndrome virus, human T lymphotropic virus-III, lymphadenopathy-associated virus, with special reference to antihemophilic factor. *J Clin Invest* 76:875–877.

1721. McElrath, M. J., L. Corey, P. D. Greenberg, T. J. Matthews, D. C. Montefiori, L. Rowen, L. Hood, and J. I. Mullins. 1996. Human immunodeficiency virus type 1 infection despite prior immunization with a recombinant envelope vaccine regimen. *Proc Natl Acad Sci USA* 93:3972–3977.

1722. McElrath, M. J., J. E. Pruett, and Z. A. Cohn. 1989. Mononuclear phagocytes of blood and bone marrow: comparative roles as viral reservoirs in human immunodeficiency virus type 1 infections. *Proc Natl Acad Sci USA* 86:675–679.

1723. McGavin, C. H., S. A. Land, K. L. Sebire, D. J. Hooker, A. D. Gurusinghe, and C. J. Birch. 1996. Syncytium-inducing phenotype and zidovudine susceptibility of HIV-1 isolated from post mortem tissue. *AIDS* 10:47–53.

1724. McGhee, J. R., J. Mestecky, M. T. Dertzbaugh, J. H. Eldridge, M. Hirasawa, and H. Kiyono. 1992. The mucosal immune system: from fundamental concepts to vaccine development. *Vaccine* 10:75–88.

1725. McGrath, M. S., B. Shiramizu, T. C. Meeker, L. D. Kaplan, and B. Herndier. 1991. AIDS-associated polyclonal lymphoma: identification of a new HIV-associated disease process. *J AIDS* **4**:408–415.

1726. McGuire, T. C., D. S. Adams, G. C. Johnson, P. Klevjer-Anderson, D. D. Barbee, and J. R. Gorham. 1986. Acute arthritis in caprine arthritis-encephalitis virus challenge exposure of vaccinated or persistently infected goats. *Am J Vet Res* **47**:537–540.

1727. McIlroy, D., B. Autran, R. Cheynier, S. Wain-Hobson, J.-P. Clauvel, E. Oksenhendler, P. Debre, and A. Hosmalin. 1995. Infection frequency of dendritic cells and CD4+ T lymphocytes in spleens of human immunodeficiency virus-positive patients. *J Virol* **69**:4737–4745.

1727a.McInerney, T. L., L. McLain, S. J. Armstrong, and N. J. Dimmock. 1997. A human IgG1 (b12) specific for the CD4 binding site of HIV-1 neutralizes by inhibiting the virus fusion entry process, but b12 Fab neutralizes by inhibiting a postfusion event. *Virol* **233**:313–326.

1728. McKeating, J., A. McKnight, and J. P. Moore. 1991. Differential loss of envelope glycoprotein gp120 from virions of human immunodeficiency virus type 1 isolates: effects on infectivity and neutralization. *J Virol* **65**:852–860.

1729. McKeating, J. A. 1996. Biological consequences of human immunodeficiency virus type 1 envelope polymorphism: does variation matter? *J Gen Virol* **77**:2905–2919.

1730. McKeating, J. A., J. Bennett, S. Zolla-Pazner, M. Schutten, S. Ashelford, A. Leigh Brown, and P. Balfe. 1993. Resistance of a human serum-selected human immunodeficiency virus type 1 escape mutant to neutralization by CD4 binding site monoclonal antibodies is conferred by a single amino acid change in gp120. *J Virol* **67**:5216–5225.

1731. McKeating, J. A., J. Cordell, C. J. Dean, and P. Balfe. 1992. Synergistic interaction between ligands binding to the CD4 binding site and V3 domain of human immunodeficiency virus type 1 gp120. *Virol* **191**:732–742.

1732. McKeating, J. A., J. Gow, J. Goudsmit, L. H. Pearl, C. Mulder, and R. A. Weiss. 1989. Characterization of HIV-1 neutralization escape mutants. *AIDS* **3**:777–784.

1733. McKeating, J. A., P. D. Griffiths, and R. A. Weiss. 1990. HIV susceptibility conferred to human fibroblasts by cytomegalovirus-induced Fc receptor. *Nature* **343**:659–661.

1734. McKeating, J. A., C. Shotton, J. Cordell, S. Graham, P. Balfe, N. Sullivan, M. Charles, M. Page, A. Bolmstedt, S. Olofsson, S. C. Kayman, Z. Wu, A. Pinter, C. Dean, J. Sodroski, and R. A. Weiss. 1993. Characterization of neutralizing monoclonal antibodies to linear and conformation-dependent epitopes within the first and second variable domains of human immunodeficiency virus type 1 gp120. *J Virol* **67**:4932–4944.

1735. McKenzie, S. W., G. Dallalio, M. North, P. Frame, and R. T. Means, Jr. 1996. Serum chemokine levels in patients with non-progressing HIV infection. *AIDS* **10**:F29-F33.

1736. McKnight, A., C. Shotton, J. Cordell, I. Jones, G. Simmons, and P. R. Clapham. 1996. Location, exposure, and conservation of neutralizing and nonneutralizing epitopes on human immunodeficiency virus type 2 SU glycoprotein. *J Virol* **70**:4598–4606.

1737. McKnight, A., R. A. Weiss, C. Shotton, Y. Takeuchi, H. Hoshino, and P. R. Clapham. 1995. Change in tropism upon immune escape by human immunodeficiency virus. *J Virol* **69**:3167–3170.

1738. McKnight, A., D. Wilkinson, G. Simmons, S. Talbot, L. Picard, M. Ahuja, M. Marsh, J. A. Hoxie, and P. R. Clapham. 1997. Inhibition of human immunodeficiency virus fusion by a monoclonal antibody to a coreceptor (CXCR4) is both cell type and virus strain dependent. *J Virol* **71**:1692–1696.

1739. McMillan, A., P. E. Bishop, D. Aw, and J. F. Peutherer. 1989. Immunohistology of the skin rash associated with acute HIV infection. *AIDS* **3**:309–312.

1740. McNearney, T., Z. Hornickova, R. Markham, A. Birdwell, M. Arens, A. Saah, and L. Ratner. 1992. Relationship of human immunodeficiency virus type 1 sequence heterogeneity to stage of disease. *Proc Natl Acad Sci USA* **89**:10247–10251.

1741. McNearney, T., P. Westervelt, B. J. Thielan, D. B. Trowbridge, J. Garcia, R. Whittier, and L. Ratner. 1990. Limited sequence heterogeneity among biologically distinct human immunodeficiency virus type 1 isolates from individuals involved in a clustered infectious outbreak. *Proc Natl Acad Sci USA* **87**:1917–1921.

1742. McNearney, T. A., C. Odell, V. M. Holers, P. G. Spear, and J. P. Atkinson. 1987. Herpes simplex virus glycoproteins gC-1 and gC-2 bind to the third component of complement and provide protection against complement-mediated neutralization of viral infectivity. *J Exp Med* **166**:1525–1535.

1743. McNeely, T. B., M. Dealy, D. J. Dripps, J. M. Orenstein, S. P. Eisenberg, and S. M. Wahl. 1995. Secretory leukocyte protease inhibitor: a human saliva protein exhibiting anti-human immunodeficiency virus 1 activity *in vitro*. *J Clin Invest* **96**:456–464.

1744. Medina, D. J., P. P. Tung, M. B. Lerner-Tung, C. J. Nelson, J. W. Mellors, and R. K. Strair. 1995. Sanctuary growth of human immunodeficiency virus in the presence of 3′-azido-3′deoxythymidine. *J Virol* **69**:1606–1611.

1745. Meeker, T. C., B. Shiramizu, L. Kaplan, B. Herndier, H. Sanchez, J. C. Grimaldi, J. Baumgartner, J. Rachlin, E. Feigal, M. Rosenblum, and M. S. McGrath. 1991. Evidence for molecular subtypes of HIV-associated lymphoma: division into peripheral monoclonal lymphoma, peripheral polyclonal lymphoma, and central nervous system lymphoma. *AIDS* **5**:669–674.

1746. Meerloo, T., H. K. Parmentier, A. D. M. E. Osterhaus, J. Goudsmit, and H. J. Schuurman. 1992. Modulation of cell surface molecules during HIV-1 infection of H9 cells. An immunoelectron microscopic study. *AIDS* **6**:1105–1116.

1747. Meerloo, T., M. A. Sheikh, A. C. Bloem, A. de Ronde, M. Schutten, C. A. C. van Els, P. J. M. Rohol, P. Joling, J. Goudsmit, and H.-J. Schuurman. 1993. Host cell membrane proteins on human immunodeficiency virus type 1 after in vitro infection of H9 cells and blood mononuclear cells. An immuno-electron microscopic study. *J Gen Virol* **74**:129–135.

1748. Meier, U.-C., P. Klenerman, P. Griffin, W. James, B. Koppe, B. Larder, A. McMichael, and R. Phillips. 1995. Cytotoxic T lymphocyte lysis inhibited by viable HIV mutants. *Science* **270**:1360–1362.

1749. Melendez-Guerrero, L. D., J. K. A. Nicholson, and J. S. McDougal. 1991. Infection of human monocytes with HIV-1$_{Ba-L}$. Effect on accessory cell function for T-cell proliferation *in vitro*. *AIDS Res Hum Retro* **7**:465–474.

1750. Mellert, W., A. Kleinschmidt, J. Schmidt, H. Festl, S. Elmer, W. K. Roth, and V. Erfle. 1990. Infection of human fibroblasts and osteoblast-like cells with HIV-1. *AIDS* **4**:527–535.

1751. Mellors, J. W., L. A. Kingsley, C. R. Rinaldo, Jr., J. A. Todd, B. S. Hoo, R. P. Kokka, and P. Gupta. 1995. Quantitation of HIV-1 RNA in plasma predicts outcome after seroconversion. *Ann Int Med* **122**:573–579.

1752. Mellors, J. W., C. R. Rinaldo, Jr., P. Gupta, R. M. White, J. A. Todd, and L. A. Kingsley. 1996. Prognosis in HIV-1 infection predicted by the quantity of virus in plasma. *Science* **272**:1167–1170.

1753. Menez-Bautista, R., S. M. Fikrig, S. Pahwa, M. G. Sarngadharan, and R. L. Stoneburner. 1986. Monozygotic twins discordant for the acquired immunodeficiency syndrome. *Am J Dis Children* **140**:678–679.

1754. Menzo, S., P. Bagnarelli, M. Giacca, A. Manzin, P. E. Varaldo, and M. Clementi. 1992. Absolute quantitation of viremia in human immunodeficiency virus infection by competitive reverse transcription and polymerase chain reaction. *J Clin Micro* **30**:1752–1757.

1755. Merigan, T. C., R. L. Hirsch, A. C. Fisher, L. A. Meyerson, G. Goldstein, and M. A. Winters. 1996. The prognostic significance of serum viral load, codon 215 reverse transcriptase mutation and CD4+ T cells on progression of HIV disease in a double-blind study of thymopentin. *AIDS* **10**:159–165.

1756. Mermin, J. H., M. Holodniy, D. A. Katzenstein, and T. C. Merigan. 1991. Detection of human immunodeficiency virus DNA and RNA in semen by the polymerase chain reaction. *J Inf Dis* **164**:769–772.

1757. Merrill, J. E. 1992. Cytokines and retroviruses. *Clin Immunol Immunopathol* **64**:23–27.

1758. Merrill, J. E., Y. Koyanagi, and I. S. Y. Chen. 1989. Interleukin-1 and tumor necrosis factor α can be induced from mononuclear phagocytes by human immunodeficiency virus type 1 binding to the CD4 receptor. *J Virol* **63**:4404–4408.

1759. Merrill, J. E., Y. Koyanagi, J. Zack, L. Thomas, F. Martin, and I. S. Y. Chen. 1992. Induction of interleukin-1 and tumor necrosis factor alpha in brain cultures by human immunodeficiency virus type 1. *J Virol* **66**:2217–2225.

1760. Merry, C., M. G. Barry, F. Mulcahy, M. Ryan, J. Heavey, J. D. Tjia, S. E. Gibbons, A. M. Breckenridge, and D. J. Back. 1997. Saquinavir pharmacokinetics alone and in combination with ritonavir in HIV-infected patients. *AIDS* **11**:F29-F33.

1761. Merson, M. H., E. A. Feldman, R. Bayer, and J. Stryker. 1996. Rapid self testing for HIV infection. *Lancet* **349**:352–353.

1762. Mestecky, J., and S. Jackson. 1994. Reassessment of the impact of mucosal immunity in infection with the human immunodeficiency virus (HIV) and design of relevant vaccines. *J Clin Immunol* **14**:259–272.

1763. Metler, R. P. (Centers for Disease Control and Prevention). Personal communication.

1764. Meyaard, L., S. A. Otto, R. R. Jonker, M. J. Mijnster, R. P. M. Keet, and F. Miedema. 1992. Programmed death of T cells in HIV-1 infection. *Science* **257**:217–219.

1765. Meyaard, L., H. Schuitemaker, and F. Miedema. 1993. T-cell dysfunction in HIV infection: anergy due to defective antigen-presenting cell function? *Immunol Today* **14**:161–164.

1766. Meyenhofer, M. F., L. G. Epstein, E.-S. Cho, and L. R. Sharer. 1987. Ultrastructural morphology and intracellular production of human immunodeficiency virus (HIV) in brain. *J Neuropath Exp Neurol* **46**:474–484.

1767. Meyerhans, A., R. Cheynier, J. Albert, M. Seth, S. Kwok, J. Sninsky, L. Morfeldt-Manson, B. Asjo, and S. Wain-Hobson. 1989. Temporal fluctuations in HIV quasispecies *in vivo* are not reflected by sequential HIV isolations. *Cell* **58**:901–910.

1768. Meyerhans, A., G. Dadaglio, J. P. Vartanian, P. Langlade-Demoyen, R. Frank, B. Asjo, F. Plata, and S. Wain-Hobson. 1991. *In vivo* persistence of an HIV-1-encoded HLA-B27-restricted cytotoxic T lymphocyte epitope despite specific *in vitro* reactivity. *Eur J Immunol* **21**:2637–2640.

1769. Meyerhans, A., J. P. Vartanian, C. Hultgren, U. Plikat, A. Karlsson, L. Wang, S. Eriksson, and S. Wain-Hobson. 1994. Restriction and enhancement of human immunodeficiency virus type 1 replication by modulation of intracellular deoxynucleoside triphosphate pools. *J Virol* **68**:535–540.

1770. Meylan, P. R. A., J. C. Guatelli, J. R. Munis, D. D. Richman, and R. S. Kornbluth. 1993. Mechanisms for the inhibition of HIV replication by interferons-alpha, -beta, and -gamma in primary human macrophages. *Virol* **193**:138–148.

1771. Meyohas, M. C., L. Morand-Joubert, P. Van de Wiel, M. Mariotti, and J. J. Lefrere. 1995. Time to HIV seroconversion after needlestick injury. *Lancet* **345**:1634–1635.

1772. Michael, N. L., A. E. Brown, R. F. Voigt, S. S. Frankel, J. R. Mascola, K. S. Brothers, M. Louder, D. L. Birx, and S. A. Cassol. 1997. Rapid disease progression without seroconversion following primary human immunodeficiency virus type 1 infection—evidence for highly susceptible human hosts. *J Inf Dis* **175**:1352–1359.

1773. Michael, N. L., G. Chang, L. A. d'Arcy, C. J. Tseng, D. L. Birx, and H. W. Sheppard. 1995. Functional characterization of human immunodeficiency virus type 1 *nef* genes in patients with divergent rates of disease progression. *J Virol* **69**:6758–6769.

1773a. Michael, N. L., L. G. Louie, A. L. Rohrbaugh, K. A. Schultz, D. E. Dayhoff, C. E. Wang, and H. W. Sheppard. 1997. The role of CCR5 and CCR2 polymorphisms in HIV-1 transmission and disease progression. *Nature Med* **3**:1160–1162.

1774. Michael, N. L., P. Morrow, J. Mosca, M. Vahey, D. S. Burke, and R. R. Redfield. 1991. Induction of human immunodeficiency virus type 1 expression in chronically infected cells is associated primarily with a shift in RNA splicing patterns. *J Virol* **65**:1291–1303.

1775. Michaelis, B., and J. A. Levy. 1989. HIV replication can be blocked by recombinant human interferon beta. *AIDS* **3**:27–31.

1776. Michaelis, B., and J. A. Levy. 1987. Recovery of human immunodeficiency virus from serum. *J Am Med Assoc* **257**:1327.

1777. Michaels, J., L. R. Sharer, and L. G. Epstein. 1988. Human immunodeficiency virus type 1 (HIV-1) infection of the nervous system: a review. *Immunodef Rev* **1**:71–104.

1778. Michel, M. L., M. Mancini, Y. Riviere, D. Dormont, and P. Tiollais. 1990. T- and B-lymphocyte responses to human immunodeficiency virus (HIV) type 1 in macaques immunized with hybrid HIV-hepatitis B surface antigen particles. *J Virol* 64:2452–2455.

1779. Michie, C. A., A. McLean, C. Alcock, and P. C. L. Beverley. 1992. Lifespan of human lymphocyte subsets defined by CD45 isoforms. *Nature* 360:264–265.

1780. Miedema, F., L. Meyaard, M. Koot, M. R. Klein, M. T. Roos, M. Groenink, R. A. Fouchier, A. B. Van't Wout, M. Tersmette, and P. T. Schellekens. 1994. Changing virus-host interactions in the course of HIV-1 infection. *Immunol Rev* 140:35–72.

1781. Miedema, F., A. J. C. Petit, F. G. Terpstra, J. K. M. Eeftinck Schattenkerk, F. de Wolf, B. J. M. Al, J. Roos, J. M. A. Lange, S. A. Danner, J. Goudsmit, and P. T. A. Schellenkens. 1988. Immunological abnormalities in human immunodeficiency virus (HIV)-infected asymptomatic homosexual men. *J Clin Invest* 82:1908–1914.

1782. Mildvan, D., U. Mathur, and R. W. Enlow. 1982. Opportunistic infections and immune deficiency in homosexual men. *Ann Int Med* 96:700–704.

1783. Miles, S. A., O. Martinez-Maza, and A. Rezai. 1992. Oncostatin M as a potent mitogen for AIDS-Kaposi's sarcoma-derived cells. *Science* 255:1432–1434.

1784. Miles, S. A., A. R. Rezai, J. F. Salazar-Gonzalez, M. Vander Mayden, R. H. Stevens, D. M. Logan, R. T. Mitsuyasu, T. Taga, T. Hirano, and T. Kishimoto. 1990. AIDS Kaposi's sarcoma-derived cells produce and respond to interleukin 6. *Proc Natl Acad Sci USA* 87:4068–4072.

1785. Milich, L., B. Margolin, and R. Swanstrom. 1993. V3 loop of the human immunodeficiency virus type 1 Env protein: interpreting sequence variability. *J Virol* 67:5623–5634.

1786. Miller, C., and M. B. Gardner. 1991. AIDS and mucosal immunity: usefulness of the SIV macaque model of genital mucosal transmission. *J AIDS* 4:1169–1172.

1787. Miller, C. J., N. J. Alexander, S. Sutjipto, A. A. Lackner, A. Gettie, A. G. Hendrickx, L. J. Lowenstine, M. Jennings, and P. A. Marx. 1989. Genital mucosal transmission of simian immunodeficiency virus: animal model for heterosexual transmission of human immunodeficiency virus. *J Virol* 63:4277–4284.

1788. Miller, C. J., N. J. Alexander, P. Vogel, J. Anderson, and P. A. Marx. 1992. Mechanism of genital transmission of SIV: a hypothesis based on transmission studies and the location of SIV in the genital tract of chronically infected female rhesus macaques. *J Med Primatol* 21:64–68.

1789. Miller, C. J., M. B. McChesney, X. Lu, P. J. Dailey, C. Chutkowski, D. Lu, P. Brosio, B. Roberts, and Y. Lu. 1997. Rhesus macaques previously infected with simian/human immunodeficiency virus are protected from vaginal challenge with pathogenic SIVmac239. *J Virol* 71:1911–1921.

1789a.Miller, G. 1993. Personal communication.

1790. Miller, G., M. O. Rigsby, L. Heston, E. Grogan, R. Sun, C. Metroka, J. A. Levy, S. J. Gao, Y. Chang, and P. Moore. 1996. Antibodies to butyrate-inducible antigens of Kaposi's sarcoma-associated herpesvirus in patients with HIV-1 infection. *N Engl J Med* 334:1292–1297.

1791. Miller, M. A., M. W. Cloyd, J. Liebmann, C. R. Rinaldo, Jr., K. R. Islam, S. Z. S. Wang, T. A. Mietzner, and R. C. Montelaro. 1993. Alterations in cell membrane permeability by the lentivirus lytic peptide (LLP-1) of HIV-1 transmembrane protein. *Virol* 196:89–100.

1792. Miller, M. A., R. F. Garry, J. M. Jaynes, and R. C. Montelaro. 1991. A structural correlation between lentivirus transmembrane proteins and natural cytolytic peptides. *AIDS Res Hum Retro* 7:511–519.

1793. Miller, M. D., M. T. Warmerdam, I. Gaston, W. C. Greene, and M. B. Feinberg. 1994. The human immunodeficiency virus-1 *nef* gene product: a positive factor for viral infection and replication in primary lymphocytes and macrophages. *J Exp Med* 179:101–113.

1794. Miller, R. A. 1996. The aging immune system: primer and prospectus. *Science* 273:70–74.

1796. Miskovsky, E. P., A. Y. Liu, W. Pavlat, R. Viveen, P. E. Stanhope, D. Finzi, W. M. Fox III, R. H. Hruban, E. R. Podack, and R. F. Siliciano. 1994. Studies of the mechanism of cytolysis by HIV-1-specific CD4+ human CTL clones induced by candidate AIDS vaccines. *J Immunol* 153:2787–2799.

1797. Mitchell, W. M., J. Torres, P. R. Johnson, V. Hirsch, T. Yilma, M. B. Gardner, and W. E. Robinson, Jr. 1995. Antibodies to the putative SIV infection-enhancing domain diminish beneficial effects of an SIV gp160 vaccine in rhesus macaques. *AIDS* **9:**27–34.

1798. Mitsuya, H., K. J. Weinhold, P. A. Furman, M. H. St. Clair, S. N. Lehrman, R. C. Gallo, D. Bolognesi, D. W. Barry, and S. Broder. 1985. 3′-azido-3′-deoxythymidine (BW A509U): an antiviral agent that inhibits the infectivity and cytopathic effect of human T-lymphotropic virus type III/lymphadenopathy-associated virus *in vitro*. *Proc Natl Acad Sci USA* **82:**7096–7100.

1799. Miyoshi, I., I. Kubonishi, S. Yoshimoto, T. Akagi, Y. Ohtsuki, Y. Shiraishi, K. Nagata, and Y. Hinuma. 1981. Type C virus particles in a cord T-cell line derived by co-cultivating normal human cord leukocytes and human leukaemic T cells. *Nature* **294:**770–771.

1800. Mizukami, T., T. R. Fuerst, E. A. Berger, and B. Moss. 1988. Binding region for human immunodeficiency virus (HIV) and epitopes for HIV-blocking monoclonal antibodies of the CD4 molecule defined by site-directed mutagenesis. *Proc Natl Acad Sci USA* **85:**9273–9277.

1803. Mocroft, A., M. Bofill, M. Lipman, E. Medina, N. Borthwick, A. Timms, L. Batista, M. Winter, C. A. Sabin, M. Johnson, C. A. Lee, A. Phillips, and G. Janossy. 1997. CD8+, CD38+ lymphocyte percent: a useful immunological marker for monitoring HIV-1-infected patients. *J AIDS Hum Retrovirol* **14:**158–162.

1804. Moebius, U., L. K. Clayton, S. Abraham, S. C. Harrison, and E. L. Reinherz. 1992. The human immunodeficiency virus gp120 binding site on CD4: delineation by quantitative equilibrium and kinetic binding studies of mutants in conjunction with a high-resolution CD4 atomic structure. *J Exp Med* **176:**507–517.

1805. Mohamed, O. A., R. Ashley, A. Goldstein, J. McElrath, J. Dalessio, and L. Corey. 1994. Detection of rectal antibodies to HIV-1 by a sensitive chemiluminescent Western blot immunodetection method. *J AIDS* **7:**375–380.

1805a. Mole, L., S. Ripich, D. Margolis, and M. Holodniy. 1997. The impact of active herpes simplex virus infection on human immunodeficiency virus load. *J Inf Dis* **176:**766–770.

1806. Molina, J.-M., D. T. Scadden, B. Sakaguchi, B. Fuller, A. Woon, and J. E. Groopman. 1990. Lack of evidence for infection of or effect on growth of hematopoietic progenitor cells after *in vivo* or *in vitro* exposure to human immunodeficiency virus. *Blood* **76:**2476–2482.

1807. Molina, J.-M., R. Schindler, R. Ferriani, M. Sakaguchi, E. Vannier, C. A. Dinarello, and J. E. Groopman. 1990. Production of cytokines by peripheral blood monocytes/macrophages infected with human immunodeficiency virus type 1 (HIV-1). *J Inf Dis* **161:**888–893.

1808. Monini, P., L. de Lellis, M. Fabris, F. Rigolin, and E. Cassai. 1996. Kaposi's sarcoma-associated herpesvirus DNA sequences in prostate tissue and human semen. *N Engl J Med* **334:**1168–1172.

1809. Monini, P., A. Rotola, L. de Lellis, A. Corallini, P. Secchiero, A. Albini, R. Benelli, C. Parravicini, G. Barbanti-Brodano, and E. Cassai. 1996. Latent BK virus infection and Kaposi's sarcoma pathogenesis. *Int J Cancer* **66:**717–722.

1810. Monroe, J. E., A. Calender, and C. Mulder. 1988. Epstein-Barr virus-positive and -negative B-cell lines can be infected with human immunodeficiency virus types 1 and 2. *J Virol* **62:**3497–3500.

1811. Montaner, L. J., A. G. Doyle, M. Collin, G. Herbein, P. Illei, W. James, A. Minty, D. Caput, P. Ferrara, and S. Gordon. 1993. Interleukin 13 inhibits human immunodeficiency virus type 1 production in primary blood-derived human macrophages in vitro. *J Exp Med* **178:**743–747.

1812. Montagnier, L., J. Chermann, F. Barre-Sinoussi, S. Chamaret, J. Gruest, M. T. Nugeyre, F. Rey, C. Dauguet, C. Axler-Blin, F. Vezinet-Brun, C. Rouzioux, A. G. Saimot, W. Rozenbaum, J. C. Gluckman, D. Klatzmann, E. Vilmer, C. Griselli, C. Gazengel, and J. B. Brunet. 1984. A new human T-lymphotropic retrovirus: characterization and possible role in lymphadenopathy and acquired immune deficiency syndromes, p. 363–379. *In* R. C. Gallo, M. E. Essex, and L. Gross (ed.), *Human T-Cell Leukemia/Lymphoma Virus*. Cold Spring Harbor Laboratory, Cold Spring Harbor.

1813. Montagnier, L., J. Gruest, S. Chamaret, C. Dauguet, C. Axler, D. Guetard, M. T. Nugeyre,

F. Barre-Sinoussi, J. C. Chermann, and J. B. Brunet. 1984. Adaption of lymphadenopathy associated virus (LAV) to replication in EBV-transformed B lymphoblastoid cell lines. *Science* 225:63–66.

1814. **Montaner, J. S. G., C. Zala, B. Conway, J. Raboud, P. Patenaude, S. Rae, M. V. O'Shaughnessy, and M. T. Schechter.** 1997. A pilot study of hydroxyurea among patients with advanced human immunodeficiency virus (HIV) disease receiving chronic didanosine therapy: Canadian HIV trials network protocol 080. *J Inf Dis* 175:801–806.

1815. **Montefiori, D. C., B. S. Graham, S. Kliks, and P. F. Wright.** 1992. Serum antibodies to HIV-1 in recombinant vaccinia virus recipients boosted with purified recombinant gp160. *J Clin Immunol* 12:429–439.

1816. **Montefiori, D. C., B. S. Graham, J. Zhou, J. Zhou, R. A. Bucco, D. H. Schwartz, L. A. Cavacini, and M. R. Posner.** 1993. V3-specific neutralizing antibodies in sera from HIV-1 gp160-immunized volunteers block virus fusion and act synergistically with human monoclonal antibody to the conformation-dependent CD4 binding site of gp120. *J Clin Invest* 92:840–847.

1817. **Montefiori, D. C., L. B. Lefkowitz, Jr., R. E. Keller, V. Holmberg, E. Sandstrom, and J. P. Phair.** 1991. Absence of a clinical correlation for complement-mediated, infection-enhancing antibodies in plasma or sera from HIV-1-infected individuals. *AIDS* 5:513–517.

1818. **Montefiori, D. C., G. Pantaleo, L. M. Fink, J. T. Zhou, J. Y. Zhou, M. Bilska, G. D. Miralles, and A. S. Fauci.** 1996. Neutralizing and infection-enhancing antibody responses to human immunodeficiency virus type 1 in long-term nonprogressors. *J Inf Dis* 173:60–67.

1819. **Montefiori, D. C., K. A. Reimann, N. L. Letvin, J. Zhou, and S.-L. Hu.** 1995. Studies of complement-activating antibodies in the SIV/macaque model of acute primary infection and vaccine protection. *AIDS Res Hum Retro* 11:963–970.

1820. **Montefiori, D. C., W. E. Robinson, Jr., V. M. Hirsch, A. Modliszewki, W. M. Mitchell, and P. R. Johnson.** 1990. Antibody dependent enhancement of simian immunodeficiency virus (SIV) infection in vitro by plasma from SIV-infected rhesus macaques. *J Virol* 64:113–119.

1821. **Montefiori, D. C., W. E. Robinson, Jr., and W. M. Mitchell.** 1988. Role of protein N-glycosylation in pathogenesis of human immunodeficiency virus type 1. *Proc Natl Acad Sci USA* 85:9248–9252.

1822. **Monteiro, J., F. Batliwalla, H. Ostrer, and P. K. Gregersen.** 1996. Shortened telomeres in clonally expanded CD28−CD8+ T cells imply a replicative history that is distinct from their CD28+CD8+ counterparts. *J Immunol* 156:3587–3590.

1823. **Montelaro, R. C., J. M. Ball, and K. E. Rushlow.** 1993. Equine retroviruses, p. 257–360. *In* J. A. Levy (ed.), *The Retroviridae,* vol. 2. Plenum Press, New York.

1824. **Montelaro, R. C., and D. P. Bolognesi.** 1995. Vaccines against retroviruses, p. 605–656. *In* J. A. Levy (ed.), *The Retroviridae,* vol. 4. Plenum Press, New York.

1825. **Moog, C., H. J. A. Fleury, I. Pellegrin, A. Kirn, and A. M. Aubertin.** 1997. Autologous and heterologous neutralizing antibody responses following initial seroconversion in human immunodeficiency virus type 1-infected individuals. *J Virol* 71:3734–3741.

1826. **Moore, J. P.** 1997. Coreceptors: implications for HIV pathogenesis and therapy. *Science* 276:51–52.

1827. **Moore, J. P.** 1993. A monoclonal antibody to the CDR-3 region of CD4 inhibits soluble CD4 binding to virions of human immunodeficiency virus type 1. *J Virol* 67:3656–3659.

1828. **Moore, J. P.** 1993. The reactivities of HIV-1+ human sera with solid-phase V3 loop peptides can be poor predictors of their reactivities with V3 loops on native gp120 molecules. *AIDS Res Hum Retro* 9:209–219.

1829. **Moore, J. P., Y. Cao, J. Leu, L. Qin, B. Korber, and D. D. Ho.** 1996. Inter- and intraclade neutralization of human immunodeficiency virus type 1: genetic clades do not correspond to neutralization serotypes but partially correspond to gp120 antigenic serotypes. *J Virol* 70:427–444.

1830. **Moore, J. P., and D. D. Ho.** 1993. Antibodies to discontinuous or conformationally sensitive epitopes on the gp120 glycoprotein of human immunodeficiency virus type 1 are highly prevalent in sera of infected humans. *J Virol* 67:863–875.

1831. **Moore, J. P., and D. D. Ho.** 1995. HIV-1 neutralization: the consequences of viral adaptation to growth on transformed T cells. *AIDS 1995* **9**(Suppl. A):S117–S136.

1832. **Moore, J. P., J. A. McKeating, Y. X. Huang, A. Ashkenazi, and D. D. Ho.** 1992. Virions of primary human immunodeficiency virus type 1 isolates resistant to soluble CD4 (sCD4) neutralization differ in sCD4 binding and glycoprotein gp120 retention from sCD4-sensitive isolates. *J Virol* **66**:235–243.

1833. **Moore, J. P., J. A. McKeating, W. A. Norton, and Q. J. Sattentau.** 1991. Direct measurement of soluble CD4 binding to human immunodeficiency virus type 1 virions: gp120 dissociation and its implications for virus-cell binding and fusion reactions and their neutralization by soluble CD4. *J Virol* **65**:1133–1140.

1834. **Moore, J. P., J. A. McKeating, R. A. Weiss, and Q. J. Sattentau.** 1990. Dissociation of gp120 from HIV-1 virions induced by soluble CD4. *Science* **250**:1139–1142.

1835. **Moore, J. P., and P. L. Nara.** 1991. The role of the V3 loop of gp120 in HIV infection. *AIDS* **5**:s21-s33.

1836. **Moore, J. P., Q. J. Sattentau, R. Wyatt, and J. Sodroski.** 1994. Probing the structure of the human immunodeficiency virus surface glycoprotein gp120 with a panel of monoclonal antibodies. *J Virol* **68**:469–484.

1837. **Moore, J. P., Q. J. Sattentau, H. Yoshiyama, M. Thali, M. Charles, N. Sullivan, S. W. Poon, M. S. Fung, F. Traincard, M. Pinkus, G. Robey, J. E. Robinson, D. D. Ho, and J. Sodroski.** 1993. Probing the structure of the V2 domain of human immunodeficiency virus type 1 surface glycoprotein gp120 with a panel of eight monoclonal antibodies: human immune response to the V1 and V2 domains. *J Virol* **67**:6136–6151.

1838. **Moore, J. P., and R. W. Sweet.** 1993. The HIV gp120-CD4 interaction: a target for pharmacological or immunological intervention? *Perspect Drug Discov Design* **1**:235–250.

1839. **Moore, J. P., H. Yoshiyama, D. D. Ho, J. E. Robinson, and J. Sodroski.** 1993. Antigenic variation in gp120s from molecular clones of HIV-1 LAI. *AIDS Res Hum Retro* **9**:1185–1193.

1840. **Moore, P. S., C. Boshoff, R. A. Weiss, and Y. Chang.** 1996. Molecular mimicry of human cytokine and cytokine response pathway genes by KSHV. *Science* **274**:1739–1744.

1840a. **Morbidity and Mortality Weekly Report.** 1995. Case-control study of HIV seroconversion in health care workers after percutaneous exposure to HIV infected blood—France, United Kingdom, and United States, January 1988–August 1994. *Morbid Mortal Weekly Rep* **44**:929–933.

1840b. **Morbidity and Mortality Weekly Report.** 1996. Update: provisional Public Health Service recommendations for chemoprophylaxis after occupational exposure to HIV. *J Am Med Assoc* **276**:90–92.

1841. **Morein, B., B. Sundquist, S. Hoglund, K. Dalsgaard, and A. Osterhaus.** 1984. ISCOM, a novel structure for antigenic presentation of membrane proteins from enveloped viruses. *Nature* **308**:457.

1842. **Moreno, P., M. J. Rebollo, F. Pulido, R. Rubio, A. R. Noriega, and R. Delgado.** 1996. Alveolar macrophages are not an important source of viral production in HIV-1 infected patients. *AIDS* **10**:682–684.

1843. **Morgan, J. R., J. M. LeDoux, R. G. Snow, R. G. Tompkins, and M. L. Yarmush.** 1995. Retrovirus infection: effect of time and target cell number. *J Virol* **69**:6994–7000.

1844. **Mori, K., D. J. Ringler, and R. C. Desrosiers.** 1993. Restricted replication of simian immunodeficiency virus strain 239 in macrophages is determined by *env* but is not due to restricted entry. *J Virol* **67**:2807–2814.

1845. **Mori, S., R. Takada, K. Shimotohno, and T. Okamoto.** 1990. Repressive effect of the *nef* cDNA of human immunodeficiency virus type 1 on the promoter activity of the viral long terminal repeat. *Jpn J Cancer Res* **81**:1124–1131.

1846. **Morikawa, Y., J. P. Moore, A. J. Wilkinson, and I. M. Jones.** 1991. Reduction in CD4 binding affinity associated with removal of a single glycosylation site in the external glycoprotein of HIV-2. *Virol* **180**:853–856.

1847. **Moriuchi, H., M. Moriuchi, C. Combadiere, P. M. Murphy, and A. S. Fauci.** 1996. CD8+

T-cell-derived soluble factor(s), but not β-chemokines RANTES, MIP-1α, and MIP-1β, suppress HIV-1 repliction in monocyte/macrophages. *Proc Natl Acad Sci USA* **93**:15341–15345.

1848. Morrow, W. J. W., D. A. Isenberg, R. E. Sobol, R. B. Stricker, and T. Kieber-Emmons. 1991. AIDS virus infection and autoimmunity: a perspective of the clinical, immunological, and molecular origins of the autoallergic pathologies associated with HIV disease. *Clin Immunol Immunopathol* **58**:163–180.

1849. Morrow, W. J. W., M. Wharton, R. B. Stricker, and J. A. Levy. 1986. Circulating immune complexes in patients with acquired immune deficiency syndrome contain the AIDS-associated retrovirus. *Clin Immunol Immunopathol* **40**:515–524.

1850. Morse, H. C. I., S. K. Chattopadhyay, M. Makino, T. N. Frederickson, A. W. Hügin, and J. W. Hartley. 1992. Retrovirus-induced immunodeficiency in the mouse: MAIDS as a model for AIDS. *AIDS* **6**:607–621.

1851. Mosca, J. D., D. P. Bednarik, N. B. K. Raj, C. A. Rosen, J. G. Sodroski, W. A. Haseltine, and P. M. Pitha. 1987. Herpes simplex virus type 1 can reactivate transcription of latent human immunodeficiency virus. *Nature* **325**:67–70.

1852. Moses, A. V., F. E. Bloom, C. D. Pauza, and J. A. Nelson. 1993. Human immunodeficiency virus infection of human brain capillary endothelial cells occurs via a CD4/galactosyl ceramide-independent mechanism. *Proc Natl Acad Sci USA* **90**:10474–10478.

1853. Moses, A. V., S. G. Stenglein, J. G. Strussenberg, K. Wehrly, B. Chesebro, and J. A. Nelson. 1996. Sequences regulating tropism of human immunodeficiency virus type 1 for brain capillary endothelial cells map to a unique region on the viral genome. *J Virol* **70**:3401–3406.

1854. Moses, A. V., S. Williams, M. L. Heneveld, J. Strussenberg, M. Rarick, M. Loveless, G. Bagby, and J. A. Nelson. 1996. Human immunodeficiency virus infection of bone marrow endothelium reduces induction of stromal hematopoietic growth factors. *Blood* **87**:919–925.

1855. Mosier, D., and H. Sieburg. 1994. Macrophage-tropic HIV: critical for AIDS pathogenesis? *Immunol Today* **15**:332–339.

1855a. Mosier, D. E. Personal communication.

1856. Mosier, D. E., R. J. Gulizia, S. M. Baird, and D. B. Wilson. 1988. Transfer of a functional human immune system to mice with severe combined immunodeficiency. *Nature* **335**:256–259.

1857. Mosier, D. E., R. J. Gulizia, S. M. Baird, D. B. Wilson, D. H. Spector, and S. A. Spector. 1991. Human immunodeficiency virus infection of human-PBL-SCID mice. *Science* **251**:791–794.

1858. Mosier, D. E., R. J. Gulizia, P. D. MacIsaac, L. Corey, and P. D. Greenberg. 1993. Resistance to human immunodeficiency virus 1 infection of SCID mice reconstituted with peripheral blood leukocytes from donors vaccinated with vaccinia-gp160 and recombinant gp160. *Proc Natl Acad Sci USA* **90**:2443–2447.

1859. Mosier, D. E., R. J. Gulizia, P. D. MacIsaac, B. E. Torbett, and J. A. Levy. 1993. Rapid loss of CD4+ T cells in human-PBL-SCID mice by noncytopathic HIV isolates. *Science* **260**:689–692.

1861. Mosmann, T. R., H. Cherwinski, M. W. Bond, M. A. Giedlin, and R. L. Coffman. 1986. Two types of murine helper T cell clones. I. Definition according to profiles of lymphokine activities and secreted proteins. *J Immunol* **136**:2348–2357.

1862. Mosmann, T. R., and S. Sad. 1996. The expanding universe of T-cell subsets: Th1, Th2 and more. *Immunol Today* **17**:138–146.

1863. Moss, A. R., K. Vranizan, R. Gorter, P. Bacchetti, J. Watters, and D. Osmond. 1994. HIV seroconversion in intravenous drug users in San Francisco, 1985–1990. *AIDS* **8**:223–231.

1864. Moss, G. B., D. Clemetson, L. D'Costa, F. A. Plummer, J. O. Ndinya-Achola, M. Reilly, K. K. Holmes, P. Piot, G. M. Maitha, S. L. Hillier, N. C. Kiviat, C. W. Cameron, I. A. Wamola, and J. K. Kreiss. 1991. Association of cervical ectopy with heterosexual transmission of human immunodeficiency virus: results of a study of couples in Nairobi, Kenya. *J Inf Dis* **164**:588–591.

1865. Moss, G. B., J. Overbaugh, M. Welch, M. Reilly, J. Bwayo, F. A. Plummer, J. O. Ndinya-Achola, M. A. Malisa, and J. K. Kreiss. 1995. Human immunodeficiency virus DNA in urethral secretions in men: association with gonococcal urethritis and CD4 cell depletion. *J Inf Dis* 172:1469–1474.

1866. Moss, P. A. H., S. L. Rowland-Jones, P. M. Frodsham, S. McAdam, P. Giangrande, A. J. McMichael, and J. I. Bell. 1995. Persistent high frequency of human immunodeficiency virus-specific cytotoxic T cells in peripheral blood of infected donors. *Proc Natl Acad Sci USA* 92:5773–5777.

1867. Mossman, S. P., F. Bex, P. Berglund, J. Arthos, S. P. O'Neil, D. Riley, D. H. Maul, C. Bruck, P. Momin, A. Burny, P. N. Fultz, J. I. Mullins, P. Liljestrom, and E. A. Hoover. 1996. Protection against lethal simian immunodeficiency virus SIVsmmPBj14 disease by a recombinant Semliki Forest virus gp160 vaccine and by a gp120 subunit vaccine. *J Virol* 70:1953–1960.

1868. Mostad, S. B., and J. K. Kreiss. 1996. Shedding of HIV-1 in the genital tract. *AIDS* 10:1305–1315.

1868a.Motti, P. G., G. A. Dallabetta, R. W. Daniel, J. K. Canner, J. D. Chiphangwi, G. N. Liomba, L. P. Yang, and K. V. Shah. 1996. Cervical abnormalities, human papillomavirus, and human immunodeficiency virus infections in women in Malawi. *J Inf Dis* 173:714–717.

1869. Moutouh, L., J. Corbeil, and D. D. Richman. 1996. Recombination leads to the rapid emergence of HIV-1 dually resistant mutants under selective drug pressure. *Proc Natl Acad Sci USA* 93:6106–6111.

1870. Moyer, M. P., R. I. Juot, A. Ramirez, Jr., S. Joe, M. S. Meltzer, and H. E. Gendelman. 1990. Infection of human gastrointestinal cells by HIV-1. *AIDS Res Hum Retro* 6:1409–1415.

1871. Muesing, M. A., D. H. Smith, C. D. Cabradilla, C. V. Benton, L. A. Lasky, and D. J. Capon. 1985. Nucleic acid structure and expression of the human AIDS/lymphadenopathy retrovirus. *Nature* 313:450–458.

1872. Mulder, C. 1988. Human AIDS virus not from monkeys. *Nature* 333:396.

1873. Mulder, J. W., P. Krijnen, J. Goudsmit, J. K. M. Eeftinck Schattenkerk, P. Reiss, and J. M. A. Lange. 1990. HIV-1 p24 antigenaemia does not predict time of survival in AIDS patients. *Genitourin Med* 66:138–141.

1874. Muller, C., S. Kukel, and R. Bauer. 1993. Relationship of antibodies against CD4+ T cells in HIV-infected patients to markers of activation and progression: autoantibodies are closely associated with CD4 cell depletion. *Immunol* 79:248–254.

1875. Mundy, D. C., R. F. Schinazi, A. Ressell-Gerber, A. J. Nahmias, and H. W. Randal. 1987. Human immunodeficiency virus isolated from amniotic fluid. *Lancet* ii:459–460.

1876. Munis, J. R., R. S. Kornbluth, J. C. Guatelli, and D. D. Richman. 1992. Ordered appearance of human immunodeficiency virus type 1 nucleic acids following high multiplicity infection of macrophages. *J Gen Virol* 73:1899–1906.

1877. Munoz, A., A. J. Kirby, Y. D. He, J. B. Margolick, B. R. Visscher, C. R. Rinaldo, R. A. Kaslow, and J. P. Phair. 1995. Long-term survivors with HIV-1 infection: incubation period and longitudinal patterns of CD4+ lymphocytes. *J AIDS Hum Retrovirol* 8:496–505.

1878. Murakami, T., T. Hattori, and K. Takatsuki. 1991. A principal neutralizing domain of human immunodeficiency virus type 1 interacts with proteinase-like molecule(s) at the surface of Molt-4 clone 8 cells. *Biochim Biophys Acta* 1079:279–284.

1879. Murakami, T., S. Matsushita, Y. Maeda, K. Takatsuki, T. Uchiyama, and T. Hattori. 1993. Applications of biotinylated V3 loop peptides of human immunodeficiency virus type 1 to flow cytometric analyses and affinity chromatographic techniques. *Biochim Biophys Acta* 1181:155–162.

1880. Muro-Cacho, C. A., G. Pantaleo, and A. S. Fauci. 1995. Analysis of apoptosis in lymph nodes of HIV-infected persons. *J Immunol* 154:5555–5566.

1881. Murphey-Corb, M., L. N. Martin, B. Davison-Fairburn, R. C. Montelaro, M. Miller, M. West, S. Ohkawa, G. B. Baskin, J.-Y. Zhang, S. D. Putney, A. C. Allison, and D. A. Eppstein. 1989. A formalin-inactivated whole SIV vaccine confers protection in macaques. *Science* 246:1293–1297.

1882. Murphey-Corb, M., R. C. Montelaro, M. A. Miller, M. West, L. N. Martin, B. Davison-Fairburn, S. Ohkawa, G. B. Baskin, J.-Y. Zhang, G. B. Miller, S. D. Putney, A. C. Allison, and D. A. Eppstein. 1991. Efficacy of SIV/deltaB670 glycoprotein-enriched and glycoprotein-depleted subunit vaccines in protecting against infection and disease in rhesus monkeys. *AIDS* **5:**655–662.

1883. Musey, L., Y. Hu, L. Eckert, M. Christensen, T. Karchmer, and M. J. McElrath. 1997. HIV-1 induces cytotoxic T lymphocytes in the cervix of infected women. *J Exp Med* **185:**293–303.

1884. Musicco, M., A. Lazzarin, A. Nicolosi, M. Gasparini, P. Costigliola, C. Arici, and A. Saracco. 1994. Antiretroviral treatment of men infected with human immunodeficiency virus type 1 reduces the incidence of heterosexual transmission. *Arch Int Med* **154:**1971–1976.

1885. Muster, T., F. Steindl, M. Purtscher, A. Trkola, A. Klima, G. Himmler, F. Ruker, and H. Katinger. 1993. A conserved neutralizing epitope on gp41 of human immunodeficiency virus type 1. *J Virol* **67:**6642–6647.

1886. Myagkikh, M., S. Alipanah, P. D. Markham, J. Tartaglia, E. Paoletti, R. C. Gallo, G. Franchini, and M. Robert-Guroff. 1996. Multiple immunizations with attenuated poxvirus HIV type 2 recombinants and subunit boosts required for protection of rhesus macaques. *AIDS Res Hum Retro* **12:**985–992.

1887. Myers, G. 1991. Analysis. Protein information summary, p. III-4. *In* G. Myers, J. A. Berzofsky, B. Korber, R. F. Smith, and G. Pavlakis (ed.), *Human Retroviruses and AIDS 1991. A Compilation and Analysis of Nucleic Acid and Amino Acid Sequences.* Theoretical Biology and Biophysics, Los Alamos National Laboratory, Los Alamos.

1888. Myers, G. 1994. Tenth anniversary perspectives on AIDS. HIV: between past and future. *AIDS Res Hum Retro* **10:**1317–1324.

1889. Myers, G., B. Korber, B. Foley, K. T. Jeang, J. W. Mellors, and S. Wain-Hobson. 1996. *Human Retroviruses and AIDS 1996.* Los Alamos National Laboratory, Los Alamos.

1890. Myers, G., B. Korber, S. Wain-Hobson, R. F. Smith, and G. N. Pavlakis. 1993. *Human Retroviruses and AIDS 1993, I-V. A Compilation and Analysis of Nucleic Acid and Amino Acid Sequences.* Los Alamos National Laboratory, Los Alamos.

1891. Myers, G., K. MacInnes, and B. Korber. 1992. The emergence of simian/human immunodeficiency viruses. *AIDS Res Hum Retro* **8:**373–386.

1892. Myers, G., and G. N. Pavlakis. 1992. Evolutionary potential of complex retroviruses, p. 51–105. *In* J. A. Levy (ed.), *The Retroviridae,* vol. 1. Plenum Press, New York.

1893. Myers, M., and J. G. Montaner. 1996. A randomized double-blinded comparative trial of the effects of zidovudine, didanosine and novirapine combinations in antiviral naive, AIDS-free, HIV-infected patients with CD4 counts 200–600/mm³, vol. 1, p. 22. Presented at the VI International Conference on AIDS, Vancouver, B.C., Canada.

1894. Nabel, E. G., L. Shum, V. J. Pompili, Z. Y. Yang, H. San, H. B. Shu, S. Liptay, L. Gold, D. Gordon, R. Derynck, and G. J. Nabel. 1993. Direct transfer of transforming growth factor beta-1 gene into arteries stimulates fibrocellular hyperplasia. *Proc Natl Acad Sci USA* **90:**10759–10763.

1895. Nabel, G., and D. Baltimore. 1987. An inducible transcription factor activates expression of human immunodeficiency virus in T cells. *Nature* **326:**711–713.

1896. Nabel, G. J., S. A. Rice, D. M. Knipe, and D. Baltimore. 1988. Alternative mechanisms for activation of human immunodeficiency virus enhancer in T cells. *Science* **239:**1299–1302.

1897. Nadji, M., A. R. Morales, J. Zieggles-Weisman, and N. S. Penneys. 1984. Kaposi's sarcoma: immunohistological evidence for an endothelial origin. *Arch Pathol Lab Med* **105:**274–275.

1898. Nagashunmugam, T., H. M. Friedman, C. Davis, S. Kennedy, L. T. Goldstein, and D. Malamud. 1997. Human submandibular saliva specifically inhibits HIV type 1. *AIDS Res Hum Retro* **13:**371–376.

1899. Nahmias, A. J., J. Weiss, X. Yao, F. Lee, R. Kodsi, M. Schanfield, T. Matthews, D. Bolognesi, D. Durack, A. Motulsky, P. Kanki, and M. Essex. 1986. Evidence for human infection with an HTLV III/LAV-like virus in Central Africa, 1959. *Lancet* **i:**1279–1280.

1900. Nair, B. C., A. L. DeVico, and S. Nakamura. 1992. Identification of a major growth factor for AIDS-Kaposi's sarcoma cells as oncostatin M. *Science* 255:1430–1432.

1901. Nakajima, K., O. Martinez-Maza, T. Hirano, E. C. Breen, P. G. Nishanian, J. F. Salazar-Gonzalez, J. L. Fahey, and T. Kishimoto. 1989. Induction of IL-6 (B cell stimulatory factor-2/IFN-beta-2) production by human immunodeficiency virus. *J Immunol* 142:531–536.

1902. Nakamura, G. R., R. Byrn, D. M. Wilkes, J. A. Fox, M. R. Hobbs, R. Hastings, H. C. Wessling, M. A. Norcross, B. M. Fendly, and P. W. Berman. 1993. Strain specificity and binding affinity requirements of neutralizing monoclonal antibodies to the CD4 domain of gp120 from human immunodeficiency virus type 1. *J Virol* 67:6179–6191.

1903. Nakamura, S., S. K. Salahuddin, and P. Biberfeld. 1988. Kaposi's sarcoma cells: long-term culture with growth factor from retrovirus-infected CD4+ T cells. *Science* 242:426–430.

1904. Namikawa, R., H. Kaneshima, M. Lieberman, I. L. Weissman, and J. M. McCune. 1988. Infection of the SCID-hu mouse by HIV-1. *Science* 242:1684–1686.

1905. Nara, P. L., R. R. Garrity, and J. Goudsmit. 1991. Neutralization of HIV-1: a paradox of humoral proportions. *FASEB J* 5:2437–2455.

1906. Nara, P. L., W. G. Robey, L. O. Arthur, D. M. Asher, A. V. Wolff, J. C. Gibbs, Jr., D. C. Gajdusek, and P. J. Fischinger. 1987. Persistent infection of chimpanzees with human immunodeficiency virus: serological responses and properties of reisolated viruses. *J Virol* 61:3173–3180.

1907. Nara, P. L., L. Smit, N. Dunlop, W. Hatch, M. Merges, D. Waters, J. Kelliher, R. C. Gallo, P. G. Fischinger, and J. Goudsmit. 1990. Emergence of viruses resistant to neutralization by V3-specific antibodies in experimental human immunodeficiency virus type 1 IIIB infection of chimpanzees. *J Virol* 64:3779–3791.

1907a. National Library of Medicine. 1997. AIDS Line Database.

1908. Navia, B. A., and R. W. Price. 1987. The acquired immunodeficiency syndrome dementia complex as the presenting or sole manifestation of human immunodeficiency virus infection. *Arch Neurol* 44:65–69.

1909. Navia, M. A., P. M. Fitzgerald, B. M. McKeever, C. T. Leu, J. C. Heimbach, W. K. Herber, I. S. Sigal, P. L. Darke, and J. P. Springer. 1989. Three-dimensional structure of aspartyl protease from human immunodeficiency virus HIV-1. *Nature* 337:615–620.

1910. Naylor, P. H., C. W. Naylor, M. Badamchian, S. Wada, A. L. Goldstein, S.-S. Wang, D. K. Sun, A. H. Thornton, and P. S. Sarin. 1987. Human immunodeficiency virus contains an epitope immunoreactive with thymosin alpha-1 and the 30-amino acid synthetic p17 group-specific antigen peptide HGP-30. *Proc Natl Acad Sci USA* 84:2951–2955.

1911. Nduati, R. W., G. C. John, B. A. Richardson, J. Overbaugh, M. Welch, J. Ndinya-Achola, S. Moses, K. Holmes, F. Onyango, and J. K. Kreiss. 1995. Human immunodeficiency virus type 1-infected cells in breast milk: association with immunosuppression and vitamin A deficiency. *J Inf Dis* 172:1461–1468.

1912. Nehete, P. N., R. B. Arlinghaus, and K. J. Sastry. 1993. Inhibition of human immunodeficiency virus type 1 infection and syncytium formation in human cells by V3 loop synthetic peptides from gp120. *J Virol* 67:6841–6846.

1913. Nelbock, P., P. J. Dillon, A. Perkins, and C. A. Rosen. 1990. A cDNA for a protein that interacts with the human immunodeficiency virus Tat transactivator. *Science* 248:1650–1653.

1914. Nelson, J. A., P. Ghazal, and C. A. Wiley. 1990. Role of opportunistic viral infections in AIDS. *AIDS* 4:1–10.

1915. Nelson, J. A., C. Reynolds-Kohler, M. B. A. Oldstone, and C. A. Wiley. 1988. HIV and HCMV coinfect brain cells in patients with AIDS. *Virol* 165:286–290.

1916. Nelson, J. A., C. A. Wiley, C. Reynolds-Kohler, C. E. Reese, W. Margaretten, and J. A. Levy. 1988. Human immunodeficiency virus detected in bowel epithelium from patients with gastrointestinal symptoms. *Lancet* i:259–262.

1917. Neumann, M., B. K. Felber, A. Kleinschmidt, B. Froese, V. Erfle, G. N. Pavlakis, and R. Brack-Werner. 1995. Restriction of human immunodeficiency virus type 1 production in a human astrocytoma cell line is associated with a cellular block in Rev function. *J Virol* 69:2159–2167.

1918. **Newburg, D. S., R. P. Viscidi, A. Ruff, and R. H. Yolken.** 1992. A human milk factor inhibits binding of human immunodeficiency virus to the CD4 receptor. *Ped Res* **31**:22–28.

1919. **Newell, M. L., D. Dunn, C. S. Peckham, A. E. Ades, G. Pardi, and A. E. Semprini.** 1992. Risk factors for mother-to-child transmission of HIV-1. *Lancet* **339**:1007–1012.

1920. **Newell, M. L., D. T. Dunn, C. S. Peckham, A. E. Semprini, and G. Pardi.** 1996. Vertical transmission of HIV-1: maternal immune status and obstetric factors. *AIDS* **10**:1675–1681.

1921. **Newman, M. J., K. J. Munroe, C. A. Anderson, C. I. Murphy, D. L. Panicali, J. R. Seals, J.-Y. Wu, M. S. Wyand, and C. R. Kensil.** 1994. Induction of antigen-specific killer T lymphocyte responses using subunit SIVmac251 gag and env vaccines containing QS-21 saponin adjuvant. *AIDS Res Hum Retro* **10**:853–861.

1922. **Newstein, M., E. J. Stanbridge, G. Casey, and P. R. Shank.** 1990. Human chromosome 12 encodes a species-specific factor which increases human immunodeficiency virus type 1 *tat*-mediated *trans* activation in rodent cells. *J Virol* **64**:4565–4567.

1923. **Ngugi, E. N., F. A. Plummer, J. N. Simonsen, D. W. Cameron, M. Bosire, P. Waiyaki, A. R. Ronald, and J. O. Ndinya-Achola.** 1988. Prevention of transmission of human immunodeficiency virus in Africa: effectiveness of condom promotion and health education among prostitutes. *Lancet* **ii**:887–890.

1924. **Nicholson, J. K., G. D. Cross, C. S. Callaway, and J. S. McDougal.** 1986. *In vitro* infection of human monocytes with human T lymphotropic virus type III/lymphadenopathy-associated virus (HTLV-III/LAV). *J Immunol* **137**:323–329.

1925. **Nick, S., J. Kalws, K. Friebel, C. Birr, G. Hunsmann, and H. Bayer.** 1990. Virus neutralizing and enhancing epitopes characterized by synthetic oligopeptides derived from the feline leukemia virus glycoprotein sequence. *J Gen Virol* **71**:77–83.

1926. **Nickoloff, B. J., and C. E. M. Griffiths.** 1989. The spindle-shaped cells in cutaneous Kaposi's sarcoma. *Am J Path* **135**:793–800.

1927. **Niederman, T. M. J., J. V. Garcia, W. R. Hastings, S. Luria, and L. Ratner.** 1992. Human immunodeficiency virus type 1 Nef protein inhibits NF-kB induction in human T cells. *J Virol* **66**:6213–6219.

1928. **Niederman, T. M. J., W. R. Hastings, S. Luria, J. C. Bandres, and L. Ratner.** 1993. HIV-1 nef protein inhibits the recruitment of AP-1 DNA-binding activity in human T-cells. *Virol* **194**:338–344.

1929. **Niederman, T. M. J., W. Hu, and L. Ratner.** 1991. Simian immunodeficiency virus negative factor suppresses the level of viral mRNA in COS cells. *J Virol* **65**:3538–3546.

1930. **Niederman, T. M. J., B. J. Thielan, and L. Ratner.** 1989. Human immunodeficiency virus type 1 negative factor is a transcriptional silencer. *Proc Natl Acad Sci USA* **86**:1128–1132.

1931. **Nielsen, C., C. Pedersen, J. D. Lundgren, and J. Gerstoft.** 1993. Biological properties of HIV isolates in primary HIV infection: consequences for the subsequent course of infection. *AIDS* **7**:1035–1040.

1932. **Nielsen, K., P. Boyer, M. Dillon, D. Wafer, L. S. Wei, E. Garratty, R. E. Dickover, and Y. J. Bryson.** 1996. Presence of human immunodeficiency virus (HIV) type 1 and HIV-1-specific antibodies in cervicovaginal secretions of infected mothers and in the gastric aspirates of their infants. *J Inf Dis* **173**:1001–1004.

1933. **Nieman, R. B., J. Fleming, R. J. Coker, J. R. W. Harris, and D. M. Mitchell.** 1993. The effect of cigarette smoking on the development of AIDS in HIV-1 seropositive individuals. *AIDS* **7**:705–710.

1934. **Niruthisard, S., R. E. Roddy, and S. Chutivongse.** 1991. The effects of frequent nonoxynol-9 use on the vaginal and cervical mucosa. *STD* **18**:176–179.

1935. **Nishioka, K., and I. Katayama.** 1978. Angiogenic activity in culture supernatant of antigen-stimulated lymph node cells. *J Pathol* **126**:63–69.

1936. **Nisini, R., A. Aiuti, P. M. Matricardi, A. Fattorossi, C. Ferlini, R. Biselli, I. Mazzaroma, E. Pinter, and R. D'Amelio.** 1994. Lack of evidence for a superantigen in lymphocytes from HIV-discordant monozygotic twins. *AIDS* **8**:443–449.

1937. **Niu, M. T., D. S. Stein, and S. M. Schnittman.** 1993. Primary human immunodeficiency virus type 1 infection: review of pathogenesis and early treatment intervention in humans and animal retrovirus infections. *J Inf Dis* **168**:1490–1501.

1938. **Nixon, D. F., K. Broliden, G. Ogg, and P. A. Broliden.** 1992. Cellular and humoral antigenic epitopes in HIV and SIV. *Immunol* **76**:515–534.

1939. **Nkengasong, J. N., W. Janssens, L. Heyndrickx, K. Fransen, P. M. Ndumbe, J. Motte, A. Leonares, M. Ngolle, J. Ayuk, P. Piot, and G. van der Groen.** 1994. Genotypic subtypes of HIV-1 in Cameroon. *AIDS* **8**:1405–1412.

1940. **Nkowane, B. M.** 1991. Prevalence and incidence of HIV infection in Africa: a review of data published in 1990. *AIDS* **5**:s7–s16.

1941. **Nolan, G. P., S. Ghosh, H. C. Liou, P. Tempst, and D. Baltimore.** 1991. DNA binding and IκB inhibition of the cloned p65 subunit of NF-κB, rel-related polypeptide. *Cell* **65**:961–969.

1942. **Norley, S., B. Beer, D. Binninger-Schinzel, C. Cosma, and R. Kurth.** 1996. Protection from pathogenic SIVmac challenge following short-term infection with a nef-deficient attenuated virus. *Virol* **219**:195–205.

1943. **Norley, S., and R. Kurth.** 1994. Immune response to retroviral infection, p. 363–464. *In* J. A. Levy (ed.), *The Retroviridae*, vol. 3. Plenum Press, New York.

1944. **Norley, S. G., U. Mikschy, A. Werner, S. Staszewski, E. B. Helm, and R. Kurth.** 1990. Demonstration of cross-reactive antibodies able to elicit lysis of both HIV-1- and HIV-2-infected cells. *J Immunol* **145**:1700–1705.

1945. **Noronha, I. L., V. Daniel, K. Schimpf, and G. Opelz.** 1992. Soluble IL-2 receptor and tumour necrosis factor-alpha in plasma of haemophilia patients infected with HIV. *Clin Exp Immunol* **87**:287–292.

1946. **Norton, S. D., L. Zuckerman, K. B. Urdahl, R. Shefner, J. Miller, and M. K. Jenkins.** 1992. The CD28 ligand, B7, enhances IL2 production by providing a costimulatory signal to T cells. *J Immunol* **149**:1556–1561.

1947. **Notkins, A., S. Mergenhagen, and R. Howard.** 1970. Effect of virus infections on the function of the immune system. *Annu Rev Microbiol* **24**:525–537.

1948. **Nottet, H. S., Y. Persidsky, V. G. Sasseville, A. N. Nukana, P. Bock, Q. H. Zhai, L. R. Sharer, R. D. McComb, S. Swindells, C. Soderland, and H. E. Gendelman.** 1996. Mechanisms for the transendothelial migration of HIV-1-infected monocytes into brain. *J Immunol* **156**:1284–1295.

1949. **Nottet, H. S. L. M., L. deGraaf, N. M. de Vos, L. J. Bakker, J. A. G. van Strijp, M. R. Visser, and J. Verhoef.** 1993. Down-regulation of human immunodeficiency virus type 1 (HIV-1) production after stimulation of monocyte-derived macrophages infected with HIV-1. *J Inf Dis* **167**:810–817.

1950. **Nottet, H. S. L. M., M. Jett, C. R. Flanagan, Q.-H. Zhai, Y. Persidsky, A. Rizzino, E. W. Bernton, P. Genis, T. Baldwin, J. Schwartz, C. J. LaBenz, and H. E. Gendelman.** 1994. A regulatory role for astrocytes in HIV-1 encephalitis. *J Immunol* **154**:3567–3581.

1951. **Novembre, F. J., M. M. Saucier, D. C. Anderson, S. A. Klumpp, S. P. O'Neill, C. R. Brown II, C. E. Hart, P. C. Guenthner, R. B. Swenson, and H. M. McClure.** 1997. Development of AIDS in a chimpanzee infected with HIV-1. *J Virol* **71**:4086–4091.

1952. **Numazaki, K., X.-Q. Bai, H. Goldman, I. Wong, B. Spira, and M. A. Wainberg.** 1989. Infection of cultured human thymic epithelial cells by human immunodeficiency virus. *Clin Immunol Immunopathol* **51**:185–195.

1953. **Nunn, M. F., and J. W. Marsh.** 1996. Human immunodeficiency virus type 1 Nef associates with a member of the p21-activated kinase family. *J Virol* **70**:6157–6161.

1954. **Nuovo, G. J., J. Becker, M. W. Burk, M. Margiotta, J. Fuhrer, and R. T. Steigbigel.** 1994. *In situ* detection of PCR-amplified HIV-1 nucleic acids in lymph nodes and peripheral blood in patients with asymptomatic HIV-1 infection and advanced stage AIDS. *J AIDS* **7**:916–923.

1955. **Nuovo, G. J., J. Becker, A. Simsir, M. Margiotta, G. Khalife, and M. Shevchuk.** 1994. HIV-1 nucleic acids localize to the spermatogonia and their progeny: a study by PCR *in situ* hybridization. *Am J Path* **145**:1–7.

1956. Nuovo, G. J., A. Forde, P. MacConnell, and R. Fahrenwald. 1993. *In situ* detection of PCR-amplified HIV-1 nucleic acids and tumor necrosis factor cDNA in cervical tissues. *Am J Path* 143:40–48.

1957. Nuovo, G. J., F. Gallery, P. MacConnell, and A. Braun. 1994. *In situ* detection of PCR-amplified HIV-1 nucleic acids and tumor necrosis factor alpha RNA in the central nervous system. *Am J Path* 144:659–666.

1958. Nyambi, P. N., J. Nkengasong, M. Peeters, F. Simon, J. Eberle, W. Janssens, K. Fransen, B. Willems, K. Vereecken, L. Heyndrickx, P. Piot, and G. van der Groen. 1995. Reduced capacity of antibodies from patients infected with human immunodeficiency virus type 1 (HIV-1) group O to neutralize primary isolates of HIV-1 group M viruses. *J Inf Dis* 172:1228–1237.

1959. Nyambi, P. N., B. Willems, W. Janssens, K. Fransen, J. Nkengasong, M. Peeters, K. Vereecken, L. Heyndrickx, P. Piot, and G. van der Groen. 1997. The neutralization relationship of HIV type 1, HIV type 2, and SIVcpz is reflected in the genetic diversity that distinguishes them. *AIDS Res Hum Retro* 13:7–17.

1960. Nygren, A., T. Bergman, T. Matthews, H. Jornvall, and H. Wigzell. 1988. 95- and 25-kDa fragments of the human immunodeficiency virus envelope glycoprotein gp120 bind to the CD4 receptor. *Proc Natl Acad Sci USA* 85:6543–6546.

1961. O'Brien, T. R., J. R. George, and S. D. Holmberg. 1992. Human immunodeficiency virus type 2 infection in the United States. *J Am Med Assoc* 267:2775–2779.

1962. O'Brien, T. R., C. Winkler, M. Dean, J. A. E. Nelson, M. Carrington, N. L. Michael, and G. C. White II. 1997. HIV-1 infection in a man homozygous for CCR5Δ32. *Lancet* 349:1219.

1963. O'Brien, W. A., I. S. Y. Chen, D. D. Ho, and E. S. Daar. 1992. Mapping genetic determinants for human immunodeficiency virus type 1 resistance to soluble CD4. *J Virol* 66:3125–3130.

1964. O'Brien, W. A., K. Grovit-Ferbas, A. Namazi, S. Ovcak-Derzic, H.-J. Wang, J. Park, C. Yeramian, S.-H. Mao, and J. Zack. 1995. Human immunodeficiency virus-type 1 replication can be increased in peripheral blood of seropositive patients after influenza vaccination. *Blood* 86:1082–1089.

1965. O'Brien, W. A., P. M. Hartigan, D. Martin, J. Esinhart, A. Hill, S. Benoit, M. Rubin, M. S. Simberkoff, and J. D. Hamilton. 1996. Changes in plasma HIV-1 RNA and CD4+ lymphocyte counts and the risk of progression to AIDS. *N Engl J Med* 334:426–431.

1966. O'Brien, W. A., Y. Koyanagi, A. Namazie, J.-Q. Zhao, A. Diagne, K. Idler, J. A. Zack, and I. S. Y. Chen. 1990. HIV-1 tropism for mononuclear phagocytes can be determined by regions of gp120 outside the CD4-binding domain. *Nature* 348:69–73.

1967. O'Brien, W. A., S.-H. Mao, Y. Cao, and J. P. Moore. 1994. Macrophage-tropic and T-cell line-adapted chimeric strains of human immunodeficiency virus type 1 differ in their susceptibilities to neutralization by soluble CD4 at different temperatures. *J Virol* 68:5264–5269.

1968. O'Brien, W. A., A. Namazi, H. Kalhor, S. H. Mao, J. A. Zack, and I. S. Y. Chen. 1994. Kinetics of human immunodeficiency virus type 1 reverse trancription in blood mononuclear phagocytes are slowed by limitations of nucleotide precursors. *J Virol* 68:1258–1263.

1969. O'Brien, W. A., M. Sumner-Smith, S.-H. Mao, S. Sadeghi, J.-Q. Zhao, and I. S. Y. Chen. 1996. Anti-human immunodeficiency virus type 1 activity of an oligocationic compound mediated via gp120 V3 interactions. *J Virol* 70:2825–2831.

1970. O'Connor, T. J., D. Kinchington, H. O. Kangro, and D. J. Jeffries. 1995. The activity of candidate virucidal agents, low pH and genital secretions against HIV-1 *in vitro*. *Int J STD AIDS* 6:267–272.

1971. O'Doherty, U., R. M. Steinman, M. Peng, P. U. Cameron, S. Gezelter, I. Kopeloff, W. J. Swiggard, M. Pope, and N. Bhardwaj. 1993. Dendritic cells freshly isolated from human blood express CD4 and mature into typical immunostimulatory dendritic cells after culture in monocyte-conditioned medium. *J Exp Med* 178:1067–1078.

1972. O'Shea, S., T. Rostron, A. S. Hamblin, S. J. Palmer, and J. E. Banatvala. 1991. Quantitation of HIV: correlation with clinical, virological, and immunological status. *J Med Virol* 35:65–69.

1973. O'Toole, C. M., S. Graham, M. W. Lowdell, D. Chargelegue, H. Marsden, and B. T. Colvin. 1992. Decline in CTL and antibody responses to HIV-1 p17 and p24 antigens in HIV-1-infected hemophiliacs irrespective of disease progression. A 5-year follow-up study. *AIDS Res Hum Retro* **8**:1361–1368.

1974. Oberlin, E., A. Amara, F. Bachelerie, C. Bessia, J. L. Virelizier, F. Arenzana-Seisdedos, O. Schwartz, J. M. Heard, I. Clark-Lewis, D. F. Legler, M. Loetscher, M. Baggiolini, and B. Moser. 1996. The CXC chemokine SDF-1 is the ligand for LESTR/fusin and prevents infection by T-cell-line adapted HIV-1. *Nature* **382**:833–835.

1975. Ohki, K., M. Kishi, K. Ohmura, Y. Morikawa, I. M. Jones, I. Azuma, and K. Ikuta. 1992. Human immunodeficiency virus type 1 (HIV-1) superinfection of a cell clone converting it from production of defective to infectious HIV-1 is mediated predominantly by CD4 regions other than the major binding site for HIV-1 glycoproteins. *J Gen Virol* **73**:1761–1772.

1976. Ojo-Amaize, E. A., P. Nishanian, D. E. Keith, Jr., R. L. Houghton, D. F. Heitjan, J. L. Fahey, and J. V. Giorgi. 1987. Antibodies to human immunodeficiency virus in human sera induce cell-mediated lysis of human immunodeficiency virus-infected cells. *J Immunol* **139**:2458–2463.

1976a. Okada, E., S. Sasaki, N. Ishii, I. Aoki, T. Yasuda, K. Nishioka, J. Fukushima, J. Miyazaki, B. Wahren, and K. Okuda. 1997. Intranasal immunization of a DNA vaccine with IL-12- and granulocyte-macrophage colony-stimulating factor (GM-CSF)-expressing plasmids in liposomes induces strong mucosal and cell-mediated immune responses against HIV-1 antigens. *J Immunol* **159**:3638–3647.

1977. Olafsson, K., M. S. Smith, P. Marshburn, S. G. Carter, and S. Haskill. 1991. Variation of HIV infectibility of macrophages as a function of donor, stage of differentiation, and site of origin. *J AIDS* **4**:154–164.

1978. Oldstone, M. B. A. 1987. Molecular mimicry and autoimmune disease. *Cell* **50**:819–820.

1979. Oleske, J., A. Minnefor, R. Cooper, Jr., K. Thomas, A. dela Cruz, H. Ahdieh, I. Guerrero, V. V. Joshi, and F. Desposito. 1983. Immune deficiency syndrome in children. *J Am Med Assoc* **249**:2345–2349.

1980. Oliver, R. E., J. R. Gorham, S. F. Parish, W. J. Hadlow, and O. Narayan. 1981. Studies on ovine progressive pneumonia. I. Pathologic and virologic studies on the naturally occurring disease. *Am J Vet Res* **42**:1554–1558.

1981. Olsen, G. P., and J. W. Shields. 1984. Seminal lymphocytes, plasma and AIDS. *Nature* **309**:116.

1982. Olshevsky, U., E. Helseth, C. Furman, J. Li, W. Haseltine, and J. Sodroski. 1990. Identification of individual human immunodeficiency virus type 1 gp120 amino acids important for CD4 receptor binding. *J Virol* **64**:5701–5707.

1983. Ometto, L., C. Zanotto, A. Maccabruni, D. Caselli, D. Truscia, C. Giaquinto, E. Ruga, L. Chieco-Bianchi, and A. De Rossi. 1995. Viral phenotype and host-cell susceptibility to HIV-1 infection as risk factors for mother-to-child HIV-1 transmission. *AIDS* **9**:427–434.

1983a. Operskalski, E. A., M. P. Busch, J. W. Mosley, and D. O. Stram. 1997. Comparative rates of disease progression among persons infected with the same or different HIV-1 strains. *J AIDS Hum Retrovirol* **15**:145–150.

1984. Oppenheim, J. J., E. J. Kovacs, K. Matsushima, and S. K. Durum. 1986. There is more than one interleukin-1. *Immunol Today* **7**:45–56.

1985. Oppenheim, J. J., C. O. C. Zachariae, N. Mukaida, and K. Matsushima. 1991. Properties of the novel proinflammatory supergene "intercrine" cytokine family. *Ann Rev Immunol* **9**:617–648.

1986. Oravecz, T., M. Pall, and M. A. Norcross. 1996. β-chemokine inhibition of monocytotropic HIV-1 infection. Interference with a postbinding fusion step. *J Immunol* **157**:1329–1332.

1987. Orenstein, J. M., S. Alkan, A. Blauvelt, K. T. Jeang, M. D. Weinstein, D. Ganem, and B. Herndier. 1997. Visualization of human herpesvirus type 8 in Kaposi's sarcoma by light and transmission electron microscopy. *AIDS* **11**:F35-F45.

1988. Orentas, R. J., J. E. K. Hildreth, E. Obah, M. Polydefkis, G. E. Smith, M. L. Clements, and

R. F. Siliciano. 1990. Induction of CD4+ human cytolytic T cells specific for HIV-infected cells by a gp160 subunit vaccine. *Science* **248**:1234–1237.

1989. Oriss, T. B., S. A. McCarthy, B. F. Morel, M. A. K. Campana, and P. A. Morel. 1997. Cross-regulation between T helper cell (Th)1 and Th2. *J Immunol* **158**:3666–3672.

1990. Orloff, G. M., M. S. Kennedy, C. Dawson, and J. S. McDougal. 1991. HIV-1 binding to CD4 T cells does not induce a Ca^{2+} influx or lead to activation of protein kinases. *AIDS Res Hum Retro* **7**:587–593.

1991. Orloff, G. M., S. L. Orloff, M. S. Kennedy, P. J. Maddon, and J. S. McDougal. 1991. The CD4 receptor does not internalize with HIV, and CD4-related signal transduction events are not required for entry. *J Immunol* **146**:2578–2587.

1992. Orloff, S. L., M. S. Kennedy, A. A. Belperron, P. J. Maddon, and J. S. McDougal. 1993. Two mechanisms of soluble CD4 (sCD4)-mediated inhibition of human immunodeficiency virus type 1 (HIV-1) infectivity and their relation to primary HIV-1 isolates with reduced sensitivity to sCD4. *J Virol* **67**:1461–1471.

1993. Oroszlan, S., and R. B. Luftig. 1990. Retroviral proteinases. *Curr Top Micro Immunol* **157**:153–185.

1994. Osborn, L., S. Kunkel, and G. J. Nabel. 1989. Tumor necrosis factor alpha and interleukin 1 stimulate the human immunodeficiency virus enhancer by activation of the nuclear factor kappa B. *Proc Natl Acad Sci USA* **86**:2336–2340.

1995. Osmond, D., P. Bacchetti, R. E. Chaisson, T. Kelly, R. Stempel, J. Carlson, and A. R. Moss. 1988. Time of exposure and risk of HIV infection in homosexual partners of men with AIDS. *Am J Pub Health* **78**:944–948.

1996. Osmond, D. H., S. Shiboski, P. Bacchetti, E. E. Winger, and A. R. Moss. 1991. Immune activation markers and AIDS prognosis. *AIDS* **5**:505–511.

1997. Ostrove, J. M., J. Leonard, K. E. Weck, A. B. Rabson, and H. E. Gendelman. 1987. Activation of the human immunodeficiency virus by herpes simplex virus type 1. *J Virol* **61**:3726–3732.

1998. Otsyula, M. G., C. J. Miller, A. F. Tarantal, M. L. Marthas, T. P. Greene, J. R. Collins, K. K. A. van Rompay, and M. B. McChesney. 1996. Fetal or neonatal infection with attenuated simian immunodeficiency virus results in protective immunity against oral challenge with pathogenic SIVmac251. *Virol* **222**:275–278.

1999. Ott, D. E., L. V. Coren, B. P. Kane, L. K. Busch, D. G. Johnson, R. C. Sowder II, E. N. Chertova, L. O. Arthur, and L. E. Henderson. 1996. Cytoskeletal proteins inside human immunodeficiency virus type 1 virions. *J Virol* **70**:7734–7743.

2000. Ou, C.-Y., C. A. Ciesielski, G. Myers, C. I. Bandea, C.-H. Luo, B. T. M. Korber, J. I. Mullins, G. Schochetman, R. L. Berkelman, A. N. Economou, J. J. Witte, L. J. Furman, G. A. Satten, K. A. MacInnes, J. W. Curran, and H. W. Jaffe. 1992. Molecular epidemiology of HIV transmission in a dental practice. *Science* **256**:1165–1171.

2001. Ou, C.-Y., S. Kwok, S. W. Mitchell, D. H. Mack, J. J. Sninsky, J. W. Krebs, P. Feorino, D. Warfield, and G. Schochetman. 1988. DNA amplification for direct detection of HIV-1 in DNA of peripheral blood mononuclear cells. *Science* **239**:295–297.

2002. Ou, C. Y., Y. Takebe, C. C. Luo, M. L. Kalish, W. Auwanit, S. Yamazaki, H. D. Gayle, N. L. Young, and G. Schochetman. 1993. Independent introduction of two major HIV-1 genotypes into distinct high-risk populations in Thailand. *Lancet* **341**:1171–1175.

2003. Ou, S. H. I., and R. B. Gaynor. 1995. Intracellular factors involved in gene expression of human retroviruses, p. 97–187. *In* J. A. Levy (ed.), *The Retroviridae*, vol. 4. Plenum Press, New York.

2004. Overbaugh, J., E. A. Hoover, J. I. Mullins, D. P. W. Burns, L. Rudensey, S. L. Quackenbush, V. Stallard, and P. R. Donohue. 1992. Structure and pathogenicity of individual variants within an immunodeficiency disease-inducing isolate of FeLV. *Virol* **188**:558–569.

2005. Owens, R. J., J. W. Dubay, E. Hunter, and R. W. Compans. 1991. Human immunodeficiency virus envelope protein determines the site of virus release in polarized epithelial cells. *Proc Natl Acad Sci USA* **88**:3987–3991.

2006. **Oxtoby, M. J.** 1990. Perinatally acquired human immunodeficiency virus infection. *Pediatr Infect Dis J* **9**:609–619.

2007. **Oyaizu, N., Y. Adachi, F. Hashimoto, T. W. McCloskey, N. Hosaka, N. Kayagaki, H. Yagita, and S. Pahwa.** 1997. Monocytes express Fas ligand upon CD4 cross-linking and induce CD4+ T cell apoptosis: a possible mechanism of bystander cell death in HIV infection. *J Immunol* **158**:2456–2463.

2008. **Oyaizu, N., N. Chirmule, V. S. Kalyanaraman, W. W. Hall, R. Pahwa, M. Shuster, and S. Pahwa.** 1990. Human immunodeficiency virus type 1 envelope glycoprotein gp120 produces immune defects in CD4+ T lymphocytes by inhibiting interleukin 2 mRNA. *Proc Natl Acad Sci USA* **87**:2379–2383.

2009. **Oyaizu, N., T. W. McCloskey, M. Coronesi, N. Chirmule, V. S. Kalyanaraman, and S. Pahwa.** 1993. Accelerated apoptosis in peripheral blood mononuclear cells (PBMCs) from human immunodeficiency virus type-1 infected patients and in CD4 cross-linked PBMCs from normal individuals. *Blood* **82**:3392–3400.

2010. **Ozel, M., G. Pauli, and H. R. Gelderblom.** 1988. The organization of the envelope projections on the surface of HIV. *Arch Virol* **100**:255–266.

2010a. **Padian, N. S., S. C. Shiboski, S. O. Glass, and E. Vittinghoff.** 1997. Heterosexual transmission of human immunodeficiency virus (HIV) in northern California: results from a ten-year study. *Am J Epidemiol* **146**:350–357.

2011. **Padian, N. S., S. Shiboski, and N. P. Jewell.** 1991. Female-to-male transmission of human immunodeficiency virus. *J Am Med Assoc* **266**:1664–1667.

2012. **Padian, N. S., S. C. Shiboski, and N. P. Jewell.** 1990. The effect of number of exposures on the risk of heterosexual HIV transmission. *J Inf Dis* **161**:883–887.

2013. **Paganin, C., D. S. Monos, J. D. Marshall, I. Frank, and G. Trinchieri.** 1997. Frequency and cytokine profile of HPRT mutant T cells in HIV-infected and healthy donors: implications for T cell proliferation in HIV disease. *J Clin Invest* **99**:663–668.

2014. **Page, J. B., S. Lai, D. D. Chitwood, N. G. Klimas, P. C. Smith, and M. A. Fletcher.** 1990. HTLV-I/II seropositivity and death from AIDS among HIV-1 seropositive intravenous drug users. *Lancet* **335**:1439–1441.

2015. **Page, K. A., S. M. Stearns, and D. R. Littman.** 1992. Analysis of mutations in the V3 domain of gp160 that affect fusion and infectivity. *J Virol* **66**:524–533.

2016. **Pahwa, S., N. Chirmule, C. Leombruno, W. Lim, R. Harper, R. Bhalla, R. Rahwa, R. P. Nelson, and R. A. Good.** 1989. *In vitro* synthesis of human immunodeficiency virus-specific antibodies in peripheral blood lympyhocytes of infants. *Proc Natl Acad Sci USA* **86**:7532–7536.

2017. **Pahwa, S., R. Pahwa, C. Saxinger, R. C. Gallo, and R. A. Good.** 1985. Influence of the human T-lymphotropic virus/lymphadenopathy-associated virus on functions of human lymphocytes: evidence for immunosuppressive effects and polyclonal B-cell activation by banded viral preparations. *Proc Natl Acad Sci USA* **82**:8198–8202.

2018. **Palamara, A. T., C.-F. Perno, S. Aquaro, M. C. Bue, L. Dini, and E. Garaci.** 1996. Glutathione inhibits HIV replication by acting at late stages of the virus life cycle. *AIDS Res Hum Retro* **12**:1537–1541.

2019. **Palasanthiran, P., J. B. Ziegler, G. J. Stewart, M. Stuckey, J. A. Armstrong, D. A. Cooper, R. Penny, and J. Gold.** 1993. Breast-feeding during primary maternal human immunodeficiency virus infection and risk of transmission from mother to infant. *J Inf Dis* **167**:441–444.

2020. **Palefsky, J. M.** 1994. Anal human papillomavirus infection and anal cancer in HIV-positive individuals: an emerging problem. *AIDS* **8**:283–295.

2021. **Palefsky, J. M., E. A. Holly, J. Gonzales, K. Lamborn, and H. Hollander.** 1992. Natural history of anal cytologic abnormalities and papillomavirus infection among homosexual men with group IV HIV disease. *J AIDS* **5**:1258–1265.

2022. **Paliard, X., A. Y. Lee, and C. M. Walker.** 1996. RANTES, MIP-1α and MIP-1β are not involved in the inhibition of HIV-1$_{SF33}$ replication mediated by CD8+ T-cell clones. *AIDS* **10**:1317–1321.

2022a. **Pan, L.-Z., and J. A. Levy.** Unpublished observations.

2023. Pan, L.-Z., A. Werner, and J. A. Levy. 1993. Detection of plasma viremia in HIV-infected individuals at all clinical stages. *J Clin Micro* 31:283–288.

2024. Pandolfi, F., M. Pierdominici, A. Oliva, G. D'Offizi, I. Mezzaroma, B. Mollicone, A. Giovannetti, L. Rainaldi, I. Quinti, and F. Aiuti. 1995. Apoptosis-related mortality in vitro of mononuclear cells from patients with HIV infection correlates with disease severity and progression. *J AIDS Hum Retrovirol* 9:450–458.

2025. Pandori, M. W., N. J. S. Fitch, H. M. Craig, D. D. Richman, C. A. Spina, and J. C. Guatelli. 1996. Producer-cell modification of human immunodeficiency virus type 1: Nef is a virion protein. *J Virol* 70:4283–4290.

2026. Pang, S., Y. Koyanagi, S. Miles, C. Wiley, H. V. Vinters, and I. S. Y. Chen. 1990. High levels of unintegrated HIV-1 DNA in brain tissue of AIDS dementia patients. *Nature* 343:85–89.

2027. Pang, S., Y. Shlesinger, E. S. Daar, T. Moudgil, D. D. Ho, and I. S. Y. Chen. 1992. Rapid generation of sequence variation during primary HIV-1 infection. *AIDS* 6:453–460.

2028. Pang, S., H. V. Vinters, T. Akashi, W. A. O'Brien, and I. S. Y. Chen. 1991. HIV-1 *env* sequence variation in brain tissue of patients with AIDS-related neurologic disease. *J AIDS* 4:1082–1092.

2029. Pantaleo, G. 1997. How immune-based interventions can change HIV therapy. *Nature Med* 3:483–490.

2030. Pantaleo, G., L. Butini, C. Graziosi, G. Poli, S. M. Schnittman, J. J. Greenhouse, J. I. Gallin, and A. S. Fauci. 1991. Human immunodeficiency virus (HIV) infection in CD4+ T lymphocytes genetically deficient in LFA-1: LFA-1 is required for HIV-mediated cell fusion but not for viral transmission. *J Exp Med* 173:511–514.

2032. Pantaleo, G., A. De Maria, S. Koenig, L. Butini, B. Moss, M. Baseler, H. C. Lane, and A. S. Fauci. 1990. CD8+ T lymphocytes of patients with AIDS maintain normal broad cytolytic function despite the loss of human immunodeficiency virus-specific cytotoxicity. *Proc Natl Acad Sci USA* 87:4818–4822.

2033. Pantaleo, G., J. F. Demarest, T. Schacker, M. Vaccarezza, O. J. Cohen, M. Daucher, C. Graziosi, S. S. Schnittman, T. C. Quinn, G. M. Shaw, L. Perrin, G. Tambussi, A. Lazzarin, R. P. Sekaly, H. Soudeyns, L. Corey, and A. S. Fauci. 1997. The qualitative nature of the primary immune response to HIV infection is a prognosticator of disease progression independent of the initial level of plasma viremia. *Proc Natl Acad Sci USA* 94:254–258.

2034. Pantaleo, G., J. F. Demarest, H. Soudeyns, C. Graziosi, F. Denis, J. W. Adelsberger, P. Borrow, M. S. Saag, G. M. Shaw, R. P. Sekaly, and A. S. Fauci. 1994. Major expansion of CD8+ T cells with a predominant Vβ usage during the primary immune response to HIV. *Nature* 370:463–467.

2035. Pantaleo, G., C. Graziosi, L. Butini, P. A. Pizzo, S. M. Schnittman, D. P. Kotler, and A. S. Fauci. 1991. Lymphoid organs function as major reservoirs for human immunodeficiency virus. *Proc Natl Acad Sci USA* 88:9838–9842.

2036. Pantaleo, G., C. Graziosi, J. F. Demarest, L. Butini, M. Montroni, C. H. Fox, J. M. Orenstein, D. P. Kotler, and A. S. Fauci. 1993. HIV infection is active and progressive in lymphoid tissue during the clinically latent stage of disease. *Nature* 362:355–358.

2037. Pantaleo, G., C. Graziosi, and A. S. Fauci. 1993. Mechanisms of disease: the immunopathogenesis of human immunodeficiency virus infection. *N Engl J Med* 328:327–336.

2038. Pantaleo, G., C. Graziosi, and A. S. Fauci. 1993. The role of lymphoid organs in the pathogenesis of HIV infection. *Sem Immunol* 5:157–163.

2039. Pantaleo, G., S. Koenig, M. Baseler, H. C. Lane, and A. S. Fauci. 1990. Defective clonogenic potential of CD8+ T-lymphocytes in patients with AIDS: expansion in vivo of a nonclonogenic CD3+CD8+CD25− T cell population. *J Immunol* 144:1696–1704.

2040. Pantaleo, G., S. Menzo, M. Vaccarezza, C. Graziosi, O. J. Cohen, J. F. Demarest, D. Montefiori, J. M. Orenstein, C. Fox, L. K. Schrager, J. B. Margolick, S. Buchbinder, J. V. Giorgi, and A. S. Fauci. 1995. Studies in subjects with long-term nonprogressive human immunodeficiency virus infection. *N Engl J Med* 332:209–216.

2041. **Pardoll, D.** 1992. New strategies for active immunotherapy with genetically engineered tumor cells. *Curr Opin Immunol* **4**:619–623.

2042. **Parekh, B. S., N. Shaffer, R. Coughlin, C. H. Hung, K. Krasinski, E. Abrams, M. Bamji, P. Thomas, D. Hutson, G. Schochetman, M. Rogers, and J. R. George.** 1993. Dynamics of maternal IgG antibody decay and HIV-specific antibody synthesis in infants born to seropositive mothers. *AIDS Res Hum Retro* **9**:907–912.

2043. **Parish, C. R., and F. Y. Liew.** 1972. Immune response to chemically modified flagellin. III. Enhanced cell-mediated immunity during high and low zone antibody tolerance to flagellin. *J Exp Med* **135**:298–311.

2044. **Parra, E., A. G. Wingren, G. Hedlund, T. Kalland, and M. Dohlsten.** 1997. The role of B7–1 and LFA-3 in costimulation of CD8+ T cells. *J Immunol* **158**:637–642.

2045. **Parravicini, C. L., D. Klatzmann, P. Jaffray, G. Costanzi, and J.-C. Gluckman.** 1988. Monoclonal antibodies to the human immunodeficiency virus p18 protein cross-react with normal human tissues. *AIDS* **2**:171–177.

2046. **Patarroyo, M. E., R. Amador, P. Clavijo, A. Moreno, F. Guzman, P. Romero, R. Tascon, A. Franco, L. A. Murillo, G. Ponton, and G. Trujillo.** 1988. A synthetic vaccine protects humans against challenge with asexual blood stages of *Plasmodium falciparum* malaria. *Nature* **332**:158–161.

2047. **Patick, A. K., H. Mo, M. Markowitz, K. Appelt, B. Wu, L. Musick, V. Kalish, S. Kaldor, S. Reich, D. Ho, and S. Webber.** 1996. Antiviral and resistance studies of AG1343, an orally bioavailable inhibitor of human immunodeficiency virus protease. *Antimicrob Agents Chemo* **40**:292–297.

2047a. **Patterson, B, and A. Landay.** Personal communication.

2048. **Patterson, B. K., M. Till, P. Otto, C. Goolsby, M. R. Furtado, L. J. McBride, and S. M. Wolinsky.** 1993. Detection of HIV-1 DNA and messenger RNA in individual cells by PCR-driven in situ hybridization and flow cytometry. *Science* **260**:976–979.

2049. **Patterson, S., and S. C. Knight.** 1987. Susceptibility of human peripheral blood dendritic cells to infection by human immunodeficiency virus. *J Gen Virol* **68**:1177–1181.

2050. **Paul, M. O., S. Tetali, M. L. Lesser, E. J. Abrams, X. P. Wang, R. Kowalski, M. Bamji, B. Napolitano, L. Gulick, S. Bakshi, and S. Pahwa.** 1996. Laboratory diagnosis of infection status in infants perinatally exposed to human immunodeficiency virus type 1. *J Inf Dis* **173**:68–76.

2051. **Paul, N. L., M. Marsh, J. A. McKeating, T. F. Schulz, P. Liljestrom, H. Garoff, and R. A. Weiss.** 1993. Expression of HIV-1 envelope glycoproteins by Semliki Forest virus vectors. *AIDS Res Hum Retro* **9**:963–970.

2052. **Pauza, C. D., J. E. Galindo, and D. D. Richman.** 1990. Reinfection results in accumulation of unintegrated viral DNA in cytopathic and persistent human immunodeficiency virus type 1 infection of CEM cells. *J Exp Med* **172**:1035–1042.

2053. **Pauza, C. D., and T. M. Price.** 1988. Human immunodeficiency virus infection of T cells and monocytes proceeds via receptor-mediated endocytosis. *J Cell Biol* **107**:959–968.

2054. **Paxton, W., R. I. Connor, and N. R. Landau.** 1993. Incorporation of Vpr into human immunodeficiency virus type 1 virions: requirement for the p6 region of gag and mutational analysis. *J Virol* **67**:7229–7237.

2055. **Pearce-Pratt, R., and D. M. Phillips.** 1993. Studies of adhesion of lymphocytic cells: implications for sexual transmission of HIV. *Biol Repro* **48**:431–435.

2056. **Peckham, C., and D. Gibb.** 1995. Mother-to-child transmission of the human immunodeficiency virus. *N Engl J Med* **333**:298–302.

2057. **Peden, K., M. Emerman, and L. Montagnier.** 1991. Changes in growth properties on passage in tissue culture of viruses derived from infectious molecular clones of HIV-1$_{LAI}$, HIV-1$_{MAL}$, and HIV-1$_{ELI}$. *Virol* **185**:661–672.

2058. **Pedersen, C., B. O. Lindhardt, B. L. Jensen, E. Lauritzen, J. Gerstoft, E. Dickmeiss, J. Gaub, E. Scheibel, and T. Karlsmark.** 1989. Clinical course of primary HIV infection: consequences for subsequent course of infection. *Brit Med J* **299**:154–157.

2059. Pedersen, N. C., and J. F. Boyle. 1980. Immunologic phenomena in the effusive form of feline infectious peritonitis. *Am J Vet Res* **44**:868–876.

2060. Pedersen, N. C., E. W. Ho, M. L. Brown, and J. K. Yamamoto. 1987. Isolation of a T-lymphotropic virus from domestic cats with an immunodeficiency-like syndrome. *Science* **235**:790–793.

2061. Peeters, M., K. Fransen, F. Delaporte, M. Van den Haesevelde, G. M. Gershy-Damet, L. Kestens, G. van der Groen, and P. Piot. 1992. Isolation and characterization of a new chimpanzee lentivirus (simian immunodeficiency virus isolate cpz-ant) from a wild-captured chimpanzee. *AIDS* **6**:447–452.

2062. Peeters, M., C.-Y. Gershy-Damet, K. Fransen, K. Koffi, M. Coulibaly, E. Delaporte, P. Piot, and G. van der Groen. 1992. Virological and polymerase chain reaction studies of HIV-1/HIV-2 dual infection in Cote d'Ivoire. *Lancet* **340**:339–340.

2063. Peeters, M., A. Gueye, S. Mboup, F. Bibollet-Ruche, E. Ekaza, C. Mulanga, R. Ouedrago, R. Gandji, P. Mpele, G. Dibanga, B. Koumare, M. Saidou, E. Esu-Williams, J.-P. Lombart, W. Badombena, N. Luo, M. Vanden Haesevelde, and E. Delaporte. 1997. Geographical distribution of HIV-1 group O viruses in Africa. *AIDS* **11**:493–498.

2064. Peeters, M., P. Piot, and G. van der Groen. 1991. Variability among HIV and SIV strains of African origin. *AIDS* **5**:S29–S36.

2065. Peiris, J. S. M., and J. S. Porterfield. 1979. Antibody-mediated enhancement of flavivirus replication in macrophage-like cell lines. *Nature* **282**:509–511.

2066. Pelicci, P.-G., D. M. Knowles, I. Magrath, and R. Dalla-Favera. 1986. Chromosomal breakpoints and structural alterations of the c-myc locus differ in endemic and sporadic forms of Burkitt's lymphoma. *Proc Natl Acad Sci USA* **83**:2984–2988.

2067. Peng, H., D. E. Callison, P. Li, and C. J. Burrell. 1997. Enhancement or inhibition of HIV-1 replication by intracellular expression of sense or antisense RNA targeted at different intermediates of reverse transcription. *AIDS* **11**:587–595.

2068. Penn, I. 1986. Cancers of the anogenital region in renal transplant recipients. Analysis of 65 cases. *Am J Obstet Gynecol* **58**:611–616.

2069. Penn, I. 1981. Depressed immunity and the development of cancer. *Clin Exp Immunol* **46**:459–474.

2070. Penn, I. 1979. Kaposi's sarcoma in organ transplant recipients: report of 20 cases. *Transplantation* **27**:8.

2071. Pepin, J., G. Morgan, D. Dunn, S. Gevao, M. Mendy, I. Gaye, N. Scollen, R. Tedder, and H. Whittle. 1991. HIV-2-induced immunosuppression among asymptomatic West African prostitutes: evidence that HIV-2 is pathogenic, but less so than HIV-1. *AIDS* **5**:1165–1172.

2072. Perelson, A. S., P. Essunger, Y. Cao, M. Vesanen, A. Hurley, K. Saksela, M. Markowitz, and D. D. Ho. 1997. Decay characteristics of HIV-1-infected compartments during combination therapy. *Nature* **387**:188–191.

2073. Perelson, A. S., A. U. Neumann, M. Markowitz, J. M. Leonard, and D. D. Ho. 1996. HIV-1 dynamics *in vivo*: virion clearance rate, infected cell life-span, and viral generation time. *Science* **271**:1582–1586.

2074. Perez, L. G., M. A. O'Donnell, and E. B. Stephens. 1992. The transmembrane glycoprotein of human immunodeficiency virus type 1 induces syncytium formation in the absence of the receptor binding glycoprotein. *J Virol* **66**:4134–4143.

2075. Perkins, H. A., S. Samsen, J. Garner, D. Echenberg, J. R. Allen, M. Cowan, and J. A. Levy. 1987. Risk of acquired immunodeficiency syndrome (AIDS) for recipients of blood components from donors who subsequently developed AIDS. *Blood* **70**:1604–1610.

2076. Perno, C.-F., M. W. Baseler, S. Broder, and R. Yarchoan. 1990. Infection of monocytes by human immunodeficiency virus type 1 blocked by inhibitors of CD4-gp120 binding, even in the presence of enhancing antibodies. *J Exp Med* **171**:1043–1056.

2077. Perotti, M. E., X. Tan, and D. M. Phillips. 1996. Directional budding of human immunodeficiency virus from monocytes. *J Virol* **70**:5916–5921.

2078. Perry, V. H., and S. Gordon. 1988. Macrophages and microglia in the nervous system. *Trends NeuroSci* **11**:273–277.

2079. Persidsky, Y., M. Stins, D. Way, M. H. Witte, M. Weinand, K. S. Kim, P. Bock, H. E. Gendelman, and M. Fiala. 1997. A model for monocyte migration through the blood-brain barrier during HIV-1 encephalitis. *J Immunol* **158**:3499–3510.

2080. Pert, C. B., C. C. Smith, M. R. Ruff, and J. M. Hill. 1988. AIDS and its dementia as a neuropeptide disorder: role of VIP receptor blockade by human immunodeficiency virus envelope. *Ann Neurol* **23**:s71–s73.

2081. Peterlin, B. M. 1995. Molecular biology of HIV, p. 185–238. *In* J. A. Levy (ed.), *The Retroviridae*, vol. 4. Plenum Press, New York.

2082. Peterman, T. A., H. W. Jaffe, and V. Beral. 1993. Epidemiologic clues to the etiology of Kaposi's sarcoma. *AIDS* **7**:605–611.

2083. Peterman, T. A., H. W. Jaffe, and P. M. Feorino. 1985. Transfusion-associated acquired immunodeficiency syndrome in the United States. *J Am Med Assoc* **254**:2913–2917.

2084. Peterson, P. K., G. Gekker, C. C. Chao, S. Hu, C. Edelman, H. H. Balfour, Jr., and J. Verhoef. 1992. Human cytomegalovirus-stimulated peripheral blood mononuclear cells induce HIV-1 replication via a tumor necrosis factor-alpha-mediated mechanism. *J Clin Invest* **89**:574–580.

2085. Peterson, P. K., G. Gekker, C. C. Chao, R. Schut, J. Verhoef, C. K. Edelman, A. Erice, and H. H. Balfour. 1992. Cocaine amplifies HIV-1 replication in cytomegalovirus-stimulated peripheral blood mononuclear cell coculture. *J Immunol* **149**:676–680.

2086. Petito, C. K., B. A. Navia, E.-S. Cho, B. D. Jordan, D. C. George, and R. W. Price. 1985. Vacuolar myelopathy pathologically resembling subacute combined degeneration in patients with the acquired immunodeficiency syndrome. *N Engl J Med* **312**:874–879.

2087. Petry, H., U. Dittmer, C. Stahl-Hennig, C. Coulibaly, B. Makoschey, D. Fuchs, H. Wachter, T. Tolle, C. Morys-Wortmann, F.-J. Kaup, E. Jurkiewicz, W. Luke, and G. Hunsmann. 1995. Reactivation of human immunodeficiency virus type 2 in macaques after simian immunodeficiency virus SIVmac superinfection. *J Virol* **69**:1564–1574.

2088. Peudenier, S., C. Hery, L. Montagnier, and M. Tardieu. 1991. Human microglial cells: characterization in cerebral tissue and in primary culture, and study of their susceptibility to HIV-1 infection. *Ann Neurol* **29**:152–161.

2088a.Phillips, A. N., C. A. Lee, J. Elford, G. Janossy, A. Timms, M. Bofill, and P. B. A. Kernoff. 1991. Serial CD4 lymphocyte counts and development of AIDS. *Lancet* **337**:389–392.

2089. Phillips, A. N., C. A. Sabin, J. Elford, M. Bofill, C. A. Lee, and G. Janossy. 1993. CD8 lymphocyte counts and serum immunoglobulin A levels early in HIV infection as predictors of CD4 lymphocyte depletion during 8 years of follow-up. *AIDS* **7**:975–980.

2089a.Phillips, D. Personal communication.

2090. Phillips, D. M., and A. S. Bourinbaiar. 1992. Mechanism of HIV spread from lymphocytes to epithelia. *Virol* **186**:261–273.

2091. Phillips, R. E., S. Rowland-Jones, D. F. Nixon, F. M. Gotch, J. P. Edwards, A. O. Ogunlesi, J. G. Elvin, J. A. Rothbard, C. R. M. Bangham, C. R. Rizza, and A. J. McMichael. 1991. Human immunodeficiency virus genetic variation that can escape cytotoxic T cell recognition. *Nature* **354**:453–459.

2092. Piatak, M., Jr., S. Saag, L. C. Yang, J. C. Kappes, K.-C. Luk, B. H. Hahn, G. M. Shaw, and J. D. Lifson. 1993. High levels of HIV-1 in plasma during all stages of infection determined by competitive PCR. *Science* **259**:1749–1754.

2093. Piazza, C., M. S. Gilardini Montani, S. Moretti, E. Cundari, and E. Piccolella. 1997. CD4+ T cells kill CD8+ T cells via Fas/Fas ligand-mediated apoptosis. *J Immunol* **158**:1503–1506.

2094. Picard, L., D. A. Wilkinson, A. McKnight, P. W. Gray, J. A. Hoxie, P. R. Clapham, and R. A. Weiss. 1997. Role of the amino-terminal extracellular domain of CXCR-4 in human immunodeficiency virus type 1 entry. *Virol* **231**:105–111.

2095. Pinter, A., W. J. Honnen, M. E. Racho, and S. A. Tilley. 1993. A potent, neutralizing human monoclonal antibody against a unique epitope overlapping the CD4-binding site of HIV-1 gp120 that is broadly conserved across North American and African virus isolates. *AIDS Res Hum Retro* **9**:985–996.

2096. Pinter, A., W. J. Honnen, and S. A. Tilley. 1993. Conformational changes affecting the V3 and CD4-binding domains of human immunodeficiency virus type 1 gp120 associated with env processing and with binding of ligands to these sites. *J Virol* **67**:5692–5697.

2097. Pinter, A., W. J. Honnen, S. A. Tilley, C. Bona, H. Zaghouani, M. K. Gorny, and S. Zolla-Pazner. 1989. Oligomeric structure of gp41, the transmembrane protein of human immunodeficiency virus type 1. *J Virol* **63**:2674–2679.

2098. Pinto, L. A., J. Sullivan, J. A. Berzofsky, M. Clerici, H. A. Kessler, A. L. Landay, and G. M. Shearer. 1995. ENV-specific cytotoxic T lymphocyte responses in HIV seronegative health care workers occupationally exposed to HIV-contaminated body fluids. *J Clin Invest* **96**:867–876.

2099. Pitrak, D. L., P. M. Bak, P. DeMarais, R. M. Novak, and B. R. Andersen. 1993. Depressed neutrophil superoxide production in human immunodeficiency virus infection. *J Inf Dis* **167**:1406–1410.

2100. Plaeger-Marshall, S., M. A. Hausner, V. Isacescu, and J. V. Giorgi. 1992. CD8 T-cell-mediated inhibition of HIV replication in HIV infected adults and children. *AIDS Res Hum Retro* **8**:1375–1376.

2101. Planz, O., P. Seiler, H. Hengartner, and R. M. Zinkernagel. 1996. Specific cytotoxic T cells eliminate B cells producing virus-neutralizing antibodies. *Nature* **382**:726–729.

2102. Plata, F. 1989. HIV-specific cytotoxic T lymphocytes. *Res Immunol* **140**:89–91.

2103. Plata, F., F. Garcia-Pons, A. Ryter, F. Lebargy, M. M. Goodenow, M. H. Q. Dat, B. Autran, and C. Mayaud. 1990. HIV-1 infection of lung alveolar fibroblasts and macrophages in humans. *AIDS Res Hum Retro* **6**:979–986.

2104. Platt, E. J., N. Madani, S. L. Kozak, and D. Kabat. 1997. Infectious properties of human immunodeficiency virus type 1 mutants with distinct affinities for the CD4 receptor. *J Virol* **71**:883–890.

2105. Pleskoff, O., C. Treboute, A. Brelot, N. Heveker, M. Seman, and M. Alizon. 1997. Identification of a chemokine receptor encoded by human cytomegalovirus as a cofactor for HIV-1 entry. *Science* **276**:1874–1878.

2106. Pluda, J. M., R. Yarchoan, E. S. Jaffe, I. M. Feuerstein, D. Solomon, S. M. Steinberg, K. M. Wyvill, A. Raubitschek, D. Katz, and S. Broder. 1990. Development of non-Hodgkin lymphoma in a cohort of patients with severe human immunodeficiency virus (HIV) infection on long-term antiretroviral therapy. *Ann Int Med* **113**:276–282.

2107. Plummer, F. A., J. N. Simonsen, D. W. Cameron, J. O. Ndinya-Achola, J. K. Kreiss, M. N. Gakinya, P. Waiyaki, M. Cheang, P. Piot, A. R. Ronald, and E. N. Ngugi. 1991. Cofactors in male-female sexual transmission of human immunodeficiency virus type 1. *J Inf Dis* **163**:233–239.

2108. Poiesz, B. J., F. W. Ruscetti, A. F. Gazdar, P. A. Bunn, J. D. Minna, and R. C. Gallo. 1980. Detection and isolation of type C retrovirus particles from fresh and cultured lymphocytes of a patient with cutaneous T cell lymphoma. *Proc Natl Acad Sci USA* **77**:7415–7418.

2109. Polacino, P., V. Stallard, J. Klaniecki, C. Brown, R. Watanabe, W. R. Morton, R. E. Benveniste, and S. L. Hu. 1996. Immunization with SIV$_{mnc}$ envelope gp160 vaccines protected macaques against intrarectal challenge by uncloned virus. Abstr. M.A103. *XI International Conference on AIDS*, Vancouver, Canada.

2110. Polak, J. M., A. G. E. Pearse, and C. M. Heath. 1975. Complete identification of endocrine cells in the gastrointestinal tract using semithin-thin sections to identify motilin cells in human and animal intestine. *Gut* **16**:225–229.

2111. Poland, S. D., G. P. A. Rice, and G. A. Dekaban. 1995. HIV-1 infection of human brain-derived microvascular endothelial cells in vitro. *J AIDS Hum Retrovirol* **8**:437–445.

2112. Poli, G., B. Bottazzi, R. Acero, L. Bersani, V. Rossi, M. Introna, A. Lazzarini, M. Galli, and A. Mantovani. 1985. Monocyte function in intravenous drug abusers with acquired immunodeficiency syndrome: selective impairment of chemotaxis. *Clin Exp Immunol* **62**:136–142.

2113. Poli, G., and A. S. Fauci. 1993. Cytokine modulation of HIV expression. *Sem Immunol* **5**:165–173.

2114. **Poli, G., and A. S. Fauci.** 1992. The effect of cytokines and pharmacologic agents on chronic HIV infection. *AIDS Res Hum Retro* **8**:191–197.

2115. **Poli, G., A. Kinter, J. S. Justement, J. H. Kehrl, P. Bressler, S. Stanley, and A. S. Fauci.** 1990. Tumor necrosis factor alpha functions in an autocrine manner in the induction of human immunodeficiency virus expression. *Proc Natl Acad Sci USA* **87**:782–785.

2116. **Pollack, H., M.-X. Zhan, J. T. Safrit, S.-H. Chen, G. Rochford, P.-Z. Tao, R. Koup, K. Krasinski, and W. Borkowsky.** 1997. CD8+ T-cell-mediated suppression of HIV replication in the first year of life: association with lower viral load and favorable early survival. *AIDS* **11**:F9-F13.

2117. **Pollack, M. S., B. Safai, and B. Dupont.** 1983. HLA-DR5 and DR2 are susceptibility factors for acquired immunodeficiency syndrome with Kaposi's sarcoma in different ethnic populations. *Dis Markers* **1**:135–139.

2117a.**Polyak, S., H. Chen, D. Hirsch, I. George, R. Hershberg, and K. Sperber.** 1997. Impaired class II expression and antigen uptake in monocytic cells after HIV-1 infection. *J Immunol* **159**:2177–2188.

2118. **Pomerantz, R. J., S. M. de la Monte, S. P. Donegan, T. R. Rota, M. W. Vogt, D. E. Craven, and M. S. Hirsch.** 1988. Human immunodeficiency virus (HIV) infection of the uterine cervix. *Ann Int Med* **108**:321–327.

2119. **Pomerantz, R. J., D. R. Kuritzkes, S. M. de la Monte, T. R. Rota, A. S. Baker, D. Albert, D. H. Bor, E. L. Feldman, R. T. Schooley, and M. S. Hirsch.** 1987. Infection of the retina by human immunodeficiency virus type 1. *N Engl J Med* **317**:1643–1647.

2120. **Pomerantz, R. J., D. Trono, M. B. Feinberg, and D. Baltimore.** 1990. Cells nonproductively infected with HIV-1 exhibit an aberrant pattern of viral RNA expression: a molecular model for latency. *Cell* **61**:1271–1276.

2120a.**Pope, M., S. S. Frankel, J. R. Mascola, A. Trkola, F. Isdell, D. L. Birx, D. S. Burke, D. D. Ho, and J. P. Moore.** 1997. Human immunodeficiency virus type 1 strains of subtypes B and E replicate in cutaneous dendritic cell-T cell mixtures without displaying subtype-specific tropism. *J Virol* **71**:8001–8007.

2120b.**Pope, M., S. Gezelter, N. Gallo, L. Hoffman, and R. M. Steinman.** 1995. Low levels of HIV-1 infection in cutaneous dendritic cells promote extensive viral replication upon binding to memory CD4+ T cells. *J Exp Med* **182**:2045–2056.

2121. **Popovic, M., and S. Gartner.** 1987. Isolation of HIV-1 from monocytes but not T lymphocytes. *Lancet* **ii**:916.

2122. **Popovic, M., M. G. Sarngadharan, E. Read, and R. C. Gallo.** 1984. Detection, isolation, and continuous production of cytopathic retroviruses (HTLV-III) from patients with AIDS and pre-AIDS. *Science* **224**:497–500.

2123. **Portegies, P.** 1994. AIDS dementia complex: a review. *J AIDS* **7**:S38-S48.

2124. **Portegies, P., J. de Gans, J. M. A. Lange, M. M. A. Derix, H. Speelman, M. Bakker, S. A. Danner, and J. Goudsmit.** 1989. Declining incidence of AIDS dementia complex after introduction of zidovudine treatment. *Brit Med J* **291**:819–821.

2125. **Porter, D. C., D. C. Ansardi, W. S. Choi, and C. D. Morrow.** 1993. Encapsidation of genetically engineered poliovirus minireplicons which express human immunodeficiency virus type 1 gag and pol proteins upon infection. *J Virol* **67**:3712–3719.

2126. **Posner, M. R., T. Hideshima, T. Cannon, M. Murkherjee, K. H. Mayer, and R. A. Byrn.** 1991. An IgG human monoclonal antibody that reacts with HIV-1/gp120, inhibits virus binding to cells, and neutralizes infection. *J Immunol* **146**:4325–4332.

2127. **Posnett, D. N., S. Kabak, A. S. Hodtsev, E. A. Goldberg, and A. Asch.** 1993. T-cell antigen receptor V-beta subsets are not preferentially deleted in AIDS. *AIDS* **7**:625–631.

2128. **Poss, M., H. L. Matrin, J. K. Kreiss, L. Granville, B. Chohan, P. Nyange, K. Mandaliya, and J. Overbaugh.** 1995. Diversity in virus populations from genital secretions and peripheral blood from women recently infected with human immunodeficiency virus type 1. *J Virol* **69**:8118–8122.

2129. **Potash, M. J., M. Zeira, Z.-B. Huang, T. E. Pearce, E. Eden, H. E. Gendelman, and D. J. Volsky.** 1992. Virus-cell membrane fusion does not predict efficient infection of alveolar macrophages by human immunodeficiency virus type 1 (HIV-1). *Virol* **188**:864–868.

2130. Potempa, S., L. Picard, J. D. Reeves, D. Wilkinson, R. A. Weiss, and S. J. Talbot. 1997. CD4-independent infection by human immunodeficiency virus type 2 strain ROD/B: the role of the N-terminal domain of CXCR-4 in fusion and entry. *J Virol* 71:4419–4424.

2131. Potts, K. E., M. L. Kalish, T. Lott, G. Orloff, C. C. Luo, M. A. Bernard, C. B. Alves, R. Badaro, J. Suleiman, O. Ferreira, G. Schochetman, W. D. Johnson, Jr., C. Y. Ou, and J. L. Ho. 1993. Genetic heterogeneity of the principal neutralizing determinant of the human immunodeficiency virus type 1 (HIV-1) in Brazil. *AIDS* 7:1191–1197.

2132. Poulin, L., L. A. Evans, S. Tang, A. Barboza, H. Legg, D. R. Littman, and J. A. Levy. 1991. Several CD4 domains can play a role in human immunodeficiency virus infection of cells. *J Virol* 65:4893–4901.

2133. Poulin, L., and J. A. Levy. 1992. The HIV-1 nef gene product is associated with phosphorylation of a 46 kD cellular protein. *AIDS* 6:787–791.

2133a. Poulin, L., and J. A. Levy. Unpublished observations.

2134. Poulsen, A. G., B. Kvinesdal, P. Aaby, K. Molbak, K. Frederiksen, F. Dias, and E. Lauritzen. 1989. Prevalence of and mortality from human immunodeficiency virus type 2 in Bissau, West Africa. *Lancet* ii:827–830.

2135. Powell, J. D., D. P. Bednarik, T. M. Folks, T. Jehuda-Cohen, F. Villinger, K. W. Sell, and A. A. Ansari. 1993. Inhibition of cellular activity of retroviral replication by CD8 T cells derived from non-human primates. *Clin Exp Immunol* 91:473–481.

2136. Powell, J. D., T. Yehuda-Cohen, F. Villinger, H. M. McClure, K. W. Sell, and A. Ahmed-Ansari. 1990. Inhibition of SIV-SMM replication *in vitro* by CD8+ cells from SIV/SMM infected seropositive clinically asymptomatic sooty mangabeys. *J Med Primatol* 19:239–249.

2137. Power, C., J. C. McArthur, R. T. Johnson, D. E. Griffin, J. D. Glass, S. Perryman, and B. Chesebro. 1994. Demented and nondemented patients with AIDS differ in brain-derived human immunodeficiency virus type 1 envelope sequences. *J Virol* 68:4643–4649.

2138. Poznansky, M. C., R. Coker, C. Skinner, A. Hill, S. Bailey, L. Whitaker, A. Renton, and J. Weber. 1995. HIV positive patients first presenting with an AIDS defining illness: characteristics and survival. *Brit Med J* 311:156–158.

2139. Prabhakar, B. S., and N. Nathanson. 1981. Acute rabies death mediated by antibody. *Nature* 290:590–591.

2140. Pratt, R. D., J. F. Shapiro, N. McKinney, S. Kwok, and S. A. Spector. 1995. Virologic characterization of primary human immunodeficiency virus type 1 infection in a health care worker following needlestick injury. *J Inf Dis* 172:851–854.

2141. Prazuck, T., J. M. V. Yameogo, B. Heylinck, L. T. Ouedraogo, A. Rochereau, J. B. Guiard-Schmid, P. Lechuga, P. Agranat, M. Cot, J. E. Malkin, O. Patey, and C. Lafaix. 1995. Mother-to-child transmission of human immunodeficiency virus type 1 and type 2 and dual infection: a cohort study in Banfora, Burkina Faso. *Pediatr Infect Dis J* 14:940–947.

2142. Preston, B. D., B. J. Poiesz, and L. A. Loeb. 1988. Fidelity of HIV-1 reverse transcriptase. *Science* 242:1168–1171.

2143. Price, D. A., P. J. R. Goulder, P. Klenerman, A. K. Sewell, P. J. Easterbrook, M. Troop, C. R. M. Bangham, and R. E. Phillips. 1997. Positive selection of HIV-1 cytotoxic T lymphocyte escape variants during primary infection. *Proc Natl Acad Sci USA* 94:1890–1895.

2144. Price, R. W. 1996. Neurological complications of HIV infection. *Lancet* 348:445–452.

2145. Price, R. W., B. Brew, J. Sidtis, M. Rosenblum, A. G. Scheck, and P. Clearly. 1988. The brain in AIDS: central nervous system HIV-1 infection and AIDS dementia complex. *Science* 239:586–592.

2145a. Prince, A. M. Personal communication.

2146. Prince, A. M., B. Horowitz, L. Baker, R. W. Shulman, H. Ralph, J. Valinsky, A. Cundell, B. Brotman, W. Boehle, F. Rey, M. Piet, H. Reesink, N. Lelie, M. Tersmette, F. Miedema, L. Barbosa, G. Nemo, C. L. Nastala, J. S. Allan, D. R. Lee, and J. W. Eichberg. 1988. Failure of a human immunodeficiency virus (HIV) immune globulin to protect chimpanzees against experimental challenge with HIV. *Proc Natl Acad Sci USA* 85:6944–6948.

2147. Prince, A. M., H. Reesink, D. Pascual, B. Horowitz, I. Hewlett, K. K. Murthy, K. E. Cobb, and J. W. Eichberg. 1991. Prevention of HIV infection by passive immunization with HIV immunoglobulin. *AIDS Res Hum Retro* **7**:971–973.

2148. Prince, H. E., and E. R. Jensen. 1991. HIV-related alterations in CD8 cell subsets defined by in vitro survival characteristics. *Cell Immunol* **134**:276–286.

2149. Psallidopoulos, M. C., S. M. Schnittman, L. M. Thompson III, M. Baseler, A. S. Fauci, H. C. Lane, and N. P. Salzman. 1989. Integrated proviral human immunodeficiency virus type 1 is present in CD4+ peripheral blood lymphocytes in healthy seropositive individuals. *J Virol* **63**:4626–4631.

2150. Pu, R., S. Okada, E. R. Little, B. Xu, W. V. Stoffs, and J. K. Yamamoto. 1995. Protection of neonatal kittens against feline immunodeficiency virus infection with passive maternal antiviral antibodies. *AIDS* **9**:235–242.

2151. Pudney, J., M. Oneta, K. Mayer, G. Seage III, and D. Anderson. 1992. Pre-ejaculatory fluid as potential vector for sexual transmission of HIV-1. *Lancet* **340**:1470.

2152. Pulakhandam, U., and H. P. Dincsoy. 1990. Cytomegaloviral adrenalitis and adrenal insufficiency in AIDS. *Am J Clin Path* **93**:651–656.

2152a. Pulliam, L. Personal communication.

2153. Pulliam, L., R. Gascon, M. Stubblebine, D. McGuire, and M. S. McGrath. 1997. Unique monocyte subset in patients with AIDS dementia. *Lancet* **349**:692–695.

2154. Pulliam, L., B. G. Herndier, N. M. Tang, and M. S. McGrath. 1991. Human immunodeficiency virus-infected macrophages produce soluble factors that cause histological and neurochemical alterations in cultured human brains. *J Clin Invest* **87**:503–512.

2155. Pulliam, L., D. West, N. Haigwood, and R. A. Swanson. 1993. HIV-1 envelope gp120 alters astrocytes in human brain cultures. *AIDS Res Hum Retro* **9**:439–444.

2156. Pumarola-Sune, T., B. A. Navia, C. Cordon-Cardo, E. S. Cho, and R. W. Price. 1987. HIV antigen in the brains of patients with the AIDS dementia complex. *Ann Neurol* **21**:490–496.

2157. Purtscher, M., A. Trkola, G. Gruber, A. Buchacher, R. Predl, F. Steindl, C. Tauer, R. Berger, N. Barrett, A. Jungbauder, and H. Katinger. 1994. A broadly neutralizing human monoclonal antibody against gp41 of human immunodeficiency virus type 1. *AIDS Res Hum Retro* **10**:1651–1658.

2158. Putkonen, P., R. Thorstensson, J. Albert, K. Hild, E. Norrby, P. Biberfeld, and G. Biberfeld. 1990. Infection of cynomolgus monkeys with HIV-2 protects against pathogenic consequences of a subsequent simian immunodeficiency virus infection. *AIDS* **4**:783–789.

2159. Putkonen, P., R. Thorstensson, L. Ghavamzadeh, J. Albert, K. Hild, G. Biberfeld, and E. Norrby. 1991. Prevention of HIV-2 and SIVsm infection by passive immunization in cynomolgus monkeys. *Nature* **352**:436–438.

2160. Putkonen, P., R. Thorstensson, L. Walther, J. Albert, L. Akerblom, O. Granquist, G. Wadell, E. Norrby, and G. Biberfeld. 1991. Vaccine protection against HIV-2 infection in cynomolgus monkeys. *AIDS Res Hum Retro* **7**:271–277.

2161. Putney, S. D., T. J. Matthews, W. G. Robey, D. D. Lynn, M. Robert-Guroff, W. T. Mueller, A. J. Langlois, J. Ghrayeb, S. R. Petteway, and K. J. Weinhold. 1986. HTLV-III/LAV-neutralizing antibodies to an E. coli-produced fragment of the virus envelope. *Science* **234**:1392–1395.

2162. Qian, J., V. Bours, J. Manischewitz, R. Blackburn, U. Siebenlist, and H. Golding. 1994. Chemically selected subclones of the CEM cell line demonstrate resistance to HIV-1 infection resulting from a selective loss of NF-κB DNA binding proteins. *J Immunol* **152**:4183–4191.

2162a. Quayle, A. J., C. Xu, K. H. Mayer, and D. J. Anderson. 1997. T lymphocytes and macrophages, but not motile spermatozoa, are a significant source of human immunodeficiency virus in semen. *J Inf Dis* **176**:960–968.

2163. Quesada-Rolander, M., B. Makitalo, R. Thorstensson, Y. J. Zhang, E. Castanos-Velez, G. Biberfeld, and P. Pukonen. 1996. Protection against mucosal SIV$_{sm}$ challenge in macaques infected with a chimeric SIV that expresses HIV type 1 envelope. *AIDS Res Hum Retro* **12**:993–999.

2164. Quinn, T. C. 1996. Global burden of the HIV pandemic. *Lancet* **348**:99–106.

2165. Quinn, T. C., R. L. Kline, N. Halsey, N. Hutton, A. Ruff, A. Butz, R. Boulos, and J. F. Modlin. 1991. Early diagnosis of perinatal HIV infection by detection of viral-specific IgA antibodies. *J Am Med Assoc* **266**:3439–3442.

2166. Qureshi, M. N., C. E. Barr, T. Seshamma, J. Reidy, R. J. Pomerantz, and O. Bagasra. 1995. Infection of oral mucosal cells by human immunodeficiency virus type 1 in seropositive persons. *J Inf Dis* **171**:190–193.

2167. Qureshi, N. M., D. H. Coy, R. F. Garry, and L. A. Henderson. 1990. Characterization of a putative cellular receptor for HIV-1 transmembrane glycoprotein using synthetic peptides. *AIDS* **4**:553–558.

2168. Rabeneck, L., M. Popovic, S. Gartner, D. M. McLean, W. A. McLeod, E. Read, K. K. Wong, and W. J. Boyko. 1990. Acute HIV infection presenting with painful swallowing and esophageal ulcers. *J Am Med Assoc* **263**:2318–2322.

2169. Rabinovich, N. R., P. McInnes, D. L. Klein, and B. F. Hall. 1994. Vaccine technologies: view to the future. *Science* **265**:1401–1404.

2170. Rabkin, C. S., J. J. Goedert, R. J. Biggar, F. Yellin, and W. A. Blattner. 1990. Kaposi's sarcoma in three HIV-1 infected cohorts. *J AIDS* **3**(Suppl. 1):S38–S43.

2171. Rabkin, C. S., S. Janz, A. Lash, A. E. Coleman, E. Musaba, L. Liotta, R. J. Biggar, and Z. Zhuang. 1997. Monoclonal origin of multicentric Kaposi's sarcoma lesions. *N Engl J Med* **336**:988–993.

2172. Rabkin, C. S., and F. Yellin. 1994. Cancer incidence in a population with a high prevalence of infection with human immunodeficiency virus type 1. *JNCI* **86**:1711–1716.

2173. Rabkin, J. G., J. B. W. Williams, R. H. Remien, R. Goetz, R. Kertzner, and J. M. Gorman. 1991. Depression, distress, lymphocyte subsets, and human immunodeficiency virus symptoms on two occasions in HIV-positive homosexual men. *Arch Gen Psychiatry* **48**:111–119.

2174. Raboud, J. M., J. S. G. Montaner, B. Conway, L. Haley, C. Sherlock, M. V. O'Shaughnessy, and M. T. Schecter. 1996. Variation in plasma RNA levels, CD4 cell counts, and p24 antigen levels in clinically stable men with human immunodeficiency virus infection. *J Inf Dis* **174**:191–194.

2175. Rabson, A., and M. Martin. 1985. Molecular organization of the AIDS retrovirus. *Cell* **40**:477–480.

2176. Racz, P., Tenner-Racz, K., C. Kahl, A. C. Feller, P. Kern, and M. Dietrich. 1986. Spectrum of morphologic changes of lymph nodes from patients with AIDS or AIDS-related complexes. *Prog Allergy* **37**:81–181.

2177. Rahman, A. A., M. Teschner, K. K. Sethi, and H. Brandis. 1976. Appearance of IgG (Fc) receptor(s) on cultured human fibroblasts infected with human cytomegalovirus. *J Immunol* **117**:253–258.

2178. Rameshwar, P., T. N. Denny, and P. Gascon. 1996. Enhanced HIV-1 activity in bone marrow can lead to myelopoietic suppression partially contributed by gag p24. *J Immunol* **157**:4244–4250.

2179. Ramilo, O., K. D. Bell, J. W. Uhr, and E. S. Vitetta. 1993. Role of CD25+ and CD25− T cells in acute HIV infection in vitro. *J Immunol* **150**:5202–5208.

2180. Rammensee, H. G., K. Falk, and O. Rotzschke. 1993. Peptides naturally presented by MHC class I molecules. *Annu Rev Immunol* **11**:213–244.

2181. Rana, S., G. Besson, D. G. Cook, J. Rucker, R. J. Smyth, Y. Yi, J. D. Turner, H. H. Guo, J. G. Du, S. C. Peiper, E. Lavi, M. Samson, F. Libert, C. Liesnard, G. Vassart, R. W. Doms, M. Parmentier, and R. G. Collman. 1997. Role of CCR5 in infection of primary macrophages and lymphocytes by macrophage-tropic strains of human immunodeficiency virus: resistance to patient-derived and prototype isolates resulting from the $\Delta ccr5$ mutation. *J Virol* **71**:3219–3227.

2182. Rando, R. F., A. Srinivasan, J. Feingold, E. Gonczol, and S. Plotkin. 1990. Characterization of multiple molecular interactions between human cytomegalovirus (HCMV) and human immunodeficiency virus type 1 (HIV-1). *Virol* **176**:87–97.

2183. Ranki, A., S. Mattinen, R. Yarchoan, S. Broder, J. Ghrayeb, J. Lahdevirta, and K. Krohn. 1989. T-cell response towards HIV in infected individuals with and without zidovudine therapy, and in HIV-exposed sexual partners. *AIDS* 3:63–69.

2184. Ranki, A., M. Nyberg, V. Ovod, M. Haltia, I. Elovaara, R. Raininko, H. Haapasalo, and K. Krohn. 1995. Abundant expression of HIV Nef and Rev proteins in brain astrocytes *in vivo* is associated with dementia. *AIDS* 9:1001–1008.

2185. Ranki, A., S.-L. Valle, M. Krohn, J. Antonen, J.-P. Allain, M. Leuther, G. Franchini, and K. Krohn. 1987. Long latency precedes overt seroconversion in sexually transmitted human-immunodeficiency-virus infection. *Lancet* ii:589–593.

2186. Rao, T. K. S., E. J. Filippone, A. D. Nicastri, S. H. Landesman, E. Frank, C. K. Chen, and E. A. Friedman. 1984. Associated focal and segmental glomerulosclerosis in the acquired immunodeficiency syndrome. *N Engl J Med* 310:669–673.

2187. Rappaport, J., J. B. Kopp, and P. E. Klotman. 1994. Host virus interactions and the molecular regulation of HIV-1: role in the pathogenesis of HIV-associated nephropathy. *Kidney Int* 46:16–27.

2188. Rappersberger, K., S. Gartner, P. Schenk, G. Stingl, V. Groh, E. Tschachler, D. L. Mann, K. Wolff, K. Konrad, and M. Popovic. 1988. Langerhans's cells are an actual site of HIV-1 replication. *Intervirol* 29:185–194.

2189. Rappersberger, K., E. Tschachler, and E. Zonzits. 1990. Endemic Kaposi's sarcoma in human immunodeficiency virus type 1-seronegative persons: demonstration of retrovirus-like particles in cutaneous lesions. *J Invest Derm* 95:371–381.

2190. Rasheed, S., A. A. Gottlieb, and R. F. Garry. 1986. Cell killing by ultraviolet-inactivated human immunodeficiency virus. *Virol* 154:395–400.

2191. Rasheed, S., Z. Li, D. Xu, and A. Kovacs. 1996. Presence of cell-free human immunodeficiency virus in cervicovaginal secretions is independent of viral load in the blood of human immunodeficiency virus-infected women. *Am J Obstet Gynecol* 175:122–129.

2192. Ratner, L. 1992. Glucosidase inhibitors for treatment of HIV-1 infection. *AIDS Res Hum Retro* 8:165–173.

2193. Ratner, L., W. Haseltine, R. Patarca, K. J. Livak, B. Starcich, S. F. Josephs, E. R. Doran, A. Rafalski, E. A. Whitehorn, K. Baumeister, L. Ivanoff, S. R. Petteway, Jr., M. L. Pearson, J. A. Lautenberger, T. S. Papas, J. Ghrayeb, N. T. Chang, R. C. Gallo, and F. Wong-Staal. 1985. Complete nucleotide sequence of the AIDS virus, HTLV-III. *Nature* 313:277–284.

2194. Rautonen, N., J. Rautonen, N. L. Martin, and D. W. Wara. 1994. HIV-1 Tat induces cytokine synthesis by uninfected mononuclear cells. *AIDS* 8:1504–1506.

2195. Rayfield, M., K. De Cock, W. Heyward, L. Goldstein, J. Krebs, S. Kwok, S. Lee, J. McCormick, J. M. Moreau, K. Odehouri, G. Schochetman, J. Sninsky, and C.-Y. Ou. 1988. Mixed human immunodeficiency virus (HIV) infection in an individual: demonstration of both HIV type 1 and type 2 proviral sequences by using polymerase chain reaction. *J Inf Dis* 158:1170–1176.

2196. Rayfield, M. A., P. Sullivan, C. I. Bandea, L. Britvan, R. A. Otten, C. P. Pau, D. Pieniazek, S. Subbarao, P. Simon, C. A. Schable, A. C. Wright, J. Ward, and G. Schochetman. 1996. HIV-1 group O virus identified for the first time in the United States. *Emerg Infect Dis* 2:209–212.

2197. Razvi, E. S., and R. M. Welsh. 1993. Programmed cell death of T lymphocytes during acute viral infection: a mechanism for virus-induced immune deficiency. *J Virol* 67:5754–5765.

2198. Re, F., D. Braaten, E. K. Franke, and J. Luban. 1995. Human immunodeficiency virus type 1 Vpr arrests the cell cycle in G$_2$ by inhibiting the activation of p34^{cdc2}-cyclin B. *J Virol* 69:6859-6864.

2199. Re, M. C., G. Furlini, G. Zauli, and M. La Placa. 1994. Human immunodeficiency virus type 1 (HIV-1) and human hematopoietic progenitor cells. *Arch Virol* 137:1–23.

2200. Re, M. C., G. Zauli, D. Gibellini, G. Furlini, E. Ramazzotti, P. Monari, S. Ranieri, S. Capitani, and M. La Placa. 1993. Uninfected haematopoietic progenitor (CD34+) cells purified from the bone marrow of AIDS patients are committed to apoptotic cell death in culture. *AIDS* 7:1049–1055.

2201. **Real, F. X., and S. E. Krown.** 1985. Spontaneous regression of Kaposi's sarcoma in patients with AIDS. *N Engl J Med* **313**:1659.

2202. **Rebai, N., G. Pantaleo, J. F. Demarest, C. Ciurli, H. Soudeyns, J. W. Adelsberger, M. Vaccarezza, R. E. Walker, R. P. Sekaly, and A. S. Fauci.** 1994. Analysis of the T-cell receptor β-chain variable region (Vβ) repertoire in monozygotic twins discordant for human immunodeficiency virus: evidence for perturbations of specific Vβ segments in CD4+ T cells of the virus-positive twins. *Proc Natl Acad Sci USA* **91**:1529–1533.

2203. **Reddy, M. M., and M. H. Grieco.** 1989. Neopterin and alpha and beta interleukin-1 levels in sera of patients with human immunodeficiency virus infection. *J Clin Micro* **27**:1919–1923.

2204. **Redfield, R. R., D. L. Birx, N. Ketter, E. Tramont, V. Polonis, C. Davis, J. F. Brundage, G. Smith, S. Johnson, A. Fowler, T. Wierzba, A. Shafferman, F. Volvovitz, C. Oster, and D. S. Burke.** 1991. A phase I evaluation of the safety and immunogenicity of vaccination with recombinant gp160 in patients with early human immunodeficiency virus infection. *N Engl J Med* **324**:1677–1684.

2205. **Reeves, J. D., and T. F. Schulz.** 1997. The CD4-independent tropism of human immunodeficiency virus type 2 involves several regions of the envelope protein and correlates with a reduced activation threshold for envelope-mediated fusion. *J Virol* **71**:1453–1465.

2206. **Reiher, W. E. I., J. E. Blalock, and T. K. Brunck.** 1986. Sequence homology between acquired immunodeficiency syndrome virus envelope protein and interleukin 2. *Proc Natl Acad Sci USA* **83**:9188–9192.

2207. **Reimann, K. A., J. T. Li, R. Veazey, M. Halloran, I.-W. Park, G. B. Karlsson, J. Sodroski, and N. L. Letvin.** 1996. A chimeric simian/human immunodeficiency virus expressing a primary patient human immunodeficiency virus type 1 isolate *env* causes an AIDS-like disease after in vivo passage in rhesus monkeys. *J Virol* **70**:6922–6928.

2208. **Reimann, K. A., K. Tenner-Racz, P. Racz, D. C. Montefiori, Y. Yasutomi, W. Lin, B. J. Ransil, and N. L. Letvin.** 1994. Immunopathogenic events in acute infection of rhesus monkeys with simian immunodeficiency virus of macaques. *J Virol* **68**:2362–2370.

2208a. **Reimer, L., S. Mottice, C. Schable, P. Sullivan, A. Nakashima, M. Rayfield, R. Den, and C. Brokopp.** 1997. Absence of detectable antibody in a patient infected with human immunodeficiency virus. *Clin Infect Dis* **25**:98–100.

2209. **Reinhardt, P. P., B. Reinhardt, J. L. Lathey, and S. A. Spector.** 1995. Human cord blood mononuclear cells are preferentially infected by non-syncytium-inducing macrophage-tropic human immunodeficiency virus type 1 isolates. *J Clin Micro* **33**:292–297.

2210. **Reinhart, T. A., M. J. Rogan, G. A. Viglianti, D. M. Rausch, L. E. Eiden, and A. T. Haase.** 1997. A new approach to investigating the relationship between productive infection and cytopathicity *in vivo*. *Nature Med* **3**:218–221.

2211. **Reiser, H., and M. J. Stadecker.** 1996. Costimulatory B7 molecules in the pathogenesis of infectious and autoimmune diseases. *N Engl J Med* **335**:1369–1377.

2212. **Reiser, J., G. Harmison, S. Kluepfel-Stahl, R. O. Brady, S. Karlsson, and M. Schubert.** 1996. Transduction of nondividing cells using pseudotyped defective high-titer HIV type 1 particles. *Proc Natl Acad Sci USA* **93**:15266–15271.

2213. **Reisinger, E. C., W. Vogetseder, D. Berzow, D. Kofler, G. Bitterlich, H. A. Lehr, H. Wachter, and M. P. Dierich.** 1990. Complement-mediated enhancement of HIV-1 infection of the monoblastoid cell line U937. *AIDS* **4**:961–965.

2214. **Reitz, M. S., Sr., C. Wilson, C. Naugle, R. C. Gallo, and M. Robert-Guroff.** 1988. Generation of a neutralization-resistant variant of HIV-1 is due to selection for a point mutation in the envelope gene. *Cell* **54**:57–63.

2215. **Renne, R., W. Zhong, B. Herndier, M. McGrath, N. Abbey, D. Kedes, and D. Ganem.** 1996. Lytic growth of Kaposi's sarcoma-associated herpesvirus (human herpesvirus 8) in culture. *Nature Med* **2**:342–346.

2216. **Resnick, D. A., A. D. Smith, S. C. Gesiler, A. Zhang, E. Arnold, and G. F. Arnold.** 1995. Chimeras from a human rhinovirus 14-human immunodeficiency virus type 1 (HIV-1) V3 loop seroprevalence library induce neutralizing responses against HIV-1. *J Virol* **69**:2406–2411.

2217. Resnick, L., J. R. Berger, P. Shapshak, and W. W. Tourtellotte. 1988. Early penetration of the blood-brain-barrier by HIV. *Neurol* **38**:9–14.

2218. Rettig, M. B., H. J. Ma, R. A. Vescio, M. Pold, G. Schiller, D. Belson, A. Savage, C. Nishikubo, C. Wu, J. Fraser, J. W. Said, and J. R. Berenson. 1997. Kaposi's sarcoma-associated herpesvirus infection of bone marrow dendritic cells from multiple myeloma patients. *Science* **276**:1851–1854.

2219. Rey, F., G. Donker, I. Hirsch, and J.-C. Chermann. 1991. Productive infection of CD4+ cells by selected HIV strains is not inhibited by anti-CD4 monoclonal antibodies. *Virol* **181**:165–171.

2220. Reyburn, H. T., O. Mandelboim, M. Vales-Gomez, D. M. Davis, L. Pazmany, and J. L. Strominger. 1997. The class I MHC homologue of human cytomegalovirus inhibits attack by natural killer cells. *Nature* **386**:514–515.

2220a.Reyes-Teran, G., and J. A. Levy. Unpublished observations.

2221. Reyes-Teran, G., J. G. Sierra-Madero, V. Martinez del Cerro, H. Arroyo-Figueroa, A. Pasquetti, J. J. Calva, and G. M. Ruiz-Palacios. 1996. Effects of thalidomide on HIV-associated wasting syndrome: a randomized, double-blind, placebo-controlled clinical trial. *AIDS* **10**:1501–1507.

2222. Rice, W. G., and J. P. Bader. 1995. Discovery and in vitro development of AIDS antiviral drugs as biopharmaceuticals. *Adv Pharmacol* **33**:389–438.

2223. Rice, W. G., J. G. Supko, L. Malspeis, R. W. Buckheit, Jr., D. Clanton, M. Bu, L. Graham, C. A. Schaeffer, J. A. Turpin, J. Domagala, R. Gogliotti, J. P. Bader, S. M. Halliday, L. Coren, R. C. Sowder II, L. O. Arthur, and L. E. Henderson. 1995. Inhibitors of HIV nucleocapsid protein zinc fingers as candidates for the treatment of AIDS. *Science* **270**:1194–1197.

2224. Rich, E. A., I. S. Y. Chen, J. A. Zack, M. L. Leonard, and W. A. O'Brien. 1992. Increased susceptibility of differentiated mononuclear phagocytes to productive infection with human immunodeficiency virus-1 (HIV-1). *J Clin Invest* **89**:176–183.

2225. Richards, R. L., M. D. Hayre, W. T. Hockmeyer, and C. R. Alving. 1988. Liposomes, lipid A, and aluminum hydroxide enhance the immune response to a synthetic malaria sporozoite antigen. *Infect Immun* **56**:682–686.

2226. Richman, D., C.-K. Shih, I. Lowy, J. Rose, P. Prodanovich, S. Goff, and J. Griffin. 1991. Human immunodeficiency virus type 1 mutants resistant to nonnucleoside inhibitors of reverse transcriptase arise in tissue culture. *Proc Natl Acad Sci USA* **88**:11241–11245.

2227. Richman, D. D. 1992. HIV drug resistance. *AIDS Res Hum Retro* **8**:1065–1071.

2228. Richman, D. D. 1990. Zidovudine resistance of human immunodeficiency virus. *Rev Inf Dis* **12**:s507-s510.

2229. Richman, D. D., and S. A. Bozzette. 1994. The impact of the syncytium-inducing phenotype of human immunodeficiency virus on disease progression. *J Inf Dis* **169**:968–974.

2230. Richman, D. D., R. S. Kornbluth, and D. A. Carson. 1987. Failure of dideoxynucleosides to inhibit human immunodeficiency virus replication in cultured human macrophages. *J Exp Med* **166**:1144–1149.

2231. Rickman, L. S., D. M. Gordon, R. Wistar, Jr., U. Krzych, M. Gross, M. R. Hollingale, J. E. Egan, J. D. Chulay, and S. L. Hoffman. 1991. Use of adjuvant containing mycobacterial cell-wall skeleton, monophosphoryl lipid A and squalene in malaria circumsporozoite protein vaccine. *Lancet* **337**:998–1001.

2231a.Riley, J. L., R. G. Carroll, B. L. Levine, W. Bernstein, D. C. St. Louis, O. S. Weislow, and C. H. June. 1997. Intrinsic resistance to T cell infection with HIV type 1 induced by CD28 costimulation. *J Immunol* **158**:5545–5553.

2232. Rinaldo, C., X. L. Huang, Z. F. Fan, M. Ding, L. Beltz, A. Logar, D. Panicali, G. Mazzara, J. Liebmann, M. Cottrill, and P. Gupta. 1995. High levels of anti-human immunodeficiency virus type 1 (HIV-1) memory cytotoxic T-lymphocyte activity and low viral load are associated with lack of disease in HIV-1-infected long-term nonprogressors. *J Virol* **69**:5838–5842.

2233. Rinaldo, C., L. Kingsley, J. Neumann, D. Reed, P. Gupta, and D. Lyter. 1989. Association of human immunodeficiency virus (HIV) p24 antigenemia with decrease in CD4+ lymphocytes and onset of acquired immunodeficiency syndrome during the early phase of HIV infection. *J Clin Micro* **27**:880–884.

2234. Rinaldo, C. R., Jr. 1994. Modulation of major histocompatibility complex antigen expression by viral infection. *Am J Path* **144**:637–650.

2235. Rinaldo, C. R., Jr., L. A. Beltz, X. L. Huang, P. Gupta, Z. Fan, and D. J. Torpey III. 1995. Anti-HIV type 1 cytotoxic T lymphocyte effector activity and disease progression in the first 8 years of HIV type 1 infection of homosexual men. *AIDS Res Hum Retro* **11**:481–489.

2236. Ritter, J., M. Sepetjan, and J. C. Monier. 1987. Lack of reactivity of anti-human immunodeficiency virus (HIV) p17/18 antibodies against alpha-1 thymosin and of anti-alpha-1 thymosin monoclonal antibody against p17/18 protein. *Immunol Let* **16**:97–100.

2237. Riviere, Y., M. B. McChesney, F. Porrot, F. Tanneau-Salvadori, P. Sansonetti, O. Lopez, G. Pialoux, V. Feuillie, M. Mollereau, S. Chamaret, F. Tekaia, and L. Montagnier. 1995. Gag-specific cytotoxic respones to HIV type 1 are associated with a decreased risk of progression to AIDS-related complex or AIDS. *AIDS Res Hum Retro* **11**:903–907.

2238. Riviere, Y., F. Tanneau-Salvadori, A. Regnault, O. Lopez, P. Sansonetti, B. Guy, M.-P. Kieny, J.-J. Fournel, and L. Montagnier. 1989. Human immunodeficiency virus-specific cytotoxic responses of seropositive individuals: distinct types of effector cells mediate killing of targets expressing *gag* and *env* proteins. *J Virol* **63**:2270–2277.

2239. Rizzardi, G. P., W. Barcellini, G. Tambussi, F. Lillo, M. Malnati, L. Perrin, and A. Lazzarin. 1996. Plasma levels of soluble CD30, tumour necrosis factor (TNF)-α and TNF receptors during primary HIV-1 infection: correlation with HIV-1 RNA and the clinical outcome. *AIDS* **10**:F45-F50.

2240. Rizzardini, G., S. Piconi, S. Ruzzante, M. L. Fusi, M. Lukwiya, S. Declich, M. Tamburini, M. L. Villa, M. Fabiani, F. Milazzo, and M. Clerici. 1996. Immunological activation markers in the serum of African and European HIV-seropositive and seronegative individuals. *AIDS* **10**:1535–1542.

2241. Rizzuto, C. D., and J. G. Sodroski. 1997. Contribution of virion ICAM-1 to human immunodeficiency virus infectivity and sensitivity to neutralization. *J Virol* **71**:4847–4851.

2242. Robbins, D. S., Y. Shirazi, B. E. Drysdale, A. Lieberman, H. S. Shin, and M. L. Shin. 1987. Production of cytotoxic factor for oligodendrocytes by stimulated astrocytes. *J Immunol* **139**:2593–2597.

2244. Robert-Guroff, M., K. Aldrich, R. Muldoon, T. L. Stern, G. P. Bansal, T. J. Matthews, P. D. Markham, R. C. Gallo, and G. Franchini. 1992. Cross-neutralization of human immunodeficiency virus type 1 and 2 and simian immunodeficiency virus isolates. *J Virol* **66**:3602–3608.

2245. Robert-Guroff, M., M. Brown, and R. Gallo. 1985. HTLV-III neutralizing antibodies in patients with AIDS and AIDS-related complex. *Nature* **316**:72–74.

2246. Robert-Guroff, M., M. Popovic, S. Gartner, P. Markham, R. C. Gallo, and M. S. Reitz. 1990. Structure and expression of Tat-, Rev-, and Nef-specific transcripts of human immunodeficiency virus type 1 in infected lymphocytes and macrophages. *J Virol* **64**:3391–3398.

2247. Robert-Guroff, M., M. S. Reitz, Jr., W. G. Robey, and R. C. Gallo. 1986. *In vitro* generation of an HTLV-III variant by neutralizing antibody. *J Immunol* **137**:3306–3309.

2248. Roberts, J. D., K. Bebenek, and T. A. Kunkel. 1988. The accuracy of reverse transcriptase from HIV-1. *Science* **242**:1171–1173.

2249. Roberts, N. A., J. A. Martin, D. Kinchington, A. V. Broadhurst, J. C. Craig, I. B. Duncan, S. A. Galpin, B. J. Handa, J. Kay, A. Krohn, R. W. Lambert, J. H. Merrett, J. S. Mills, K. E. B. Parkes, S. Redshaw, A. J. Ritchie, D. L. Taylor, G. J. Thomas, and P. J. Machin. 1990. Rational design of peptide-based HIV proteinase inhibitors. *Science* **248**:358–361.

2250. Robertson, D. L., P. M. Sharp, F. E. McCutchan, and B. H. Hahn. 1995. Recombination in HIV-1. *Nature* **374**:124–126.

2251. Rovinski, B., L. Rodrigues, S. X. Cao, F. L. Yao, U. McGuinness, C. Sia, G. Cates, S. Zolla-Pazner, S. Karwowska, T. J. Matthews, C. B. McDanal, J. Mascola, and M. H. Klein. 1995. Induction of HIV type 1 neutralizing and *env*-CD4 blocking antibodies by immunization with genetically engineered HIV type 1-like particles containing unprocessed gp160 glycoproteins. *AIDS Res Hum Retro* **11**:1187–1195.

2251a. Robinson, H. L. 1997. DNA vaccines for immunodeficiency viruses. *AIDS 1997* **11**:s109-s119.

2252. Robinson, H. L., and D. M. Zinkus. 1990. Accumulation of human immunodeficiency virus type 1 DNA in T cells: results of multiple infection events. *J Virol* **64**:4836–4841.

2253. Robinson, W. E., Jr., M. K. Gorny, J.-Y. Xu, W. M. Mitchell, and S. Zolla-Pazner. 1991. Two immunodominant domains of gp41 bind antibodies which enhance human immunodeficiency virus type 1 infection *in vitro*. *J Virol* **65**:4169–4176.

2254. Robinson, W. E., Jr., T. Kawamura, M. K. Gorny, D. Lake, J.-Y. Xu, Y. Matsumoto, T. Sugano, Y. Masuho, W. M. Mitchell, E. Hersh, and S. Zolla-Pazner. 1990. Human monoclonal antibodies to the human immunodeficiency virus type 1 (HIV-1) transmembrane glycoprotein gp41 enhance HIV-1 infection *in vitro*. *Proc Natl Acad Sci USA* **87**:3185–3189.

2255. Robinson, W. E., Jr., and W. M. Mitchell. 1990. Neutralization and enhancement of *in vitro* and *in vivo* HIV and simian immunodeficiency virus infections. *AIDS* **4**:S151-S162.

2256. Robinson, W. E., Jr., D. C. Montefiori, and W. M. Mitchell. 1988. Antibody-dependent enhancement of human immunodeficiency virus type 1 infection. *Lancet* **i**:790–794.

2257. Robinson, W. E., Jr., D. C. Montefiori, and W. M. Mitchell. 1990. Complement-mediated antibody-dependent enhancement of HIV-1 infection requires CD4 and complement receptors. *Virol* **175**:600–604.

2258. Rocha, B., N. Dautigny, and P. Pereira. 1989. Peripheral T lymphocytes: expansion potential and homeostatic regulation of pool sizes and CD4/CD8 ratios *in vivo*. *Eur J Immunol* **19**:905–911.

2259. Rodriguez, E. M., L. M. Mofenson, B.-H. Chang, K. C. Rich, M. G. Fowler, V. Smeriglio, S. Landesman, H. E. Fox, C. Diaz, K. Green, and I. C. Hanson. 1996. Association of maternal drug use during pregnancy with maternal HIV culture positivity and perinatal HIV transmission. *AIDS* **10**:273–282.

2260. Rodriguez, E. R., S. Nasim, J. Hsia, R. L. Sandin, A. Ferreira, B. A. Hilliard, A. M. Ross, and C. T. Garrett. 1991. Cardiac myocytes and dendritic cells harbor human immunodeficiency virus in infected patients with and without cardiac dysfunction: detection by multiplex, nested, polymerase chain reaction in individually microdissected cells from right ventricular endomyocardial biopsy tissue. *Am J Cardiol* **68**:1511–1520.

2261. Rodriguez, M., K. D. Pavelko, M. K. Njenga, W. C. Logan, and P. J. Wettstein. 1996. The balance between persistent virus infection and immune cells determines demyelination. *J Immunol* **157**:5699–5709.

2262. Roederer, M., J. G. Dubs, M. T. Anderson, P. A. Raju, L. A. Herzenberg, and L. A. Herzenberg. 1995. CD8 naive T cell counts decrease progressively in HIV-infected adults. *J Clin Invest* **95**:2061–2066.

2263. Roederer, M., P. A. Raju, D. K. Mitra, L. A. Herzenberg, and L. A. Herzenberg. 1997. HIV does not replicate in naive CD4 T cells stimulated with CD3/CD28. *J Clin Invest* **99**:1555–1564.

2264. Roederer, M., F. J. T. Staal, P. A. Raju, S. W. Ela, L. A. Herzenberg, and L. A. Herzenberg. 1990. Cytokine-stimulated human immunodeficiency virus replication is inhibited by N-acetyl-L-cysteine. *Proc Natl Acad Sci USA* **87**:4884–4888.

2265. Rogers, M. F., C.-Y. Ou, B. Kilbourne, and G. Schochetman. 1991. Advances and problems in the diagnosis of human immunodeficiency virus infection in infants. *Pediatr Infect Dis J* **10**:523–531.

2266. Rogers, M. F., C. R. White, R. Sanders, C. Schable, T. E. Ksell, R. L. Wasserman, J. A. Bellanti, S. M. Peters, and B. B. Wray. 1990. Lack of transmission of human immunodeficiency virus from infected children to their household contacts. *Pediatrics* **85**:210–214.

2267. Rogge, L., L. Barberis-Maino, M. Biffi, N. Passini, D. H. Presky, U. Gubler, and F. Sinigaglia. 1997. Selective expression of an interleukin-12 receptor component by human T helper 1 cells. *J Exp Med* **185**:825–831.

2268. Roglic, M., R. D. MacPhee, S. R. Duncan, F. R. Sattler, and A. N. Theofilopoulos. 1997. T cell receptor (TCR) BV gene repertoires and clonal expansions of CD4 cells in patients with HIV infections. *Clin Exp Immunol* **107**:21–30.

2269. Rojko, J. L., R. M. Fulton, L. J. Rezanka, L. L. Williams, E. Copelan, C. M. Cheney, G. S. Reichel, J. C. Neil, L. E. Mathes, T. G. Fisher, and M. W. Cloyd. 1992. Lymphocytotoxic strains of feline leukemia virus induce apoptosis in feline T4-thymic lymphoma cells. *Lab Invest* **66**:418–426.

2269a. Roman, M., E. Martin-Orozco, J. S. Goodman, M. D. Nguyen, Y. Sato, A. Ronaghy, R. S. Kornbluth, D. D. Richman, D. A. Carson, and E. Raz. 1997. Immunostimulatory DNA sequences function as T helper-1-promoting adjuvants. *Nature Med* **3**:849–854.

2270. Romagnani, S. 1992. Human TH1 and TH2 subsets: regulation of differentiation and role in protection and immunopathology. *Int Arch Allergy Immunol* **98**:279–285.

2271. Romagnani, S. 1992. Induction of TH1 and TH2 responses: a key role for the 'natural' immune response? *Immunol Today* **13**:379-381.

2272. Rook, A. H., H. C. Lane, T. Folks, S. McCoy, H. Alter, and A. S. Fauci. 1987. Sera from HTLV-III/LAV antibody-positive individuals mediate antibody-dependent cellular cytotoxicity against HTLV-III/LAV-infected T cells. *J Immunol* **138**:1064–1067.

2273. Rooke, R., M. A. Parniak, M. Tremblay, H. Soudeyns, X. G. Li, Q. Gao, X. J. Yao, and M. A. Wainberg. 1991. Biological comparison of wild-type and zidovudine-resistant isolates of human immunodeficiency virus type 1 from the same subjects: susceptibility and resistance to other drugs. *Antimicrob Agents Chemo* **35**:988–991.

2274. Roos, M. T. L., J. M. A. Lange, R. E. Y. de Goede, R. A. Coutinho, P. T. A. Schellenkens, F. Miedema, and M. Termsette. 1992. Viral phenotype and immune response in primary human immunodeficiency virus type 1 infection. *J Inf Dis* **165**:427–432.

2275. Roos, M. T. L., F. Miedema, M. Koot, M. Tersmette, W. P. Schaasberg, R. A. Coutinho, and P. T. A. Schellekens. 1995. T cell function *in vitro* is an independent progression marker for AIDS in human immunodeficiency virus-infected asymptomatic subjects. *J Inf Dis* **171**:531–536.

2276. Roos, M. T. L., F. Miedema, A. P. Meinesz, N. A. S. M. De Leeuw, N. G. Pakker, J. M. A. Lange, R. A. Coutinho, and P. T. A. Schellekens. 1996. Low T cell reactivity to combined CD3 plus CD28 stimulation is predictive for progression to AIDS: correlation with decreased CD28 expression. *Clin Exp Immunol* **105**:409–415.

2277. Roques, P. A., G. Gras, F. Parnet-Mathieu, A. M. Mabondzo, C. Dollfus, R. Narwa, D. Marce, J. Tranchot-Diallo, F. Herve, G. Lasfargues, C. Courpotin, and D. Dormont. 1995. Clearance of HIV infection in 12 perinatally infected children: clinical, virological and immunological data. *AIDS* **9**:F19-F26.

2278. Rose, R. E., Y. F. Gong, J. A. Greytok, C. M. Bechtold, B. J. Terry, B. S. Robinson, M. Alam, R. J. Colonno, and P. F. Lin. 1996. Human immunodeficiency virus type 1 viral background plays a major role in development of resistance to protease inhibitors. *Proc Natl Acad Sci USA* **93**:1648–1653.

2279. Rose, T. M., K. B. Strand, E. R. Schultz, G. Schaefer, G. W. Randkin, Jr., M. E. Thouless, C. C. Tsai, and M. L. Bosch. 1997. Identification of two homologs of the Kaposi's sarcoma-associated herpesvirus (human herpesvirus 8) in retroperitoneal fibromatosis of different macaque species. *J Virol* **71**:4138–4144.

2280. Rosen, C. A., E. Terwilliger, A. Dayton, J. G. Sodroski, and W. A. Haseltine. 1988. Intragenic cis-acting *art* gene-responsive sequences of the human immunodeficiency virus. *Proc Natl Acad Sci USA* **85**:2071–2075.

2281. Rosenberg, Y. J., M. G. Lewis, E. C. Leon, A. Cafaro, G. A. Eddy, and J. J. Greenhouse. 1994. Viral DNA burden and decline in percentage of CD4-positive cells in the lymphoid compartment of SIV-infected macaques. *AIDS Res Hum Retro* **10**:1269–1277.

2282. Rosenberg, Y. J., P. M. Zack, E. C. Leon, B. D. White, S. F. Papermaster, E. Hall, J. J. Greenhouse, G. A. Eddy, and M. G. Lewis. 1994. Immunological and virological changes associated with decline in CD4/CD8 ratios in lymphoid organs of SIV-infected macaques. *AIDS Res Hum Retro* **10**:863–872.

2283. Rosenberg, Y. J., P. M. Zack, B. D. White, S. F. Papermaster, W. R. Elkins, G. A. Eddy, and M. G. Lewis. 1993. Decline in the CD4+ lymphocyte population in the blood of SIV-infected macaques is not reflected in lymph nodes. *AIDS Res Hum Retro* 9:639–646.

2284. Rosenberg, Z. F., and A. S. Fauci. 1990. Immunopathogenic mechanisms of HIV infection: cytokine induction of HIV expression. *Immunol Today* 11:176–180.

2284a.Rosenthal, K. Personal communication.

2284b.Rosok, B., J. E. Brinchmann, P. Voltersvik, J. Olofsson, L. Bostad, and B. Asjo. 1997. Correlates of latent and productive HIV type-1 infection in tonsillar CD4+ T cells. *Proc Natl Acad Sci USA* 94:9332–9336.

2285. Rosok, B., P. Voltersvik, B.-M. Larsson, J. Albert, J. E. Brinchmann, and B. Asjo. 1997. CD8+ T cells from HIV type 1-seronegative individuals suppress virus replication in acutely infected cells. *AIDS Res Hum Retro* 13:79–85.

2286. Rosok, B. I., L. Bostad, P. Voltersvik, R. Bjerknes, J. Olofsson, B. Asjo, and J. E. Brinchmann. 1996. Reduced CD4 cell counts in blood do not reflect CD4 cell depletion in tonsillar tissue in asymptomatic HIV-1 infection. *AIDS* 10:F35-F38.

2287. Rossi, J. J., D. Elkins, J. A. Zaia, and S. Sullivan. 1992. Ribozymes as anti-HIV-1 therapeutic agents: principles, applications, and problems. *AIDS Res Hum Retro* 8:183–189.

2288. Rossi, P. 1992. Maternal factors involved in mother-to-child transmission of HIV-1. Report of a Consensus Workshop, Siena, Italy, January 1992. *J AIDS* 5:1019–1029.

2289. Rossi, P., V. Moschese, P. A. Broliden, C. Fundaro, I. Quinti, A. Plebani, C. Giaquinto, P. A. Tovo, K. Ljunggren, J. Rosen, H. Wigzell, M. Jondal, and B. Wahren. 1989. Presence of maternal antibodies to human immunodeficiency virus 1 envelope glycoprotein gp120 epitopes correlates with the uninfected status of children born to seropositive mothers. *Proc Natl Acad Sci USA* 86:8055–8058.

2290. Roth, W. K. 1991. HIV-associated Kaposi's sarcoma: new developments in epidemiology and molecular pathology. *J Cancer Res Clin Oncol* 117:186–191.

2291. Roth, W. K., H. Brandstetter, and M. Sturzl. 1992. Cellular and molecular features of HIV-associated Kaposi's sarcoma. *AIDS* 6:895–913.

2292. Roth, W. K., S. Werner, W. Risau, K. Remberger, and P. H. Hofschneider. 1988. Cultured, AIDS-related Kaposi's sarcoma cells express endothelial cell markers and are weakly malignant in vitro. *Int J Cancer* 42:767–773.

2293. Rouse, B. T., and D. W. Horohov. 1986. Immunosuppression in viral infections. *Rev Inf Dis* 8:850–873.

2294. Rouzioux, C., J. Puel, H. Agut, F. Brun-Vezinet, F. Ferchal, C. Tamalet, P. Descamps, and H. Fleury. 1992. Comparative assessment of quantitative HIV viraemia assays. *AIDS* 6:373–377.

2295. Rowland-Jones, S., and A. McMichael. 1993. Cytotoxic T lymphocytes in HIV infection. *Sem Virol* 4:83–94.

2296. Rowland-Jones, S., J. Sutton, K. Ariyoshi, T. Dong, F. Gotch, S. McAdam, D. Whitby, S. Sabally, A. Gallimore, T. Corrah, M. Takiguchi, T. Schultz, A. McMichael, and H. Whittle. 1995. HIV-specific cytotoxic T-cells in HIV-exposed but uninfected Gambian women. *Nature Med* 1:59–64.

2297. Rowland-Jones, S. L., and A. McMichael. 1995. Immune responses in HIV-exposed seronegatives: have they repelled the virus? *Curr Opin Immunol* 7:448–455.

2298. Roy, M. J., J. J. Damato, and D. S. Burke. 1993. Absence of true seroreversion of HIV-1 antibody in seroreactive individuals. *J Am Med Assoc* 269:2876–2879.

2299. Roy, S., L. Fitz-Gibbon, L. Poulin, and M. A. Wainberg. 1988. Infection of human monocytes/macrophages by HIV-1: effect on secretion of IL-1 activity. *Immunol* 64:233–239.

2300. Royce, R. A., A. Sena, W. Cates, Jr., and M. S. Cohen. 1997. Sexual tranmission of HIV. *N Engl J Med* 336:1072–1078.

2301. Rubbert, A., D. Weissman, C. Combadiere, K. A. Pettrone, J. A. Daucher, P. M. Murphy, and A. S. Fauci. 1997. Multifactorial nature of noncytolytic CD8+ T cell-mediated suppression of HIV replication: β-chemokine-dependent and -independent effects. *AIDS Res Hum Retro* 13:63–69.

2302. Rubsamen-Waigmann, H., E. Huguenel, A. Paessens, J. P. Kleim, M. A. Wainberg, and A. Shah. 1997. Second-generation non-nucleosidic reverse transcriptase inhibitor HBY097 and HIV-1 viral load. *Lancet* **349:**1517.

2303. Rucker, J., M. Samson, B. J. Doranz, F. Libert, J. F. Berson, Y. Yi, R. J. Smyth, R. G. Collman, C. C. Broder, G. Vassart, R. W. Doms, and M. Parmentier. 1996. Regions in β-chemokine receptors CCR5 and CCR2b that determine HIV-1 cofactor specificity. *Cell* **87:**437–446.

2304. Rudbach, J. A., J. L. Cantrell, and J. T. Ulrich. 1988. Molecularly engineered microbial immunostimulators, p. 443–454. *In* L. Lasky (ed.), *Technological Advances in Vaccine Development.* Alan R. Liss, Inc., New York.

2305. Ruegg, C. L., C. R. Monell, and M. Strand. 1989. Inhibition of lymphoproliferation by a synthetic peptide with sequence identity to gp41 of human immunodeficiency virus type 1. *J Virol* **63:**3257–3260.

2306. Ruegg, C. L., and M. Strand. 1991. A synthetic peptide with sequence identity to the transmembrane protein gp41 of HIV-1 inhibits distinct lymphocyte activation pathways dependent on protein kinase C and intracellular calcium influx. *Cell Immunol* **137:**1–13.

2307. Ruff, A. J., J. Coberly, N. A. Halsey, R. Boulos, J. Desormeaux, A. Burnley, D. J. Joseph, M. McBrien, T. Quinn, P. Losikoff, K. L. O'Brien, M. A. Louis, and H. Farzadegan. 1994. Prevalence of HIV-1 DNA and p24 antigen in breast milk and correlation with maternal factors. *J AIDS* **7:**68–73.

2308. Rusche, J. R., K. Javaherian, C. McDanal, J. Petro, D. L. Lynn, R. Grimaila, A. Langlois, R. C. Gallo, L. O. Arthur, P. J. Fischinger, D. P. Bolognesi, S. D. Putney, and T. J. Matthews. 1988. Antibodies that inhibit fusion of human immunodeficiency virus-infected cells bind a 24-amino acid sequence of the viral envelope, gp120. *Proc Natl Acad Sci USA* **85:**3198–3202.

2309. Russell-Jones, R., and E. Wilson-Jones. 1988. The histogenesis of Kaposi's sarcoma. *Am J Dermatopathol* **8:**369–370.

2310. Russo, J. J., R. A. Bohenzky, M. C. Chien, J. Chen, M. Yan, D. Maddalena, J. P. Parry, D. Peruzzi, I. S. Edelman, Y. Chang, and P. S. Moore. 1996. Nucleotide sequence of Kaposi sarcoma-associated herpesvirus (HHV8). *Proc Natl Acad Sci USA* **93:**14862–14867.

2311. Rutherford, G. W., A. R. Lifson, and N. A. Hessol. 1990. Course of HIV-1 infection in a cohort of homosexual and bisexual men: an 11 year follow up study. *Brit Med J* **301:**1183–1188.

2312. Rutka, J. T., J. R. Giblin, M. E. Berens, E. Bar-Shiva, K. Tokuda, J. R. McCulloch, M. L. Rosenblum, T. E. Eessalu, B. B. Aggarwal, and W. J. Bodell. 1988. The effects of human recombinant tumor necrosis factor on glioma-derived cell lines: cellular proliferation, cytotoxicity, morphological and radioreceptor studies. *Int J Cancer* **41:**573–582.

2313. Ryan-Graham, M. A., and K. W. C. Peden. 1995. Both virus and host components are important for the manifestation of Nef− phenotype in HIV-1 and HIV-2. *Virol* **213:**158–168.

2314. Ryu, S. E., P. D. Kwong, A. Truneh, T. G. Porter, J. Arthos, M. Rosenberg, X. Dai, N. Xuong, R. Axel, R. W. Sweet, and W. A. Hendrickson. 1990. Crystal structure of an HIV-binding recombinant fragment of human CD4. *Nature* **348:**419–426.

2315. Saag, M. S., M. J. Crain, W. D. Decker, S. Campbell-Hill, S. Robinson, W. E. Brown, M. Leuther, R. J. Whitley, B. H. Hahn, and G. M. Shaw. 1991. High-level viremia in adults and children infected with human immunodeficiency virus: relation to disease stage and CD4+ lymphocyte levels. *J Inf Dis* **164:**72–80.

2316. Saag, M. S., E. A. Emini, O. L. Laskin, J. Douglas, W. I. Lapidus, W. A. Schleif, R. J. Whitley, C. Hildebrand, V. W. Byrnes, J. C. Kappes, K. W. Anderson, F. Massari, and G. M. Shaw. 1993. A short-term clinical evaluation of L-697,661, a non-nucleoside inhibitor of HIV-1 reverse transcriptase. *N Engl J Med* **329:**1065–1072.

2317. Saag, M. S., B. H. Hahn, J. Gibbons, Y. Li, E. S. Parks, W. P. Parks, and G. M. Shaw. 1988. Extensive variation of human immunodeficiency virus type-1 *in vivo. Nature* **334:**440–444.

2318. Saag, M. S., S. M. Hammer, and J. M. A. Lange. 1994. Pathogenicity and diversity of HIV and implications for clinical management: a review. *J AIDS* **7:**S2-S10.

2319. Saarloos, M.-N., B. L. Sullivan, M. A. Czerniewski, K. D. Parameswar, and G. T. Spear. 1997. Detection of HLA-DR associated with monocytotropic, primary, and plasma isolates of human immunodeficiency virus type 1. *J Virol* **71**:1640–1643.

2320. Sabatier, J.-M., E. Vives, K. Mabrouk, A. Benjouad, H. Rochat, A. Duval, B. Hue, and E. Bahraoui. 1991. Evidence for neurotoxic activity of *tat* from human immunodeficiency virus type 1. *J Virol* **65**:961–967.

2321. Sabin, E. A., M. I. Araujo, E. M. Carvalho, and E. J. Pearce. 1996. Impairment of tetanus toxoid-specific Th1-like immune responses in humans infected with *Schistosoma mansoni*. *J Inf Dis* **173**:269–272.

2322. Sabino, E., L. Z. Pan, C. Cheng-Mayer, and A. Mayer. 1994. Comparison of in vivo plasma and peripheral blood mononuclear cell HIV-1 quasispecies to short-term tissue culture isolates: an analysis of Tat and C2-V3 Env regions. *AIDS* **8**:901–909.

2323. Sabri, F., F. Chiodi, and E. M. Fenyo. 1996. Lack of correlation between V3 amino acid sequence and syncytium-inducing capacity of some HIV type 1 isolates. *AIDS Res Hum Retro* **12**:855–858.

2324. Sad, S., and T. R. Mosmann. 1995. Interleukin (IL) 4, in the absence of antigen stimulation, induces an anergy-like state in differentiated CD8+ TC1 cells: loss of IL-2 synthesis and autonomous proliferation but retention of cytotoxicity and synthesis of other cytokines. *J Exp Med* **182**:1505–1515.

2325. Sadat-Sowti, B., P. Debre, T. Idziorek, J. M. Guillon, F. Hadida, E. Oksenhendler, C. Katlama, C. Mayaud, and B. Autran. 1991. A lectin-binding soluble factor released by CD8+CD57+ lymphocytes from AIDS patients inhibits T cell cytotoxicity. *Eur J Immunol* **21**:737–741.

2326. Saeland, S., V. Duvert, D. Pandrau, C. Caux, I. Durand, N. Wrighton, J. Wideman, F. Lee, and J. Banchereau. 1991. Interleukin-7 induces the proliferation of normal B cell precursors. *Blood* **78**:2229–2238.

2327. Safai, B., and R. A. Good. 1981. Kaposi's sarcoma: a review and recent developments. *CA Cancer J Clin (New York)* **335**:2–12.

2328. Said, W., K. Chien, S. Takeuchi, T. Tasaka, H. Asou, S. K. Cho, S. de Vos, E. Cesarman, D. M. Knowles, and H. P. Koeffler. 1996. Kaposi's sarcoma-associated herpesvirus (KSHV or HHV8) in primary effusion lymphoma: ultrastructural demonstration of herpesvirus in lymphoma cells. *Blood* **87**:4937–4943.

2329. Saito, Y., L. R. Sharer, L. G. Epstein, J. Michaels, M. Mintz, M. Louder, K. Golding, T. A. Cvetkovich, and B. M. Blumberg. 1994. Overexpression of nef as a marker for restricted HIV-1 infection of astrocytes in postmortem pediatric central nervous system tissues. *Neurol* **44**:474–481.

2330. Sakaguchi, M., T. Sato, and J. E. Groopman. 1991. Human immunodeficiency virus infection of megakaryocytic cells. *Blood* **77**:481–485.

2331. Sakai, H., M. Kawamura, J.-I. Sakuragi, S. Sakuragi, R. Shibata, A. Ishimoto, N. Ono, S. Ueda, and A. Adachi. 1993. Integration is essential for efficient gene expression of human immunodeficiency virus type 1. *J Virol* **67**:1169–1174.

2332. Sakai, K., S. Dewhurst, X. Ma, and D. J. Volsky. 1988. Differences in cytopathogenicity and host cell range among infectious molecular clones of human immunodeficiency virus type 1 simultaneously isolated from an individual. *J Virol* **62**:4078–4085.

2333. Sakai, K., X. Ma, I. Gordienko, and D. J. Volsky. 1991. Recombinational analysis of a natural noncytopathic human immunodeficiency virus type 1 (HIV-1) isolate: role of the *vif* gene in HIV-1 infection kinetics and cytopathicity. *J Virol* **65**:5765–5773.

2334. Saksela, K., E. Muchmore, M. Girard, P. Fultz, and D. Baltimore. 1993. High viral load in lymph nodes and latent human immunodeficiency virus (HIV) in peripheral blood cells of HIV-1-infected chimpanzees. *J Virol* **67**:7423–7427.

2335. Saksela, K., C. Stevens, P. Rubinstein, and D. Baltimore. 1994. Human immunodeficiency virus type 1 mRNA expression in peripheral blood cells predicts disease progression independently of the numbers of CD4+ lymphocytes. *Proc Natl Acad Sci USA* **91**:1104–1108.

2336. Sala, M., G. Zambruno, J.-P. Vartanian, A. Marconi, U. Bertazzoni, and S. Wain-Hobson.

1994. Spatial discontinuities in human immunodeficiency virus type 1 quasispecies derived from epidermal Langerhans cells of a patient with AIDS and evidence for double infection. *J Virol* **68**:5280–5283.

2337. Salahuddin, S. Z., P. D. Markham, M. Popovic, M. G. Sarngadharan, S. Orndorff, A. Fladagar, A. Patel, J. Gold, and R. C. Gallo. 1985. Isolation of infectious human T-cell leukemia/lymphotropic virus type III (HTLV-III) from patients with acquired immunodeficiency syndrome (AIDS) or AIDS-related complex (ARC) and from healthy carriers: a study of risk groups and tissue sources. *Proc Natl Acad Sci USA* **82**:5530–5534.

2338. Salahuddin, S. Z., S. Nakamura, and P. Biberfeld. 1988. Angiogenic properties of Kaposi's sarcoma-derived cells after long-term culture in vitro. *Science* **242**:430–433.

2339. Salahuddin, S. Z., A. G. Palestine, E. Heck, D. Ablashi, M. Luckenbach, J. P. McCulley, and R. B. Nussenblatt. 1986. Isolation of the human T-cell leukemia/lymphotropic virus type III from the cornea. *Am J Ophthalmol* **101**:149–152.

2340. Salim, Y. S., V. Faber, A. Wiik, P. L. Andersen, M. Hoier-Madsen, and S. Mouritsen. 1988. Anti-corticosteroid antibodies in AIDS patients. *APMIS* **96**:889–894.

2341. Salinovich, O., S. L. Payne, R. C. Montelaro, K. A. Hussain, C. J. Issel, and K. L. Schnoor. 1986. Rapid emergence of novel antigenic and genetic variants of equine infectious anemia virus during persistent infection. *J Virol* **57**:71–80.

2342. Salk, J. 1987. Prospects for the control of AIDS by immunizing seropositive individuals. *Nature* **327**:473–476.

2343. Salk, J., P. A. Bretscher, P. L. Salk, M. Clerici, and G. M. Shearer. 1993. A strategy for prophylactic vaccination against HIV. *Science* **260**:1270–1272.

2343a. Sallusto, F., C. R. Mackay, and A. Lanzavecchia. 1997. Selective expression of the exotaxin receptor CCR3 by human T helper 2 cells. *Science* **277**:2005–2007.

2344. Salmon, P., R. Olivier, Y. Riviere, E. Brisson, J.-C. Gluckman, M.-P. Kieny, L. Montagnier, and D. Klatzmann. 1988. Loss of CD4 membrane expression and CD4 mRNA during acute human immunodeficiency virus replication. *J Exp Med* **168**:1953–1969.

2345. Sampaio, E. P., E. N. Sarno, R. Galilly, Z. A. Cohn, and G. Kaplan. 1991. Thalidomide selectively inhibits tumor necrosis factor-alpha production by stimulated human monocytes. *J Exp Med* **173**:699–703.

2346. Samson, M., F. Libert, B. J. Doranz, J. Rucker, C. Liesnard, C. M. Farber, S. Saragosti, C. Lapoumeroulie, J. Cognaux, C. Forceille, G. Muyldermans, C. Verhofstede, G. Burtonboy, M. Georges, T. Imai, S. Rana, Y. Yi, R. J. Smyth, R. G. Collman, R. W. Doms, G. Vassart, and M. Parmentier. 1996. Resistance to HIV-1 infection in Caucasian individuals bearing mutant alleles of the CCR-5 chemokine receptor gene. *Nature* **382**:722–725.

2347. Samuel, K. P., A. Seth, A. Konopka, J. A. Lautenberger, and T. S. Papas. 1987. The 3'-orf protein of human immunodeficiency virus shows structural homology with the phosphorylation domain of human interleukin-2 receptor and the ATP-binding site of the protein kinase family. *FEBS Letters* **218**:81–86.

2348. Samuel, M. C., N. Hessol, S. Shiboski, R. R. Engel, T. P. Speed, and W. Winkelstein, Jr. 1993. Factors associated with human immunodeficiency virus seroconversion in homosexual men in three San Francisco cohort studies, 1984–1989. *J AIDS* **6**:303–312.

2349. Sanchez, G., X. Xu, J. C. Chermann, and I. Hirsch. 1997. Accumulation of defective viral genomes in peripheral blood mononuclear cells of human immunodeficiency virus type 1-infected individuals. *J Virol* **71**:2233–2240.

2350. Sanchez-Palomino, S., J. M. Rohas, M. A. Martinez, E. M. Fenyo, R. Najera, E. Domingo, and C. Lopez-Galindez. 1993. Dilute passage promotes expression of genetic and phenotypic variants of human immunodeficiency virus type 1 in cell culture. *J Virol* **67**:2938–2943.

2351. Sanchez-Pescador, R., M. D. Power, P. J. Barr, K. S. Steimer, M. M. Stempien, S. L. Brown-Shimer, W. W. Gee, A. Renard, A. Randolph, J. A. Levy, D. Dina, and P. A. Luciw. 1985. Nucleotide sequence and expression of an AIDS-associated retrovirus (ARV-2). *Science* **227**:484–492.

2352. Sande, M. A., C. C. J. Carpenter, C. G. Cobbs, K. K. Holmes, and J. P. Sanford. 1993. Antiretroviral therapy for adult HIV-infected patients. *J Am Med Assoc* **270**:2583–2589.

2353. Sandstrom, P. A., D. Pardi, C. S. Goldsmith, D. Chengying, A. M. Diamond, and T. M. Folks. 1996. *bcl-2* expression facilitates human immunodeficiency virus type 1-mediated cytopathic effects during acute spreading infections. *J Virol* **70**:4617–4622.

2354. Sankale, J. L., R. S. De La Tour, R. G. Marlink, R. Scheib, S. Mboup, M. E. Essex, and P. J. Kanki. 1996. Distinct quasi-species in the blood and the brain of an HIV-2-infected individual. *Virol* **226**:418–423.

2355. Sankale, J. L., R. S. De La Tour, B. Renjifo, T. Siby, S. Mboup, R. G. Marlink, M. E. Essex, and P. J. Kanki. 1995. Intrapatient variability of the human immunodeficiency virus type 2 envelope V3 loop. *AIDS Res Hum Retro* **11**:617–623.

2356. Saracco, A., M. Musicco, A. Nicolosi, G. Angarano, C. Arici, G. Gavazzeni, P. Costigliola, S. Gafa, C. Gervasoni, F. Luzzati, F. Piccinino, F. Puppo, B. Salassa, A. Sinicco, R. Stellini, U. Tirelli, G. Turbessi, G. M. Vigevani, G. Visco, R. Zerboni, and A. Lazzarin. 1993. Man-to-woman sexual transmission of HIV: longitudinal study of 343 steady partners of infected men. *J AIDS* **6**:497–502.

2357. Saravolatz, L. D., D. L. Winslow, G. Collins, J. S. Hodges, C. Pettinelli, D. S. Stein, N. Markowitz, R. Reves, M. O. Loveless, L. Crane, M. Thompson, and D. Abrams. 1996. Zidovudine alone or in combination with didanosine or zalcitabine in HIV-infected patients with the acquired immunodeficiency syndrome or fewer than 200 CD4 cells per cubic millimeter. *N Engl J Med* **335**:1099–1106.

2358. Sarin, P. S., D. K. Sun, A. H. Thornton, P. H. Naylor, and A. L. Goldstein. 1986. Neutralization of HTLV-III/LAV replication by antiserum to thymosin alpha 1. *Science* **232**:1135–1137.

2359. Sarngadharan, M. G., M. Popovic, L. Bruch, J. Schupbach, and R. C. Gallo. 1984. Antibodies reactive with human T-lymphotropic retroviruses (HTLV-III) in the serum of patients with AIDS. *Science* **224**:506–508.

2360. Sato, A. I., F. B. Balamuth, K. E. Ugen, W. V. Williams, and D. B. Weiner. 1994. Identification of CD7 glycoprotein as an accessory molecule in HIV-1-mediated syncytium formation and cell-free infection. *J Immunol* **152**:5142–5152.

2361. Sato, H., J. Orenstein, D. Dimitrov, and M. Martin. 1992. Cell-to-cell spread of HIV-1 occurs within minutes and may not involve the participation of virus particles. *Virol* **186**:712–724.

2362. Satow, Y.-I., M. Hashido, K.-I. Ishikawa, H. Honda, M. Mizuno, T. Kawana, and M. Hayami. 1991. Detection of HTLV-I antigen in peripheral and cord blood lymphocytes from carrier mothers. *Lancet* **338**:915–916.

2363. Sattentau, Q. J., A. G. Dalgleish, R. A. Weiss, and P. C. L. Beverley. 1986. Epitopes of the CD4 antigen and HIV infection. *Science* **234**:1120–1123.

2364. Sattentau, Q. J., and J. P. Moore. 1991. Conformational changes induced in the human immunodeficiency virus envelope glycoprotein by soluble CD4 binding. *J Exp Med* **174**:407–415.

2365. Sattentau, Q. J., and J. P. Moore. 1995. Human immunodeficiency virus type 1 neutralization is determined by epitope exposure on the gp120 oligomer. *J Exp Med* **182**:185–196.

2366. Sattentau, Q. J., J. P. Moore, F. Vignaux, F. Traincard, and P. Poignard. 1993. Conformational changes induced in the envelope glycoproteins of the human and simian immunodeficiency viruses by soluble receptor binding. *J Virol* **67**:7383–7393.

2367. Saulsbury, F. T. 1997. The clinical course of human immunodeficiency virus infection in genetically identical children. *Clin Infect Dis* **24**:971–974.

2368. Sawai, E. T., A. Baur, H. Struble, B. M. Peterlin, J. A. Levy, and C. Cheng-Mayer. 1994. Human immunodeficiency virus type 1 Nef associates with a cellular serine kinase in T lymphocytes. *Proc Natl Acad Sci USA* **91**:1539–1543.

2369. Sawai, E. T., I. H. Khan, P. M. Montbriand, B. M. Peterlin, C. Cheng-Mayer, and P. A. Luciw. 1996. Activation of PAK by HIV and SIV Nef: importance for AIDS in rhesus macaques. *Curr Biol* **6**:1519–1527.

2370. Sawyer, L. A., D. A. Katzenstein, R. M. Hendry, E. J. Boone, L. K. Vujcic, C. C. Williams, S.

L. Zeger, A. J. Saah, C. R. Rinaldo, Jr., J. P. Phair, J. V. Giorgi, and G. V. Quinnan, Jr. 1990. Possible beneficial effects of neutralizing antibodies and antibody-dependent cell mediated cytotoxicity in human immunodeficiency virus infection. *AIDS Res Hum Retro* 6:341–356.

2371. Sawyer, L. S. W., M. T. Wrin, L. Crawford-Miksza, B. Potts, Y. Wu, P. A. Weber, R. D. Alfonso, and C. V. Hanson. 1994. Neutralization sensitivity of human immunodeficiency virus type 1 is determined in part by the cells in which the virus is propagated. *J Virol* 68:1342–1349.

2372. Sayers, M. H., P. G. Beatty, and J. A. Hansen. 1986. HLA antibodies as a cause of false-positive reactions in screening enzyme immunoassays for antibodies to human T-lymphotropic virus type III. *Transfusion* 26:113–115.

2373. Scadden, D. T., O. Pickus, S. M. Hammer, B. Stretcher, J. Bresnahan, J. Gere, J. McGrath, and J. M. Agosti. 1996. Lack of *in vivo* effect of granuloycte-macrophage colony-stimulating factor on human immunodeficiency virus type 1. *AIDS Res Hum Retro* 12:1151–1159.

2374. Scadden, D. T., M. Zeira, A. Woon, Z. Wang, L. Schieve, K. Ikeuchi, B. Lim, and J. E. Groopman. 1990. Human immunodeficiency virus infection of human bone marrow stromal fibroblasts. *Blood* 76:317–322.

2375. Scarlatti, G. 1996. Paediatric HIV infection. *Lancet* 348:863–868.

2376. Scarlatti, G., J. Albert, P. Rossi, V. Hodara, P. Biraghi, L. Muggiasca, and E. M. Fenyo. 1993. Mother-to-child transmission of human immunodeficiency virus type 1: correlation with neutralizing antibodies against primary isolates. *J Inf Dis* 168:207–210.

2377. Scarlatti, G., V. Hodara, P. Rossi, L. Muggiasca, A. Bucceri, J. Albert, and E. M. Fenyo. 1993. Transmission of human immunodeficiency virus type 1 (HIV-1) from mother to child correlates with viral phenotype. *Virol* 197:624–629.

2378. Scarlatti, G., T. Leitner, E. Halapi, J. Wahlberg, P. Marchisio, M. A. Clerici-Schoeller, H. Wigzell, E. M. Fenyo, J. Albert, M. Uhlen, and R. P. 1993. Comparison of variable region 3 sequences of human immunodeficiency virus type 1 from infected children with the RNA and DNA sequences of the virus populations of their mothers. *Proc Natl Acad Sci USA* 90:1721–1725.

2379. Scarlatti, G., T. Leitner, V. Hodara, E. Halapi, P. Rossi, J. Albert, and E. M. Fenyo. 1993. Neutralizing antibodies and viral characteristics in mother-to-child transmission of HIV-1. *AIDS* 7:s45–s48.

2380. Scarlatti, G., V. Lombardi, A. Plebani, N. Principi, C. Vegni, G. Ferraris, A. Bucceri, E. M. Fenyo, H. Wigzell, P. Rossi, and J. Albert. 1991. Polymerase chain reaction, virus isolation and antigen assay in HIV-1-antibody-positive mothers and their children. *AIDS* 5:1173–1178.

2381. Schable, C., L. Zekeng, C. P. Pau, D. Hu, L. Kaptue, L. Gurtler, T. Dondero, J. M. Tsague, G. Schochetman, H. Jaffe, and J. R. George. 1994. Sensitivity of United States HIV antibody tests for detection of HIV-1 group O infections. *Lancet* 344:1333–1334.

2382. Schacker, T., A. C. Collier, J. Hughes, T. Shea, and L. Corey. 1996. Clinical and epidemiologic features of primary HIV infection. *Ann Int Med* 125:257–264.

2383. Schattner, A., and B. Rager-Zisman. 1990. Virus-induced autoimmunity. *Rev Inf Dis* 12:204–222.

2384. Schechter, M., L. H. Harrison, N. A. Halsey, G. Trade, M. Santino, L. H. Moulton, and T. C. Quinn. 1994. Coinfection with human T-cell lymphotropic virus type 1 and HIV in Brazil. *J Am Med Assoc* 271:353–357.

2385. Schechter, M. T., K. J. P. Craib, T. N. Le, J. S. G. Montaner, B. Douglas, P. Sestak, B. Willoughby, and M. V. O'Shaughnessy. 1990. Susceptibility to AIDS progression appears early in HIV infection. *AIDS* 4:185–190.

2386. Scheffner, M., K. Munger, J. M. Huibregtse, and P. M. Howley. 1992. Targeted degradation of the retinoblastoma protein by human papillomavirus E7-E6 fusion proteins. *EMBO J* 11:2425–2431.

2387. Scheffner, M., B. A. Werness, J. M. Huibregtse, A. J. Levine, and P. M. Howley. 1990. The E6 oncoprotein encoded by human papillomavirus types 16 and 18 promotes the degradation of p53. *Cell* 63:1129–1136.

2388. Schellekens, P. T., M. Tersmette, M. T. Roos, R. P. Koot, F. De Wolf, R. A. Coutinho, and F. Miedema. 1992. Biphasic rate of CD4+ cell count decline during progression to AIDS correlates with HIV-1 phenotype. *AIDS* **6**:665–670.

2389. Schenk, P. 1986. Retroviruses in Kaposi's sarcoma in acquired immune deficiency syndrome (AIDS). *Acta Otolaryngol (Stockholm)* **101**:295–298.

2390. Scheppler, J. A., J. K. A. Nicholson, D. C. Swan, A. Ahmed-Ansari, and J. S. McDougal. 1989. Down-modulation of MHC-I in a CD4+ T cell line, CEM-E5, after HIV-1 infection. *J Immunol* **143**:2858–2866.

2390a. Schinazi, R. F. 1992. Progress in the development of natural products for human immunodeficiency virus infections, p. 1–29. *In* C. K. Chu and H. G. Cutler (ed.), *Natural Products as Antiviral Agents*. Plenum Press, New York.

2391. Schlienger, K., M. Mancini, Y. Riviere, D. Dormont, P. Tiollais, and M. L. Michel. 1992. Human immunodeficiency virus type 1 major neutralizing determinant exposed on hepatitis B surface antigen particles is highly immunogenic in primates. *J Virol* **66**:2570–2576.

2392. Schlienger, K., D. C. Montefiori, M. Mancini, Y. Riviere, P. Tiollais, and M. L. Michel. 1994. Vaccine-induced neutralizing antibodies directed in part to the simian immunodeficiency virus (SIV) V2 domain were unable to protect rhesus monkeys from SIV experimental challenge. *J Virol* **68**:6578–6588.

2393. Schmidtmayerova, H., C. Bolmont, S. Baghdiguian, I. Hirsch, and J. C. Chermann. 1992. Distinctive pattern of infection and replication of HIV-1 strains in blood-derived macrophages. *Virol* **190**:124–133.

2394. Schmidtmayerova, H., H. S. L. Nottet, G. Nuovo, T. Raabe, C. R. Flanagan, L. Dubrovsky, H. E. Gendelman, A. Cerami, M. Bukrinsky, and B. Sherry. 1996. Human immunodeficiency virus type 1 infection alters chemokine beta peptide expression in human monocytes: implications for recruitment of leukocytes into brain and lymph nodes. *Proc Natl Acad Sci USA* **93**:700–704.

2395. Schmidtmayerova, H., B. Sherry, and M. Bukrinsky. 1996. Chemokines and HIV replication. *Nature* **382**:767.

2396. Schmit, J.-C., J. Cogniaux, P. Hermans, C. Van Vaeck, S. Sprecher, B. Van Remoortel, M. Witvrouw, J. Balzarini, J. Desmyter, E. De Clercq, and A.-M. Vandamme. 1996. Multiple drug resistance to nucleoside analogues and nonnucleoside reverse transcriptase inhibitors in an efficiently replicating human immunodeficiency virus type 1 patient strain. *J Inf Dis* **174**:962–968.

2397. Schmitt, M. P., J. L. Gendrault, C. Schweitzer, A. M. Steffan, C. Beyer, C. Royer, D. Jaeck, J. L. Pasquali, A. Kirn, and A. M. Aubertin. 1990. Permissivity of primary cultures of human Kupffer cells for HIV-1. *AIDS Res Hum Retro* **6**:987–991.

2398. Schmitz, J., J. van Lunzen, K. Tenner-Racz, G. Großschupff, P. Racz, H. Schmitz, M. Dietrich, and F. T. Hufert. 1994. Follicular dendritic cells retain HIV-1 particles on their plasma membrane, but are not productively infected in asymptomatic patients with follicular hyperplasia. *J Immunol* **153**:1352–1359.

2399. Schmitz, J., J. P. Zimmer, B. Kluxen, S. Aries, M. Bogel, I. Gigli, and H. Schmitz. 1995. Antibody-dependent complement-mediated cytotoxicity in sera from patients with HIV-1 infection is controlled by CD55 and CD59. *J Clin Invest* **96**:1520–1526.

2400. Schmitz, T., R. Underwood, R. Khiroya, W. W. Bachovchin, and B. T. Huber. 1996. Potentiation of the immune response in HIV-1+ individuals. *J Clin Invest* **97**:1545–1549.

2401. Schneider, J., O. Kaaden, T. D. Copeland, S. Oroszlan, and G. Hunsmann. 1986. Shedding and interspecies type sero-reactivity of the envelope glycopolypeptide gp120 of the human immunodeficiency virus. *J Gen Virol* **67**:2533–2538.

2402. Schneider, T., A. Beck, C. Ropke, R. Ullrich, H.-P. Harthis, M. Broker, and G. Pauli. 1993. The HIV-1 Nef protein shares an antigenic determinant with a T-cell surface protein. *AIDS* **7**:647–654.

2403. Schneider-Schaulies, J., S. Schneider-Schaulies, R. Brinkman, P. Tas, M. Halbrugge, U. Walter, H. C. Holmes, and V. Ter Meulen. 1992. HIV-1 gp120 receptor on CD4-negative brain cells activates a tyrosine kinase. *Virol* **191**:765–772.

2404. Schnittman, S. M., J. J. Greenhouse, M. C. Psallidopoulos, M. Baseler, N. P. Salzman, A. S. Fauci, and H. C. Lane. 1990. Increasing viral burden in CD4+ T cells from patients with human immunodeficiency virus (HIV) infection reflects rapidly progressive immunosuppression and clinical disease. *Ann Int Med* 113:438–443.

2405. Schnittman, S. M., H. C. Lane, J. Greenhouse, J. S. Justement, M. Baseler, and A. S. Fauci. 1990. Preferential infection of CD4+ memory T cells by human immunodeficiency virus type 1: evidence for a role in the selective T-cell functional defects observed in infected individuals. *Proc Natl Acad Sci USA* 87:6058–6062.

2406. Schnittman, S. M., H. C. Lane, S. E. Higgins, T. Folks, and A. S. Fauci. 1986. Direct polyclonal activation of human B lymphocytes by the acquired immune deficiency syndrome virus. *Science* 233:1084–1086.

2407. Schnittman, S. M., M. C. Psallidopoulos, H. C. Lane, L. Thompson, M. Baseler, F. Massari, C. H. Fox, N. P. Salzman, and A. S. Fauci. 1989. The reservoir for HIV-1 in human peripheral blood is a T cell that maintains expression of CD4. *Science* 245:305–308.

2408. Schnittman, S. M., S. Vogel, M. Baseler, H. C. Lane, and R. T. Davery, Jr. 1994. A phase I study of interferon-alpha 2b in combination with interleukin-2 in patients with human immunodeficiency virus infection. *J Inf Dis* 169:981–989.

2409. Schochetman, G., J. S. Epstein, and T. F. Zuck. 1989. Serodiagnosis of infection with the AIDS virus and other human retroviruses. *Annu Rev Microbiol* 43:629–659.

2410. Schols, D., and E. De Clercq. 1996. Human immunodeficiency virus type 1 gp120 induces anergy in human peripheral blood lymphocytes by inducing interleukin-10 production. *J Virol* 70:4953–4960.

2411. Schols, D., R. Pauwels, J. Desmyter, and E. De Clercq. 1992. Presence of class II histocompatibility DR proteins on the envelope of human immunodeficiency virus demonstrated by FACS analysis. *Virol* 189:374–376.

2412. Schreiber, G. B., M. P. Busch, S. H. Kleinman, and J. J. Korelitz. 1996. The risk of transfusion-transmitted viral infections. *N Engl J Med* 334:1685–1690.

2413. Schrier, R. D., J. A. McCutchan, J. C. Venable, J. A. Nelson, and C. A. Wiley. 1990. T-cell-induced expression of human immunodeficiency virus in macrophages. *J Virol* 64:3280–3288.

2414. Schrier, R. D., J. A. McCutchan, and C. A. Wiley. 1993. Mechanisms of immune activation of human immunodeficiency virus in monocytes/macrophages. *J Virol* 67:5713–5720.

2415. Schrier, R. D., C. A. Wiley, C. Spina, J. A. McCutchan, and I. Grant. 1996. Pathogenic and protective correlates of T cell proliferation in AIDS. *J Clin Invest* 98:731–740.

2416. Schrum, S., P. Probst, B. Fleischer, and P. F. Zipfel. 1996. Synthesis of the CC-chemokines MIP-1α, MIP-1β, and RANTES is associated with a type 1 immune response. *J Immunol* 157:3598–3604.

2417. Schuitemaker, H., M. Groenink, L. Meyaard, N. A. Kootstra, R. A. M. Fouchier, R. A. Gruters, H. G. Huisman, M. Tersmette, and F. Miedema. 1993. Early replication steps but not cell type-specific signalling of the viral long terminal repeat determine HIV-1 monocytotropism. *AIDS Res Hum Retro* 9:669–675.

2418. Schuitemaker, H., M. Koot, N. A. Kootstra, M. W. Dercksen, R. E. Y. de Goede, R. P. van Steenwijk, J. M. A. Lange, J. K. M. Schattenkerk, F. Miedema, and M. Tersmette. 1992. Biological phenotype of human immunodeficiency virus type 1 clones at different stages of infection: progression of disease is associated with a shift from monocytotropic to T-cell-tropic virus populations. *J Virol* 66:1354–1360.

2419. Schuitemaker, H., N. A. Kootstra, R. E. Y. de Goede, F. de Wolf, F. Miedema, and M. Tersmette. 1991. Monocytotropic human immunodeficiency virus type-1 (HIV-1) variants detectable in all stages of HIV-1 infection lack T-cell line tropism and syncytium-inducing ability in primary T-cell culture. *J Virol* 65:356–363.

2420. Schuitemaker, H., N. A. Kootstra, M. H. G. M. Koppelman, S. M. Bruisten, H. G. Huisman, M. Tersmette, and F. Miedema. 1992. Proliferation-dependent HIV-1 infection of monocytes occurs during differentiation into macrophages. *J Clin Invest* 89:1154–1160.

2421. Schuitemaker, H., L. Meyaard, J. A. Kootstra, R. Dubbes, S. A. Otto, M. Tersmette, J. L.

Heeney, and F. Miedema. 1993. Lack of T cell dysfunction and programmed cell death in human immunodeficiency virus type 1-infected chimpanzees correlates with absence of monocytotropic variants. *J Inf Dis* **168**:1140–1147.

2422. Schulz, T. F., B. A. Jameson, L. Lopalco, A. G. Siccardi, R. A. Weiss, and J. P. Moore. 1992. Conserved structural features in the interaction between retroviral surface and transmembrane glycoproteins. *AIDS Res Hum Retro* **8**:1571–1580.

2423. Schulz, T. F., J. D. Reeves, J. G. Hoad, C. Tailor, P. Stephens, G. Clements, S. Ortlepp, K. A. Page, J. P. Moore, and R. A. Weiss. 1993. Effect of mutations in the V3 loop of HIV-1 gp120 on infectivity and susceptibility to proteolytic cleavage. *AIDS Res Hum Retro* **9**:159–166.

2424. Schulz, T. F., D. Whitby, J. G. Hoad, T. Corrah, H. Whittle, and R. A. Weiss. 1990. Biological and molecular variability of human immunodeficiency virus type 2 isolates from The Gambia. *J Virol* **64**:5177–5182.

2425. Schupbach, J., M. Popovic, R. V. Gilden, M. A. Gonda, M. G. Sarngadharan, and R. C. Gallo. 1984. Serological analysis of a subgroup of human T-lymphotropic retroviruses (HTLV-III) associated with AIDS. *Science* **224**:503–505.

2426. Schwartz, D. H., G. Gorse, M. L. Clements, R. Belshe, A. Izu, A.-M. Duliege, P. Berman, T. Twaddell, D. Stablein, R. Sposto, R. Siliciano, and T. Matthews. 1993. Induction of HIV-1-neutralising and syncytium-inhibiting antibodies in uninfected recipients of HIV-1IIIB rgp120 subunit vaccine. *Lancet* **342**:69–73.

2427. Schwartz, O., V. Marechal, O. Danos, and J.-M. Heard. 1995. Human immunodeficiency virus type 1 Nef increases the efficiency of reverse transcription in the infected cell. *J Virol* **69**:4053–4059.

2428. Schwartz, O., V. Marechal, S. Le Gall, F. Lemonnier, and J. M. Heard. 1996. Endocytosis of major histocompatibility complex class I molecules is induced by the HIV-1 Nef protein. *Nature Med* **2**:338–342.

2429. Schwartz, S., B. K. Felber, E.-M. Fenyo, and G. N. Pavlakis. 1989. Rapidly and slowly replicating human immunodeficiency virus type 1 isolates can be distinguished according to target-cell tropism in T-cell and monocyte cell lines. *Proc Natl Acad Sci USA* **86**:7200–7203.

2430. Schwarz, A., G. Offermann, F. Keller, I. Bennhold, J. L'Age-Stehr, P. H. Krause, and M. J. Mihatsch. 1993. The effect of cyclosporine on the progression of human immunodeficiency virus type 1 infection transmitted by transplantation—data on four cases and review of the literature. *Transplantation* **55**:95–103.

2431. Scinicariello, F., P. Rady, M. W. Cloyd, and S. K. Tyring. 1991. HPV 18 in HIV-associated Kaposi's sarcoma. *Lancet* **337**:501.

2432. Scoazec, J.-Y., and G. Feldmann. 1990. Both macrophages and endothelial cells of the human hepatic sinusoid express the CD4 molecule, a receptor for the human immunodeficiency virus. *Hepatol* **12**:505–510.

2433. Scott, P. 1993. IL-12: initiation cytokine for cell-mediated immunity. *Science* **260**:496–497.

2434. Scott, W. A., D. Brambilla, E. Siwak, C. Beatty, J. Bremer, R. W. Coombs, H. Farzadegen, S. A. Fiscus, S. M. Hammer, F. B. Hollinger, N. Khan, S. Rasheed, and P. S. Reichelderfer. 1996. Evaluation of an infectivity standard for real-time quality control of human immunodeficiency virus type 1 quantitative microcococulture assays. *J Clin Micro* **34**:2312–2315.

2435. Scott-Algara, D., F. Vuillier, A. Cayota, V. Rame, D. Guetard, M. L. J. Moncany, M. Marasescu, C. Dauguet, and G. Dighiero. 1993. In vitro non-productive infection of purified natural killer cells by the BRU isolate of the human immunodeficiency virus type 1. *J Gen Virol* **74**:725–731.

2436. Seder, R. A., R. Gazzinelli, A. Sher, and W. E. Paul. 1993. Interleukin 12 acts directly on CD4+ T cells to enhance priming for interferon gamma production and diminishes interleukin 4 inhibition of such priming. *Proc Natl Acad Sci USA* **90**:10188–10192.

2437. Sei, S., S. K. Stewart, M. Farley, B. U. Mueller, J. R. Lane, M. L. Robb, P. Brouwers, and P. A. Pizzo. 1996. Evaluation of human imunodeficiency virus (HIV) type 1 RNA levels in cerebrospinal fluid and viral resistance to zidovudine in children with HIV encephalopathy. *J Inf Dis* **174**:1200–1206.

2438. Sei, Y., P. H. Tsang, F. N. Chu, I. Wallace, J. P. Roboz, P. S. Sarin, and J. G. Bekesi. 1989.

Inverse relationship between HIV-1 p24 antigenemia, anti-p24 antibody and neutralizing antibody response in all stages of HIV-1 infection. *Immunol Let* **20**:223–230.

2439. Sei, Y., P. H. Tsang, J. P. Roboz, P. S. Sarin, J. I. Wallace, and J. G. Bekesi. 1988. Neutralizing antibodies as a prognostic indicator in the progression of acquired immune deficiency syndrome (AIDS)-related disorders: a double-blind study. *J Clin Immunol* **8**:464–472.

2440. Seidman, R., N. S. Peress, and G. J. Nuovo. 1994. In situ detection of polymerase chain reaction-amplified HIV-1 nucleic acids in skeletal muscle in patients with myopathy. *Mod Path* **7**:369–375.

2441. Seligmann, M., D. A. Warrell, J. P. Aboulker, C. Carbon, J. H. Darbyshire, J. Dormont, E. Eschwege, D. J. Girling, D. R. James, J. P. Levy, T. E. A. Peto, D. Schwarz, A. B. Stone, I. V. D. Weller, and R. Withnall. 1994. Concorde: MRT/ANRS randomized double-blind controlled trial of immediate and deferred zidovudine in symptom-free HIV infection. *Lancet* **343**:871–881.

2442. Selmaj, K., C. S. Raine, M. Farooq, W. T. Norton, and C. F. Brosnan. 1991. Cytokine cytotoxicity against oligodendrocytes. *J Immunol* **147**:1522–1529.

2443. Selmaj, K. W., M. Farooq, W. T. Norton, C. S. Raine, and C. F. Brosnan. 1990. Proliferation of astrocytes in vitro in response to cytokines. *J Immunol* **144**:129–135.

2444. Selmaj, K. W., and C. S. Raine. 1988. Tumor necrosis factor mediates myelin and oligodendrocyte damage *in vitro. Ann Neurol* **23**:339–346.

2445. Selwyn, P. A., P. Alcabes, D. Hartel, D. Buono, E. E. Schoenbaum, R. S. Klein, K. Davenny, and G. H. Friedland. 1992. Clinical manifestations and predictors of disease progression in drug users with human immunodeficiency virus infection. *N Engl J Med* **327**:1697–1703.

2446. Semba, R. D., P. G. Miotti, J. D. Chiphangwi, A. J. Saah, J. K. Canner, G. A. Dallabetta, and D. R. Hoover. 1994. Maternal vitamin A deficiency and mother-to-child transmission of HIV-1. *Lancet* **343**:1593–1597.

2447. Semenzato, G., C. Agostini, L. Ometto, R. Zambello, L. Trentin, L. Chieco-Bianchi, and A. De Rossi. 1995. CD8+ T lymphocytes in the lung of acquired immunodeficiency syndrome patients harbor human immunodeficiency virus type 1. *Blood* **85**:2308–2314.

2448. Semple, M., C. Loveday, I. Weller, and R. Tedder. 1991. Direct measurement of viraemia in patients infected with HIV-1 and its relationship to disease progression and zidovudine therapy. *J Med Virol* **35**:38–45.

2449. Semple, M. G., C. Loveday, E. Preston, and R. S. Tedder. 1991. Detection of HIV-1 RNA in factor VIII concentrate. *AIDS* **5**:597–598.

2450. Semprini, A., P. Levy-Setti, M. Bozzo, M. Ravizza, A. Taglioretti, P. Sulpizio, E. Albani, M. Oneta, and G. Pardi. 1992. Insemination of HIV-negative women with processed semen of HIV-positive partners. *Lancet* **340**:1317–1319.

2451. Seremetis, S., L. M. Aledort, G. E. Bergman, R. Bona, G. Bray, D. Brettler, M. E. Eyster, C. Kessler, T. S. Lau, J. Lusher, and F. Rickles. 1993. Three-year randomised study of high-purity or intermediate-purity factor VIII concentrates in symptom-free HIV-seropositive haemophiliacs: effects on immune status. *Lancet* **342**:700–703.

2452. Serwadda, D., R. D. Mugerwa, N. K. Sewankambo, A. Lwegaba, J. W. Carswell, G. B. Kirya, A. C. Bayley, R. G. Downing, R. S. Tedder, S. A. Clayden, R. A. Weiss, and A. G. Dalgleish. 1985. Slim disease: a new disease in Uganda and its association with HTLV-III infection. *Lancet* **ii**:849–852.

2453. Seshamma, T., O. Bagasra, D. Trono, D. Baltimore, and R. J. Pomerantz. 1992. Blocked early-stage latency in the peripheral blood cells of certain individuals infected with human immunodeficiency virus type 1. *Proc Natl Acad Sci USA* **89**:10663–10667.

2454. Shadduck, P. P., J. B. Weinberg, A. F. Haney, J. A. Bartlett, A. J. Langlois, D. P. Bolognesi, and T. J. Matthews. 1991. Lack of enhancing effect of human anti-human immunodeficiency virus type 1 (HIV-1) antibody on HIV-1 infection of human blood monocytes and peritoneal macrophages. *J Virol* **65**:4309–4316.

2455. Shafer, R. W., A. K. N. Iversen, M. A. Winters, E. Aguiniga, D. A. Katzenstein, and T. C. Merigan. 1995. Drug resistance and heterogeneous long-term virologic responses of human immunodeficiency virus type 1-infected subjects to zidovudine and didanosine combination therapy. *J Inf Dis* **172**:70–78.

2456. **Shafferman, A., P. B. Jahrling, R. E. Benveniste, M. G. Lewis, T. J. Phipps, F. Eden-Mc-Cutchan, J. Sadoff, G. A. Eddy, and D. S. Burke.** 1991. Protection of macaques with a simian immunodeficiency virus envelope peptide vaccine based on conserved human immunodeficiency virus type 1 sequences. *Proc Natl Acad Sci USA* **88**:7126–7130.

2457. **Shahabuddin, M., B. Volsky, M. C. Hsu, and D. J. Volsky.** 1992. Restoration of cell surface CD4 expression in human immunodeficiency virus type 1-infected cells by treatment with a Tat antagonist. *J Virol* **66**:6802–6805.

2458. **Shang, F., H. Huang, K. Revesz, H.-C. Chen, R. Herz, and A. Pinter.** 1991. Characterization of monoclonal antibodies against the human immunodeficiency virus matrix protein, p17^{gag}: identification of epitopes exposed at the surfaces of infected cells. *J Virol* **65**:4798–4804.

2459. **Shannon, K., M. J. Cowan, E. Ball, D. Abrams, P. Volberding, and A. J. Ammann.** 1985. Impaired mononuclear-cell proliferation in patients with the acquired immune deficiency syndrome results from abnormalities of both T lymphocytes and adherent mononuclear cells. *J Clin Immunol* **5**:239–245.

2459a. **Shao, Y.** Personal communication.

2460. **Sharer, L. R.** 1992. Pathology of HIV-1 infection of the central nervous system. A review. *J Neuropath Exp Neurol* **51**:3–11.

2461. **Sharer, L. R., C. Eun-Sook, and L. G. Epstein.** 1985. Multinucleated giant cells and HTLV-III in AIDS encephalopathy. *Human Path* **16**:760.

2462. **Sharma, D. P., M. Anderson, M. C. Zink, R. J. Adams, A. D. Donnenberg, J. E. Clements, and O. Narayan.** 1992. Pathogenesis of acute infection in rhesus macaques with a lymphocyte-tropic strain of simian immunodeficiency virus. *J Inf Dis* **166**:738–746.

2463. **Sharma, D. P., M. C. Zink, M. Anderson, R. Adams, J. E. Clements, S. V. Joag, and O. Narayan.** 1992. Derivation of neurotropic simian immunodeficiency virus from exclusively lymphocytotropic parental virus: pathogenesis of infection in macaques. *J Virol* **66**:3550–3556.

2464. **Sharp, P. M., D. L. Robertson, F. Gao, and B. H. Hahn.** 1994. Origins and diversity of human immunodeficiency viruses. *AIDS* **8**:S27-S42.

2465. **Sharpless, N. E., W. A. O'Brien, E. Verdin, C. V. Kufta, I. S. Y. Chen, and M. Dubois-Dalcq.** 1992. Human immunodeficiency virus type 1 tropism for brain microglial cells is determined by a region of the *env* glycoprotein that also controls macrophage tropism. *J Virol* **66**:2588–2593.

2466. **Shaw, G. M., B. H. Hahn, S. K. Arya, J. E. Groopman, R. C. Gallo, and F. Wong-Staal.** 1984. Molecular characterization of human T-cell leukemia (lymphotropic) virus type III in the acquired immune deficiency syndrome. *Science* **226**:1165–1171.

2467. **Shaw, G. M., M. E. Harper, B. H. Hahn, L. G. Epstein, D. C. Gajdusek, R. W. Price, B. A. Navia, C. K. Petito, C. J. O'Hara, J. E. Groopman, E.-S. Cho, J. Oleske, M., F. Wong-Staal, and R. C. Gallo.** 1985. HTLV-III infection in brains of children and adults with AIDS encephalopathy. *Science* **227**:177–182.

2467a. **Shearer, G.** Personal communication.

2468. **Shearer, G. M., and M. Clerici.** 1993. Abnormalities of immune regulation in human immunodeficiency virus infection. *Ped Res* **33**:S71-S74.

2469. **Shearer, G. M., and M. Clerici.** 1991. Early T-helper cell defects in HIV infection. *AIDS* **5**:245–253.

2470. **Shearer, G. M., and M. Clerici.** 1996. Protective immunity against HIV infection: has nature done the experiment for us? *Immunol Today* **17**:21–24.

2470a. **Shearer, W. T., T. C. Quinn, P. La Russa, J. F. Lew, L. Mofenson, S. Almy, K. Rich, E. Handlesman, C. Diaz, M. Pagano, V. Smeriglio, and L. A. Kalish.** 1997. Viral load and disease progression in infants infected with human immunodeficiency virus type 1. *N Engl J Med* **336**:1337–1342.

2471. **Shen, L., G. P. Mazzara, S. O. DiSciullo, D. L. Panicali, and N. L. Letvin.** 1993. Immunization with lentivirus-like particles elicits a potent SIV-specific recall cytotoxic T-lymphocyte response in rhesus monkeys. *AIDS Res Hum Retro* **9**:129–132.

2472. Shepp, D. H., and A. Ashraf. 1993. Effect of didanosine on human immunodeficiency virus viremia and antigenemia in patients with advanced disease: correlation with clinical response. *J Inf Dis* **167**:30–35.

2473. Sheppard, H. W., M. S. Ascher, B. McRae, R. E. Anderson, W. Lang, and J. P. Allain. 1991. The initial immune response to HIV and immune system activation determine the outcome of HIV disease. *J AIDS* **4**:704–712.

2474. Sheppard, H. W., W. Lang, M. S. Ascher, E. Vittinghoff, and W. Winkelstein. 1993. The characterization of non-progressors: long-term HIV-1 infection with stable CD4+ T-cell levels. *AIDS* **7**:1159–1166.

2475. Sher, A., R. T. Gazzinelli, I. P. Oswald, M. Clerici, M. Kullberg, E. J. Pearce, J. A. Berzofsky, T. R. Mosmann, S. L. James, H. C. Morse III, and G. M. Shearer. 1992. Role of T cell derived cytokines in the downregulation of immune responses in parasitic and retroviral infection. *Immunol Rev* **127**:183–204.

2476. Shi, B., U. De Girolami, J. He, S. Wang, A. Lorenzo, J. Busciglio, and D. Gabuzda. 1996. Apoptosis induced by HIV-1 infection of the central nervous system. *J Clin Invest* **98**:1979–1990.

2477. Shibata, D., R. K. Brynes, B. Nathwani, S. Kwok, J. Sninsky, and N. Arnheim. 1989. Human immunodeficiency viral DNA is readily found in lymph node biopsies from seropositive individuals. *Am J Path* **135**:697–702.

2478. Shibata, D., L. M. Weiss, A. M. Hernandez, B. N. Nathwani, L. Bernstein, and A. M. Levine. 1993. Epstein-Barr virus-associated non-Hodgkin's lymphoma in patients infected with the human immunodeficiency virus. *Blood* **8**:2102–2109.

2479. Shibata, R., H. Sakai, T. Kiyomasu, A. Ishimoto, M. Hayami, and A. Adachi. 1990. Generation and characterization of infectious chimeric clones between human immunodeficiency virus type 1 and simian immunodeficiency virus from an African green monkey. *J Virol* **64**:5861–5868.

2480. Shibata, R., C. Siemon, M. W. Cho, L. O. Arthur, S. M. Nigida, Jr., T. Matthews, L. A. Sawyer, A. Schultz, K. K. Murthy, Z. Israel, A. Javadian, P. Frost, R. C. Kennedy, H. C. Lane, and M. A. Martin. 1996. Resistance of previously infected chimpanzees to successive challenges with a heterologous intraclade B strain of human immunodeficiency virus type 1. *J Virol* **70**:4361–4369.

2481. Shibuya, H., K. Irie, J. Ninomiya-Tsuji, M. Goebl, T. Taniguchi, and K. Matsumoto. 1992. New human gene encoding a positive modulator of HIV Tat-mediated transactivation. *Nature* **357**:700–702.

2482. Shih, C.-K., J. M. Rose, G. L. Hansen, J. C. Wu, A. Bacolla, and J. A. Griffin. 1991. Chimeric human immunodeficiency virus type 1/type 2 reverse transcriptase display reversed sensitivity to nonnucleoside analog inhibitors. *Proc Natl Acad Sci USA* **88**:9878–9882.

2483. Shimizu, N. S., N. G. Shimizu, Y. Takeuchi, and H. Hoshino. 1994. Isolation and characterization of human immunodeficiency virus type 1 variants infectious to brain-derived cells: detection of common point mutations in the V3 region of the env gene of the variants. *J Virol* **68**:6130–6135.

2484. Shioda, T., J. A. Levy, and C. Cheng-Mayer. 1991. Macrophage and T-cell line tropisms of HIV-1 are determined by specific regions of the envelope gp120 gene. *Nature* **349**:167–169.

2485. Shioda, T., J. A. Levy, and C. Cheng-Mayer. 1992. Small amino acid changes in the V3 hypervariable region of gp120 can affect the T cell line and macrophage tropisms of human immunodeficiency virus type 1. *Proc Natl Acad Sci USA* **89**:9434–9438.

2486. Shioda, T., and H. Shibuta. 1990. Production of human immunodeficiency virus (HIV)-like particles from cells infected with recombinant vaccinia viruses carrying the *gag* gene of HIV. *Virol* **175**:139–148.

2487. Shirai, A., M. Cosentino, S. F. Leitman-Klinman, and D. M. Klinman. 1992. Human immunodeficiency virus infection induces both polyclonal and virus-specific B cell activation. *J Clin Invest* **89**:561–566.

2488. Shiramizu, B., B. Herndier, T. Meeker, L. D. Kaplan, and M. McGrath. 1992. Molecular and immunophenotypic characterization of AIDS-associated EBV-negative polyclonal lymphoma. *J Clin Oncol* **10**:383–389.

2489. Shiramizu, B., B. G. Herndier, and M. S. McGrath. 1994. Identification of a common clonal human immunodeficiency virus integration site in human immunodeficiency virus-associated lymphomas. *Cancer Res* **54**:2069–2072.

2490. Shore, S. L., T. L. Cromeons, and T. J. Romano. 1976. Immune destruction of virus-infected cells early in the infection cycle. *Nature* **262**:695–696.

2491. Shotton, C., C. Arnold, Q. Sattentau, J. Sodroski, and J. A. McKeating. 1995. Identification and characterization of monoclonal antibodies specific for polymorphic antigenic determinants within the V2 region of the human immunodeficiency virus type 1 envelope glycoprotein. *J Virol* **69**:222–230.

2493. Shrikant, P., D. J. Benos, L. P. Tang, and E. N. Benveniste. 1996. HIV glycoprotein 120 enhances intercellular adhesion molecule-1 gene expression in glial cells. *J Immunol* **156**:1307–1314.

2494. Shrikant, P., and E. N. Benveniste. 1996. The central nervous system as an immunocompetent organ. Role of glial cells in antigen presentation. *J Immunol* **157**:1819–1882.

2495. Siddiqui, A. 1983. Hepatitis B virus DNA in Kaposi's sarcoma. *Proc Natl Acad Sci USA* **80**:4861–4864.

2496. Siddiqui, A., R. Gaynor, A. Srinivasan, J. Mapoles, and R. W. Farr. 1989. Trans-activation of viral enhancers including long terminal repeat of the human immunodeficiency virus by the hepatitis B virus X protein. *Virol* **169**:479–484.

2497. Siddiqui, M. A., M. Tachibana, S. Ohta, Y. Ikegami, S. Tahara-Hanaoka, Y. Y. Huang, and N. Shinohara. 1997. Comparative analysis of the gp120-binding area of murine and human CD4 molecules. *J AIDS Hum Retrovirol* **14**:7–12.

2498. Siebelink, K. H. J., E. Tijhaar, R. C. Huisman, W. Huisman, A. de Ronde, I. H. Darby, M. J. Francis, G. F. Rimmelzwaan, and A. D. M. E. Osterhaus. 1995. Enhancement of feline immunodeficiency virus infection after immunization with envelope glycoprotein subunit vaccines. *J Virol* **69**:3704–3711.

2499. Siegal, B., S. Levinton-Kriss, and A. Schiffer. 1990. Kaposi's sarcoma in immunosuppression. *Cancer* **65**:492–498.

2500. Siegal, F. P., C. Lopez, and G. S. Hammer. 1981. Severe acquired immunodeficiency in male homosexuals, manifested by chronic perianal ulcerative herpes simplex lesions. *N Engl J Med* **305**:1439–1444.

2501. Siegal, F. P., C. Lopez, P. A. Fitzgerald, K. Shah, P. Baron, I. Z. Liederman, D. Imperato, and S. Landesman. 1986. Opportunistic infections in acquired immune deficiency syndrome result from synergistic defects of both the natural and adaptive components of cellular immunity. *J Clin Invest* **78**:115–123.

2502. Siegel, F., R. Kurth, and S. Norley. 1995. Neither whole inactivated virus immunogen nor passive immunoglobulin transfer protects against SIVagm infection in the African green monkey natural host. *J AIDS Hum Retrovirol* **8**:217–226.

2503. Siegel, J. P., J. Y. Djeu, N. I. Stocks, H. Mazur, E. P. Gelman, and G. V. Quinnan. 1985. Sera from patients with the acquired immune deficiency syndrome inhibit production of interleukin-2 by normal lymphocytes. *J Clin Invest* **75**:1957–1964.

2504. Sieling, P. A., J. S. Abrams, M. Yamamura, P. Salgame, B. R. Bloom, T. H. Rea, and R. L. Modlin. 1993. Immunosuppressive roles for IL-10 and IL-4 in human infection: *in vitro* modulation of T-cell response in leprosy. *J Immunol* **150**(12):5501–5510.

2505. Siliciano, R. F., T. Lawton, C. Knall, R. W. Karr, P. Berman, T. Gregory, and E. L. Reinherz. 1988. Analysis of host-virus interactions in AIDS with anti-gp120 T cell clones: effect of HIV sequence variation and a mechanism for CD4+ cell depletion. *Cell* **54**:561–575.

2506. Silvestris, F., P. Cafforio, M. A. Frassanito, M. Tucci, A. Romito, S. Nagata, and F. Dammacco. 1996. Overexpression of Fas antigen on T cells in advanced HIV-1 infection: differential ligation constantly induces apoptosis. *AIDS* **10**:131–141.

2507. Simmonds, P., P. Balfe, J. F. Peutherer, C. A. Ludlam, J. O. Bishop, and A. J. Leigh Brown. 1990. Human immunodeficiency virus-infected individuals contain provirus in small numbers of peripheral mononuclear cells and at low copy numbers. *J Virol* **64**:864–872.

2508. Simmonds, P., L. Q. Zhang, F. McOmish, P. Balfe, C. A. Ludlam, and A. J. L. Brown. 1991.

Discontinuous sequence change of human immunodeficiency virus (HIV) type 1 *env* sequences in plasma viral and lymphocyte-associated proviral populations *in vivo*: implications for models of HIV pathogenesis. *J Virol* 65:6266–6276.

2509. Simmons, G., P. R. Clapham, L. Picard, R. E. Offord, M. M. Rosenkilde, T. W. Schwartz, R. Buser, T. N. C. Wells, and A. E. I. Proudfoot. 1997. Potent inhibition of HIV-1 infectivity in macrophages and lymphocytes by a novel CCR5 antagonist. *Science* 276:276–279.

2509a. Simmons, G., D. Wilkinson, J. D. Reeves, M. Dittmar, S. Beddows, J. Weber, G. Carnegie, U. Desselberger, P. W. Gray, R. A. Weiss, and P. R. Clapham. 1996. Primary syncytium-inducing human immunodeficiency virus type 1 isolates are dual-tropic and most can use either Lestr or CCR5 as coreceptors for virus entry. *J Virol* 70:8355–8360.

2510. Simon, F., S. Matheron, C. Tamalet, I. Loussert-Ajaka, S. Bartczak, J. M. Pepin, C. Dhiver, E. Gamba, C. Elbim, J. A. Gastaut, A. G. Saimot, and F. Brun-Vezinet. 1993. Cellular and plasma viral load in patients infected with HIV-2. *AIDS* 7:1411–1417.

2511. Simpson, G. R., T. F. Schulz, D. Whitby, P. M. Cook, C. Boshoff, L. Rainbow, M. R. Howard, S. J. Gao, R. A. Bohenzky, P. Simmonds, C. Lee, A. de Ruiter, A. Hatzakis, R. S. Tedder, I. V. D. Weller, R. A. Weiss, and P. S. Moore. 1996. Prevalence of Kaposi's sarcoma associated herpesvirus infection measured by antibodies to recombinant capsid protein and latent immunofluorescence antigen. *Lancet* 348:1133–1138.

2512. Sinangil, F., A. Loyter, and D. J. Volsky. 1988. Quantitative measurement of fusion between human immunodeficiency virus and cultured cells using membrane fluorescence dequenching. *FEBS Letters* 239:88–92.

2513. Singh, M. K., and C. D. Pauza. 1992. Extrachromosomal human immunodeficiency virus type 1 sequences are methylated in latently infected U937 cells. *Virol* 188:451–458.

2514. Sinicco, A., R. Fora, R. Raiteri, M. Sciandra, G. Bechis, M. M. Calvo, and P. Gioannini. 1997. Is the clinical course of HIV-1 changing? Cohort study. *Brit Med J* 314:1232–1237.

2515. Sinicco, A., R. Fora, M. Sciandra, A. Lucchini, P. Caramello, and P. Gioannini. 1993. Risk of developing AIDS after primary acute HIV-1 infection. *J AIDS* 6:575–581.

2515a. Sipsas, N. V., S. A. Kalams, A. Trocha, S. He, W. A. Blattner, B. D. Walker, and R. P. Johnson. 1997. Identification of type-specific cytotoxic T lymphocyte responses to homologous viral proteins in laboratory workers accidentally infected with HIV-1. *J Clin Invest* 99:752–762.

2516. Sirianni, M. C., S. Soddu, W. Malorni, G. Arancia, and F. Aiuti. 1988. Mechanism of defective natural killer cell activity in patients with AIDS is associated with defective distribution of tubulin. *J Immunol* 140:2565–2568. (Erratum, 141:709.)

2517. Sirianni, M. C., S. Uccini, A. Angeloni, A. Faggioni, F. Cottoni, and B. Ensoli. 1997. Circulating spindle cells: correlation with human herpesvirus-8 (HHV-8) infection and Kaposi's sarcoma. *Lancet* 349:255.

2518. Skinner, M. A., A. J. Langlois, C. B. McDanal, J. S. McDougal, D. P. Bolognesi, and T. J. Matthews. 1988. Neutralizing antibodies to an immunodominant envelope sequence do not prevent gp120 binding to CD4. *J Virol* 62:4195–4200.

2519. Skolnik, P. R., B. R. Kosloff, L. J. Bechtel, K. R. Huskins, T. Flynn, N. Karthas, K. McIntosh, and M. S. Hirsch. 1989. Absence of infectious HIV-1 in the urine of seropositive viremic subjects. *J Inf Dis* 160:1056–1060.

2520. Skolnik, P. R., B. R. Kosloff, and M. S. Hirsch. 1988. Bidirectional interactions between human immunodeficiency virus type 1 and cytomegalovirus. *J Inf Dis* 157:508–514.

2521. Skowronski, J., D. Parks, and R. Mariani. 1993. Altered T cell activation and development in transgenic mice expressing the HIV-1 nef gene. *EMBO J* 12:703–713.

2522. Slepushkin, V. A., G. V. Kornilaeva, S. M. Andreev, M. V. Sidorova, A. O. Petrukhina, G. R. Matsevich, S. V. Raduk, V. B. Grigoriev, T. V. Makarova, V. V. Lukashov, and E. V. Karamov. 1993. Inhibition of human immunodeficiency virus type 1 (HIV-1) penetration into target cells by synthetic peptides mimicking the N-terminus of the HIV-1 transmembrane glycoprotein. *Virol* 194:294–301.

2522a. Smith, M. W., M. Dean, M. Carrington, C. Winkler, G. A. Huttley, D. A. Lomb, J. J. Goedert, T. R. O'Brien, L. P. Jacobson, R. Kaslow, S. Buchbinder, E. Vittinghoff, D. Vlahov, K. Hoots, M. W. Hilgartner, and S. J. O'Brien. 1997. Contrasting genetic influence of CCR2 and CCR5 variants on HIV-1 infection and disease progression. *Science* 277:959–965.

2523. Smith, A. J., N. Srinivasakumar, M.-L. Hammarskjöld, and D. Rekosh. 1993. Requirements for incorporation of Pr160$^{gag-pol}$ from human immunodeficiency virus type 1 into virus-like particles. *J Virol* 67:2266–2275.

2524. Smith, D. K., J. J. Neal, and S. D. Holmberg. 1993. Unexplained opportunistic infections and CD4+ T-lymphocytopenia without HIV infection. *N Engl J Med* 328:373–379.

2525. Smith, P. D., K. Ohura, H. Masur, H. C. Lane, A. S. Fauci, and S. M. Wahl. 1984. Monocyte function in the acquired immune deficiency syndrome: defective chemotaxis. *J Clin Invest* 74:2121–2128.

2526. Smithgall, M. D., J. G. P. Wong, P. S. Linsley, and O. K. Haffar. 1995. Costimulation of CD4+ T cells via CD28 modulates human immundeficiency virus type 1 infection and replication *in vitro*. *AIDS Res Hum Retro* 11:885–892.

2527. Snider, W. D., D. M. Simpson, K. E. Aronyk, and S. L. Nielsen. 1983. Primary lymphoma of the nervous system associated with acquired immune-deficiency syndrome. *N Engl J Med* 308:45.

2528. Snijders, F., P. C. Wever, S. A. Danner, C. E. Hack, F. J. W. ten Kate, and I. J. M. ten Berge. 1996. Increased numbers of granzyme-B-expressing cytotoxic T-lymphocytes in the small intestine of HIV-infected patients. *J AIDS Hum Retrovirol* 12:276–281.

2529. So, Y. T., J. H. Beckstead, and R. L. Davis. 1986. Primary central nervous system lymphoma in acquired immune deficiency syndrome: a clinical and pathological study. *Ann Neurol* 20:566.

2530. Sodroski, J., W. C. Goh, C. Rosen, K. Campbell, and W. A. Haseltine. 1986. Role of the HTLV-III/LAV envelope in syncytium formation and cytopathicity. *Nature* 322:470–474.

2531. Sodroski, J. G., W. C. Goh, C. Rosen, A. Dayton, E. Terwilliger, and W. A. Haseltine. 1986. A second posttranscriptional transactivator gene required for HTLV-III replication. *Nature* 321:412–417.

2532. Soeiro, R., A. Rubinstein, W. K. Rashbaum, and W. D. Lyman. 1992. Maternofetal transmission of AIDS: frequency of human immunodeficiency virus type 1 nucleic acid sequences in human fetal DNA. *J Inf Dis* 166:699–703.

2533. Solder, B. M., T. F. Schulz, P. Hengster, J. Lower, C. Larcher, G. Bitterlich, R. Kurth, H. Wachter, and M. P. Dierich. 1989. HIV and HIV-infected cells differentially activate the human complement system independent of antibody. *Immunol Let* 22:135–145.

2534. Somasundaran, M., and H. L. Robinson. 1987. A major mechanism of human immunodeficiency virus-induced cell killing does not involve cell fusion. *J Virol* 61:3114–3119.

2535. Song, S. K., H. Li, and M. W. Cloyd. 1996. Rates of shutdown of HIV-1 into latency: roles of the LTR and *tat/rev/vpu* gene region. *Virol* 225:377–386.

2536. Sonnerborg, A., B. Johansson, and O. Strannegard. 1991. Detection of HIV-1 DNA and infectious virus in cerebrospinal fluid. *AIDS Res Hum Retro* 7:369–373.

2537. Sonnerborg, A. B., A. C. Ehrnst, S. K. M. Bergdahl, P. O. Pehrson, B. R. Skoldenberg, and O. O. Strannegard. 1988. HIV isolation from cerebrospinal fluid in relation to immunological deficiency and neurological symptoms. *AIDS Res Hum Retro* 2:89–93.

2538. Sonza, S., A. Maerz, N. Deacon, J. Meanger, J. Mills, and S. Crowe. 1996. Human immunodeficiency virus type 1 replication is blocked prior to reverse transcription and integration in freshly isolated peripheral blood monocytes. *J Virol* 70:3863–3869.

2539. Soto-Ramirez, L. E., B. Renjifo, M. F. McLane, R. Marlink, C. O'Hara, R. Sutthent, C. Wasi, P. Vithayasai, V. Vithayasai, C. Apichartpiyakul, P. Auewarakul, V. Pena Cruz, D. S. Chui, R. Osathanondh, K. Mayer, T. H. Lee, and M. Essex. 1996. HIV-1 Langerhans' cell tropism associated with heterosexual transmission of HIV. *Science* 271:1291–1293.

2540. Soulier, J., L. Grollet, E. Oksenhendler, P. Cacoub, D. Cazals-Hatem, P. Babinet, M. F. d'Agay, J. P. Clauvel, M. Raphael, L. Degos, and F. Sigaux. 1995. Kaposi's sarcoma-associated herpesvirus-like DNA sequences in multicentric Castleman's disease. *Blood* 86:1276–1280.

2541. Spear, G. T. 1993. Interaction of non-antibody factors with HIV in plasma. *AIDS* 7:1149–1157.

2541a. Spear, G. T., L. Al-Harthi, B. Sha, M. N. Saarloos, M. Hayden, L. S. Massad, C. Benson, K. A. Roebuck, N. R. Glick, and A. Landay. 1997. A potent activator of HIV-1 replication is present in the genital tract of a subset of HIV-1-infected and uninfected women. *AIDS* 11:1319–1326.

2542. Spear, G. T., J. R. Carlson, M. B. Jennings, D. M. Takefman, and A. L. Landay. 1992. Complement-mediated neutralizing activity of antibody from HIV-infected persons and HIV-vaccinated macaques. *AIDS* 6:1047. (Letter.)

2543. Spear, G. T., B. L. Sullivan, A. L. Landay, and T. F. Lint. 1990. Neutralization of human immunodeficiency virus type 1 by complement occurs by viral lysis. *J Virol* 64:5869–5873.

2544. Spear, G. T., D. M. Takefman, B. L. Sullivan, A. L. Landay, and S. Zolla-Pazner. 1993. Complement activation by human monoclonal antibodies to human immunodeficiency virus. *J Virol* 67:53–59.

2545. Spearman, P., J. J. Wang, N. Vander Heyden, and L. Ratner. 1994. Identification of human immunodeficiency virus type 1 Gag protein domains essential to membrane binding and particle assembly. *J Virol* 68:3232–3242.

2545a. Speck, R. F., K. Wehrly, E. J. Platt, R. E. Atchison, I. F. Charo, D. Kabat, B. Chesebro, and M. A. Goldsmith. 1997. Selective employment of chemokine receptors as human immunodeficiency virus type 1 coreceptors determined by individual amino acids within the envelope V3 loop. *J Virol* 71:7136–7139.

2546. Spector, D. H., E. Wade, D. A. Wright, V. Koval, C. Clark, D. Jaquish, and S. A. Spector. 1990. Human immunodeficiency virus pseudotypes with expanded cellular and species tropism. *J Virol* 64:2298–2308.

2546a. Spehar, T., and M. Strand. 1994. Cross-reactivity of anti-human immunodeficiency virus type 1 gp41 antibodies with human astrocytes and astrocytoma cell lines. *J Virol* 68:6262–6269.

2547. Spencer, L. T., M. T. Ogino, W. M. Dankner, and S. A. Spector. 1994. Clinical significance of human immunodeficiency virus type 1 phenotypes in infected children. *J Inf Dis* 169:491–495.

2548. Sperduto, A. R., Y. J. Bryson, and I. S. Y. Chen. 1993. Increased susceptibility of neonatal monocyte/macrophages to HIV-1 infection. *AIDS Res Hum Retro* 9:1277–1285.

2549. Sperlagh, M., K. Stefano, F. Gonzalez-Scarano, S. Liang, J. Hoxie, H. Maruyama, M. Prewett, S. Matsuchita, and D. Herlyn. 1993. Monoclonal anti-idiotypic antibodies that mimic the epitope on gp120 defined by anti-HIV-1 monoclonal antibody 0.5-beta. *AIDS* 7:1553–1559.

2550. Spiegel, H., H. Berbst, G. Niedobitek, H. D. Foss, and H. Stein. 1992. Follicular dendritic cells are a major reservoir for human immunodeficiency virus type 1 in lymphoid tissues facilitating infection of CD4+ T-helper cells. *Am J Path* 140:15–22.

2551. Spijkerman, I. J. B., M. Koot, M. Prins, I. P. M. Keet, A. J. A. R. van den Hoek, F. Miedema, and R. A. Coutinho. 1995. Lower prevalence and incidence of HIV-1 syncytium-inducing phenotype among injecting drug users compared with homosexual men. *AIDS* 9:1085–1092.

2552. Spina, C. A., T. J. Kwoh, M. Y. Chowers, J. C. Guatelli, and D. D. Richman. 1994. The importance of Nef in the induction of human immunodeficiency virus type 1 replication from primary quiescent CD4 lymphocytes. *J Exp Med* 179:115–123.

2553. Spina, C. A., H. E. Prince, and D. D. Richman. 1997. Preferential replication of HIV-1 in the CD45RO memory cell subset of primary CD4 lymphcytes *in vitro. J Clin Invest* 99:1774–1785.

2554. Spira, A. I., P. A. Marx, B. K. Patterson, J. Mahoney, R. A. Koup, S. M. Wolinsky, and D. D. Ho. 1996. Cellular targets of infection and route of viral dissemination after an intravaginal inoculation of simian immunodeficiency virus into rhesus macaques. *J Exp Med* 183:215–225.

2556. Sprecher, S., G. Soumenkoff, F. Puissant, and M. Deguildre. 1986. Vertical transmission of HIV in 15-week fetus. *Lancet* ii:288–289.

2557. Sprent, J., and D. F. Tough. 1994. Lymphocyte life-span and memory. *Science* 265:1395–1400.

2558. Spruance, S. L., A. T. Pavia, J. W. Mellors, R. Murphy, J. Gathe, Jr., E. Stool, J. G. Jemsek, P. Dellamonica, A. Cross, and L. Dunkle. 1997. Clinical efficacy of monotherapy with stavudine compared with zidovudine in HIV-infected, zidovudine experienced patients. *Ann Int Med* 126:355–363.

2559. St. Clair, M. H., J. L. Martin, G. Tudor-Williams, M. C. Bach, C. L. Vavro, D. M. King, P. Kellam, S. D. Kemp, and B. A. Larder. 1991. Resistance to ddI and sensitivity to AZT induced by a mutation in HIV-1 reverse transcriptase. *Science* 253:1557–1559.

2560. St. Louis, M. E., M. Kamenga, C. Brown, A. M. Nelson, T. Manzila, V. Batter, F. Behets, U. Kabagabo, R. W. Ryder, M. Oxtoby, T. C. Quinn, and W. L. Heyward. 1993. Risk for perinatal HIV-1 transmission according to maternal immunologic, virologic, and placental factors. *J Am Med Assoc* 269:2853–2859.

2561. Staak, K., S. Prosch, J. Stein, C. Priemer, R. Ewert, W. D. Docke, D. H. Kruger, H. D. Volk, and P. Reinke. 1997. Pentoxifylline promotes replication of human cytomegalovirus *in vivo* and *in vitro*. *Blood* 89:3682–3690.

2562. Stahl, R. E., A. Friedman-Kien, R. Dubin, M. Marmor, and S. Zolla-Pazner. 1982. Immunologic abnormalities in homosexual men. *Am J Med* 73:171–178.

2563. Stahl-Hennig, C., U. Dittmer, T. Nißlein, H. Petry, E. Jurkiewicz, D. Fuchs, H. Wachter, K. Matz-Rensing, E.-M. Kuhn, F.-J. Kaup, E. W. Rud, and G. Hunsmann. 1996. Rapid development of vaccine protection in macaques by live-attenuated simian immunodeficiency virus. *J Gen Virol* 77:2969–2981.

2564. Stahl-Hennig, C., G. Voss, S. Nick, H. Petry, D. Fuchs, H. Wachter, C. Coulibaly, W. Luke, and G. Hunsmann. 1992. Immunization with Tween-ether-treated SIV adsorbed onto aluminum hydroxide protects monkeys against experimental SIV infection. *Virol* 186:588–596.

2565. Stahmer, I., J. P. Zimmer, M. Ernst, T. Fenner, R. Finnern, H. Schmitz, H.-D. Flad, and J. Gerdes. 1991. Isolation of normal human follicular dendritic cells and CD4-independent *in vitro* infection by human immunodeficiency virus (HIV-1). *Eur J Immunol* 21:1873–1878.

2566. Stamatatos, L., and C. Cheng-Mayer. 1993. Evidence that the structural conformation of envelope gp120 affects human immunodeficiency virus type 1 infectivity, host range, and syncytium-forming ability. *J Virol* 67:5635–5639.

2567. Stamatatos, L., and C. Cheng-Mayer. 1995. Structural modulations of the envelope gp120 glycoprotein of human immunodeficiency virus type 1 upon oligomerization and differential V3 loop epitope exposure of isolates displaying distinct tropism upon virion-soluble receptor binding. *J Virol* 69:6191–6198.

2568. Stamatatos, L., and N. Duzgunes. 1993. Simian immunodeficiency virus (SIVmac251) membrane lipid mixing with human CD4+ and CD4-cell lines in vitro does not necessarily result in internalization of the viral core proteins and productive infection. *J Gen Virol* 74:1043–1054.

2569. Stamatatos, L., and J. A. Levy. 1994. CD26 is not involved in infection of peripheral blood mononuclear cells by HIV-1. *AIDS* 8(12):1727–1728.

2569a. Stamatatos, L., and J. A. Levy. Unpublished observations.

2570. Stamatatos, L., A. Werner, and C. Cheng-Mayer. 1994. Differential regulation of cellular tropism and sensitivity to sCD4 neutralization by the envelope gp120 of human immunodeficiency virus type 1. *J Virol* 68(8):4973–4979.

2571. Stamatatos, L., S. Zolla-Pazner, M. K. Gorny, and C. Cheng-Mayer. 1997. Binding of antibodies to virion-associated gp120 molecules of primary-like human immunodeficiency virus type 1 (HIV-1) isolates: effect on HIV-1 infection of macrophages and peripheral blood mononuclear cells. *Virol* 229:360–369.

2572. Stanley, S. K., T. M. Folks, and A. S. Fauci. 1989. Induction of expression of human immunodeficiency virus in a chronically infected promonocytic cell line by ultraviolet irradiation. *AIDS Res Hum Retro* 5:375–384.

2573. Stanley, S. K., S. W. Kessler, J. S. Justement, S. M. Schnittman, J. J. Greenhouse, C. C. Brown, L. Musongela, K. Musey, B. Kapita, and A. S. Fauci. 1992. CD34+ bone marrow cells are infected with HIV in a subset of seropositive individuals. *J Immunol* **149**:689–697.

2574. Stanley, S. K., J. M. McCune, H. Kaneshima, J. S. Justement, M. Sullivan, M. Baseler, J. Adelsberger, M. Bonyhadi, J. Orenstein, C. H. Fox, and A. S. Fauci. 1993. Human immunodeficiency virus infection of the human thymus and disruption of the thymic microenvironment in the SCID-hu mouse. *J Exp Med* **178**:1151–1163.

2575. Stanley, S. K., M. A. Ostrowski, J. S. Justement, K. Gantt, S. Hedayati, M. Mannix, K. Roche, D. J. Schwartzentruber, C. H. Fox, and A. S. Fauci. 1996. Effect of immunization with a common recall antigen on viral expression in patients infected with human immunodeficiency virus type 1. *N Engl J Med* **334**:1222–1230.

2576. Staprans, S. I., B. L. Hamilton, S. E. Follansbee, T. Elbeik, P. Barbosa, R. M. Grant, and M. B. Feinberg. 1995. Activation of virus replication after vaccination of HIV-1-infected individuals. *J Exp Med* **182**:1727–1737.

2577. Starcich, B. R., B. H. Hahn, G. M. Shaw, R. D. McNeely, S. Morrow, H. Wolf, E. S. Parks, W. P. Parks, S. F. Josephs, and R. C. Gallo. 1986. Identification and characterization of conserved and variable regions in the envelope gene of HTLV-III/LAV, the retrovirus of AIDS. *Cell* **45**:637–648.

2578. Staskus, K. A., W. Zhong, K. Gebhard, B. Herndier, H. Wang, R. Renne, J. Beneke, J. Pudney, D. J. Anderson, D. Ganem, and A. T. Haase. 1997. Kaposi's sarcoma-associated herpesvirus gene expression in the endothelial (spindle) tumor cells. *J Virol* **71**:715–719.

2579. Steck, F. T., and H. Rubin. 1966. The mechanism of interference between an avian leukosis virus and Rous sarcoma virus. I. Establishment of interference. *Virol* **29**:628–641.

2579a. Steel, C. M., D. Beatson, R. J. G. Cuthbert, H. Morrison, C. A. Ludlam, J. F. Peutherer, P. Simmonds, and M. Jones. 1988. HLA haplotype A1 B8 DR3 as a risk factor for HIV-related disease. *Lancet* **i**:1185–1188.

2580. Steffan, A. M., M. E. Lafon, J. L. Gendrault, C. Schweitzer, C. Royer, D. Jaeck, J. P. Arnaud, M. P. Schmitt, A. M. Aubertin, and A. Kirn. 1992. Primary cultures of endothelial cells from the human liver sinusoid are permissive for human immunodeficiency virus type 1. *Proc Natl Acad Sci USA* **89**:1582–1586.

2581. Steffen, M., H. C. Reinecker, H. C. Petersen, C. Doehn, I. Pfluger, A. Voss, and A. Raedler. 1993. Differences in cytokine secretion by intestinal mononuclear cells, peripheral blood monocytes and alveolar macrophages from HIV-infected patients. *Clin Exp Immunol* **91**:30–36.

2582. Steffy, K. R., G. Kraus, D. J. Looney, and F. Wong-Staal. 1992. Role of the fusogenic peptide sequence in syncytium induction and infectivity of human immunodeficiency virus type 2. *J Virol* **66**:4532–4535.

2583. Steimer, K. S., P. J. Klasse, and J. A. McKeating. 1991. HIV-1 neutralization directed to epitopes other than linear V3 determinants. *AIDS* **1991**:S135-S143.

2584. Steimer, K. S., C. J. Scandella, P. V. Skiles, and N. L. Haigwood. 1991. Neutralization of divergent HIV-1 isolates by conformation-dependent human antibodies to gp120. *Science* **254**:105–108.

2585. Stein, B., M. Kramer, H. J. Rahmsdorf, H. Ponta, and P. Herrlich. 1989. UV-induced transcription from the human immunodeficiency virus type 1 (HIV-1) long terminal repeat and UV-induced secretion of an extracellular factor that induces HIV-1 transcription in non-irradiated cells. *J Virol* **63**:4540–4544.

2586. Stein, B. S., S. F. Gowda, J. D. Lifson, R. C. Penhallow, K. G. Bensch, and E. G. Engleman. 1987. pH-independent HIV entry into CD4-positive T cells via virus envelope fusion to the plasma membrane. *Cell* **49**:659–668.

2587. Stein, D. S., and G. L. Drusano. 1997. Modeling of the change in CD4 lymphocyte counts in patients before and after administration of the human immunodeficiency virus protease inhibitor indinavir. *Antimicrob Agents Chemo* **41**:449–453.

2588. Stein, D. S., J. A. Korvick, and S. H. Vermund. 1992. CD4+ lymphocyte cell enumeration for prediction of clinical course of human immunodeficiency virus disease: a review. *J Inf Dis* **165**:352–363.

2589. Steinberg, H. N., J. Anderson, C. S. Crumpacker, and P. A. Chatis. 1993. HIV infection of the BS-1 human stroma cell line: effect on murine hematopoiesis. *Virol* **193**:524–527.

2590. Steinberg, H. N., C. S. Crumpacker, and P. A. Chatis. 1991. *In vitro* suppression of normal human bone marrow progenitor cells by human immunodeficiency virus. *J Virol* **65**:1765–1769.

2591. Steinman, L. 1993. Connections between the immune system and the nervous system. *Proc Natl Acad Sci USA* **90**:7912–7914.

2592. Steinman, R. M., and M. D. Witmer. 1978. Lymphoid dendritic cells are potent stimulators of the primary mixed leukocyte reaction in mice. *Proc Natl Acad Sci USA* **75**:5132–5135.

2593. Steketee, R. W., E. J. Abrams, D. M. Thea, T. M. Brown, G. Lambert, S. Orloff, J. Weedon, M. Bamji, E. E. Schoenbaum, J. Rapier, and M. L. Kalish. 1997. Early detection of perinatal human immunodeficiency virus (HIV) type 1 infection using HIV RNA amplification and detection. *J Inf Dis* **175**:707–711.

2593a. Stellbrink, H. J., J. van Lunzen, F. T. Hufert, G. Froschle, G. Wolf-Vorbeck, B. Zollner, H. Albrecht, H. Greten, P. Racz, and K. Tenner-Racz. 1997. Asymptomatic HIV infection is characterized by rapid turnover of HIV RNA in plasma and lymph nodes but not of latently infected lymph-node CD4+ T cells. *AIDS 1997* **11**:1103–1110.

2593b. Stephens, E. B., H. M. McClure, and O. Narayan. 1995. The proteins of lymphocyte- and macrophage-tropic strains of simian immunodeficiency virus are processed differently in macrophages. *Virol* **206**:535–544.

2594. Steuler, H., B. Storch-Hagenlocher, and B. Wildemann. 1992. Distinct populations of human immunodeficiency virus type 1 in blood and cerebrospinal fluid. *AIDS Res Hum Retro* **8**:53–59.

2594a. Stevenson, M. 1997. Molecular mechanisms for the regulation of HIV replication, persistence and latency. *AIDS* **11**:s25-s33.

2595. Stevenson, M., S. Haggerty, C. Lamonica, A. M. Mann, C. Meier, and A. Wasiak. 1990. Cloning and characterization of human immunodeficiency virus type 1 variants diminished in the ability to induce syncytium-independent cytolysis. *J Virol* **64**:3792–3803.

2596. Stevenson, M., C. Meier, A. M. Mann, N. Chapman, and A. Wasiak. 1988. Envelope glycoprotein of HIV induces interference and cytolysis resistance in CD4+ cells: mechanism for persistence in AIDS. *Cell* **53**:483–496.

2597. Stevenson, M., T. L. Stanwick, M. P. Dempsey, and C. A. Lamonica. 1990. HIV-1 replication is controlled at the level of T cell activation and proviral integration. *EMBO J* **9**:1551-1560.

2598. Stevenson, M., X. H. Zhang, and D. J. Volsky. 1987. Downregulation of cell surface molecules during noncytopathic infection of T cells with human immunodeficiency virus. *J Virol* **61**:3741–3748.

2599. Stewart, G. J., J. P. P. Tyler, A. L. Cunningham, J. A. Barr, G. L. Driscoll, J. Gold, and B. J. Lamont. 1985. Transmission of human T-cell lymphotropic virus type III (HTLV-III) by artificial insemination by donor. *Lancet* **ii**:581–585.

2600. Stingl, G., K. Rappersberger, E. Tschachler, S. Gartner, V. Groh, D. L. Mann, K. Wolff, and M. Popovic. 1990. Langerhans cells in HIV-1 infection. *J Am Acad Derm* **22**:1210–1217.

2601. Stott, E. J. 1991. Anti-cell antibody in macaques. *Nature* **353**:393.

2601a. Stranford, S., and J. A. Levy. Unpublished observations.

2602. Street, N. E., J. H. Schumacher, A. T. Fong, H. Bass, D. F. Fiorentino, J. A. Leverah, and T. R. Mosmann. 1990. Heterogeneity of mouse helper T cells. Evidence from bulk cultures and limiting dilution cloning for precursors of Th1 and Th2 cells. *J Immunol* **144**:1629–1639.

2603. Strieter, R. M., T. J. Standiford, G. B. Huffnagle, L. M. Colletti, N. W. Lukacs, and S. L. Kunkel. 1996. "The good, the bad, and the ugly." The role of chemokines in models of human disease. *J Immunol* **156**:3583–3586.

2604. Strizki, J. M., A. V. Albright, H. Sheng, M. O'Connor, L. Perrin, and F. Gonzalez-Scarano. 1996. Infection of primary human microglia and monocyte-derived macrophages with human immunodeficiency virus type 1 isolates: evidence of differential tropism. *J Virol* **70**:7654–7662.

2605. Stromberg, K., R. E. Benveniste, L. O. Arthur, H. Rabin, W. E. Giddens, Jr., H. D. Ochs, W. R. Morton, and C.-C. Tsai. 1984. Characterization of exogenous type D retrovirus from a fibroma of a macaque with simian AIDS and fibromatosis. *Science* 224:289–292.

2606. Stryker, J., and T. J. Coates. 1997. Home access HIV testing. What took so long? *Arch Int Med* 157:261–262.

2607. Su, H., and R. J. Boackle. 1991. Interaction of the envelope glycoprotein of human immunodeficiency virus with C1q and fibronectin under conditions present in human saliva. *Molec Immunol* 28:811–817.

2608. Subar, M., A. Neri, G. Inghirami, D. M. Knowles, and R. Dalla-Favera. 1988. Frequent c-myc oncogene activation and infrequent presence of Epstein-Barr virus genome in AIDS-associated lymphoma. *Blood* 72:667–672.

2609. Subramanyam, M., W. G. Gutheil, W. W. Bachovchin, and B. T. Huber. 1993. Mechanism of HIV-1 tat induced inhibition of antigen-specific T cell responsiveness. *J Immunol* 150:2544–2553.

2610. Sugamura, K., and Y. Hinuma. 1993. Human retroviruses: HTLV-I and HTLV-II, p. 399–436. *In* J. A. Levy (ed.), *The Retroviridae*, vol. 2. Plenum Press, New York.

2611. Sugiura, K., N. Oyaizu, R. Pahwa, V. S. Kalyanaraman, and S. Pahwa. 1992. Effect of human immunodeficiency virus-1 envelope glycoprotein on *in vitro* hematopoiesis of umbilical cord blood. *Blood* 80:1463–1469.

2612. Sullivan, B. L., E. J. Knopoff, M. Saifuddin, D. M. Takefman, M. N. Saarloos, B. E. Sha, and G. T. Spear. 1996. Susceptibility of HIV-1 plasma virus to complement-mediated lysis. *J Immunol* 157:1791–1798.

2613. Sullivan, N., Y. Sun, J. Li, W. Hofmann, and J. Sodroski. 1995. Replicative function and neutralization sensitivity of envelope glycoproteins from primary and T-cell line-passaged human immunodeficiency virus type 1 isolates. *J Virol* 69:4413–4422.

2614. Sullivan, N., M. Thali, C. Furman, D. D. Ho, and J. Sodroski. 1993. Effect of amino acid changes in the V1/V2 region of the human immunodeficiency virus type 1 gp120 glycoprotein on subunit association, syncytium formation, and recognition by a neutralizing antibody. *J Virol* 67:3674–3679.

2614a. Sullivan, P. S., A. N. Do, K. Robbins, M. Kalish, S. Subbarao, D. Pieniazek, C. Schable, G. Afaq, J. Markowitz, R. Myers, J. M. Joseph, and G. Benjamin. 1997. Surveillance for variant strains of HIV: subtype G and group O HIV-1. *J Am Med Assoc* 278:292.

2615. Sun, N.-C., D. D. Ho, C. R. Y. Sun, R.-S. Liou, W. Gordon, M. S. C. Fung, X.-L. Li, R. C. Ting, T.-H. Lee, N. T. Chang, and T.-W. Chang. 1989. Generation and characterization of monoclonal antibodies to the putative CD4-binding domain of human immunodeficiency virus type 1 gp120. *J Virol* 63:3579–3585.

2616. Sun, S., L. M. Pinchuk, M. B. Agy, and E. A. Clark. 1997. Nuclear import of HIV-1 DNA in resting CD4+ T cells requires a cyclosporin A-sensitive pathway. *J Immunol* 158:512–517.

2617. Susal, C., M. Kirschfink, M. Kropelin, V. Daniel, and G. Opelz. 1994. Complement activation by recombinant HIV-1 glycoprotein gp120. *J Immunol* 152:6028–6034.

2618. Sutjipto, S., N. C. Pedersen, C. J. Miller, M. B. Gardner, C. V. Hanson, A. Gettie, M. Jennings, J. Higgins, and P. Marx. 1990. Inactivated simian immunodeficiency virus vaccine failed to protect rhesus macaques from intravenous or genital mucosal infection but delayed disease in intravenously exposed animals. *J Virol* 64:2290–2297.

2619. Svansson, L., and I. Kvarnstrom. 1991. Synthesis of 2′,3′-dideoxy-3′-C-hydroxymethyl nucleosides as potential inhibitors of HIV. *J Org Chem* 56:2993–2997.

2620. Swart, P. J., M. E. Kuipers, C. Smit, R. Pauwels, M. P. deBethune, E. de Clercq, D. K. F. Meijer, and J. G. Huisman. 1996. Antiviral effects of milk proteins: acylation results in polyanionic compounds with potent activity against human immunodeficiency virus types 1 and 2 *in vitro*. *AIDS Res Hum Retro* 12:769–775.

2621. Sweet, R. W., A. Truneh, and W. A. Hendrickson. 1991. CD4: its structure, role in immune function and AIDS pathogenesis, and potential as a pharmacological target. *Curr Opin Biotech* 2:622–633.

2622. Swingler, S., A. Easton, and A. Morris. 1992. Cytokine augmentation of HIV-1 LTR-driven gene expression in neural cells. *AIDS Res Hum Retro* **8**:487–493.

2623. Szabo, S. J., A. S. Dighe, U. Gubler, and K. M. Murphy. 1997. Regulation of the interleukin (IL)-12R β2 subunit expression in developing T helper 1 (Th1) and Th2 cells. *J Exp Med* **185**:817–824.

2624. Szawlowski, P. W. S., T. Hanke, and R. E. Randall. 1993. Sequence homology between HIV-1 gp120 and the apoptosis mediating protein Fas. *AIDS* **7**:1018.

2625. Szelc, C. M., C. Mitcheltree, R. L. Roberts, and E. R. Stiehm. 1992. Deficient polymorphonuclear cell and mononuclear cell antibody-dependent cellular cytotoxicity in pediatric and adult human immunodeficiency virus infection. *J Inf Dis* **166**:486–493.

2626. Taddeo, B., M. Federico, F. Titti, G. B. Rossi, and P. Verani. 1993. Homologous superinfection of both producer and nonproducer HIV-infected cells is blocked at a late retrotranscription step. *Virol* **194**:441–452.

2627. Takahashi, H., Y. Nakagawa, C. D. Pendleton, R. A. Houghten, K. Yokomuro, R. N. Germain, and J. A. Berzofsky. 1992. Induction of broadly cross-reactive cytotoxic T cells recognizing an HIV-1 envelope determinant. *Science* **255**:333–336.

2628. Takahashi, H., Y. Nakagawa, K. Yokomuro, and J. A. Berzofsky. 1993. Induction of CD8+ CTL by immunization with syngeneic irradiated HIV-1 envelope derived peptide-pulsed dendritic cells. *Int Immunol* **5**:849–857.

2629. Takahashi, H., T. Takeshita, B. Morein, S. Putney, R. N. Germain, and J. A. Berzofsky. 1990. Induction of CD8+ cytotoxic T cells by immunization with purified HIV-1 envelope protein in ISCOMs. *Nature* **344**:873–875.

2630. Takamizawa, M., A. Rivas, F. Fagnoni, C. Benike, J. Kosek, H. Hyakawa, and E. G. Engleman. 1997. Dendritic cells that process and present nominal antigens to naive T lymphocytes are derived from CD2+ precursors. *J Immunol* **158**:2134–2142.

2631. Takeda, A., J. E. Robinson, D. D. Ho, C. Debouck, N. L. Haigwood, and F. A. Ennis. 1992. Distinction of human immunodeficiency virus type 1 neutralization and infection enhancement by human monoclonal antibodies to glycoprotein 120. *J Clin Invest* **89**:1952–1957.

2632. Takeda, A., R. W. Sweet, and F. A. Ennis. 1990. Two receptors are required for antibody-dependent enhancement of human immunodeficiency virus type 1 infection: CD4 and FcγR. *J Virol* **64**:5605–5610.

2633. Takeda, A., C. V. Tuazon, and F. A. Ennis. 1988. Antibody-enhanced infection by HIV-1 via Fc receptor-mediated entry. *Science* **242**:580–583.

2634. Takehisa, J., L. Zekeng, T. Miura, E. Ido, M. Yamashita, I. Mboudjeka, L. G. Gurtler, M. Hayami, and L. Kaptue. 1997. Triple HIV-1 infection with group O and group M of different clades in a single Cameroonian AIDS patient. *J AIDS Hum Retrovirol* **14**:81–82.

2635. Takeuchi, Y., M. Akutsu, K. Murayama, N. Shimizu, and H. Hoshino. 1991. Host range mutant of human immunodeficiency virus type 1: modification of cell tropism by a single point mutation at the neutralization epitope in the *env* gene. *J Virol* **65**:1710–1718.

2636. Takeuchi, Y., T. Nagumo, and H. Hoshino. 1988. Low fidelity of cell-free DNA synthesis by reverse transcriptase of human immunodeficiency virus. *J Virol* **62**:3900–3902.

2637. Tamalet, C., A. Lafeuillade, C. Tourres, N. Yahi, C. Vignoli, and P. De Micco. 1994. Inefficacy of neutralizing antibodies against lymph-node HIV-1 isolates in patients with early-stage HIV infection. *AIDS* **8**:388–389.

2638. Tan, X., R. Pearce-Pratt, and D. M. Phillips. 1993. Productive infection of a cervical epithelial cell line with human immunodeficiency virus: implications for sexual transmission. *J Virol* **67**:6447–6452.

2639. Tanaka, T., J. Hu-Li, R. A. Seder, B. F. De St. Groth, and W. E. Paul. 1993. Interleukin 4 suppresses interleukin 2 and interferon gamma production by naive T cells stimulated by accessory cell-dependent receptor engagement. *Proc Natl Acad Sci USA* **90**:5914–5918.

2640. Tanaka, Y., Y. Koyanagi, R. Tanaka, Y. Kumazawa, T. Nishimura, and N. Yamamoto. 1997. Productive and lytic infection of human CD4+ type 1 helper T cells with macrophage-tropic human immunodeficiency virus type 1. *J Virol* **71**:465–470.

2641. Tang, S., and J. A. Levy. 1990. Parameters involved in the cell fusion induced by HIV. *AIDS* 4:409–414.

2642. Tang, S., B. Patterson, and J. A. Levy. 1995. Highly purified quiescent human peripheral blood CD4+ T cells are infectible by human immunodeficiency virus but do not release virus after activation. *J Virol* 69:5659–5665.

2643. Tang, S., L. Poulin, and J. A. Levy. 1992. Lack of human immunodeficiency virus type-1 (HIV-1) replication and accumulation of viral DNA in HIV-1-infected T cells blocked in cell replication. *J Gen Virol* 73:933–939.

2645. Tardieu, M., C. Hery, S. Peudenier, O. Boespflug, and L. Montagnier. 1992. Human immunodeficiency virus type 1-infected monocytic cells can destroy human neural cells after cell-to-cell adhesion. *Ann Neurol* 32:11–17.

2646. Tasaka, T., J. W. Said, and H. P. Koeffler. 1996. Absence of HHV-8 in prostate and semen. *N Engl J Med* 335:1237–1238.

2647. Tascini, C., F. Baldelli, C. Monari, C. Retini, D. Pietrella, D. Francisci, F. Bistoni, and A. Vecchiarelli. 1996. Inhibition of fungicidal activity of polymorphonuclear leukocytes from HIV-infected patients by interleukin (IL)-4 and IL-10. *AIDS* 10:477–483.

2648. Tateno, M., F. Gonzalez-Scarano, and J. A. Levy. 1989. The human immunodeficiency virus can infect CD4-negative human fibroblastoid cells. *Proc Natl Acad Sci USA* 86:4287–4290.

2649. Tateno, M., and J. A. Levy. 1988. MT-4 plaque formation can distinguish cytopathic subtypes of the human immunodeficiency virus (HIV). *Virol* 167:299–301.

2650. Taylor, J. P., R. Pomerantz, O. Bagasra, M. Chowdhury, J. Rappaport, K. Khalili, and S. Amini. 1992. TAR-independent transactivation by Tat in cells derived from the CNS: a novel mechanism of HIV-1 gene regulation. *EMBO J* 11:3395–3403.

2651. Tedla, N., P. Palladinetti, M. Kelly, R. K. Kumar, N. DiGirolamo, U. Chattophadhay, B. Cooke, P. Truskett, J. Dwyer, D. Wakefield, and A. Lloyd. 1996. Chemokines and T lymphocyte recruitment to lymph nodes in HIV infection. *Am J Path* 148:1367–1373.

2652. Tenner-Racz, K., P. Racz, M. Dietrich, and P. Kern. 1985. Altered follicular dendritic cells and virus-like particles in AIDS and AIDS-related lymphadenopathy. *Lancet* i:105–106.

2653. Teppler, H., G. Kaplan, K. Smith, P. Cameron, A. Montana, P. Meyn, and Z. Cohn. 1993. Efficacy of low doses of polyethylene glycol derivative of interleukin-2 in modulating the immune response of patients with human immunodeficiency virus type 1 infection. *J Inf Dis* 167:291–298.

2654. Ter-Grigorov, V. S., O. Krifuks, E. Liubashevsky, A. Nyska, Z. Trainin, and V. Toder. 1997. A new transmissible AIDS-like disease in mice induced by alloimmune stimuli. *Nature Med* 3:37–41.

2655. Terai, C., R. S. Kornbluth, C. D. Pauza, D. D. Richman, and D. A. Carson. 1991. Apoptosis as a mechanism of cell death in cultured T lymphoblasts acutely infected with HIV-1. *J Clin Invest* 87:1710–1715.

2656. Tereskerz, P. M., M. Bentley, and J. Jagger. 1996. Risk of HIV-1 infection after human bites. *Lancet* 348:1512.

2657. Tersmette, M., R. E. Y. de Goede, B. J. M. Al, I. N. Winkel, R. A. Gruters, H. T. Cuypers, H. G. Huisman, and F. Miedema. 1988. Differential syncytium-inducing capacity of human immunodeficiency virus isolates: frequent detection of syncytium-inducing isolates in patients with acquired immunodeficiency syndrome (AIDS) and AIDS-related complex. *J Virol* 62:2026–2032.

2658. Tersmette, M., R. A. Gruters, F. de Wolf, R. E. Y. de Goede, J. M. A. Lange, P. T. A. Schellekens, J. Goudsmit, H. G. Huisman, and F. Miedema. 1989. Evidence for a role of virulent human immunodeficiency virus (HIV) variants in the pathogenesis of acquired immunodeficiency syndrome: studies on sequential HIV isolates. *J Virol* 63:2118–2125.

2659. Tersmette, M., J. M. A. Lange, R. E. Y. deGoede, F. deWolf, J. K. M. Eeftink-Schattenkerk, P. T. A. Schellekens, R. A. Coutinho, H. G. Huisman, J. Goudsmit, and F. Miedema. 1989. Association between biological properties of human immunodeficiency virus variants and risk for AIDS and AIDS mortality. *Lancet* i:983-985.

2660. Tersmette, M., J. J. M. Van Dongen, P. R. Clapham, R. E. Y. De Goede, I. L. M. Wolvers-

Tettero, A. G. Van Kessel, J. G. Huisman, R. A. Weiss, and F. Miedema. 1989. Human immunodeficiency virus infection studied in CD4-expressing human-murine T-cell hybrids. *Virol* **168**:267–273.

2661. Terwilliger, E., J. G. Sodroski, C. A. Rosen, and W. A. Haseltine. 1986. Effects of mutations within the 3' *orf* open reading frame region of human T-cell lymphotropic virus type III (HTLV-III/LAV) on replication and cytopathogenicity. *J Virol* **60**:754–760.

2662. Terwilliger, E. F., E. Langhoff, D. Gabuzda, E. Zazopoulos, and W. A. Haseltine. 1991. Allelic variation in the effects of the *nef* gene on replication of human immunodeficiency virus type 1. *Proc Natl Acad Sci USA* **88**:10971–10975.

2663. Thali, M., A. Bukovsky, E. Kondo, B. Rosenwirth, C. T. Walsh, J. Sodroski, and H. G. Gottlinger. 1994. Functional association of cyclophilin A with HIV-1 virions. *Nature* **372**:363–365.

2664. Thali, M., M. Charles, C. Furman, L. Cavacini, M. Posner, J. Robinson, and J. Sodroski. 1994. Resistance to neutralization by broadly reactive antibodies to the human immunodeficiency virus type 1 gp120 glycoprotein conferred by a gp41 amino acid change. *J Virol* **68**:674–680.

2665. Thali, M., C. Furman, E. Helseth, H. Repke, and J. Sodroski. 1992. Lack of correlation between soluble CD4-induced shedding of the human immunodeficiency virus type 1 exterior envelope glycoprotein and subsequent membrane fusion events. *J Virol* **66**:5516–5524.

2666. Thali, M., C. Furman, D. D. Ho, J. Robinson, S. Tilley, A. Pinter, and J. Sodroski. 1992. Discontinuous, conserved neutralization epitopes overlapping the CD4-binding region of human immunodeficiency virus type 1 gp120 envelope glycoprotein. *J Virol* **66**:5635–5641.

2667. Thali, M., C. Furman, B. Wahren, M. Posner, D. D. Ho, J. Robinson, and J. Sodroski. 1992. Cooperativity of neutralizing antibodies directed against the V3 and CD4 binding regions of the human immunodeficiency virus gp120 envelope glycoprotein. *J AIDS* **5**:591–599.

2668. Thali, M., J. P. Moore, C. Furman, M. Charles, D. D. Ho, J. Robinson, and J. Sodroski. 1993. Characterization of conserved human immunodeficiency virus type 1 gp120 neutralization epitopes exposed upon gp120-CD4 binding. *J Virol* **67**:3978–3988.

2669. Theodorou, I., L. Meyer, M. Magierowska, C. Katlama, and C. Rouzioux. 1997. HIV-1 infection in an individual homozygous for CCR5Δ32. *Lancet* **349**:1219–1220.

2670. Thieblemont, N., N. Haeffner-Cavaillon, A. Ledur, J. L'Age-Stehr, H. W. Ziegler-Heitbrock, and M. D. Kazatchkine. 1993. CR1 (CD35) and CR3 (CD11b/CD18) mediate infection of human monocytes and monocytic cell lines with complement-opsonized HIV independently of CD4. *Clin Exp Immunol* **92**:106–113.

2671. Thielens, N. M., I. M. Bally, C. F. Ebenbichler, M. P. Dierich, and G. J. Arlaud. 1993. Further characterization of the interaction between the C1q subcomponent of human C1 and the transmembrane envelope glycoprotein gp41 of HIV-1. *J Immunol* **151**:6583–6592.

2672. Thiriart, C., J. Goudsmit, P. Schellekens, F. Barin, D. Zagury, M. De Wilde, and C. Bruck. 1988. Antibodies to soluble CD4 in HIV-1 infected individuals. *AIDS* **2**:345–351.

2673. Thiry, L., S. Sprecher-Goldberger, T. Jonckheer, J. Levy, P. Van de Perre, P. Henrivaux, J. Cogniaux-LeClerc, and N. Clumeck. 1985. Isolation of AIDS virus from cell-free breast milk of three healthy virus carriers. *Lancet* **ii**:891–892.

2674. Tian, H., E. T. Donoghue, F. Fang, J. W. Newport, and D. I. Cohen. 1994. Cells expressing mutated CDC2 kinase undergo programmed cell death with striking similarities to HIV-directed cytopathicity. *J Cell Biochem* **18B**(Suppl.):143.

2675. Tian, H., R. Lempicki, L. King, E. Donoghue, L. E. Samelson, and D. I. Cohen. 1996. HIV envelope-directed aberrancies and cell death of CD4+ T cells in the absence of TCR costimulation. *Int Immunol* **8**:65–74.

2676. Tilley, S., W. Honnen, M. Racho, T.-C. Chou, and A. Pinter. 1992. Synergistic neutralization of HIV-1 by human monoclonal antibodies against the V3 loop and the CD4-binding site of gp120. *AIDS Res Hum Retro* **8**:461–467.

2676a. Tilney, L. G., and D. A. Portnoy. 1989. Actin filaments and the growth, movements, and spread of the intracellular bacterial parasite *Listeria monocytogenes*. *J Cell Biol* **109**:1597–1608.

2677. Tindall, B., S. Barker, B. Donovan, T. Barnes, J. Roberts, C. Kronenberg, J. Gold, R. Penny, and D. Cooper. 1988. Characterization of the acute clinical illness associated with human immunodeficiency virus infection. *Arch Int Med* **148**:945–949.

2678. Tindall, B., A. Carr, D. Goldstein, R. Penny, and D. A. Cooper. 1993. Administration of zidovudine during primary HIV-1 infection may be associated with a less vigorous immune response. *AIDS* **7**:127–128.

2679. Tindall, B., and D. A. Cooper. 1991. Primary HIV infection: host responses and intervention strategies. *AIDS* **5**:1–14.

2680. Tindall, B., J. Elford, T. Sharkey, A. Carr, J. Kaldor, and D. A. Cooper. 1993. CD4+ lymphocytopenia in HIV-seronegative homosexual men. *AIDS* **7**:1272–1273.

2681. Tindall, B., L. Evans, P. Cunningham, P. McQueen, L. Hurren, E. Vasak, J. Mooney, and D. A. Cooper. 1992. Identification of HIV-1 in seminal fluid following primary HIV-1 infection. *AIDS* **6**:949–952.

2682. Tindall, B., H. Gaines, I. Imrie, M. A. E. von Sydow, L. A. Evans, O. Strannegard, M. L. Tsang, S. Lindback, and D. A. Cooper. 1991. Zidovudine in the management of primary HIV infection. *AIDS* **5**:477–484.

2683. Todd, B. J., P. Kedar, and J. H. Pope. 1995. Syncytium induction in primary CD4+ T-cell lines from normal donors by human immunodeficiency virus type 1 isolates with non-syncytium-inducing genotype and phenotype in MT-2 cells. *J Virol* **69**:7099–7105.

2684. Toggas, S. M., E. Masliah, E. M. Rockenstein, G. F. Rall, C. R. Abraham, and L. Mucke. 1994. Central nervous system damage produced by expression of the HIV-1 coat protein gp120 in transgenic mice. *Nature* **367**:188–193.

2685. Tokars, J. I., R. Marcus, D. H. Culver, C. A. Schabler, P. S. McKibben, C. I. Bandea, and D. M. Bell. 1993. Surveillance of HIV infection and zidovudine use among health care workers after occupational exposure to HIV-infected blood. *Ann Int Med* **118**:913–919.

2686. Tong-Starksen, S., and B. M. Peterlin. 1990. Mechanisms of retroviral transcriptional activation. *Sem Virol* **1**:215–227.

2687. Tong-Starksen, S. E., P. A. Luciw, and B. M. Peterlin. 1989. Signaling through T lymphocyte surface proteins, TCR/CD3 and CD28, activates the HIV-1 long terminal repeat. *J Immunol* **142**:702–707.

2688. Toniolo, A., C. Serra, P. G. Conaldi, F. Basolo, V. Falcone, and A. Dolei. 1995. Productive HIV-1 infection of normal human mammary epithelial cells. *AIDS* **9**:859–866.

2689. Toohey, K., K. Wehrly, J. Nishio, S. Perryman, and B. Chesebro. 1995. Human immunodeficiency virus envelope V1 and V2 regions influence replication efficiency in macrophages by affecting virus spread. *Virol* **213**:70–79.

2690. Tornatore, C., K. Meyers, W. Atwood, K. Conant, and E. Major. 1994. Temporal patterns of human immunodeficiency virus type 1 transcripts in human fetal astrocytes. *J Virol* **68**:93–102.

2691. Tornatore, C., A. Nath, K. Amemiya, and E. O. Major. 1991. Persistent human immunodeficiency virus type 1 infection in human fetal glial cells reactivated by T cell factor(s) or by the cytokines tumor necrosis factor alpha and interleukin-1 beta. *J Virol* **65**:6094–6100.

2692. Tornatore, C., R. Chandra, J. R. Berger, and E. O. Major. 1994. HIV-1 infection of subcortical astrocytes in the pediatric central nervous system. *Neurol* **44**:481–487.

2693. Torres, C. A. T., A. Iwasaki, B. H. Barber, and H. L. Robinson. 1997. Differential dependence on target site tissue for gene gun and intramuscular DNA immunizations. *J Immunol* **158**:4529–4532.

2694. Toso, J. F., C. H. Chen, J. R. Mohr, L. Piglia, C. Oei, G. Ferrari, M. L. Greenberg, and K. J. Weinhold. 1995. Oligoclonal CD8 lymphocytes from persons with asymptomatic human immunodeficiency virus (HIV) type 1 infection inhibit HIV-1 replication. *J Inf Dis* **172**:964–973.

2695. Toth, F. D., P. Mosborg-Petersen, J. Kiss, G. Aboagye-Mathiesen, M. Zdravkovic, H. Hager, J. Aranyosi, L. Lampe, and P. Ebbesen. 1994. Antibody-dependent enhancement of HIV-1 infection in human term syncytiotrophoblast cells cultured *in vitro*. *Clin Exp Immunol* **95**:389–394.

2696. Tovo, P.-A., M. de Martino, C. Gabiano, L. Galli, C. Tibaldi, A. Vierucci, and F. Veglia. 1994. AIDS appearance in children is associated with the velocity of disease progression in their mothers. *J Inf Dis* **170**:1000–1002.

2697. Tovo, P. A., M. de Martino, C. Gabiano, L. Galli, N. Cappello, E. Ruga, S. Tulisso, A. Vierucci, A. Loy, G. V. Zuccotti, A. M. Bucceri, A. Plebani, P. Marchisio, D. Caselli, S. Livi-adotti, and P. Dallacasa. 1996. Mode of delivery and gestational age influence perinatal HIV-1 transmission. *J AIDS Hum Retrovirol* **11**:88–94.

2698. Tovo, P. A., M. deMartino, C. Gabiano, N. Cappello, R. D'Elia, A. Loy, A. Plebani, G. V. Zuccotti, P. Dallacasa, G. Ferraris, D. Caselli, C. Fundarò, P. D'Argenio, L. Galli, N. Principi, M. Stegagno, E. Ruga, and E. Palomba. 1992. Prognostic factors and survival in children with perinatal HIV-1 infection. *Lancet* **339**:1249–1253.

2700. Trauger, R. J., F. Ferre, A. E. Diagle, F. C. Jensen, R. B. Moss, S. H. Mueller, S. P. Richieri, H. B. Slade, and D. J. Carlo. 1994. Effect of immunization with inactivated gp120-depleted human immunodeficiency virus type 1 (HIV-1) immunogen on HIV-1 immunity, viral DNA, and percentage of CD4 cells. *J Inf Dis* **169**:1256–1264.

2701. Travers, K., S. Mboup, R. Marlink, A. Gueye-Ndiaye, T. Siby, I. Thior, I. Traore, A. Dieng-Sarr, J.-L. Sankale, C. Mullins, I. Ndoye, C.-C. Hsieh, M. Essex, and P. Kanki. 1995. Natural protection against HIV-1 infection provided by HIV-2. *Science* **268**:1612–1615.

2702. Tremblay, M., S. Meloche, R.-P. Sekaly, and M. A. Wainberg. 1990. Complement receptor 2 mediates enhancement of human immunodeficiency virus 1 infection in Epstein-Barr virus-carrying B cells. *J Exp Med* **171**:1791–1796.

2703. Tremblay, M., K. Numazaki, X. G. Li, M. Gornitsky, J. Hiscott, and M. A. Wainberg. 1990. Resistance to infection by HIV-1 of peripheral blood mononuclear cells from HIV-1-infected patients is probably mediated by neutralizing antibodies. *J Immunol* **145**:2896–2901.

2704. Tremblay, M., and M. A. Wainberg. 1990. Neutralization of multiple HIV-1 isolates from a single subject by autologous sequential sera. *J Inf Dis* **162**:735–737.

2705. Trial, J., H. H. Birdsall, J. A. Hallum, M. L. Crane, M. C. Rodriguez-Barradas, A. L. de Jong, B. Krishnan, C. E. Lacke, C. G. Figdor, and R. D. Rossen. 1995. Phenotypic and functional changes in peripheral blood monocytes during progression of human immunodeficiency virus infection. *J Clin Invest* **95**:1690–1701.

2706. Trinchieri, G. 1994. Interleukin-12: a cytokine produced by antigen-presenting cells with immunoregulatory functions in the generation of T-helper cells type 1 and cytotoxic lymphocytes. *Blood* **84**:4008–4027.

2707. Trinchieri, G., and P. Scott. 1994. The role of interleukin 12 in the immune response, disease and therapy. *Immunol Today* **15**:460–463.

2708. Trischmann, H., D. Davis, and P. J. Lachmann. 1995. Lymphocytotropic strains of HIV type 1 when complexed with enhancing antibodies can infect macrophages via FcγRIII, independently of CD4. *AIDS Res Hum Retro* **11**:343–352.

2709. Tristem, M., C. Marshall, A. Karpas, and F. Hill. 1992. Evolution of the primate lentiviruses: evidence from vpx and vpr. *EMBO J* **11**:3405–3412.

2710. Trkola, A., T. Dragic, J. Arthos, J. M. Binley, W. C. Olson, G. P. Allaway, C. Cheng-Mayer, J. Robinson, P. J. Maddon, and J. P. Moore. 1996. CD4-dependent, antibody-sensitive interactions between HIV-1 and its co-receptor CCR-5. *Nature* **384**:184–187.

2711. Trkola, A., A. B. Pomales, H. Yuan, B. Korber, P. J. Maddon, G. P. Allaway, H. Katinger, C. F. Barbas III, D. R. Burton, D. D. Ho, and J. P. Moore. 1995. Cross-clade neutralization of primary isolates of human immunodeficiency virus type 1 by human monoclonal antibodies and tetrameric CD4-IgG. *J Virol* **69**:6609–6617.

2712. Trkola, A., M. Purtscher, T. Muster, C. Ballaun, A. Buchacher, N. Sullivan, K. Srinivasan, J. Sodroski, J. P. Moore, and H. Katinger. 1996. Human monoclonal antibody 2G12 defines a distinctive neutralization epitope on the gp120 glycoprotein of human immunodeficiency virus type 1. *J Virol* **70**:1100–1108.

2713. Trono, D. 1992. Partial reverse trancripts in virions from human immunodeficiency and murine leukemia viruses. *J Virol* **66**:4893–4900.

2714. Trono, D., and C. Aiken. 1994. Nef induces CD4 endocytosis: requirement for a critical motif in the membrane-proximal CD4 cytoplasmic domain. *J Cell Biochem* **18B**(Suppl.):143.

2715. Trono, D., and D. Baltimore. 1990. A human cell factor is essential for HIV-1 *rev* action. *EMBO J* 9:4155–4160.

2716. Trujillo, J. R., M. F. McLane, T. H. Lee, and M. Essex. 1993. Molecular mimicry between the human immunodeficiency virus type 1 gp120 V3 loop and human brain proteins. *J Virol* 67:7711–7715.

2717. Truneh, A., D. Buck, D. R. Cassatt, R. Juszczak, S. Kassis, S. E. Ryu, D. Healey, R. Sweet, and Q. Sattentau. 1991. A region in domain 1 of CD4 distinct from the primary gp120 binding site is involved in HIV infection and virus-mediated fusion. *J Biol Chem* 266:5942–5948.

2718. Tsai, C. C., K. E. Follis, A. Sabo, T. W. Beck, R. F. Grant, N. Bischofberger, R. E. Benveniste, and R. Black. 1995. Prevention of SIV infection in macaques by (R)-9-(2-phosphonyl-methoxypropyl)adenine. *Science* 270:1197–1199.

2719. Tsai, C. C., T. F. C. S. Warner, H. Uno, W. E. Giddens, Jr., and H. D. Ochs. 1985. Subcutaneous fibromatosis associated with an acquired immune deficiency syndrome in pig-tailed macaques. *Am J Path* 120:30–37.

2720. Tsang, M. L., L. A. Evans, P. McQueen, L. Hurren, C. Byrne, R. Penny, B. Tindall, and D. A. Cooper. 1994. Neutralizing antibodies against sequential autologous human immunodeficiency virus type 1 isolates after seroconversion. *J Inf Dis* 170:1141–1147.

2721. Tschlachler, E., V. Groh, M. Popovic, D. L. Mann, K. Konrad, B. Safai, L. Eron, F. D. M. Veronese, K. Wolff, and G. Stingl. 1987. Epidermal Langerhans cells—a target for HTLV-III/LAV infection. *J Invest Derm* 88:233–237.

2722. Tsubota, H., D. J. Ringler, M. Kannagi, N. W. King, K. R. Solomon, J. J. MacKey, D. G. Walsh, and N. L. Letvin. 1989. CD8+CD4− lymphocyte lines can harbor the AIDS virus *in vitro*. *J Immunol* 143:858–863.

2722a. Tsuji, T., K. Hamajima, J. Fukushima, K. Q. Zin, N. Ishii, I. Aoki, Y. Ishigatsubo, K. Tani, S. Kawamoto, Y. Nitta, J. Miyazaki, W. C. Koff, T. Okubo, and K. Okuda. 1997. Enhancement of cell-mediated immunity against HIV-1 induced by coinoculation of plasmid-encoded HIV-1 antigen with plasmid expressing IL-12. *J Immunol* 158:4008–4013.

2722b. Tsuji, T., K. Hamajima, N. Ishii, I. Aoki, J. Fukushima, K. Q. Xin, S. Kawamoto, S. Sasaki, K. Matsunaga, Y. Ishigatsubo, K. Tani, T. Okubo, and K. Okuda. 1997. Immunomodulatory effects of a plasmid expressing B7-2 on human immunodeficiency virus-1-specific cell-mediated immunity induced by a plasmid encoding the viral antigen. *Eur J Immunol* 27:782–787.

2723. Tsujimoto, H., A. Hasegawa, N. Maki, M. Fukasawa, T. Miura, S. Speidel, R. W. Cooper, E. N. Moriyama, T. Gojobori, and M. Hayami. 1989. Sequence of a novel simian immunodeficiency virus from a wild-caught African mandrill. *Nature* 341:539–541.

2724. Tsunetsugu-Yokota, Y., K. Akagawa, H. Kimoto, K. Suzuki, M. Iwasaki, S. Yasuda, G. Hausser, C. Hultgren, A. Meyerhans, and T. Takemori. 1995. Monocyte-derived cultured dendritic cells are susceptible to human immunodeficiency virus infection and transmit virus to resting T cells in the process of nominal antigen presentation. *J Virol* 69:4544–4547.

2725. Tsunetsugu-Yokota, Y., S. Matsuda, M. Maekawa, T. Saito, T. Takemori, and Y. Takebe. 1992. Constitutive expression of the *nef* gene suppresses human immunodeficiency virus type 1 (HIV-1) replication in monocytic cell lines. *Virol* 191:960–963.

2726. Tsunoda, R., K. Hashimoto, M. Baba, S. Shigeta, and N. Sugai. 1996. Follicular dendritic cells *in vitro* are not susceptible to infection by HIV-1. *AIDS* 10:595–602.

2727. Tummino, P. J., J. D. Scholten, P. J. Harvey, T. P. Holler, L. Maloney, R. Gogliotti, J. Domagala, and D. Hupe. 1996. The *in vitro* ejection of zinc from human immunodeficiency virus (HIV) type 1 nucleocapsid protein by disulfide benzamides with cellular anti-HIV activity. *Proc Natl Acad Sci USA* 93:969–973.

2728. Turner, S., R. Tizard, J. DeMarinis, R. B. Pepinsky, J. Zullo, R. Schooley, and R. Fisher. 1992. Resistance of primary isolates of human immunodeficiency virus type 1 to neutralization by soluble CD4 is not due to lower affinity with the viral envelope glycoprotein gp120. *Proc Natl Acad Sci USA* 89:1335–1339.

2729. Twigg, H. L., III, D. M. Soliman, and B. A. Spain. 1994. Impaired alveolar macrophage accessory cell function and reduced incidence of lymphocytic alveolitis in HIV-infected patients who smoke. *AIDS* 8:611–618.

2730. Tyler, D. S., S. D. Stanley, C. A. Nastala, A. A. Austin, J. A. Bartlett, K. C. Stine, H. K. Lyerly, D. P. Bolognesi, and K. J. Weinhold. 1990. Alterations in antibody-dependent cellular cytotoxicity during the course of HIV-1 infection. *J Immunol* 144:3375–3384.

2731. Tyndall, M. W., A. R. Ronald, E. Agoki, W. Malisa, J. J. Bwayo, J. O. Ndinya-Achola, S. Moses, and F. A. Plummer. 1996. Increased risk of infection with human immunodeficiency virus type 1 among uncircumcised men presenting with genital ulcer disease in Kenya. *Clin Infect Dis* 23:449–453.

2732. Tyor, W. R., J. D. Glass, J. W. Griffin, B. P.S., J. C. McArthur, L. Bezman, and D. E. Griffin. 1991. Cytokine expression in the brain during the acquired immunodeficiency syndrome. *Ann Neurol* 31:349–360.

2733. Tyor, W. R., C. Power, H. E. Gendelman, and R. B. Markham. 1993. A model of human immunodeficiency virus encephalitis in SCID mice. *Proc Natl Acad Sci USA* 90:8658–8662.

2734. Uehara, T., T. Miyawaki, K. Ohta, Y. Tamaru, T. Yokio, S. Nakamura, and N. Taniguchi. 1992. Apoptotic cell death of primed CD45RO+ T lymphocytes in Epstein-Barr virus-induced infectious mononucleosis. *Blood* 80:452–458.

2735. Ugen, K. E., V. Srikantan, J. J. Goedert, R. P. Nelson, Jr., W. V. Williams, and D. B. Weiner. 1997. Vertical transmission of human immunodeficiency virus type 1: seroreactivity by maternal antibodies to the carboxy region of the gp41 envelope glycoprotein. *J Inf Dis* 175:63–69.

2736. Uittenbogaart, C. H., D. J. Anisman, B. D. Jamieson, S. Kitchen, I. Schmid, J. A. Zack, and E. F. Hays. 1996. Differential tropism of HIV-1 isolates for distinct thymocyte subsets *in vitro. AIDS* 10:F9-F16.

2737. Ullum, H., J. Palmo, J. Halkjaer-Kristensen, M. Diamant, M. Klokker, A. Kruuse, A. LaPerriere, and B. K. Pedersen. 1994. The effect of acute exercise on lymphocyte subsets, natural killer cells, proliferative responses, and cytokines in HIV-seropositive persons. *J AIDS* 7:1122–1133.

2738. Urdea, M. S. 1993. Synthesis and characterization of branched DNA (bDNA) for the direct and quantitative detection of CMV, HBV, HCV, and HIV. *Clin Chem* 39:725–726.

2739. Vaishnav, Y., and F. Wong-Staal. 1992. The biochemistry of AIDS. *Annu Rev Biochem* 60:578–630.

2740. Valentin, A., J. Albert, E. M. Fenyo, and B. Asjo. 1994. Dual tropism for macrophages and lymphocytes is a common feature of primary human immunodeficiency virus type 1 and 2 isolates. *J Virol* 68:6684–6689.

2741. Valentin, A., J. Albert, E. M. Fenyo, and B. Asjo. 1990. HIV-1 infection of normal human macrophage cultures: implication for silent infection. *Virol* 177:790–794.

2742. Valentin, A., K. Lundin, M. Patarroyo, and B. Asjo. 1990. The leukocyte adhesion glycoprotein CD18 participates in HIV-1-induced syncytia formation in monocytoid and T cells. *J Immunol* 144:934–937.

2743. Valentin, A., A. von Gegerfelt, S. Matsuda, K. Nilsson, and B. Asjo. 1991. *In vitro* maturation of mononuclear phagocytes and susceptibility to HIV-1 infection. *J AIDS* 4:751–759.

2744. Valentin, H., M. T. Nugeyre, F. Vuillier, L. Boumsell, and M. Schmid. 1994. Two subpopulations of human triple-negative thymic cells are susceptible to infection by human immunodeficiency virus type 1 in vitro. *J Virol* 68:3041–3050.

2745. Valeriano-Marcet, J., L. Ravichandran, and L. D. Kerr. 1990. HIV associated systemic necrotizing vasculitis. *J Rheumatol* 17:1091–1093.

2746. Valerie, K., A. Delers, C. Bruck, C. Thiriart, H. Rosenberg, C. Debouck, and C. M. Rosenberg. 1988. Activation of human immunodeficiency virus type 1 by DNA damage in human cells. *Nature* 333:78–81.

2747. Vallee, H., and H. Carre. 1904. Sur l'anémie infectieuse du cheval. *CR Acad Sci* 139:1239–1241.

2748. Van de Perre, P., A. Simonon, D. G. Hitimana, F. Dabis, P. Msellati, B. Mukamabano, J.-B. Butera, C. Van Goethem, E. Karita, and P. Lepage. 1993. Infective and anti-infective properties of breastmilk from HIV-1-infected women. *Lancet* 341:914–918.

2749. Van de Perre, P., A. Simonon, P. Msellati, D.-G. Hitimana, D. Vaira, A. Bazubagira, C. Van Goethem, A.-M. Stevens, E. Karita, D. Sondag-Thull, F. Dabis, and P. Lepage. 1991. Postnatal transmission of human immunodeficiency virus type 1 from mother to infant. *N Engl J Med* **325**:593–598.

2750. van der Hoek, L., R. Boom, J. Goudsmit, F. Snijders, and C. J. A. Sol. 1995. Isolation of human immunodeficiency virus type 1 (HIV-1) RNA from feces by a simple method and difference between HIV-1 subpopulations in feces and serum. *J Clin Micro* **33**:581–588.

2751. van Kerckhoven, I., K. Fransen, M. Peeters, H. De Beenhouwer, P. Piot, and G. van der Groen. 1994. Quantification of human immunodeficiency virus in plasma by RNA PCR, viral culture, and p24 antigen detection. *J Clin Micro* **32**:1669–1673.

2752. Van Lint, C., S. Emiliani, M. Ott, and E. Verdin. 1996. Transcriptional activation and chromatin remodeling of the HIV-1 promoter in response to histone acetylation. *EMBO J* **15**:1112–1120.

2753. Van Nest, G. A., K. S. Steimer, N. L. Haigwood, R. L. Burke, and G. Ott. 1992. Advanced adjuvant formulations for use with recombinant subunit vaccines, p. 57–62. *In* R. M. Chanock, R. A. Lerner, F. Brown, and H. Ginsburg (ed.), *Vaccines 92: Modern Approaches to New Vaccines.* Cold Spring Harbor Laboratory, Cold Spring Harbor.

2754. van Noesel, C. J. M., R. A. Gruters, F. G. Terpstra, P. T. A. Schellekens, R. A. W. van Lier, and F. Miedema. 1990. Functional and phenotypic evidence for a selective loss of memory T cells in asymptomatic human immunodeficiency virus-infected men. *J Clin Invest* **86**:293–299.

2755. Van Rompay, K. K. A., J. M. Cherrington, M. L. Marthas, C. J. Berardi, A. S. Mulato, A. Spinner, R. P. Tarara, D. R. Canfield, S. Telm, N. Bischofberger, and N. C. Pedersen. 1996. 9-[2-(Phosphonomethoxy)propyl]adenine therapy of established simian immunodeficiency virus infection in infant rhesus macaques. *Antimicrob Agents Chemo* **40**:2586–2591.

2756. Van Rompay, K. K. A., M. G. Otsyula, M. L. Marthas, C. J. Miller, M. B. McChesney, and N. C. Pedersen. 1995. Immediate zidovudine treatment protects simian immunodeficiency virus-infected newborn macaques against rapid onset of AIDS. *Antimicrob Agents Chemo* **39**:125–131.

2757. Van Rompay, K. K. A., M. G. Otsyula, R. P. Tarara, D. R. Canfield, C. J. Berardi, M. B. McChesney, and M. L. Marthas. 1996. Vaccination of pregnant macaques protects newborns against mucosal simian immunodeficiency virus infection. *J Inf Dis* **173**:1327–1335.

2758. Van Voorhis, B. J., A. Martinez, K. Mayer, and D. J. Anderson. 1991. Detection of human immunodeficiency virus type 1 in semen from seropositive men using culture and polymerase chain reaction deoxyribonucleic acid amplification techniques. *Fert Steril* **55**:588–594.

2759. VanCott, T. C., F. R. Bethke, V. R. Polonis, M. K. Gorny, S. Zolla-Pazner, R. R. Redfield, and D. L. Birx. 1994. Dissociation rate of antibody-gp120 binding interactions is predictive of V3-mediated neutralization of HIV-1. *J Immunol* **153**:449–459.

2760. Vanden Haesevelde, M. M., M. Peeters, G. Jannes, W. Janssens, G. van der Groen, P. M. Sharp, and E. Saman. 1996. Sequence analysis of a highly divergent HIV-1-related lentivirus isolated from a wild captured chimpanzee. *Virol* **221**:346–350.

2761. Vanham, G., L. Kestens, I. De Meester, J. Vingerhoets, G. Penne, G. Vanhoof, S. Scharpe, H. Heyligen, E. Bosmans, J. L. Ceuppens, and P. Gigase. 1993. Decreased expression of the memory marker CD26 on both CD4+ and CD8+ lymphocytes of HIV-infected subjects. *J AIDS* **6**:749–757.

2762. Veenstra, J., I. G. Williams, R. Colebunders, L. Dorrell, S. E. Tchamouroff, G. Patou, J. M. A. Lange, I. V. D. Weller, J. Goeman, S. Uthayakumar, I. R. Gow, J. N. Weber, and R. A. Coutinho. 1996. Immunization with recombinant p17/p24: Ty virus-like particles in human immunodeficiency virus-infected persons. *J Inf Dis* **174**:862–866.

2763. Vega, M. A., R. Guigdo, and T. F. Smith. 1990. Autoimmune response in AIDS. *Nature* **345**:26.

2764. Vella, S., M. Giuliano, M. Floridia, A. Chiesi, C. Tomino, A. Seeber, S. Barcherini, R. Bucciardini, and S. Mariotti. 1995. Effect of sex, age and transmission category on the progression to AIDS and survival of zidovudine-treated symptomatic patients. *AIDS* **9**:51–56.

2765. Vendrell, J. P., M. Segondy, J. Ducos, J. Reynes, M. F. Huguet, J. C. Nicolas, and A. Serre. 1991. Analysis of the spontaneous *in vitro* anti-HIV-1 antibody secretion by peripheral blood mononuclear cells in HIV-1 infection. *Clin Exp Immunol* **83**:197–202.

2765a. Vento, S., T. Garofano, C. Renzini, F. Casali, T. Ferraro, and E. Concia. 1997. Enhancement of hepatitis C virus replication and liver damage in HIV coinfected patients on antiretroviral combination therapy. *AIDS* in press.

2766. Verani, A., G. Scarlatti, M. Comar, E. Tresoldi, S. Polo, M. Giacca, P. Lusso, A. G. Siccardi, and D. Vercelli. 1997. C-C chemokines released by lipopolysaccharide (LPS)-stimulated human macrophages suppress HIV-1 infection in both macrophages and T cells. *J Exp Med* **185**:805–816.

2767. Verhofstede, C., S. Reniers, F. Van Wanzeele, and J. Plum. 1994. Evaluation of proviral copy number and plasma RNA level as early indicators of progression in HIV-1 infection: correlation with virological and immunological markers of disease. *AIDS* **8**:1421–1427.

2767a. Vermund, S. 1993. Rising HIV-related mortality in young Americans. *J Am Med Assoc* **269**:3034–3035.

2768. Vernazza, P. L., and J. J. Eron, Jr. 1997. Probability of heterosexual transmission of HIV. *J AIDS Hum Retrovirol* **14**:85–86.

2769. Vernazza, P. L., J. J. Eron, M. S. Cohen, C. M. van der Horst, L. Troiani, and S. A. Fiscus. 1994. Detection and biologic characterization of infectious HIV-1 in semen of seropositive men. *AIDS* **8**:1325–1329.

2770. Veugelers, P. J., J. M. Kaldor, S. A. Strathdee, K. A. Page-Shafer, M. T. Schechter, R. A. Coutinho, I. P. M. Keet, and G. J. P. van Griensven. 1997. Incidence and prognostic significance of symptomatic primary human immunodeficiency virus type 1 infection in homosexual men. *J Inf Dis* **176**:112–117.

2771. Veugelers, P. J., S. A. Strathdee, B. Tindall, K. A. Page, A. R. Moss, M. T. Schechter, J. S. G. Montaner, and G. J. P. van Griensven. 1994. Increasing age is associated with faster progression to neoplasms but not opportunistic infections in HIV-infected homosexual men. *AIDS* **8**:1471–1475.

2772. Vicenzi, E., P. Bagnarelli, E. Santagostino, S. Ghezzi, M. Alfano, M. S. Sinnons, G. Fabio, L. Turchetto, G. Moretti, A. Lazzarin, A. Mantovani, P. M. Mannucci, M. Clementi, A. Gringeri, and G. Poli. 1997. Hemophilia and nonprogressing human immunodeficiency virus type 1 infection. *Blood* **89**:191–200.

2773. Vidmar, L., M. Poljak, J. Tomazic, K. Seme, and I. Klavs. 1996. Transmission of HIV-1 by human bite. *Lancet* **347**:1762–1763.

2774. Villinger, F., T. M. Folks, S. Lauro, J. D. Powell, J. B. Sundstrom, A. Mayne, and A. A. Ansari. 1996. Immunological and virological studies of natural SIV infection of disease-resistant nonhuman primates. *Immunol Let* **51**:59–68.

2775. Viscidi, R. P., K. Mayur, H. M. Lederman, and A. D. Frankel. 1989. Inhibition of antigen-induced lymphocyte proliferation by *tat* protein from HIV-1. *Science* **246**:1606–1608.

2776. Visconti, A., L. Visconti, R. Bellocco, N. Binkin, G. Colucci, L. Vernocchi, M. Amendola, and D. Ciaci. 1993. HTLV-II/HIV-1 coinfection and risk for progression to AIDS among intravenous drug users. *J AIDS* **6**:1228–1237.

2777. Vittecoq, D., B. Mattlinger, F. Barre-Sinoussi, A. M. Courouce, C. Rouzioux, J. Doinel, M. Bary, J. P. Viard, J. F. Bach, P. Rouger, and J. J. Lefrere. 1992. Passive immunotherapy in AIDS: a randomized trial of serial human immunodeficiency virus-positive transfusions of plasma rich in p24 antibodies versus transfusions of seronegative plasma. *J Inf Dis* **165**:364–368.

2778. Viviano, E., F. Vitale, F. Ajello, A. M. Perna, M. R. Villafrate, F. Bonura, M. Arico, G. Mazzola, and N. Romano. 1997. Human herpesvirus type 8 DNA sequences in biological samples of HIV-positive and negative individuals in Sicily. *AIDS* **11**:607–612.

2779. Vlach, J., and P. M. Pitha. 1992. Herpes simplex virus type 1-mediated induction of human immunodeficiency virus type 1 provirus correlates with binding of nuclear proteins to the NF-κB enhancer and leader sequence. *J Virol* **66**:3616–3623.

2780. Vogel, J., S. H. Hinrichs, and R. K. Reynolds. 1988. The HIV Tat gene induces dermal lesions resembling Kaposi's sarcoma in transgenic mice. *Nature* **335**:606–611.

2781. Vogel, M., K. Cichutek, S. Norley, and R. Kurth. 1993. Self-limiting infection by int/nef-double mutants of simian immunodeficiency virus. *Virol* **193**:115–123.

2782. Vogt, M. W., D. J. Witt, D. E. Craven, R. Byington, D. F. Crawford, M. S. Hutchinson, R. T. Schooley, and M. S. Hirsch. 1987. Isolation patterns of the human immunodeficiency virus from cervical secretions during the menstrual cycle of women at risk for the acquired immunodeficiency syndrome. *Ann Int Med* **106**:380–382.

2783. Vogt, M. W., D. J. Witt, D. E. Craven, R. Byington, D. F. Crawford, R. T. Schooley, and M. S. Hirsch. 1986. Isolation of HTLV-III/LAV from cervical secretions of women at risk for AIDS. *Lancet* **i**:525–527.

2784. Vogt, P. K., and R. Ishizaki. 1966. Patterns of viral interference in the avian leukosis and sarcoma complex. *Virol* **30**:368–374.

2785. Volberding, P. A., S. W. Lagakos, J. M. Grimes, D. S. Stein, J. Rooney, T.-C. Meng, M. A. Fischl, A. C. Collier, J. P. Phair, M. S. Hirsch, W. D. Hardy, H. H. Balfour, Jr., and R. C. Reichman. 1995. A comparison of immediate with deferred zidovudine therapy for asymptomatic HIV-infected adults with CD4 cell counts of 500 or more per cubic millimeter. *N Engl J Med* **333**:401–407.

2786. Volberding, P. A., S. W. Lagakos, M. A. Koch, C. Pettinelli, M. W. Myers, D. K. Booth, H. H. Balfour, R. C. Reichman, J. A. Bartlett, M. S. Hirsch, R. L. Murphy, W. D. Hardy, R. Soeiro, M. A. Fischl, J. G. Bartlett, T. C. Merigan, N. E. Hyslop, D. D. Richman, F. T. Valentine, and L. Corey. 1990. Zidovudine in asymptomatic human immunodeficiency virus infection: a controlled trial in persons with fewer than 500 CD4-positive cells per cubic millimeter. *N Engl J Med* **322**:941–949.

2787. Volsky, D. J., M. Simm, M. Shahabuddin, G. Li, W. Chao, and M. J. Potash. 1996. Interference to human immunodeficiency virus type 1 infection in the absence of downmodulation of the principal virus receptor, CD4. *J Virol* **70**:3823–3833.

2788. von Briesen, H., R. Andreesen, and H. Rubsamen-Waigmann. 1990. Systematic classification of HIV biological subtypes on lymphocytes and monocytes/macrophages. *Virol* **178**:597–602.

2789. von Gegerfelt, A., J. Albert, L. Morfeldt-Manson, K. Broliden, and E. M. Fenyo. 1991. Isolate-specific neutralizing antibodies in patients with progressive HIV-1-related disease. *Virol* **185**:162–168.

2790. von Gegerfelt, A., F. Chiodi, B. Keys, G. Norkrans, L. Hagberg, E.-M. Fenyo, and K. Broliden. 1992. Lack of autologous neutralizing antibodies in the cerebrospinal fluid of HIV-1 infected individuals. *AIDS Res Hum Retro* **8**:1133–1138.

2791. von Gegerfelt, A., C. Diaz-Pohl, E. M. Fenyo, and K. Broliden. 1993. Specificity of antibody-dependent cellular cytotoxicity in sera from human immunodeficiency virus type 1-infected individuals. *AIDS Res Hum Retro* **9**:883–889.

2792. von Laer, D., F. T. Hufert, T. E. Fenner, S. Schwander, M. Dietrich, H. Schmitz, and P. Kern. 1990. CD34+ hematopoietic progenitor cells are not a major reservoir of the human immunodeficiency virus. *Blood* **76**:1281–1286.

2793. von Schwedler, U., J. Song, C. Aiken, and D. Trono. 1993. Vif is crucial for human immunodeficiency virus type 1 proviral DNA synthesis in infected cells. *J Virol* **67**:4945–4955.

2794. von Sydow, M., H. Gaines, A. Sonnerborg, M. Forsgren, P. O. Pehrson, and O. Strannegard. 1988. Antigen detection in primary HIV infection. *Brit Med J* **296**:238–240.

2795. von Sydow, M., A. Sonnerborg, H. Gaines, and O. Strannegard. 1991. Interferon-α and tumor necrosis factor-α in serum of patients in various stages of HIV-1 infection. *AIDS Res Hum Retro* **7**:375–380.

2796. Voss, T. G., C. D. Fermin, J. A. Levy, S. Vigh, B. Choi, and R. F. Garry. 1996. Alteration of intracellular potassium and sodium concentrations correlates with induction of cytopathic effects by human immunodeficiency virus. *J Virol* **70**:5447–5454.

2797. Vyakarnam, A., P. M. Matear, S. J. Martin, and M. Wagstaff. 1995. Th1 cells specific for HIV-1 gag p24 are less efficient than Th0 cells in supporting HIV replication, and inhibit virus replication in Th0 cells. *Immunol* **86**:85–96.

2798. Vyakarnam, A., J. McKeating, A. Meager, and P. C. Beverley. 1990. Tumor necrosis factors (alpha, beta) induced by HIV-1 in peripheral blood mononuclear cells potentiate virus replication. *AIDS* **4**:21–27.

2799. Wahl, L. M., M. L. Corcoran, S. W. Pyle, L. O. Arthur, A. Harel-Bellan, and W. L. Farrar. 1989. Human immunodeficiency virus glycoprotein (gp120) induction of monocyte arachidonic acid metabolites and interleukin 1. *Proc Natl Acad Sci USA* **86**:621–625.

2800. Wahl, S. M., J. B. Allen, S. Gartner, J. M. Ornstein, M. Popovic, D. E. Chenoweth, L. O. Arthur, W. L. Farrar, and L. M. Wahl. 1989. HIV-1 and its envelope glycoprotein down-regulate chemotactic ligand receptors and chemotactic function of peripheral blood monocytes. *J Immunol* **142**:3553–3559.

2801. Wahl, S. M., J. B. Allen, N. McCartney-Francis, M. C. Morganti-Kossmann, T. Kossmann, L. Ellingsworth, U. E. H. Mai, S. E. Mergenhagen, and J. M. Orenstein. 1991. Macrophage- and astrocyte-derived transforming growth factor beta as a mediator of central nervous system dysfunction in acquired immune deficiency syndrome. *J Exp Med* **173**:981–991.

2802. Wahman, A., S. L. Melnick, F. S. Rhame, and J. D. Potter. 1991. The epidemiology of classic, African and immunosuppressed Kaposi's sarcoma. *Epidemiol Rev* **13**:178–199.

2803. Wahren, B., L. Morfeldt-Mansson, G. Biberfeld, L. Moberg, A. Sonnerborg, P. Ljungman, A. Werner, R. Kurth, R. Gallo, and D. Bolognesi. 1987. Characteristics of the specific cell-mediated immune response in human immunodeficiency virus infection. *J Virol* **61**:2017–2023.

2804. Wain-Hobson, S., P. Sonigo, O. Danos, S. Cole, and M. Alizon. 1985. Nucleotide sequence of the AIDS virus, LAV. *Cell* **40**:9–17.

2805. Wain-Hobson, S., J.-P. Vartanian, M. Henry, N. Chenciner, R. Cheynier, S. Delassus, L. P. Martins, M. Sala, M.-T. Nugeyre, D. Guitard, D. Klatzmann, J.-C. Gluckman, W. Rozenbaum, F. Barre-Sinoussi, and L. Montagnier. 1991. LAV revisited: origins of the early HIV-1 isolates from Institut Pasteur. *Science* **252**:961–965.

2806. Wainberg, M., R. Beaulieu, C. Tsoukas, and R. Thomas. 1993. Detection of zidovudine-resistant variants of HIV-1 in genital fluids. *AIDS* **7**:433–444.

2807. Wainberg, M. A., W. C. Drosopoulos, H. Salomon, M. Hsu, G. Borkow, M. A. Parniak, Z. Gu, Q. Song, J. Manne, S. Islam, G. Castriota, and V. R. Prasad. 1996. Enhanced fidelity of 3TC-selected mutant HIV-1 reverse transcriptase. *Science* **271**:1282–1285.

2808. Wakrim, L., R. Le Grand, B. Vaslin, A. Cheret, F. Matheux, F. Theodoro, P. Roques, I. Nicol-Jourdain, and D. Dormont. 1996. Superinfection of HIV-2-preinfected macaques after rectal exposure to a primary isolate of SIVmac251. *Virol* **221**:260–270.

2809. Walker, B. D., C. Flexner, T. J. Paradis, T. C. Fuller, M. S. Hirsch, R. T. Schooley, and B. Moss. 1988. HIV-1 reverse transcriptase is a target for cytotoxic T lymphocytes in infected individuals. *Science* **240**:64–66.

2809a. Walker, C. Personal communication.

2810. Walker, C. M., A. L. Erikson, F. C. Hsueh, and J. A. Levy. 1991. Inhibition of human immunodeficiency virus replication in acutely infected CD4+ cells by CD8+ cells involves a noncytotoxic mechanism. *J Virol* **65**:5921–5927.

2811. Walker, C. M., and J. A. Levy. 1989. A diffusible lymphokine produced by CD8+ T lymphocytes suppresses HIV replication. *Immunol* **66**:628–630.

2811a. Walker, C. M., and J. A. Levy. Unpublished observations.

2812. Walker, C. M., D. J. Moody, D. P. Stites, and J. A. Levy. 1986. CD8+ lymphocytes can control HIV infection *in vitro* by suppressing virus replication. *Science* **234**:1563–1566.

2813. Walker, C. M., D. J. Moody, D. P. Stites, and J. A. Levy. 1989. CD8+ T lymphocyte control of HIV replication in cultured CD4+ cells varies among infected individuals. *Cell Immunol* **119**:470–475.

2814. Walker, C. M., G. A. Thomson-Honnebier, F. C. Hsueh, A. L. Erickson, L.-Z. Pan, and J. A. Levy. 1991. CD8+ T cells from HIV-1-infected individuals inhibit acute infection by human and primate immunodeficiency viruses. *Cell Immunol* **137**:420–428.

2815. Walker, L., D. Wilks, J. O'Brien, J. Habeshaw, and A. Dalgleish. 1992. Localized conformational changes in the N-terminal domain of CD4 identified in competitive binding assay of monoclonal antibodies and HIV-1 envelope glycoprotein. *AIDS Res Hum Retro* 8:1083–1090.

2816. Wallis, R. S., M. Vjecha, M. Amir-Tahmasseb, A. Okwera, F. Byekwaso, S. Nyole, S. Kabengera, R. D. Mugerwa, and J. J. Ellner. 1993. Influence of tuberculosis on human immunodeficiency virus (HIV-1): enhanced cytokine expression and elevated β2-microglobulin in HIV-1-associated tuberculosis. *J Inf Dis* 167:43–48.

2817. Wang, B., J. Boyer, V. Srikantan, K. Ugen, L. Gilbert, C. Phan, K. Dang, M. Merva, M. G. Agadjanyan, M. Newman, R. Carrano, D. McCallus, L. Coney, W. V. Williams, and D. B. Weiner. 1995. Induction of humoral and cellular immune responses to the human immunodeficiency type 1 virus in nonhuman primates by in vivo DNA inoculation. *Virol* 211:102–112.

2818. Wang, B., K. E. Ugen, V. Srikantan, M. G. Agadjanyan, K. Dang, Y. Refaeli, A. I. Sato, J. Boyer, W. V. Williams, and D. B. Weiner. 1993. Gene inoculation generates immune responses against human immunodeficiency virus type 1. *Proc Natl Acad Sci USA* 90:4156–4160.

2819. Wang, J., Y. Yan, T. P. J. Garrett, J. Liu, D. W. Rodgers, R. L. Garlick, G. E. Tarr, Y. Husain, E. L. Reinherz, and S. C. Harrison. 1990. Atomic structure of a fragment of human CD4 containing two immunoglobulin-like domains. *Nature* 348:411–418.

2820. Wang, N., T. Zhu, and D. D. Ho. 1995. Sequence diversity of V1 and V2 domains of gp120 from human immunodeficiency virus type 1: lack of correlation with viral phenotype. *J Virol* 69:2708–2715.

2821. Wang, R., S. I. Abrams, D. Y. Loh, C. S. Shieh, K. M. Murphy, and J. H. Russell. 1993. Separation of CD4+ functional responses by peptide dose in Th1 and Th2 subsets expressing the same transgenic antigen receptor. *Cell Immunol* 148:357–370.

2822. Wang, S. Z. S., K. E. Rushlow, C. J. Issel, R. F. Cook, S. J. Cook, M. L. Raabe, Y. H. Chong, L. Costa, and R. C. Montelaro. 1994. Enhancement of EIAV replication and disease by immunization with a baculovirus-expressed recombinant envelope surface glycoprotein. *Virol* 199:247–251.

2823. Ward, J. W., T. J. Bush, H. A. Perkins, L. E. Lieb, J. R. Allen, D. Goldfinger, S. M. Samson, S. H. Pepkowitz, L. P. Fernando, P. V. Holland, S. H. Kleinman, A. J. Grindon, J. L. Garner, G. W. Rutherford, and S. D. Holmberg. 1989. The natural history of transfusion-associated infection with human immunodeficiency virus: factors influencing the rate of progression to disease. *N Engl J Med* 321:947–952.

2824. Warren, M. K., W. L. Rose, J. L. Cone, W. G. Rice, and J. A. Turpin. 1997. Differential infection of CD34+ cell-derived dendritic cells and monocyte with lymphocyte-tropic and monocyte-tropic HIV-1 strains. *J Immunol* 158:5035–5042.

2825. Warren, R. Q., S. A. Anderson, W. M. M. M. Nkya, J. F. Shao, C. W. Hendrix, G. P. Melcher, R. R. Redfield, and R. C. Kennedy. 1992. Examination of sera from human immunodeficiency virus type 1 (HIV-1)-infected individuals for antibodies reactive with peptides corresponding to the principal neutralizing determinant of HIV-1 gp120 and for in vitro neutralizing activity. *J Virol* 66:5210–5215.

2826. Wasik, T. J., P. P. Jagodzinski, E. M. Hyjek, J. Wustner, G. Trinchieri, H. W. Lischner, and D. Kozbor. 1997. Diminished HIV-specific CTL activity is associated with lower type 1 and enhanced type 2 responses to HIV-specific peptides during perinatal HIV infection. *J Immunol* 158:6029–6036.

2827. Watkins, B. A., H. H. Dorn, W. B. Kelly, R. C. Armstrong, B. J. Potts, F. Michaels, C. V. Kufta, and M. Dubois-Dalcq. 1990. Specific tropism of HIV-1 for microglial cells in primary human brain cultures. *Science* 249:549–553.

2828. Watkins, B. A., M. S. Reitz, Jr., C. A. Wilson, K. Aldrich, A. E. Davis, and M. Robert-Guroff. 1993. Immune escape by human immunodeficiency virus type 1 from neutralizing antibodies: evidence for multiple pathways. *J Virol* 67:7493–7500.

2829. Watret, K. C., J. A. Whitelaw, K. S. Froebel, and A. G. Bird. 1993. Phenotypic characterization of CD8+ T cell populations in HIV disease and in anti-HIV immunity. *Clin Exp Immunol* 92:93–99.

2830. Watson, A., J. McClure, J. Ranchalis, M. Scheibel, A. Schmidt, B. Kennedy, W. R. Morton, N. L. Haigwood, and S. L. Hu. 1997. Early post-infection antiviral treatment reduces viral load and prevents CD4+ cell decline in HIV-2 infected macaques. *AIDS Res Hum Retro.* 13:1375–1381.

2831. Weber, J., P. Clapham, J. McKeating, M. Stratton, E. Robey, and R. Weiss. 1989. Infection of brain cells by diverse human immunodeficiency virus isolates: role of CD4 as receptor. *J Gen Virol* 70:2653–2660.

2832. Weber, J., E. M. Fenyo, S. Beddows, P. Kaleebu, and A. Bjorndal. 1996. Neutralization serotypes of human immunodeficiency virus type 1 field isolates are not predicted by genetic subtype. *J Virol* 70:7827–7832.

2832a. Weber, J. N., P. R. Clapham, R. A. Weiss, D. Parker, C. Roberts, J. Duncan, I. Weller, C. Carne, R. S. Tedder, A. J. Pinching, and P. Cheingsong-Popov. 1987. Human immunodeficiency virus infection in two cohorts of homosexual men: neutralizing sera and association of anti-*gag* antibody with prognosis. *Lancet* i:119–122.

2833. Webster, A., C. A. Lee, D. G. Cook, J. E. Grundy, V. C. Emery, P. B. A. Kernoff, and P. D. Griffiths. 1989. Cytomegalovirus infection and progression towards AIDS in haemophiliacs with human immunodeficiency virus infection. *Lancet* ii:63–66.

2834. Wei, X., S. K. Ghosh, M. E. Taylor, V. A. Johnson, E. A. Emini, P. Deutsch, J. D. Lifson, S. Bonhoeffer, M. A. Nowak, B. H. Hahn, M. S. Saag, and G. M. Shaw. 1995. Viral dynamics in human immunodeficiency virus type 1 infection. *Nature* 373:117–122.

2835. Weiblen, B. J., F. K. Lee, E. R. Cooper, S. H. Landesman, K. McIntosh, J. A. Harris, S. Nieshman, H. Mendez, S. I. Pelton, and A. J. Nahmias. 1990. Early diagnosis of HIV infection in infants by detection of IgA HIV antibodies. *Lancet* 335:988–990.

2836. Weimer, R., V. Daniel, R. Zimmermann, K. Schimpf, and G. Opelz. 1991. Autoantibodies against CD4 cells are associated with CD4 helper defects in human immunodeficiency virus-infected patients. *Blood* 77:133–140.

2837. Weinberg, A. D., M. English, and S. L. Swain. 1990. Distinct regulation of lymphokine production is found in fresh versus *in vitro* primed murine helper T-cells. *J Immunol* 144:1800–1807.

2838. Weinberg, J. B., T. J. Matthews, B. R. Cullen, and M. H. Malim. 1991. Productive human immunodeficiency virus type 1 (HIV-1) infection of nonproliferating human monocytes. *J Exp Med* 174:1477–1482.

2839. Weinhold, K. J., H. K. Lyerly, T. J. Matthews, D. S. Tyler, P. M. Ahearne, K. C. Stine, A. J. Langlois, D. T. Durack, and D. P. Bolognesi. 1988. Cellular anti-gp120 cytolytic reactivities in HIV-1 seropositive individuals. *Lancet* i:902–905.

2840. Weinhold, K. J., H. K. Lyerly, S. D. Stanley, A. A. Austin, T. J. Matthews, and D. P. Bolognesi. 1989. HIV-1 gp120-mediated immune suppression and lymphocyte destruction in the absence of viral infection. *J Immunol* 142:3091–3097.

2841. Weiss, A., R. L. Wiskocil, and J. D. Stobo. 1984. The role of T3 surface molecules in the activation of human T cells: a two-stimulus requirement for IL-2 production reflects events occurring at a pretranslational level. *J Immunol* 133:123–128.

2842. Weiss, C. D., S. W. Barnett, N. Cacalano, N. Killeen, D. R. Littman, and J. M. White. 1996. Studies of HIV-1 envelope glycoprotein-mediated fusion using a simple fluorescence assay. *AIDS* 10:241–246.

2842a. Weiss, C. D., and J. A. Levy. Unpublished observations.

2843. Weiss, C. D., J. A. Levy, and J. M. White. 1990. Oligomeric organization of gp120 on infectious human immunodeficiency virus type 1 particles. *J Virol* 64:5674–5677.

2844. Weiss, L., N. Okada, N. Haeffner-Cavaillon, T. Hattori, C. Faucher, M. D. Kazatchkine, and H. Okada. 1992. Decreased expression of the membrane inhibitor of complement-mediated cytolysis CD59 on T-lymphocytes of HIV-infected patients. *AIDS* 6:379–385.

2845. Weiss, R. A. 1988. Receptor molecule blocks HIV. *Nature* 331:15.

2846. Weiss, R. A., P. R. Clapham, J. N. Weber, A. G. Dalgleish, L. A. Lasky, and P. W. Berman. 1986. Variable and conserved neutralization antigens of human immunodeficiency virus. *Nature* 324:572–575.

2847. Weiss, R. A., P. R. Clapham, J. N. Weber, D. Whitby, R. S. Tedder, T. O'Connor, S. Chamaret, and L. Montagnier. 1988. HIV-2 antisera cross-neutralize HIV-1. *AIDS* **2**:95–100.

2848. Weiss, S. H., J. Lombardo, J. Michaels, L. R. Sharer, M. Rayyarah, J. Leonard, A. Mangia, P. Kloser, S. Sathe, R. Kapila, N. M. Williams, R. Altman, J. French, and W. E. Parkin. 1988. AIDS due to HIV-2 infection—New Jersey. *Morbid Mortal Weekly Rep* **259**:969–972.

2849. Weissenhorn, W., A. Dessen, S. C. Harrison, J. J. Skehel, and D. C. Wiley. 1997. Atomic structure of the ectodomain from HIV-1 gp41. *Nature* **387**:426–430.

2850. Weissman, D., Y. Li, J. Ananworanich, L. J. Zhou, J. Adelsberger, T. F. Tedder, M. Baseler, and A. S. Fauci. 1995. Three populations of cells with dendritic morphology exist in peripheral blood only one of which is infectable with human immunodeficiency virus type 1. *Proc Nat Acad Sci USA* **92**:826–830.

2851. Weissman, D., Y. Li, J. M. Orenstein, and A. S. Fauci. 1995. Both a precursor and a mature population of dendritic cells can bind HIV. *J Immunol* **155**:4111–4117.

2852. Weissman, D., G. Poli, and A. S. Fauci. 1995. IL-10 synergizes with multiple cytokines in enhancing HIV production in cells of monocytic lineage. *J AIDS Hum Retrovirol* **9**:442–449.

2853. Weissman, D., G. Poli, and A. S. Fauci. 1994. Interleukin 10 blocks HIV replication in macrophages by inhibiting the autocrine loop of tumor necrosis factor α and interleukin 6 induction of virus. *AIDS Res Hum Retro* **10**:1199–1206.

2854. Wekerle, H., C. Unington, H. Lassmann, and R. Meyermann. 1986. Cellular immune reactivity within the CNS. *Trends Neurosci* **9**:271–277.

2855. Welker, R., H. Kottler, H. R. Kalbitzer, and H.-G. Krausslich. 1996. Human immunodeficiency virus type 1 Nef protein is incorporated into virus particles and specifically cleaved by the viral proteinase. *Virol* **219**:228–236.

2856. Wendler, I., V. Bienzle, and G. Hunsman. 1987. Neutralizing antibodies and the course of HIV-induced disease. *AIDS Res Hum Retro* **3**:157–163.

2857. Weniger, B. G., Y. Takebe, C.-Y. Ou, and S. Yamazaki. 1994. The molecular epidemiology of HIV in Asia. *AIDS* **8**:S13-S28.

2858. Wenner, C. A., M. L. Guler, S. E. Macatonia, A. O'Garra, and K. M. Murphy. 1996. Roles of IFN-γ and IFN-α in IL-12 induced T helper cell-1 development. *J Immunol* **1156**:1442–1447.

2859. Werner, A., and J. A. Levy. 1993. Human immunodeficiency virus type 1 envelope gp120 is cleaved after incubation with recombinant soluble CD4. *J Virol* **67**:2566–2574.

2860. Werner, A., G. Winskowsky, and R. Kurth. 1990. Soluble CD4 enhances simian immunodeficiency virus SIV_{agm} infection. *J Virol* **64**:6252–6256.

2861. Werner, T., S. Ferroni, T. Saermark, R. Brack-Werner, R. B. Banati, R. Mager, L. Steinaa, G. W. Kreutzberg, and V. Erfle. 1991. HIV-1 *nef* protein exhibits structural and functional similarity to scorpion peptides interacting with K+ channels. *AIDS* **5**:1301–1308.

2862. Werness, B. A., A. J. Levine, and P. M. Howley. 1990. Association of human papillomavirus types 16 and 18 E6 proteins with p53. *Science* **248**:76–79.

2863. Wesselingh, S. L., C. Power, J. D. Glass, W. R. Tyor, J. C. McArthur, J. M. Farber, J. W. Griffin, and D. E. Griffin. 1993. Intracerebral cytokine messenger RNA expression in acquired immunodeficiency syndrome dementia. *Ann Neurol* **33**:576–582.

2864. Westby, M., F. Manca, and A. G. Dalgleish. 1996. The role of host immune responses in determining the outcome of HIV infection. *Immunol Today* **17**:120–126.

2865. Westermann, J., and R. Pabst. 1990. Lymphocyte subsets in the blood: a diagnostic window on the lymphoid system? *Immunol Today* **11**:406–410.

2866. Westervelt, P., T. Henkel, D. B. Trowbridge, J. Orenstein, J. Heuser, H. E. Gendelman, and L. Ratner. 1992. Dual regulation of silent and productive infection in monocytes by distinct human immunodeficiency virus type 1 determinants. *J Virol* **66**:3925–3931.

2867. Westervelt, P., D. B. Trowbridge, L. G. Epstein, B. M. Blumberg, Y. Li, B. H. Hahn, G. M. Shaw, R. W. Price, and L. Ratner. 1992. Macrophage tropism determinants of human immunodeficiency virus type 1 in vivo. *J Virol* **66**:2577–2582.

2868. Westmoreland, S. V., D. Kolson, and F. Gonzalez-Scarano. 1996. Toxicity of TNF-α and platelet activating factor for human NT2N neurons: a tissue culture model for human immunodeficiency virus dementia. *J NeuroVirol* 2:118–126.

2869. Whalen, R. G. 1996. DNA vaccines for emerging infectious diseases: what if? *Emerg Infect Dis* 2:168–175.

2870. Whitby, D., M. R. Howard, M. Tenant-Flowers, N. S. Brink, A. Copas, C. Boshoff, T. Hatzioannou, F. E. A. Suggett, D. M. Aldam, A. S. Denton, R. F. Miller, I. V. D. Weller, R. A. Weiss, R. S. Tedder, and T. F. Schulz. 1995. Detection of Kaposi's sarcoma associated herpesvirus in peripheral blood of HIV-infected individuals and progression to Kaposi's sarcoma. *Lancet* 346:799–802.

2871. White, J. M. 1990. Viral and cellular membrane fusion proteins. *Annu Rev Physiol* 52:675–697.

2872. Whittle, H., A. Egboga, J. Todd, T. Corrah, A. Wilkins, E. Demba, G. Morgan, M. Rolfe, N. Berry, and R. Tedder. 1992. Clinical and laboratory predictors of survival in Gambian patients with symptomatic HIV-1 and HIV-2 infection. *AIDS* 6:685–689.

2873. Whittle, H., J. Morris, J. Todd, T. Corrah, S. Sabally, J. Bangali, P. T. Ngom, M. Rolfe, and A. Wilkins. 1994. HIV-2-infected patients survive longer than HIV-1-infected patients. *AIDS* 8:1617–1620.

2874. Wigdahl, B., R. Guyton, and P. S. Sarin. 1987. Human immunodeficiency virus infection of the developing human nervous system. *Virol* 159:440–445.

2875. Wild, C., T. Oas, C. McDanal, D. Bolognesi, and T. Matthews. 1992. A synthetic peptide inhibitor of human immunodeficiency virus replication: correlation between solution structure and viral inhibition. *Proc Natl Acad Sci USA* 89:10537–10541.

2876. Wildemann, B., J. Haas, K. Ehrhart, H. Wagner, N. Lynen, and B. Storch-Hagenlocher. 1993. *In vivo* comparison of zidovudine resistance mutations in blood and CSF of HIV-1-infected patients. *Neurol* 43:2659–2663.

2877. Wiley, C. A., C. L. Achim, R. D. Schrier, M. P. Heyes, J. A. McCutchan, and I. Grant. 1992. Relationship of cerebrospinal fluid immune activation associated factors to HIV encephalitis. *AIDS* 6:1299–1307.

2877a. Wiley, C. A. and J. A. Nelson. 1988. Role of human immunodeficiency virus and cytomegalovirus in AIDS encephalitis. *Am J Path* 133:73–81.

2878. Wiley, C. A., R. D. Schrier, D. D. Richman, J. A. Nelson, P. W. Lambert, and M. B. A. Oldstone. 1986. Cellular localization of human immunodeficiency virus infection within the brains of acquired immune deficiency syndrome patients. *Proc Natl Acad Sci USA* 83:7089–7093.

2879. Wiley, C. A., R. D. Schrier, F. J. Denaro, J. A. Nelson, P. W. Lampert, and M. B. A. Oldstone. 1986. Localization of cytomegalovirus proteins and genome during fulminant central nervous system infection in an AIDS patient. *J Neuropath Exp Neurol* 45:127–139.

2880. Wilfert, C. M., C. Wilson, K. Luzuriaga, and L. Epstein. 1994. Pathogenesis of pediatric human immunodeficiency virus type 1 infection. *J Inf Dis* 170:286–292.

2881. Wilks, D., L. Walker, J. O'Brien, J. Habeshaw, and A. Dalgleish. 1990. Differences in affinity of anti-CD4 monoclonal antibodies predict their effects on syncytium induction by human immunodeficiency virus. *Immunol* 71:10–15.

2882. Willems, F., A. Marchant, J. P. Delville, C. Gerard, A. Delvaux, T. Velu, M. de Boer, and M. Goldman. 1994. Interleukin-10 inhibits B7 and intercellular adhesion molecule-1 expression on human monocytes. *Eur J Immunol* 24:1007–1009.

2883. Willey, R. L., E. K. Ross, A. J. Buckler-White, T. S. Theodore, and M. A. Martin. 1989. Functional interaction of constant and variable domains of HIV-1 gp120. *J Virol* 63:3595–3600.

2884. Willey, R. L., F. Maldarelli, M. A. Martin, and K. Strebel. 1992. Human immunodeficiency virus type 1 *vpu* protein regulates the formation of intracellular gp160-CD4 complexes. *J Virol* 66:226–234.

2885. Willey, R. L., and M. A. Martin. 1993. Association of human immunodeficiency virus type 1 envelope glycoprotein with particles depends on interactions between the third variable and conserved regions of gp120. *J Virol* 67:3639–3643.

2886. Willey, R. L., M. A. Martin, and K. W. C. Peden. 1994. Increase in soluble CD4 binding to and CD4-induced dissociation of gp120 from virions correlates with infectivity of human immunodeficiency virus type 1. *J Virol* **68**:1029–1039.

2887. Willey, R. L., R. A. Rutledge, S. Dias, T. Folks, T. Theodore, C. E. Buckler, and M. A. Martin. 1986. Identification of conserved and divergent domains within the envelope gene of the acquired immunodeficiency syndrome retrovirus. *Proc Natl Acad Sci USA* **83**:5038–5042.

2888. Willey, R. L., R. Shibata, E. O. Freed, M. W. Cho, and M. A. Martin. 1996. Differential glycosylation, virion incorporation, and sensitivity to neutralizing antibodies of human immunodeficiency virus type 1 envelope produced from infected primary T-lymphocyte and macrophage cultures. *J Virol* **70**:6431–6436.

2889. Willey, R. L., D. H. Smith, L. A. Lasky, T. S. Theodore, P. L. Earl, B. Moss, D. J. Capon, and M. A. Martin. 1988. In vitro mutagenesis identifies a region within the envelope gene of the human immunodeficiency virus that is critical for infectivity. *J Virol* **62**:139–147.

2890. Willey, R. L., T. S. Theodore, and M. A. Martin. 1994. Amino acid substitutions in the human immunodeficiency virus type 1 gp120 V3 loop that change viral tropism also alter physical and functional properties of the virion envelope. *J Virol* **68**:4409–4419.

2891. Williams, M. E., T. L. Chang, S. K. Burke, A. H. Lichtman, and A. K. Abbas. 1991. Activation of functionally distinct subsets of CD4+ T lymphocytes. *Res Immunol* **142**:23–27.

2891a. Williams, N. S., and V. H. Engelhard. 1997. Perforin-dependent cytotoxic activity and lymphokine secretion by CD4+ T cells are regulated by CD8+ T cells. *J Immunol* **159**:2091–2099.

2892. Wilson, C., M. S. Reitz, K. Aldrich, P. J. Klasse, J. Blomberg, R. C. Gallo, and M. Robert-Guroff. 1990. The site of an immune-selected point mutation in the transmembrane protein of human immunodeficiency virus type 1 does not constitute the neutralization epitope. *J Virol* **64**:3240–3248.

2893. Wilson, C. C., S. A. Kalams, B. M. Wilkes, D. J. Ruhl, F. Gao, B. H. Hahn, I. C. Hanson, K. Luzuriaga, S. Wolinsky, R. Koup, S. P. Buchbinder, R. P. Johnson, and B. D. Walker. 1997. Overlapping epitopes in human immunodeficiency virus type 1 gp120 presented by HLA A, B, and C molecules: effects of viral variation on cytotoxic T-lymphocyte recognition. *J Virol* **71**:1256–1264.

2894. Winkelstein, W., Jr., D. M. Lyman, N. Padian, R. Grant, M. Samuel, J. A. Wiley, R. E. Anderson, W. Lang, J. Riggs, and J. A. Levy. 1987. Sexual practices and risk of infection by the human immunodeficiency virus: the San Francisco Men's Health Study. *J Am Med Assoc* **257**:321–325.

2895. Winslow, B. J., R. J. Pomerantz, O. Bagasra, and D. Trono. 1993. HIV-1 latency due to the site of proviral integration. *Virol* **196**:849–854.

2896. Winslow, B. J., and D. Trono. 1993. The blocks to human immunodeficiency virus type 1 *tat* and *rev* functions in mouse cell lines are independent. *J Virol* **67**:2349–2354.

2897. Winslow, D. L., and M. J. Otto. 1995. HIV protease inhibitors. *AIDS* **9**:S183–S192.

2898. Wiskerchen, M., and M. A. Muesing. 1995. Human immunodeficiency virus type 1 integrase: effects of mutations on viral ability to integrate, direct viral gene expression from unintegrated viral DNA templates, and sustain viral propagation in primary cells. *J Virol* **69**:376–386.

2899. Withrington, R. H., P. Cornes, J. R. W. Harris, M. H. Seifert, E. Berrie, D. Taylor-Robinson, and D. J. Jeffries. 1987. Isolation of human immunodeficiency virus from synovial fluid of a patient with reactive arthritis. *Brit Med J* **294**:484.

2900. Wiviott, L. D., C. M. Walker, and J. A. Levy. 1990. CD8+ lymphocytes suppress HIV production by autologous CD4+ cells without eliminating the infected cells from culture. *Cell Immunol* **128**:628–634.

2901. Wlodawer, A., M. Miller, M. Jaskolski, B. K. Sathyanarayana, E. Baldwin, I. T. Weber, L. M. Selk, L. Clawson, J. Schneider, and S. B. H. Kent. 1989. Conserved folding in retroviral proteases: crystal structure of a synthetic HIV-1 protease. *Science* **245**:616–621.

2902. Wofsy, C. B., J. B. Cohen, L. B. Hauer, N. S. Padian, B. A. Michaelis, L. A. Evans, and J. A. Levy. 1986. Isolation of the AIDS-associated retrovirus from genital secretions from women with antibodies to the virus. *Lancet* **i**:527–529.

2903. Wolber, V., H. Rensland, B. Brandmeier, M. Sagemann, R. Hoffmann, H. R. Kalbitzer, and A. Wittinghofer. 1992. Expression, purification and biochemical characterization of the human immunodeficiency virus 1 *nef* gene product. *Eur J Biochem* **205**:1115–1121.

2904. Wolff, H., and D. J. Anderson. 1988. Immunohistologic characterization and quantitation of leukocyte subpopulations in human semen. *Fert Steril* **49**:497–504.

2905. Wolff, H., and D. J. Anderson. 1988. Potential human immunodeficiency virus-host cells in human semen. *AIDS Res Hum Retro* **4**:1–2.

2906. Wolff, J. A., R. W. Malone, P. Williams, W. Chong, G. Acsadi, A. Jani, and P. L. Felgner. 1990. Direct gene transfer into mouse muscle in vivo. *Science* **247**:1465–1468.

2907. Wolfs, T. F. W., G. Zwart, M. Bakker, and J. Goudsmit. 1992. HIV-1 genomic RNA diversification following sexual and parenteral virus transmission. *Virol* **189**:103–110.

2908. Wolfs, T. F. W., G. Zwart, M. Bakker, M. Valk, C. L. Kuiken, and J. Goudsmit. 1991. Naturally occurring mutations within HIV-1 V3 genomic RNA lead to antigenic variation dependent on a single amino acid substitution. *Virol* **185**:195–205.

2909. Wolinsky, S. M., C. R. Rinaldo, S. Kwok, J. J. Sninsky, P. Gupta, D. Imagawa, H. Farzadegan, L. P. Jacobson, K. S. Grovit, M. H. Lee, J. S. Chmiel, H. Ginzburg, R. A. Kaslow, and J. P. Phair. 1989. Human immunodeficiency virus type 1 (HIV-1) infection a median of 18 months before a diagnostic western blot. *Ann Int Med* **111**:961–972.

2910. Wolinsky, S. M., C. M. Wike, B. T. M. Korber, C. Hutto, W. P. Parks, L. L. Rosenblum, K. J. Kunstman, M. R. Furtado, and J. L. Munoz. 1992. Selective transmission of human immunodeficiency virus type 1 variants from mothers to infants. *Science* **255**:1134–1137.

2911. Wolthers, K. C., G. Bea, A. Wisman, S. A. Otto, A. M. de Roda Husman, N. Schaft, F. de Wolf, J. Goudsmit, R. A. Coutinho, A. G. J. van der Zee, L. Meyaard, and F. Miedema. 1996. T cell telomere length in HIV-1 infection: no evidence for increased CD4+ T cell turnover. *Science* **274**:1543–1547.

2912. Wong, J. K., C. C. Ignacio, F. Torriani, D. Havlir, N. J. S. Fitch, and D. D. Richman. 1997. In vivo compartmentalization of human immunodeficiency virus: evidence from the examination of *pol* sequences from autopsy tissues. *J Virol* **71**:2059–2071.

2913. Woodland, D. L., M. P. Happ, K. J. Gollob, and E. Palmer. 1991. An endogenous retrovirus mediating deletion of alpha beta T cells? *Nature* **349**:529–532.

2914. Woods, T. C., B. D. Roberts, S. T. Butera, and T. M. Folks. 1997. Loss of inducible virus in CD45RA naive cells after human immunodeficiency virus-1 entry accounts for preferential viral replication in CD45RO memory cells. *Blood* **89**:1635–1641.

2915. Wormser, G. P., S. Bittker, G. Forester, I. K. Hewlett, I. Argani, B. Joshi, J. S. Epstrin, and D. Bucher. 1992. Absence of infectious human immunodeficiency virus type 1 in "natural" eccrine sweat. *J Inf Dis* **165**:155–158.

2916. Wright, S. C., A. Jewett, R. Mitsuyasu, and B. Bonavida. 1988. Spontaneous cytotoxicity and tumor necrosis factor production by peripheral blood monocytes from AIDS patients. *J Immunol* **141**:99–104.

2917. Wrin, T., L. Crawford, L. Sawyer, P. Weber, H. W. Sheppard, and C. V. Hanson. 1994. Neutralizing antibody responses to autologous and heterologous isolates of human immunodeficiency virus. *J AIDS* **7**:211–219.

2918. Wu, F., J. Garcia, D. Sigman, and R. Gaynor. 1991. *Tat* regulates binding of the human immunodeficiency virus trans-activating region RNA loop-binding protein TRP-185. *Genes Develop* **5**:2128–2140.

2919. Wu, J.-Y., B. H. Gardner, C. I. Murphy, J. R. Seals, C. R. Kensil, J. Recchia, G. A. Beltz, G. W. Newman, and M. J. Newman. 1992. Saponin adjuvant enhancement of antigen-specific immune responses to an experimental HIV-1 vaccine. *J Immunol* **148**:1519–1525.

2920. Wu, L., N. P. Gerard, R. Wyatt, H. Choe, C. Parolin, N. Ruffing, A. Borsetti, A. A. Cardoso, E. Desjardin, W. Newman, C. Gerard, and J. Sodroski. 1996. CD4-induced interaction of primary HIV-1 gp120 glycoproteins with the chemokine receptor CCR-5. *Nature* **384**:179–183.

2921. Wyand, M. S., K. H. Manson, M. Garcia-Moll, D. Montefiori, and R. C. Desrosiers. 1996.

Vaccine protection by a triple deletion mutant of simian immunodeficiency virus. *J Virol* 70:3724–3733.

2922. Wyatt, R., M. Thali, S. Tilley, A. Pinter, M. Posner, D. Ho, J. Robinson, and J. Sodroski. 1992. Relationship of the human immunodeficiency virus type 1 gp120 third variable loop to a component of the CD4 binding site in the fourth conserved region. *J Virol* 66:6997–7004.

2923. Wynn, T. A., A. W. Cheever, D. Jankovic, R. W. Poindexter, P. Caspar, F. A. Lewis, and A. Sher. 1995. An IL-12-based vaccination method for preventing fibrosis induced by schistosome infection. *Nature* 376:594–596.

2924. Yaginuma, Y., and H. Westphal. 1991. Analysis of the p53 gene in human uterine carcinoma cell lines. *Cancer Res* 51:6506–6509.

2925. Yagita, H., M. Nakata, A. Kawasaki, Y. Shinkai, and K. Okumura. 1992. Role of perforin in lymphocyte-mediated cytolysis. *Adv Immunol* 51:215–242.

2926. Yahi, N., S. Baghdiguian, H. Moreau, and J. Fantini. 1992. Galactosyl ceramide (or a closely related molecule) is the receptor for human immunodeficiency virus type 1 on human colon epithelial HT29 cells. *J Virol* 66:4848–4854.

2927. Yahi, N., J.-M. Sabatier, S. Baghdiguian, F. Gonzalez-Scarano, and J. Fantini. 1995. Synthetic multimeric peptides derived from the principal neutralization domain (V3 loop) of human immunodeficiency virus type 1 (HIV-1) gp120 bind to galactosylceramide and block HIV-1 infection in a human CD4-negative mucosal epithelial cell line. *J Virol* 69:320–325.

2928. Yahi, N., S. L. Spitalnik, K. A. Stefano, P. De Micco, F. Gonzalez-Scarano, and J. Fantini. 1994. Interferon-gamma decreases cell surface expression of galactosyl ceramide, the receptor for HIV-1 gp120 on human colonic epithelial cells. *Virol* 204:550–557.

2929. Yamada, M., A. Zurbriggen, M. B. A. Oldstone, and R. S. Fujinami. 1991. Common immunologic determinant between human immunodeficiency virus type 1 gp41 and astrocytes. *J Virol* 65:1370–1376.

2930. Yamamoto, J. K., T. Hohdatsu, R. A. Olmsted, R. Pu, H. Louie, H. A. Zochlinski, V. Acevedo, H. M. Johnson, G. A. Soulds, and M. B. Gardner. 1993. Experimental vaccine protection against homologous and heterologous strains of feline immunodeficiency virus. *J Virol* 67:601–605.

2931. Yang, O. O., S. A. Kalams, M. Rosenzweig, A. Trocha, N. Jones, M. Koziel, B. D. Walker, and R. P. Johnson. 1996. Efficient lysis of human immunodeficiency virus type 1-infected cells by cytotoxic T lymphocytes. *J Virol* 70:5799–5806.

2932. Yarchoan, R., C. F. Perno, R. V. Thomas, R. W. Klecker, J.-P. Allain, R. J. Wills, N. McAtee, M. A. Fischl, R. Dubinsky, M. C. McNeely, H. Mitsuya, J. M. Pluda, T. J. Lawley, M. Leuther, B. Safai, J. M. Collins, C. E. Myers, and S. Broder. 1988. Phase I studies of 2′,3′-dideoxycytidine in severe human immunodeficiency virus infection as a single agent and alternating with zidovudine (AZT). *Lancet* i:76–81.

2933. Yarchoan, R., K. J. Weinhold, H. K. Lyerly, E. Gelmann, R. M. Blum, G. M. Shearer, H. Mitsuya, J. M. Collins, C. E. Myers, R. W. Klecker, P. D. Markham, D. T. Durack, S. N. Lehrman, D. W. Barry, M. A. Fischl, R. C. Gallo, D. P. Bolognesi, and S. Broder. 1986. Administration of 3′-azido-3′-deoxythymidine, an inhibitor of HTLV-III/LAV replication, to patients with AIDS or AIDS-related complex. *Lancet* i:575–580.

2934. Yasutomi, Y., K. A. Keimann, C. I. Lord, M. D. Miller, and N. L. Letvin. 1993. Simian immunodeficiency virus-specific CD8+ lymphocyte response in acutely infected rhesus monkeys. *J Virol* 67:1707–1711.

2935. Yasutomi, Y., S. Koenig, R. M. Woods, J. Madsen, N. M. Wassef, C. R. Alving, H. J. Klein, T. E. Nolan, L. J. Boots, J. A. Kessler, E. A. Emini, A. J. Conley, and N. L. Letvin. 1995. A vaccine-elicited, single viral epitope-specific cytotoxic T lymphocyte response does not protect against intravenous, cell-free simian immunodeficiency virus challenge. *J Virol* 69:2279–2284.

2936. Yasutomi, Y., H. L. Robinson, S. Lu, F. Mustafa, C. Lekutis, J. Arthos, J. I. Mullins, G. Voss, K. Manson, M. Wyand, and N. L. Letvin. 1996. Simian immunodeficiency virus-specific cytotoxic T-lymphocyte induction through DNA vaccination of rhesus monkeys. *J Virol* 70:678–681.

2937. Yee, C., A. Biondi, X. H. Wang, N. N. Iscove, J. deSousa, L. A. Aarden, G. G. Wong, S. C. Clark, H. A. Messner, and M. D. Minden. 1989. A possible autocrine role of IL-6 in two lymphoma cell lines. *Blood* 74:789.

2938. Yefenof, E., B. Asjo, and E. Klein. 1991. Alternative complement pathway activation by HIV infected cells: C3 fixation does not lead to complement lysis but enhances NK sensitivity. *Int Immunol* 3:395–401.

2939. Yeung, M. C., L. Pulliam, and A. S. Lau. 1995. The HIV envelope protein gp120 is toxic to human brain-cell cultures through the induction of interleukin-6 and tumor necrosis factor-alpha. *AIDS* 9:137–143.

2940. Yeung, S. C. H., F. Kazazi, C. G. M. Randle, R. C. Howard, N. Rizvi, J. C. Downie, B. J. Donovan, D. A. Cooper, H. Sekine, D. E. Dwyer, and A. L. Cunningham. 1993. Patients infected with human immunodeficiency virus type 1 have low levels of virus in saliva even in the presence of periodontal disease. *J Inf Dis* 163:803–809.

2941. Yolken, R. H., S. Li, J. Perman, and R. Viscidi. 1991. Persistent diarrhea and fecal shedding of retroviral nucleic acids in children infected with human immunodeficiency virus. *J Inf Dis* 164:61–66.

2942. Yoo, J., H. Chen, T. Kraus, D. Hirsch, S. Polyak, I. George, and K. Sperber. 1996. Altered cytokine production and accessory cell function after HIV-1 infection. *J Immunol* 157:1313–1320.

2943. York-Higgins, D., C. Cheng-Mayer, D. Bauer, J. A. Levy, and D. Dina. 1990. Human immunodeficiency virus type 1 cellular host range, replication, and cytopathicity are linked to the envelope region of the viral genome. *J Virol* 64:4016–4020.

2944. Yoshiyama, H., H. Mo, J. P. Moore, and D. D. Ho. 1994. Characterization of mutants of human immunodeficiency virus type 1 that have escaped neutralization by a monoclonal antibody to the gp120 V2 loop. *J Virol* 68:974–978.

2945. Yu, G., and R. L. Felsted. 1992. Effect of myristoylation on p27 *nef* subcellular distribution and suppression of HIV-LTR transcription. *Virol* 187:46–55.

2946. Yu, X., Z. Matsuda, Q.-C. Yu, T.-H. Lee, and M. Essex. 1993. Vpx of simian immunodeficiency virus is localized primarily outside the virus core in mature virions. *J Virol* 67:4386–4390.

2947. Yu, X., M. F. McLane, L. Ratner, W. O'Brien, R. Collman, M. Essex, and T. H. Lee. 1994. Killing of primary CD4+ T cells by non-syncytium-inducing macrophage-tropic human immunodeficiency virus type 1. *Proc Natl Acad Sci USA* 91:10237–10241.

2948. Yu, X., Y. Xin, Z. Matsuda, T. H. Lee, and M. Essex. 1992. The matrix protein of human immunodeficiency virus type 1 is required for incorporation of viral envelope protein into mature virions. *J Virol* 66:4966–4971.

2949. Yuen, M. H., M. P. Protti, O. B. Diethelm-Okita, L. Moiola, I. F. Howard, Jr., and B. M. Conti-Fine. 1995. Immunoregulatory CD8+ cells recognize antigen-activated CD4+ cells in myasthenia gravis patients and in healthy control. *J Immunol* 154:1508–1520.

2950. Yuille, M., A. M. Hugunin, P. John, L. Peer, L. V. Sacks, B. Poiesz, R. H. Tomar, and A. E. Silverstone. 1988. HIV-1 infection abolishes CD4 biosynthesis but not CD4 mRNA. *J AIDS* 1:131–137.

2951. Yusibov, V., A. Modelska, K. Steplewski, M. Agadjanyan, D. Weiner, D. C. Hooper, and H. Koprowski. 1997. Antigens produced in plants by infection with chimeric plant viruses immunize against rabies virus and HIV-1. *Proc Natl Acad Sci USA* 94:5784–5788.

2952. Zachar, V., B. Spire, I. Hirsch, J. C. Chermann, and P. Ebbesen. 1991. Human transformed trophoblast-derived cells lacking CD4 receptor exhibit restricted permissiveness for human immunodeficiency virus type 1. *J Virol* 65:2102–2107.

2953. Zack, J., A. M. Haislip, P. Krogstad, and I. S. Y. Chen. 1992. Incompletely reverse-transcribed human immunodeficiency virus type 1 genomes in quiescent cells can function as intermediates in the retroviral life cycle. *J Virol* 66:1717–1725.

2954. Zack, J. A., S. J. Arrigo, S. R. Weitsman, A. S. Go, A. Haislip, and I. S. Y. Chen. 1990. HIV-1 entry into quiescent primary lymphocytes: molecular analysis reveals a labile, latent viral structure. *Cell* **61**:213–222.

2955. Zack, J. A., A. J. Cann, J. P. Lugo, and I. S. Y. Chen. 1988. HIV-1 production from infected peripheral blood T cells after HTLV-I induced mitogenic stimulation. *Science* **240**:1026–1029.

2956. Zagury, D., J. Bernard, R. Cheynier, I. Desportes, R. Leonard, M. Fouchard, B. Reveil, D. Ittele, Z. Lurhuma, K. Mbayo, J. Wane, J.-J. Salaun, B. Goussard, L. Dechazal, A. Burny, P. Nara, and R. C. Gallo. 1988. A group specific anamnestic immune reaction against HIV-1 induced by a candidate vaccine against AIDS. *Nature* **332**:728–731.

2957. Zagury, D., J. Bernard, J. Leibowitch, B. Safai, J. E. Groopman, M. Feldman, M. G. Sarngadharan, and R. C. Gallo. 1984. HTLV-III in cells cultured from semen of two patients with AIDS. *Science* **226**:449–451.

2958. Zagury, D., J. Bernard, R. Leonard, R. Cheynier, M. Feldman, P. S. Sarin, and R. C. Gallo. 1986. Long-term cultures of HTLV-III-infected T cells: a model of cytopathology of T-cell depletion in AIDS. *Science* **231**:850–853.

2959. Zaki, S. R., R. Judd, L. M. Coffield, P. Greer, F. Rolston, and B. L. Evatt. 1992. Human papillomavirus infection and anal carcinoma. Retrospective analysis by in situ hybridization and the polymerase chain reaction. *Am J Path* **140**:1345–1355.

2960. Zamarchi, R., M. Panozzo, A. Del Mistro, A. Barelli, A. Borri, A. Amadori, and L. Chieco-Bianchi. 1994. B and T cell function parameters during zidovudine treatment of human immunodeficiency virus-infected patients. *J Inf Dis* **170**:1148–1156.

2961. Zambruno, G., L. Mori, A. Marconi, N. Mongiardo, B. De Rienzo, U. Bertazzoni, and A. Giannetti. 1991. Detection of HIV-1 in epidermal Langerhans cells of HIV-infected patients using the polymerase chain reaction. *J Invest Derm* **96**:979–982.

2962. Zanussi, S., M. D'Andrea, C. Simonelli, U. Tirelli, and P. De Paoli. 1996. Serum levels of RANTES and MIP-1α in HIV-positive long-term survivors and progressor patients. *AIDS* **10**:1431–1432.

2963. Zarling, J. M., J. A. Ledbetter, J. Sias, P. Fultz, J. Eichberg, G. Gjerset, and P. A. Moran. 1990. HIV-infected humans, but not chimpanzees, have circulating cytotoxic T lymphocytes that lyse uninfected CD4+ cells. *J Immunol* **144**:2992–2998.

2964. Zarling, J. M., P. A. Moran, O. Haffar, J. Sias, D. D. Richman, C. A. Spina, D. E. Myers, V. Kuebelbeck, J. A. Ledbetter, and F. M. Uckun. 1990. Inhibition of HIV replication by pokeweed antiviral protein targeted to CD4+ cells by monoclonal antibodies. *Nature* **347**:92–95.

2965. Zauli, G., D. Gibellini, C. Celeghini, C. Mischiati, A. Bassini, M. La Placa, and S. Capitani. 1996. Pleiotropic effects of immobilized versus soluble recombinant HIV-1 Tat protein on CD3-mediated activation, induction of apoptosis, and HIV-1 long terminal repeat transactivation in purified CD4+ T lymphocytes. *J Immunol* **157**:2216–2224.

2966. Zauli, G., D. Gibellini, D. Milani, M. Mazzoni, P. Borgatti, M. La Placa, and S. Capitani. 1993. Human immunodeficiency virus type 1 Tat protein protects lymphoid, epithelial, and neuronal cell lines from death by apoptosis. *Cancer Res* **53**:4481–4485.

2967. Zauli, G., M. C. Re, G. Visani, G. Furlini, and M. La Placa. 1992. Inhibitory effect of HIV-1 envelope glycoproteins gp120 and gp160 on the *in vitro* growth of enriched (CD34+) hematopoietic progenitor cells. *Arch Virol* **122**:271–280.

2968. Zazopoulos, E., and W. A. Haseltine. 1993. Effect of nef alleles on replication of human immunodeficiency virus type 1. *Virol* **194**:20–27.

2969. Zazopoulos, E., and W. A. Haseltine. 1992. Mutational analysis of the human immunodeficiency virus type 1 Eli Nef function. *Proc Natl Acad Sci USA* **89**:6634–6638.

2970. Zeballos, R. S., N. Cavalcante, C. A. R. Freire, H. J. Hernandez, I. M. Longo, Z. F. Peixinho, N. C. Moura, and N. F. Mendes. 1992. Delayed hypersensitivity skin tests in prognosis of human immunodeficiency virus infection. *J Clin Lab Anal* **6**:119–122.

2971. Zeira, M., R. A. Byrn, and J. E. Groopman. 1990. Inhibition of serum-enhanced HIV-1 infection of U937 monocytoid cells by recombinant soluble CD4 and anti-CD4 monoclonal antibody. *AIDS Res Hum Retro* **6**:629–639.

2972. Zhang, H., Y. Zhang, T. P. Spicer, L. Z. Abbott, M. Abbott, and B. J. Poiesz. 1993. Reverse transcription takes place within extracellular HIV-1 virions: potential biological significance. *AIDS Res Hum Retro* **9**:1287–1296.

2973. Zhang, L., Y. Huang, T. He, Y. Cao, and D. D. Ho. 1996. HIV-1 subtype and second-receptor use. *Nature* **383**:768.

2974. Zhang, L., Y. Huang, H. Yuan, B. K. Chen, J. Ip, and D. D. Ho. 1997. Identification of a replication-competent pathogenic human immunodeficiency virus type 1 with a duplication in the TCF-1α region but lacking NF-κB binding sites. *J Virol* **71**:1651–1656.

2975. Zhang, L., Y. Huang, H. Yuan, S. Tuttleton, and D. D. Ho. 1997. Genetic characterization of *vif, vpr,* and *vpu* sequences from long-term survivors of human immunodeficiency virus type 1 infection. *Virol* **228**:340–349.

2976. Zhang, L. Q., P. MacKenzie, A. Cleland, E. C. Holmes, A. J. Leigh Brown, and P. Simmonds. 1993. Selection of specific sequences in the external envelope protein of human immunodeficiency virus type 1 upon primary infection. *J Virol* **67**:3345–3356.

2977. Zhang, L. Q., P. Simmonds, C. A. Ludlam, and A. J. L. Brown. 1991. Detection, quantification and sequencing of HIV-1 from the plasma of seropositive individuals and from factor VIII concentrates. *AIDS* **5**:675–681.

2978. Zhang, R. D., M. Guan, Y. Park, R. Tawadros, J. Y. Yang, B. Gold, B. Wu, and E. E. Henderson. 1997. Synergy between human immunodeficiency virus type 1 and Epstein-Barr virus in T lymphoblastoid cell lines. *AIDS Res Hum Retro* **13**:161–171.

2979. Zhang, Y. M., S. C. Dawson, D. Landsman, H. C. Lane, and N. P. Salzman. 1994. Persistence of four related human immunodeficiency virus subtypes during the course of zidovudine therapy: relationship between virion RNA and proviral DNA. *J Virol* **68**:425–432.

2979a. Zhong, W., H. Wang, B. Herndier, and D. Ganem. 1996. Restricted expression of Kaposi sarcoma-associated herpesvirus (human herpesvirus 8) genes in Kaposi sarcoma. *Proc Natl Acad Sci USA* **93**:6641–6646.

2980. Zhou, E.-M., K. L. Lohman, and R. C. Kennedy. 1990. Administration of noninternal image monoclonal anti-idiotypic antibodies induces idiotype-restricted responses specific for human immunodeficiency virus envelope glycoprotein epitopes. *Virol* **174**:9–17.

2981. Zhou, J. Y., and D. C. Montefiori. 1997. Antibody-mediated neutralization of primary isolates of human immunodeficiency virus type 1 in peripheral blood mononuclear cells is not affected by the initial activation state of the cells. *J Virol* **71**:2512–2517.

2982. Zhu, G. W., Z. Q. Liu, S. V. Joag, D. M. Pinson, I. Adany, O. Narayan, H. M. McClure, and E. B. Stephens. 1995. Pathogenesis of lymphocyte-tropic and macrophage-tropic SIVmac infection in the brain. *J NeuroVirol* **1**:78–91.

2983. Zhu, T., H. Mo, N. Wang, D. S. Nam, Y. Cao, R. A. Koup, and D. D. Ho. 1993. Genotypic and phenotypic characterization of HIV-1 in patients with primary infection. *Science* **261**:1179–1181.

2984. Zhu, T., N. Wang, A. Carr, D. S. Nam, R. Moor-Jankowski, D. A. Cooper, and D. D. Ho. 1996. Genetic characterization of human immunodefiency virus type 1 in blood and genital secretions: evidence for viral compartmentalization and selection during sexual transmission. *J Virol* **70**:3098–3107.

2985. Zhu, T., N. Wang, A. Carr, S. Wolinsky, and D. D. Ho. 1995. Evidence for coinfection by multiple strains of human immunodeficiency virus type 1 subtype B in an acute seroconvertor. *J Virol* **69**:1324–1327.

2986. Zhu, Z. H., S. S. L. Chen, and A. S. Huang. 1990. Phenotypic mixing between human immunodeficiency virus and vesicular stomatitis virus or herpes simplex virus. *J AIDS* **3**:215–219.

2987. Ziegler, J. B., D. A. Cooper, R. O. Johnson, and J. Gold. 1985. Postnatal transmission of AIDS-associated retrovirus from mother to infant. *Lancet* **i**:896–898.

2988. Ziegler, J. L. 1993. Endemic Kaposi's sarcoma in Africa and local volcanic soils. *Lancet* **342**:1348–1351.

2989. Ziegler, J. L., J. A. Beckstead, P. A. Volberding, D. I. Abrams, A. M. Levine, R. J. Lukes, P.

Gill, S., R. L. Burkes, P. R. Meyer, C. E. Metroka, J. Mouradian, A. Moore, S. A. Riggs, J. J. Butler, F. C. Caranillas, E. Hersh, G. R. Newell, L. J. Laubenstein, D. Knowles, C. Odajnyk, B. Raphael, B. Koziner, C. Urmacher, and B. D. Clarkson. 1984. Non-Hodgkin's lymphoma in 90 homosexual men. Relation to generalized lymphadenopathy and the acquired immunodeficiency syndrome. *N Engl J Med* 311:565–570.

2990. Ziegler, J. L., W. L. Drew, and R. C. Miner. 1982. Outbreak of Burkitt's-like lymphoma in homosexual men. *Lancet* ii:631–633.

2991. Ziegler, J. L., and D. P. Stites. 1986. Hypothesis: AIDS is an autoimmune disease directed at the immune system and triggered by a lymphotropic retrovirus. *Clin Immunol Immunopathol* 41:305–313.

2992. Ziegler, J. L., A. C. Templeton, and G. L. Voegel. 1984. Kaposi's sarcoma: a comparison of classical, endemic, and epidemic forms. *Semin Oncol* 11:47–52.

2993. Zinkernagel, R. M., and H. Hengartner. 1994. T-cell-mediated immunopathology versus direct cytolysis by virus: implications for HIV and AIDS. *Immunol Today* 15:262–268.

2994. Ziza, J. M., F. Brun-Vezinet, A. Venet, C. H. Rouzioux, J. Traversat, B. Israel-Biet, F. Barre-Sinoussi, J. C. Chermann, and P. Godeau. 1985. Lymphadenopathy virus isolated from bronchoalveolar lavage fluid in AIDS-related complex with lymphoid interstitial pneumonitis. *N Engl J Med* 313:183–186.

2995. Zolla-Pazner, S., C. Alving, R. Belshe, P. Berman, S. Burda, P. Chigurupati, M. L. Clements, A. M. Duliege, J. L. Excler, C. Hoie, J. Kahn, M. J. McElrath, S. Sharpe, F. Sinangil, K. Steimer, M. C. Walker, N. Wassef, and S. Xu. 1997. Neutralization of a clade B primary isolate by sera from human immunodeficiency virus-uninfected recipients of candidate AIDS vaccines. *J Inf Dis* 175:764–774.

2996. Zolla-Pazner, S., and M. K. Gorny. 1992. Passive immunization for the prevention and treatment of HIV infection. *AIDS* 6:1235–1247.

2997. Zolla-Pazner, S., and S. Sharpe. 1995. A resting cell assay for improved detection of antibody-mediated neutralization of HIV type 1 primary isolates. *AIDS Res Hum Retro* 11:1449–1458.

2998. Zou, W., A. Dulioust, R. Fior, I. Durand-Gasselin, F. Boue, P. Galanaud, and D. Emilie. 1997. Increased T-helper-type 2 cytokine production in chronic HIV infection is due to interleukin (IL)-13 rather than IL-4. *AIDS* 11:533–534.

2999. Zou, W., A. A. Lackner, M. Simon, I. Durand-Gasselin, P. Galanaud, R. C. Desrosiers, and D. Emilie. 1997. Early cytokine and chemokine gene expression in lymph nodes of macaques infected with simian immunodeficiency virus is predictive of disease outcome and vaccine efficacy. *J Virol* 71:1227–1236.

3000. Zubiaga, A. M., E. Munoz, and B. T. Huber. 1992. IL-4 and IL-2 selectively rescue Th cell subsets from glucocorticoid-induced apoptosis. *J Immunol* 149:107–112.

3001. Zucker-Franklin, D., and Y. Z. Cao. 1989. Megakaryocytes of human immunodeficiency virus-infected individuals express viral RNA. *Proc Natl Acad Sci USA* 86:5595–5599.

3002. zur Hausen, H. 1991. Human papillomaviruses in the pathogenesis of anogenital cancer. *Virol* 184:9–13.

3003. Zwart, G., H. Langedijk, L. van der Hoek, J.-J. de Jong, T. F. W. Wolfs, C. Ramautarsing, M. Bakker, A. de Ronde, and J. Goudsmit. 1991. Immunodominance and antigenic variation of the principal neutralization domain of HIV-1. *Virol* 181:481–489.

3004. Zylberberg, H., and S. Pol. 1996. Reciprocal interactions between human immunodeficiency virus and hepatitis C virus infections. *Clin Infect Dis* 23:1117–1125.

Index[†]

[†] Figures and tables are indicated by an *f* or a *t*, respectively, after the page number.